U0348691

心血管药物学
Braunwald心脏病学姊妹篇

Opie's Cardiovascular Drugs: A Companion
to Braunwald's Heart Disease

第9版 | ninth edition

中文精要·英文影印版

◎ 主编

[美] 迪帕克·L. 巴特 （Deepak L. Bhatt）

◎ 编译

张　健　编译委员会主任委员
张宇辉

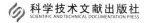

科学技术文献出版社
SCIENTIFIC AND TECHNICAL DOCUMENTATION PRESS

·北京·

图书在版编目（CIP）数据

心血管药物学：Braunwald心脏病学姊妹篇：第9版 /（美）迪帕克·L.巴特（Deepak L. Bhatt）主编；张健，张宇辉编译. —北京：科学技术文献出版社，2024.12

书名原文：Opie's Cardiovascular Drugs: A Companion to Braunwald's Heart Disease，ninth edition

ISBN 978-7-5189-9611-7

Ⅰ.①心… Ⅱ.①迪…②张…③张… Ⅲ.①心脏血管疾病—药物疗法 Ⅳ.① R540.5

中国版本图书馆 CIP 数据核字（2022）第 177291 号

著作权合同登记号 图字：01-2022-5270

中文简体字版权专有权归科学技术文献出版社所有

Elsevier (Singapore) Pte Ltd.
3 Killiney Road,
#08-01 Winsland House I,
Singapore 239519
Tel: (65) 6349-0200; Fax: (65) 6733-1817

心血管药物学：Braunwald心脏病学姊妹篇（第9版）

策划编辑：张 蓉	责任编辑：张 蓉 危文慧	责任校对：王瑞瑞	责任出版：张志平

出 版 者　科学技术文献出版社
地　　址　北京市复兴路15号　邮编 100038
编 务 部　（010）58882938，58882087（传真）
发 行 部　（010）58882868，58882870（传真）
邮 购 部　（010）58882873
官 方 网 址　www.stdp.com.cn
发 行 者　科学技术文献出版社发行　全国各地新华书店经销
印 刷 者　北京地大彩印有限公司
版　　次　2024 年 12 月第 1 版　2024 年 12 月第 1 次印刷
开　　本　787×960　1/32
字　　数　569千
印　　张　22.125
书　　号　ISBN 978-7-5189-9611-7
定　　价　498.00元

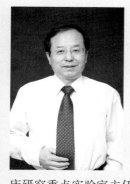

张 健

博士研究生导师，中国医学科学院北京协和医学院长聘教授

【社会任职】

现任美国心脏病学会会员、欧洲心脏病学会会员、美国心力衰竭学会会员、国家卫生健康委员会心血管药物临床研究重点实验室主任、中国医学科学院阜外医院药物与实验伦理委员会主任委员、心血管疾病国家重点实验室首席研究员、国家心血管病中心专家委员会心力衰竭专业委员会常务副主任委员、中国医师协会心力衰竭专业委员会主任委员；担任《中华心力衰竭和心肌病杂志（中英文）》总编辑、*Circulation：Heart Failure*（中文版）杂志主编。

【专业特长】

擅长对各类危急重症心力衰竭的救治、各种疑难心肌病的规范化和精准治疗。

【工作经历】

1998年至今于中国医学科学院阜外医院工作。

【学术成果】

主持完成国家和省部级重大项目及国内外多中心临床研究共20余项；主持撰写国内外指南和共识多部，发表论文100余篇，主编专著10余部；获省部级奖10余项。

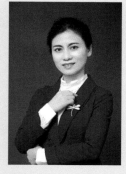

张宇辉

教授，博士研究生导师，中国医学科学院阜外医院心力衰竭中心主任

【社会任职】

现任欧洲心脏病学会会员、国家心血管病中心专家委员会心力衰竭专业委员会秘书长、中华医学会心血管病学分会心力衰竭学组副组长、中国医师协会心力衰竭专业委员会总干事、中国临床肿瘤学会肿瘤心脏病学专家委员会常务委员、中国抗癌协会整合肿瘤心脏病学分会常务委员；担任 *JACC：CardioOncology* 杂志国际编委、《中华心力衰竭和心肌病杂志（中英文）》编辑部主任。

【专业特长】

擅长各类心力衰竭、心肌病的规范化和精准治疗，肿瘤性心脏病及心脏淀粉样变的规范化诊治。

【工作经历】

1998年至今于中国医学科学院阜外医院工作。

【学术成果】

主持参与国家和省部级重大项目及国内外多中心临床研究共10余项；主持撰写国内外指南和共识多部，发表论文40余篇；获省部级奖多项。

原书编者名单

George L. Bakris, MD
Professor and Director
AHA Comprehensive Hypertension Center
Department of Medicine
The University of Chicago Medicine
Chicago, Illinois
Chapter 2. Antihypertensive Therapies

Christie M. Ballantyne, MD
Professor of Medicine and Genetics
Chief, Section of Cardiovascular Research
Chief, Section of Cardiology
Department of Medicine
Director, Center for Cardiometabolic Disease Prevention
Baylor College of Medicine
Houston, Texas
Chapter 6. Lipid-Modifying Drugs

Richard C. Becker, MD, FAHA
Professor of Medicine
Director, Heart, Lung, and Vascular Institute
University of Cincinnati College of Medicine
Cincinnati, Ohio
Chapter 8. Antithrombotic Drugs

Michael J. Blaha, MD, MPH
Director of Clinical Research
Department of Cardiology
Johns Hopkins Ciccarone Center for the Prevention of Heart Disease
Baltimore, Maryland
Chapter 4. Drugs for Diabetes

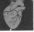
William E. Boden, MD
Scientific Director, Clinical Trials Network
Department of Medicine
VA Boston Healthcare System;
Physician Research Lead
VISN 1—VA New England Healthcare System
VA New England Healthcare System;
Professor of Medicine
Boston University School of Medicine;
Lecturer in Medicine
Harvard Medical School
Boston, Massachusetts
Chapter 1. Drugs for Ischemic Heart Disease

Marc P. Bonaca, MD, MPH
Professor of Medicine
Cardiology and Vascular Medicine
Director of Vascular Research
University of Colorado School of Medicine
Aurora, Colorado
Chapter 10. Vascular Medicine Drugs

Stephen Y. Chan, MD, PhD
Professor of Medicine
Director, Vascular Medicine Institute
Director, Center for Pulmonary Vascular Biology and Medicine
Division of Cardiology, Department of Medicine
University of Pittsburgh School of Medicine and UPMC
Pittsburgh, Pennsylvania
Chapter 11. Drugs for Pulmonary Hypertension

Vlad Cotarlan, MD
Division of Cardiovascular Health and Disease
Heart, Lung, and Vascular Institute
University of Cincinnati College of Medicine
Cincinnati, Ohio
Chapter 8. Antithrombotic Drugs

Omar Dzaye, MD, PhD
Research Fellow
Cicarrone Center for the Prevention of Cardiovascular Disease
Johns Hopkins University
Baltimore, Maryland
Chapter 4. Drugs for Diabetes

Robert H. Eckel, MD
Professor of Medicine
Department of Medicine
University of Colorado Anschutz Medical Campus
Aurora, Colorado
Chapter 4. Drugs for Diabetes

Mohammed A. Effat, MD
Division of Cardiovascular Health and Disease
Heart, Lung, and Vascular Institute
University of Cincinnati College of Medicine
Cincinnati, Ohio
Chapter 8. Antithrombotic Drugs

Michael V. Genuardi, MD, MS
Assistant Professor of Clinical Medicine
Division of Cardiology
Perelman School of Medicine
University of Pennsylvania
Pittsburgh, Pennsylvania
Chapter 11. Drugs for Pulmonary Hypertension

Ahmed A.K. Hasan, MD, PhD, FACC, FAHA
Program Director and Medical Officer
National Heart, Lung, and Blood Institute
National Institutes of Health
Bethesda, Maryland;
Professor of Medicine and Cardiology (adjunct)
University of Maryland School of Medicine
Baltimore, Maryland
Chapter 7. Drugs Targeting Inflammation

Aliza Hussain, MD
Fellow Physician
Department of Medicine
Baylor College of Medicine
Houston, Texas
Chapter 6. Lipid-Modifying Drugs

Luke J. Laffin, MD
Staff Physician
Medical Director of Cardiac Rehabilitation
Department of Cardiovascular Medicine
Cleveland Clinic Foundation
Cleveland, Ohio
Chapter 2. Antihypertensive Therapies

Peter Libby, MD
Division of Cardiovascular Medicine
Department of Medicine
Brigham and Women's Hospital
Harvard Medical School
Boston, Massachusetts
Chapter 7. Drugs Targeting Inflammation

Mandeep R. Mehra, MD
Medical Director
Heart and Vascular Center
Brigham and Women's Hospital
Boston, Massachusetts
Chapter 3. Heart Failure

Anju Nohria, MD
Assistant Professor in Internal Medicine
Division of Cardiovascular Medicine
Department of Medicine
Brigham and Women's Hospital
Harvard Medical School
Boston, Massachusetts
Chapter 7. Drugs Targeting Inflammation

Cara Reiter-Brennan
Ciccarone Center for the Prevention of Heart Disease
  Johns Hopkins School of Medicine
Baltimore, Maryland;
Department of Radiology and Neuroradiology
Charite
Berlin, Germany
Chapter 4. Drugs for Diabetes

Benjamin M. Scirica, MD, MPH
Senior Investigator
TIMI Study Group;
Director, Innovation
Cardiovascular Division
Brigham and Women's Hospital
Boston, Massachusetts;
Associate Professor of Medicine
Harvard Medical School
Cambridge, Massachusetts
Chapter 5. Drugs for Obesity

Sreekanth Vemulapalli, MD
Division of Cardiology
Duke University Medical Center
Durham, North Carolina
Chapter 8. Antithrombotic Drugs

Atul Verma, MD, FRCPC, FHRS
Associate Professor
University of Toronto
Southlake Regional Health Centre
Ontario, Canada
Chapter 9. Antiarrhythmic Drugs

Jefferson L. Vieira, MD, PhD
Post-Doctoral Research Fellow
Heart and Vascular Center
Brigham and Women's Hospital
Boston, Massachusetts
Chapter 3. Heart Failure

编译委员会名单

Lionel Opie 博士是一位"文艺复兴"式的人士，也是一位才华横溢、富有创造力的科学家。其对心脏代谢，以及交感神经系统在心力衰竭和心肌缺血中作用的研究，深受生理学家和心脏病学家的尊重和赞赏。Opie 博士亦是一位领导者，其在南非开普敦心血管研究所获得的成绩得到了全世界的关注和赞誉。与其研究能力同样出色的是，Opie 博士在患者床旁的沟通能力和在演讲台上的表达能力也十分突出，并极具感染力。在 Opie 博士的 31 部著作中，最著名的是先后出版的 8 个版本的 *Drugs for the Heart*，其具有非常广泛的世界影响力。Opie 博士用出色的图表、相对简洁的语言充分阐释了心血管药物的作用机制。伴随着心血管疾病药物的不断发展和进步，该书为临床医师提供了坚实的理解和应用基础。

当许多朋友和成千上万的学生在哀悼 Opie 博士的去世时，*Braunwald's Heart Disease* 的编者们也希望能够将 Opie 博士成功的教育方法延续，以获得良好的培训效果。幸运的是，*Drugs for the Heart* 和 *Braunwald's Heart Disease* 这两套书的出版方都是 Elsevier，出版总监都是 Dolores Meloni。为了促成本次"联姻"，*Braunwald's Heart Disease* 的编者们邀请 Deepak L. Bhatt 博士作为 *Drugs for the Heart*（ninth edition）的主编，并将本书命名为 *Opie's Cardio-vascular Drugs*。Bhatt 博士和 Opie 博士一样，为临床医师理解和使用各种当代心血管疾病的药物进行治疗做出了巨大贡献。本书不仅是建立在前作的优势之上，还是由一批有才华的多学科专家重新编撰的，包括心脏病学、内分泌学、血液病学、肾病学和血管医学等学科的专家。这些编者都是由 Bhatt 博士精心挑选，具有深厚学术造诣的专家，Bhatt 博士也对全书做了十分认真且强有力的统筹。本书还得到出色的医学插画家 Bernard Bulwer 博士的帮助，保留了解释性的图表，这些图表使得复杂的概念变得更加容易理解。

我们以极大的热情欢迎 *Opie's Cardiovascular Drugs* 成为 *Braunwald's Heart Disease* 的新成员。

Eugene Braunwald, MD

Douglas L. Mann, MD

Peter Libby, MD

Gordon F. Tomaselli, MD

Robert O. Bonow, MD

Scott Solomon, MD

曾经，作为一名医学生，我怀揣Opie博士主编的 *Drugs for the Heart*（*second edition*）度过了我的学生时代，本书是心脏药物学领域的经典教材。因此，当 Braunwald 博士邀请我担任本书第9版的主编时，我感到十分荣幸。因为本书已经成为 *Braunwald's Heart Disease* 家族的一员。

在本版图书中，书名从 *Drugs for the Heart* 更改为 *Opie's Cardiovascular Drugs*，并继承了 Opie 博士的丰富遗产，同时从仅关注心脏演变为关注整个心血管系统。本书关于治疗心绞痛、心力衰竭、高血压、心律失常、血栓形成和血脂异常药物的内容仍然有增无减，同时还扩展了肥胖症、血管医学、肺动脉高压、炎症和心脏代谢疾病全谱，反映了心脏病学在临床范围和试验调查方面的转变。

高度专业的研究者往往跨越不同的学科，不仅包括心脏病学及其亚专科，还包括血管医学、肾病学、内分泌学和血液学。这种多学科方法说明了医学的相互联系。实际上，正是这种思路导致了大规模的糖尿病心血管结局试验，使该领域超越了仅通过降低血糖来检查心血管终点的固定范式——不仅是缺血性终点，还包括心力衰竭，我们已经了解到，在糖尿病患者中，心力衰竭与心肌梗死一样令人困扰。只有通过这种知识的交叉融合，一个领域才能真正取得进步，而本书正式试图采用这种哲学理念。

本书除展示和解释数据外，杰出的编者们还以"Opiegrams"为模型，使用了大量的图表。在之前的版本中，"Opiegrams"不仅在学生中非常流行，在医学经验丰富的从业者中也很受欢迎。这些图表不仅对印刷版的著作非常有价值，在 *Braunwald's Heart Disease* 系列丛书的网络版中也将发挥重要作用。希望读者认为本书有趣、有料且有教育意义，也希望读者在面对日益复杂、快速变化的心血管药物时，能把本书作为有重要价值的参考书。

Deepak L. Bhatt, MD, MPH

首先，我必须感谢 Lionel Opie 博士，其创作了一部不朽的教科书，对医学界的同仁们都大有裨益。同时，也要感谢 Bernard Gersh 博士作为前一版的主编为本书所做的贡献。其次，我想对 Eugene Braunwald 博士表示深深的感谢，他不仅把我带进了 *Braunwald's Heart Disease* 家族，还对我进行了多年的指导，并且，我们发展了深厚的友谊。我还要感谢 Peter Libby 博士的指导，以及 *Braunwald's Heart Disease* 的其他编者（如 Robert O. Bonow 博士、Douglas L. Mann 博士、Gordon F. Tomaselli 博士和 Scott Solomon 博士）的伟大贡献。Elsevier 的高质量印刷和在线作品亦值得称赞。感谢出版总监 Dolores Meloni 将本书引入 *Braunwald's Heart Disease*。另外，来自 Elsevier 的 Robin Carter、Sara Watkins 和 Beula Christopher，也因出版这部著作并将之发扬光大而值得大家的尊敬。Bernard Bulwer 博士作为一位才华出众的医学插画家，对继承和发扬 Opie 医师的著作（这个卓越遗产）也做出了至关重要的贡献。最后，感谢我的家人允许我从事各种临床和学术工作，包括花费必要的时间来担任这本经典著作的主编。

致我的妻子

Shanthala

我们的四个儿子

Vinayak、Arjun、Ram和Raj

作为医学生，笔者一直期待能拥有一套传说中的 *Braunwald's Heart Disease* 系列丛书。在中国医学科学院北京协和医学院读硕士研究生和博士研究生时，笔者几乎每天课后都会去北京王府井外文书店影印版部寻觅佳著，那也是笔者当时最大的乐趣。然而，直到 1999 年，笔者才买到了 *Braunwald's Cardiovascular Disease* 的第五版，当时感觉如获至宝。此次，十分荣幸受邀联合主持编译 *Opie's Cardiovascular Drugs*。几十年来，笔者从比较封闭的世界走到全球化广泛交流的时代，并有幸从这些著名教科书中学到渴望已久的知识，十分令人感慨。

由 Deepak L. Bhatt 主编的 *Opie's Cardiovascular Drugs*（*ninth edition*）是一本传承了 *Opie's Heart Drugs* 精髓并在此基础上根据当今心血管疾病药物研究进展而更新、拓展的著作。本书内容既涵盖经典的冠心病、心力衰竭、高血压、心律失常、血栓形成和血脂异常等疾病的药物治疗，也拓展到了肥胖症、血管病变、肺动脉高压、炎症及心血管代谢等疾病的药物进展。本书通过对药物的作用机制、药理学特性、药物效果和不良反应等的介绍，为临床医师提供了清晰的用药指导原则。

随着对疾病的深入研究，人们对心血管疾病的认识已经超越了"系统"的概念，并拓展到了心血管疾病之外的系统改变及其相互影响。因此本书的编者不仅有心血管疾病及其亚专科的专家，还加入了血管医学、神经病学、内分泌学和血液病学等专科的专家，书中知识涵盖多个学科。例如，鉴于"强化降糖和目标降糖治疗未明显改善糖尿病患者的心血管结局"这个事实，2008 年美国食品药品监督管理局提出了新的降糖药需要有心血管疾病结局保护的要求。之后的临床试验相继验证了一些药物在降低血糖的同时，还可以改善心血管结局。这个改善作用不仅独立于降糖效果，还降低了心血管疾病的死亡率，减少了因心力衰竭住院的患者数，同时也有肾脏保护的效果，反映了多学科交叉学习和提高的结果。

本书图文并茂，沿用了传统的"Opiegrams"模式，使读者在学习时非常方便。本书既包括深刻的理论分析，还包括形象的配图描述，便于读者理解和记忆。本书的内容贴近实际，趣味性和可读性强。在理论上，本书叙述清晰；在临床上，本书便于读者参考和应用。感谢每位编委所做的工作，同时也希望读者通过阅读原文得到真传。总之，希望本书能够成为医学生学习、临床医师应用、科研人员参考的有关心血管疾病药物治疗的教科书。

张　健　张宇辉

中文目录

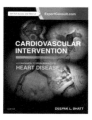

BHATT
Cardiovascular Intervention

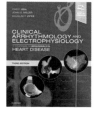

ISSA, MILLER, AND ZIPES
Clinical Arrhythmology and Electrophysiology

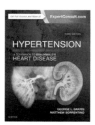

BAKRIS AND SORRENTINO
Hypertension

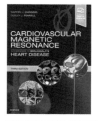

MANNING AND PENNELL
Cardiovascular Magnetic Reson

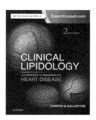

BALLANTYNE
Clinical Lipidology

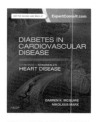

MCGUIRE AND MARX
Diabetes in Cardiovascular Disease

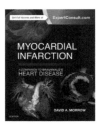

MORROW
Myocardial Infarction

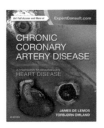

DE LEMOS AND OMLAND
Chronic Coronary Artery Disease

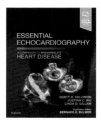

SOLOMON, WU, AND GILLAM
Essential Echocardiography

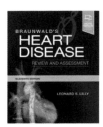

LILLY
*Braunwald's Heart Disease
Review and Assessment*

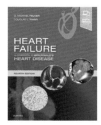

FELKER AND MANN
Heart Failure

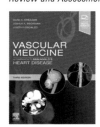

CREAGER
Vascular Medicine

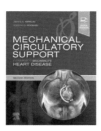

KIRKLIN AND ROGERS
Mechanical Circulatory Support

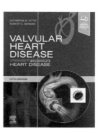

OTTO AND BONOW
Valvular Heart Disease

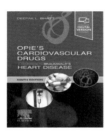

BHATT
Opie's Cardiovascular Drugs

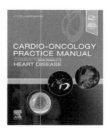

HERRMANN
Cardio-Oncology Practice Manual

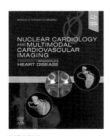

DICARLI
Nuclear Cardiology and Multimodal Cardiovascular Imaging

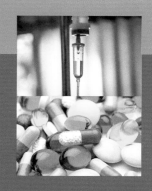

第1章
缺血性心脏病的药物治疗

　　本章的缺血性心脏病用药主要是指改善心肌缺血、减轻疾病症状的药物，包括β受体阻滞剂、硝酸酯类药物、钙通道阻滞剂三大传统类药物，以及雷诺嗪、伊伐布雷定、尼可地尔、曲美他嗪等非传统类抗心绞痛药物。本章从药物选择（不同类别药物的选择、同类不同种药物的选择、同种不同剂型药物的选择）、剂量滴定、药物相互作用、常见不良反应等多个方面对上述各类药物进行了非常全面且详细的介绍。

　　与常见药物手册不同，本章的药物介绍尤其注重用药所涉及的病理生理及药理机制的解释，并"引经据典"，每一条用药决策都有相关的循证医学证据和等级说明，从基础医学、临床医学、流行病与统计学等多方面帮助读者建立全面客观的用药认知。

　　β受体阻滞剂属于缺血性心脏病的标准治疗药物，既能有效改善心肌的缺血症状，又能作为二级预防用药，可降低急性心肌梗死的病死率，适用于其他多种心血管疾病，包括高血压、心律失常、心力衰竭等。根据β受体的选择性、药代动力学特性、临床证据充分性等的不同，可选择对应的β受体阻滞剂以应对不同的临床需求，如半衰期极短的艾司洛尔更适用于围手术期的静脉给药、心肌梗死后保护证据充分的美托洛尔更适用于心肌梗死后的二级预防等。当然，从肾上腺素能信号系统的生理机制出发，β受体阻滞剂无可避免地存在一些不良反应，尤其是对新发糖尿病患者，其在心血管疾病的管理过程中是需要重点监测的项目。

钙通道阻滞剂在缓解静息或劳力性心绞痛方面非常有效，尤其适用于血管痉挛性心绞痛，且在减轻心肌缺血的有效性和安全性方面与β受体阻滞剂相近。其中，二氢吡啶类钙通道阻滞剂更具有血管选择性，更适用于对高血压的治疗，如硝苯地平、氨氯地平；非二氢吡啶类钙通道阻滞剂对窦房结、房室结有抑制作用，更适用于对心律失常的治疗。

硝酸酯类药物主要通过扩张静脉（减轻前负荷）和冠状动脉（改善缺血）来缓解心绞痛症状，部分硝酸酯类药物也可扩张动脉（减轻后负荷）。舌下含服硝酸甘油仍然是劳力性心绞痛基本的缓解方法，但作用时间仅持续数分钟；而硝酸异山梨酯因具有肝脏转化的特性，起效延迟且作用时间更长。硝酸酯类药物也可用于劳力性心绞痛的预防。该类药物在使用过程中尤其要注意硝酸盐耐受的发生，且禁止与磷酸二酯酶-5抑制剂联合使用。

舟　君

Drugs for Ischemic Heart Disease

WILLIAM E. BODEN

Introduction

The contemporary management of patients with ischemic heart disease demands a sound understanding of the pathophysiologic precipitants of both angina pectoris and myocardial ischemia from which the principles of pharmacotherapy can be applied and tailored to the specific causes underlying these perturbations of myocardial oxygen supply and demand. This chapter details several broad classes of drug therapies directed at both symptom relief and ameliorating the consequences of reduced coronary blood flow and myocardial supply-demand imbalances for which specific treatments are targeted, including the traditional agents (β-blockers, nitrates, calcium channel blockers) as well as newer, non-traditional antianginal agents such as ranolazine as well as agents (ivabradine, nicorandil, and trimetazidine) that are not available for use in the US, but are in use internationally. These drugs are discussed comprehensively for both acute and chronic coronary syndromes, with particular attention to drug selection, dosing considerations, drug interactions, and common side effects that may influence treatment considerations.

β-Blockers

Introduction

β-adrenergic receptor antagonist agents remain a therapeutic mainstay in the management of ischemic heart disease with the exception of variant angina or myocardial ischemia due to coronary vasospasm. β-blockade is still widely regarded as standard therapy in cardiology professional society guidelines for exertional angina, unstable angina, and for variable threshold angina (or mixed angina), particularly where increases in heart rate and/or blood pressure (BP) (including the rate-pressure product rise that occurs during exercise or stress) results in an increase in myocardial oxygen consumption. β-blockers have an important role in reducing mortality when used as secondary prevention after acute myocardial infarction (MI), though outcomes data are lacking to support a beneficial role of β-blockers in ischemic heart disease patients without prior MI. And while β-blockers exert a markedly beneficial effect on outcomes in patients with heart failure, particularly in those with reduced EF, and have an important role as antiarrhythmic agents and to control the ventricular rate in chronic atrial fibrillation, as well as to adjunctively treat hypertension, the therapeutic applications of β-blockers in these other disease states will not be discussed in this chapter. Established and approved indications for β-blockers in the United States are shown in Table 1.1.

The extraordinary complexity of the β-adrenergic signaling system probably evolved millions of years ago when rapid activation was required for hunting and resisting animals, with the need for rapid inactivation during the period of rest and recovery. These mechanisms are now analyzed.[1]

Table 1.1

Indications for β-blockade and US FDA-approved drugs	
Indications for β-blockade	**FDA-approved drugs**
1. Ischemic heart disease	
Angina pectoris	Atenolol, metoprolol, nadolol, propranolol
Silent ischemia	None
AMI, early phase	Atenolol, metoprolol
AMI, follow-up	Propranolol, timolol, metoprolol, carvedilol
Perioperative ischemia	Bisoprolol[a], atenolol[a]
2. Hypertension	
Hypertension, systemic	Acebutolol, atenolol, bisoprolol, labetalol, metoprolol, nadolol, nebivolol, pindolol, propranolol, timolol
Hypertension, severe, urgent	Labetalol
Hypertension with LVH	Prefer ARB
Hypertension, isolated systolic	No outcome studies, prefer diuretic, CCB
Pheochromocytoma (already receiving alpha-blockade)	Propranolol
Hypertension, severe perioperative	Esmolol

Table 1.1

Indications for β-blockade and US FDA-approved drugs (Continued)	
Indications for β-blockade	**FDA-approved drugs**
3. Arrhythmias	
Excess urgent sinus tachycardia	Esmolol
Tachycardias (sinus, SVT, and VT)	Propranolol
Supraventricular, perioperative	Esmolol
Recurrences of Afib, Afl	Sotalol
Control of ventricular rate in Afib, Afl	Propranolol
Digitalis-induced tachyarrhythmias	Propranolol
Anesthetic arrhythmias	Propranolol
PVC control	Acebutolol, propranolol
Serious ventricular tachycardia	Sotalol
4. Congestive heart failure	Carvedilol, metoprolol, bisoprolol[a]
5. Cardiomyopathy	
Hypertrophic obstructive cardiomyopathy	Propranolol
6. Other cardiovascular indications	
POTS	Propranolol low dose[a]
Aortic dissection, Marfan syndrome, mitral valve prolapse, congenital QT prolongation, tetralogy of Fallot, fetal tachycardia	All?[a] Only some tested[a]
7. Central indications	
Anxiety	Propranolol [a]
Essential tremor	Propranolol
Migraine prophylaxis	Propranolol, nadolol, timolol
Alcohol withdrawal	Propranolol,[a] atenolol[a]
8. Endocrine	
Thyrotoxicosis (arrhythmias)	Propranolol
9. Gastrointestinal	
Esophageal varices? (data not good)	Propranolol?[a] Timolol negative study[a]
10. Glaucoma (local use)	Timolol, betaxolol, carteolol, levobunolol, metipranolol

[a]Well tested but not FDA approved.
Afib, Atrial fibrillation; *Afl*, atrial flutter; *AMI*, acute myocardial infarction; *ARB*, angiotensin receptor blocker; *CCB*, calcium channel blocker; *FDA*, Food and Drug Administration; *LVH*, left ventricular hypertrophy; *POTS*, postural tachycardia syndrome; *PVC*, premature ventricular contraction; *SVT*, supraventricular tachycardia; *VT*, ventricular tachycardia.

Mechanism of Action

The β_1-adrenoceptor and signal transduction. Situated on the cardiac sarcolemma, the β_1-receptor is part of the adenylyl (= adenyl) cyclase system (Fig. 1.1) and is one of the group of G protein–coupled receptors. The G protein system links the receptor to adenylyl cyclase (AC) when the G protein is in the stimulatory configuration (G_s, also called $G\alpha s$). The link is interrupted by the inhibitory form (G_i or $G\alpha i$), the formation of which results from muscarinic stimulation following vagal activation. When activated, AC produces cyclic adenosine monophosphate (cAMP) from adenosine triphosphate (ATP). The intracellular second messenger of β_1-stimulation is cAMP; among its actions is the "opening" of calcium channels to increase the rate and force of myocardial contraction (the positive inotropic effect) and increased reuptake of cytosolic calcium into the sarcoplasmic reticulum (SR; relaxing or lusitropic effect, see Fig. 1.1). In the sinus node the pacemaker current is increased (positive chronotropic effect), and the rate of conduction is accelerated (positive dromotropic effect). The effect of a given β-blocking agent depends on the way it is absorbed, the binding to plasma proteins, the generation of metabolites, and the extent to which it inhibits the β-receptor (lock-and-key fit).

β_2-receptors. The β-receptors classically are divided into the β_1-receptors found in heart muscle and the β_2-receptors of bronchial and vascular smooth muscle. If the β-blocking drug selectively interacts better with the β_1- than the β_2-receptors, then such a *β_1-selective blocker* is less likely to interact with the β_2-receptors in the bronchial tree, thereby giving a degree of protection from the tendency of nonselective β-blockers to cause pulmonary complications.

β_3-receptors. Endothelial β_3-receptors mediate the vasodilation induced by nitric oxide in response to the vasodilating β-blocker nebivolol (see Fig. 1.2).[2,3]

Secondary effects of β-receptor blockade. During physiologic β-adrenergic stimulation, the increased contractile activity resulting from the greater and faster rise of cytosolic calcium (Fig. 1.3) is coupled to increased breakdown of ATP by the myosin adenosine triphosphatase (ATPase). The increased rate of relaxation is linked to increased activity of the sarcoplasmic/endoplasmic reticulum calcium uptake pump. Thus, the uptake of calcium is enhanced with a more rapid rate of fall of cytosolic calcium, thereby accelerating relaxation. Increased cAMP also increases the phosphorylation of troponin-I, so that the interaction between the myosin heads and actin ends more rapidly. Therefore, the β-blocked heart not only beats more slowly by inhibition of the depolarizing currents

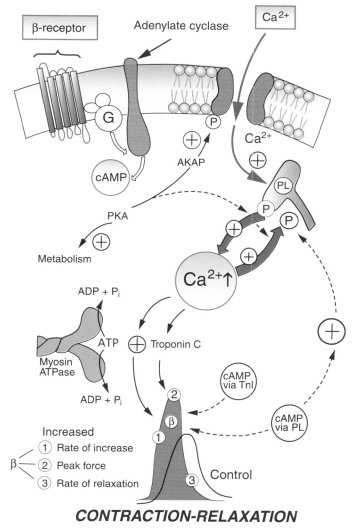

Fig. 1.1 See legend on opposite page

in the sinoatrial (SA) node but has a decreased force of contraction and decreased rate of relaxation. Metabolically, β-blockade switches the heart from using oxygen-wasting fatty acids toward oxygen-conserving glucose.[4] All these *oxygen-conserving properties* are of special importance in the therapy of ischemic heart disease. Inhibition of lipolysis in adipose tissue explains why gain of body mass may be a side effect of chronic β-blocker therapy.

Cardiovascular Effects of β-Blockade

β-blockers were originally designed by the Nobel prize winner Sir James Black to counteract the adverse cardiac effects of adrenergic stimulation. The latter, he reasoned, increased myocardial oxygen demand and worsened angina. His work led to the design of the prototype β-blocker, *propranolol*. By blocking the cardiac β-receptors, he showed that these agents could induce the now well-known inhibitory effects on the sinus node, atrioventricular (AV) node, and on myocardial contraction. These are the negative chronotropic, dromotropic, and inotropic effects, respectively (Fig. 1.4). Of these, it is especially bradycardia and the negative inotropic effects that are relevant to the therapeutic effect in angina pectoris and in patients with ischemic heart disease because these changes decrease the myocardial oxygen demand (Fig. 1.5). The inhibitory effect on the AV node is of special relevance in the therapy of supraventricular tachycardias (SVTs; see Chapter 9), or when β-blockade is used to control the ventricular response rate in atrial fibrillation.

Fig. 1.1, Cont'd β-adrenergic signal systems involved in positive inotropic and lusitropic (enhanced relaxation) effects. These can be explained in terms of changes in the cardiac calcium cycle. When the β-adrenergic agonist interacts with the β-receptor, a series of G protein-mediated changes lead to activation of adenylate cyclase and formation of the adrenergic second messenger, cyclic adenosine monophosphate *(cAMP)*. The latter acts via protein kinase A *(PKA)* to stimulate metabolism and to phosphorylate *(P)* the calcium channel protein, thus increasing the opening probability of this channel. More Ca^{2+} ions enter through the sarcolemmal channel, to release more Ca^{2+} ions from the sarcoplasmic reticulum (SR). Thus the cytosolic Ca^{2+} ions also increase the rate of breakdown of adenosine triphosphate (ATP) to adenosine diphosphate *(ADP)* and inorganic phosphate (P_i). Enhanced myosin adenosine triphosphatase *(ATPase)* activity explains the increased rate of contraction, with increased activation of troponin-C explaining increased peak force development. An increased rate of relaxation (lusitropic effect) follows from phosphorylation of the protein phospholamban *(PL)*, situated on the membrane of the SR, that controls the rate of calcium uptake into the SR. *AKAP*, A-kinase-anchoring protein. (Figure © L. H. Opie, 2012.)

VASODILATORY β-BLOCKERS

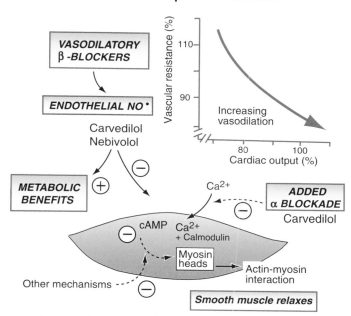

Fig. 1.2 Vasodilatory mechanisms and effects. Vasodilatory β-blockers tend to decrease the cardiac output less as the systemic vascular resistance falls. Vasodilatory mechanisms include α-blockade (carvedilol), formation of nitric oxide (nebivolol and carvedilol), and intrinsic sympathomimetic activity (ISA). ISA, as in pindolol, has a specific effect in increasing sympathetic tone when it is low, as at night, and increasing nocturnal heart rate, which might be disadvantageous in nocturnal angina or unstable angina. *cAMP,* Cyclic adenosine monophosphate; *NO,* nitric oxide. (Figure © L. H. Opie, 2012.)

Effects on coronary flow and myocardial perfusion. Enhanced β-adrenergic stimulation, as in exercise, leads to β-mediated coronary vasodilation. The signaling system in vascular smooth muscle again involves the formation of cAMP, but whereas the latter agent increases cytosolic calcium in the heart, it paradoxically decreases calcium levels in vascular muscle cells (see Fig. 1.6). Thus, during exercise, the heart pumps faster and more forcefully while coronary flow is augmented to meet the increased demand imposed by the increment in external workload. Conversely, while β-blockade

BETA-RECEPTOR BLOCKADE

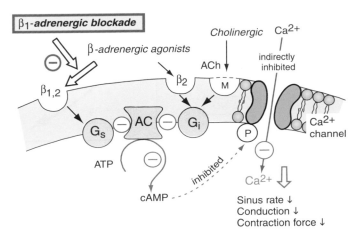

Fig. 1.3 The β-adrenergic receptor is coupled to adenyl (= adenylyl) cyclase *(AC)* via the activated stimulatory G-protein, G_s. Consequent formation of the second messenger, cyclic adenosine monophosphate *(cAMP)* activates protein kinase A (PKA) to phosphorylate *(P)* the calcium channel to increase calcium ion *(Ca^{2+})* entry. Activity of AC can be decreased by the inhibitory subunits of the acetylcholine *(ACh)*–associated inhibitory G-protein, G_i. cAMP is broken down by phosphodiesterase (PDE) so that PDE-inhibitor drugs have a sympathomimetic effect. The PDE is type 3 in contrast to the better-known PDE type 5 that is inhibited by sildenafil (see Fig. 2.6). A current hypothesis is that the $β_2$–receptor stimulation additionally signals via the inhibitory G-protein, G_i, thereby modulating the harm of excess adrenergic activity. (Figure © L. H. Opie, 2012.)

should have a coronary vasoconstrictive effect with a rise in coronary vascular resistance, the longer diastolic filling time resulting from a decreased heart rate during exercise leads to more nutritive coronary blood flow and better diastolic myocardial perfusion.

Pharmacokinetic Properties of β-Blockers

Plasma half-lives. Esmolol, given intravenously, has the shortest of all half-lives at only 9 minutes. Esmolol may therefore be preferable in unstable angina and threatened infarction when hemodynamic changes may call for withdrawal of β-blockade.

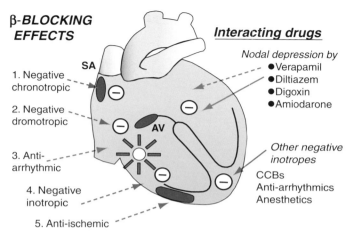

β-BLOCKING EFFECTS

1. Negative chronotropic
2. Negative dromotropic
3. Anti-arrhythmic
4. Negative inotropic
5. Anti-ischemic

Interacting drugs

Nodal depression by
- Verapamil
- Diltiazem
- Digoxin
- Amiodarone

Other negative inotropes
CCBs
Anti-arrhythmics
Anesthetics

Fig. 1.4 Cardiac effects of β-adrenergic blocking drugs at the levels of the sinoatrial *(SA)* node, atrioventricular *(AV)* node, conduction system, and myocardium. Major pharmacodynamic drug interactions are shown on the right. (Figure © L. H. Opie, 2012.)

The half-life of propranolol (Table 1.2) is only 3 hours, but continued administration saturates the hepatic process that removes propranolol from the circulation; the active metabolite 4-hydroxypropranolol is formed, and the effective half-life then becomes longer. The biological half-life of propranolol and metoprolol (and all other β-blockers) exceeds the plasma half-life considerably, so that twice-daily dosages of standard propranolol are effective even in angina pectoris. Clearly, the higher the dose of any β-blocker, the longer the biologic effects. Longer-acting compounds such as nadolol, sotalol, atenolol, and slow-release propranolol (Inderal-LA) or extended-release metoprolol (Toprol-XL) should be better for hypertension and effort angina.

Protein binding. Propranolol is highly bound, as are pindolol, labetalol, and bisoprolol. Hypoproteinemia calls for lower doses of such compounds.

First-pass hepatic metabolism. First-pass liver metabolism is found especially with the highly lipid-soluble compounds, such as propranolol, labetalol, and oxprenolol. Major hepatic clearance is also found with acebutolol, nebivolol, metoprolol, and timolol. First-pass metabolism varies greatly among patients and alters the

ISCHEMIC OXYGEN BALANCE

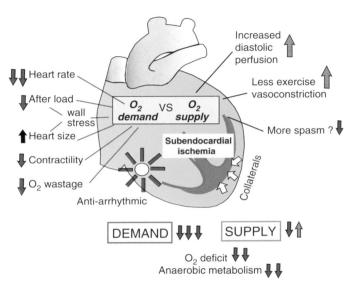

Fig. 1.5 Effects of β-blockade on ischemic heart. β-blockade has a beneficial effect on the ischemic myocardium, unless there is vasospastic angina when spasm may be promoted in some patients. Note unexpected proposal that β-blockade diminishes exercise-induced vasoconstriction. (Figure © L. H. Opie, 2012.)

dose required. In liver disease or low-output states the dose should be decreased. First-pass metabolism produces active metabolites with, in the case of propranolol, properties different from those of the parent compound. Metabolism of metoprolol occurs predominantly via cytochrome (CY) P450 2D6–mediated hydroxylation and is subject to marked genetic variability.[5] Acebutolol produces large amounts of diacetolol, and is also cardioselective with intrinsic sympathomimetic activity (ISA), but with a longer half-life and chiefly excreted by the kidneys (Fig. 1.7). Lipid-insoluble hydrophilic compounds (atenolol, sotalol, nadolol) are excreted only by the kidneys (see Fig. 1.7) and have low brain penetration. In patients with renal or liver disease, the simpler pharmacokinetic patterns of lipid-insoluble agents make dosage easier. As a group, these agents have low protein binding (see Table 1.2).

Pharmacokinetic interactions. Those drugs metabolized by the liver and hence prone to hepatic interactions are metoprolol,

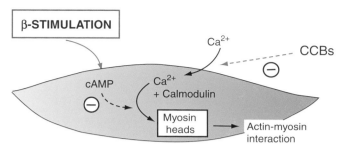

SMOOTH MUSCLE
β-blockade promotes contraction

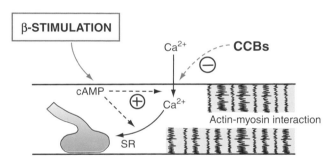

HEART MUSCLE
β-blockade inhibits contraction

Fig. 1.6 Proposed comparative effects of β-blockade and calcium channel blockers *(CCBs)* on smooth muscle and myocardium. The opposing effects on vascular smooth muscle are of critical therapeutic importance. *cAMP,* Cyclic adenosine monophosphate; *SR,* sarcoplasmic reticulum. (Figure © L.H. Opie, 2012.)

carvedilol, labetalol, and propranolol, of which metoprolol and carvedilol are more frequently used. Both are metabolized by the hepatic CYP2D6 system that is inhibited by paroxetine, a widely used antidepressant that is a selective serotonin reuptake inhibitor. To avoid such hepatic interactions, it is simpler to use those β-blockers not metabolized by the liver (see Fig. 1.7). β-blockers, in turn, depress hepatic blood flow so that the blood levels of lidocaine increase with greater risk of lidocaine toxicity.

Table 1.2

Properties of various β-adrenoceptor antagonist agents, nonselective versus cardioselective and vasodilatory agents

Generic name (trade name)	Extra mechanism	Plasma half-life (h)	Lipid solubility	First-pass effect	Loss by liver or kidney	Plasma protein binding (%)	Usual dose for angina (other indications)	Usual doses as sole therapy for mild or moderate hypertension	Intravenous dose (as licensed in United States)
Noncardioselective									
Propranolol[a,b] (Inderal)	—	1–6	+++	++	Liver	90	80 mg 2 × daily usually adequate (may give 160 mg 2 × daily)	Start with 10–40 mg 2 × daily. Mean 160–320 mg/day, 1–2 doses	1–6 mg
(Inderal-LA)	—	8–11	+++	++	Liver	90	80–320 mg 1 × daily	80–320 mg	—
Carteolol[a] (Cartrol)	ISA +	5–6	0/+	0	Kidney	20–30	(Not evaluated)	2.5–10 mg single dose	—
Nadolol[a,b] (Corgard)	—	20–24	0	0	Kidney	30	40–80 mg 1 × daily; up to 240 mg	40–80 mg/day 1 × daily; up to 320 mg	—
Penbutolol (Levatol)	ISA +	20–25	+++	++	Liver	98	(Not studied)	10–20 mg daily	—

Drug									
Sotalol[c] (Betapace; Betapace AF)	—	0	7–18 (mean 12)	0	Kidney	5	(80–240 mg 2× daily in two doses for serious ventricular arrhythmias; up to 160 mg 2× daily for atrial fib, flutter)	80–320 mg/day; mean 190 mg	—
Timolol[a] (Blocadren)	—	+	4–5	+	L, K	60	(post-AMI 10 mg 2× daily)	10–20 mg 2× daily	—
Cardioselective									
Acebutolol[a] (Sectral)	ISA ++	0 (diacetolol)	8–13 (diacetolol)	++	L, K	15	(400–1200 mg/day in 2 doses for PVC)	400–1200 mg/day; can be given as a single dose	—
Atenolol[a,b] (Tenormin)	—	0	6–7	0	Kidney	10	50–200 mg 1× daily	50–100 mg/day 1× daily	5 mg over 5 min; repeat 5 min later
Betaxolol[a] (Kerlone)	—	++	14–22	++	L, then K	50	—	10–20 mg 1× daily	—
	—	+	9–12	0	L, K	30			—

Continued on following page

Table 1.2

Properties of various β-adrenoceptor antagonist agents, nonselective versus cardioselective and vasodilatory agents (Continued)

Generic name (trade name)	Extra mechanism	Plasma half-life (h)	Lipid solubility	First-pass effect	Loss by liver or kidney	Plasma protein binding (%)	Usual dose for angina (other indications)	Usual doses as sole therapy for mild or moderate hypertension	Intravenous dose (as licensed in United States)
Bisoprolol[a] (Zebeta)	—						10 mg 1 × daily (not in US) (HF, see Table 1.2)	2.5–40 mg 1 × daily (see also Ziac)	
Metoprolol[a,b] (Lopressor)	—	3–7	+	++	Liver	12	50–200 mg 2 × daily (HF, see Table 1.2)	50–400 mg/day in 1 or 2 doses	5 mg 3 × at 2 min intervals
Vasodilatory β-blockers, nonselective									
Labetalol[a] (Trandate) (Normodyne)	—	6–8	+++	++	L, some K	90	As for hypertension	300–600 mg/ day in 3 doses; top dose 2400 mg/day	Up to 2 mg/ min, up to 300 mg for severe HT
Pindolol[a] (Visken)	ISA +++	4	+	+	L, K	55	2.5–7.5 mg 3 × daily (In UK, not US)	5–30 mg/day 2 × daily	—
Carvedilol[a] (Coreg)	β₁-, β₂-, α-block; metabolic	6	+	++	Liver	95	(US, UK for heart failure) Angina in UK: up to 25 mg 2 × daily	12.5–25 mg 2 × daily	—

Vasodilatory β-blockers, selective

| Nebivolol (Bystolic in USA; Nebilet in UK) | NO-vaso-dilation; metabolic | +++ | 10 (24 h, metabolites) | +++ (genetic variation) | L, K | 98 | Not in UK or US (in UK, heart failure, adjunct in older adults) | 5 mg once daily; 2.5 mg in renal disease or older adults | — |

[a]Approved by FDA for hypertension.
[b]Approved for angina pectoris.
[c]Approved for life-threatening ventricular tachyarrhythmias.

Octanol-water distribution coefficient (pH 7.4, 37°C) where $0 = <0.5$; $+ = 0.5$-2; $++ = 2$-10; $+++ = >10$ (Metabolic, insulin sensitivity increased.) *AMI*, Acute myocardial infarction; *FDA*, Food and Drug Administration; *fib*, fibrillation; *HF*, heart failure; *HT*, hypertension; *ISA*, intrinsic sympathomimetic activity; *K*, kidney; *L*, liver; *NO*, nitric oxide; *PVC*, premature ventricular contractions.

ROUTE OF ELIMINATION

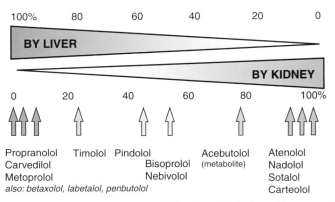

Fig. 1.7   Comparative routes of elimination of β-blockers. Those most hydrophilic and least lipid-soluble are excreted unchanged by the kidneys. Those most lipophilic and least water-soluble are largely metabolized by the liver. Note that the metabolite of acebutolol, diacetolol, is largely excreted by the kidney, in contrast to the parent compound. (For derivation of data in figure, see third edition. Estimated data points for acebutolol and newer agents added.) (Figure © L. H. Opie, 2012.)

Data for Use: Clinical Indications for β-Blockers

Angina Pectoris

Symptomatic reversible myocardial ischemia often reflects classical effort angina. Here the fundamental problem is inadequacy of coronary vasodilation in the face of increased myocardial oxygen demand, typically resulting from exercise-induced tachycardia (see Fig. 1.8). However, in many patients, there is also a variable element of associated coronary (and possibly systemic) vasoconstriction that may account for the precipitation of symptoms by cold exposure combined with exercise in patients with "mixed-pattern" angina. The choice of prophylactic antianginal agents should reflect the presumptive mechanisms of precipitation of ischemia.

β-blockade reduces the oxygen demand of the heart (see Fig. 1.5) by reducing the double product (heart rate × BP) and by limiting exercise-induced increases in contractility. Of these, the most important and easiest to measure is the reduction in heart rate. In addition, an aspect frequently neglected is the increased

EFFORT ANGINA

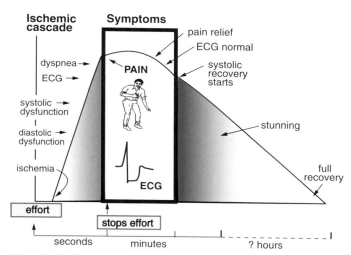

Ischemic cascade

dyspnea →
ECG →

systolic → dysfunction

diastolic → dysfunction

ischemia

effort

Symptoms

pain relief
ECG normal

PAIN

systolic recovery starts

stunning

full recovery

ECG

stops effort

seconds   minutes   ? hours

Fig. 1.8 The ischemic cascade leading to the chest pain of effort angina followed by the period of mechanical stunning with slow recovery of full function. *ECG,* Electrocardiogram. (Figure © L. H. Opie, 2012.)

oxygen demand resulting from left ventricular (LV) dilation, so that any accompanying ventricular failure needs active therapy.

All β-blockers are potentially equally effective in angina pectoris (see Table 1.1), and the choice of drug matters little in those who do not have concomitant diseases. *But a minority of patients do not respond to any β-blocker* because of (1) underlying severe obstructive coronary artery disease, responsible for angina even at low levels of exertion and at heart rates of 100 beats/min or lower; or (2) an abnormal increase in LV end-diastolic pressure resulting from an excess negative inotropic effect and a consequent decrease in subendocardial blood flow. Although it is conventional to adjust the dose of a β-blocker to secure a resting heart rate of 55 to 60 beats/min, in individual patients, heart rates less than 50 beats/min may be acceptable provided that heart block is avoided and there are no symptoms. The reduced heart rate at rest reflects the relative increase in vagal tone as adrenergic stimulation decreases. A major benefit is the restricted increase in the *heart rate during exercise,* which ideally should not exceed 100 beats/min in patients with angina. The effectiveness of medical therapy for stable angina pectoris, in which the use of β-blockers is a central component, is similar to that of percutaneous coronary intervention with stenting.[6]

Combination antiischemic therapy of angina pectoris. β-blockers are often combined with nitrate vasodilators and calcium channel blockers (CCBs) in the therapy of angina (see Table 1.3). However, the combined use of β-blockers with nondihydropyridine calcium antagonists (e.g., verapamil, diltiazem) should in general be avoided because of the risks of excess bradycardia and precipitation of heart failure, whereas the combination with long-acting dihydropyridines (DHPs) is well documented.[7]

Combination therapy in angina. Angina is basically a vascular disease that needs specific therapy designed to give long-term vascular protection. The following agents should be considered for every patient with angina: (1) aspirin and/or clopidogrel for antiplatelet protection, (2) statins and a lipid-lowering diet to decrease lipid-induced vascular damage, and (3) an angiotensin converting enzyme (ACE) inhibitor that has proven protection from MI and with the doses tested. Combinations of prophylactic antianginal agents are necessary in some patients to suppress symptoms but have less clear-cut prognostic implications.

Vasospastic angina. β-blockade is commonly held to be ineffective and even harmful because of lack of efficacy. On the other

Table 1.3

Factors limiting responsiveness to organic nitrates		
Anomaly	Principal mechanisms	Effects
NO resistance	"Scavenging" of NO Dysfunction of soluble guanylate cyclase	*De novo* hyporesponsiveness
"True" nitrate tolerance	(1) Impaired bioactivation of nitrates (2) Increased clearance of NO by O_2	Progressive attenuation of nitrate effect Worsening of endothelial dysfunction
Nitrate pseudotolerance	Increased release of vasoconstrictors (angiotensin II catecholamines, endothelin)	"Rebound" during nitrate-free periods

NO, Nitric oxide; *O_2*, oxygen.

hand, there is excellent evidence for the benefit of CCB therapy, which is the standard treatment. In the case of *exercise-induced anginal attacks in patients with variant angina,* a small prospective randomized study in 20 patients showed that nifedipine was considerably more effective than propranolol.[8]

Cold intolerance and angina. During exposure to severe cold, effort angina may occur more easily (the phenomenon of mixed-pattern angina). Conventional β-blockade by propranolol is not as good as vasodilatory therapy by a CCB[9] and may reflect failure to protect from regional coronary vasoconstriction in such patients.[10]

Silent myocardial ischemia. Episodes of myocardial ischemia, for example detected by continuous electrocardiographic recordings, may be precipitated by minor elevations of heart rate, probably explaining why β-blockers are very effective in reducing the frequency and number of episodes of silent ischemic attacks. In patients with silent ischemia and mild or no angina, atenolol given for 1 year lessened new events (angina aggravation, revascularization) and reduced combined endpoints.[11]

Acute Coronary Syndrome

Acute coronary syndrome (ACS) is an all-purpose term, including unstable angina and acute myocardial infarction (AMI), so that management is based on risk stratification (see Fig. 1.9). Plaque fissuring in the wall of the coronary artery with partial coronary thrombosis or platelet aggregation on an area of endothelial disruption is the basic pathologic condition. Urgent antithrombotic therapy with heparin (unfractionated or low molecular weight) or other antithrombotics, plus aspirin is the basic treatment (see Chapter 8). Currently, early multiple platelet–receptor blockade is standard in high-risk patients.

β-blockade is a part of conventional in-hospital quadruple therapy, the other three agents being statins, antiplatelet agents, and ACE inhibitors, a combination that reduces 6-month mortality by 90% compared with treatment by none of these.[12] β-blockade is usually started early, especially in patients with elevated BP and heart rate, to reduce the myocardial oxygen demand and to lessen ischemia (see Fig. 1.5). The major argument for early β-blockade is that threatened infarction, into which unstable angina merges, may be prevented from becoming overt.[13] Logically, the lower the heart rate, the less the risk of recurrent ischemia. However, the actual objective evidence favoring the use of β-blockers in unstable angina itself is limited to borderline results in one placebo-controlled trial,[14] plus only indirect evidence from two observational studies.[12,15]

ACUTE CORONARY SYNDROMES: TRIAGE

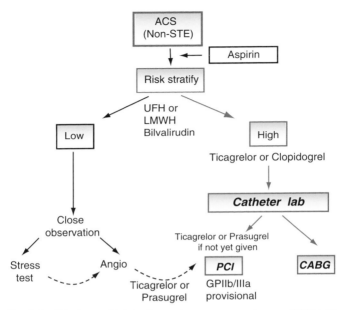

Fig. 1.9 Principles of triage for acute coronary syndromes *(ACS)* with non–ST-elevation *(non-STE)*. All receive aspirin. Patients are stratified according to the risk are given unfractionated heparin *(UFH)* or low-molecular-weight heparin *(LMWH)* and bivalirudin (no glycoprotein [GP] IIb/IIIa, as below). Those *at high risk* are given ticagrelor or clopidogrel and taken to the catheter laboratory. Then they either undergo coronary artery bypass grafting *(CABG)* or percutaneous coronary intervention *(PCI)*. Those undergoing PCI are given ticagrelor (or prasugrel), if not yet given, and some are selected to be given GPIIb/IIIa inhibitors. Those *at low risk* are closely observed and, if requiring an angiogram *(angio)*, given ticagrelor or prasugrel to be followed by PCI. Those at lower risk and stable are subject to an effort stress test. (Figure © B.J. Gersh, 2012.)

Acute ST-Elevation Myocardial Infarction

Early ST-elevation myocardial infarction. There are no good trial data on the early use of β-blockade in the reperfusion era. Logically, β-blockade should be of most use in the presence of ongoing pain,[16] inappropriate tachycardia, hypertension, or ventricular rhythm instability.[17] In the COMMIT trial, early intravenous metoprolol given to more than 45,000 Asiatic patients, about half of whom were treated by lytic agents and without primary percutaneous coronary intervention, followed by oral dosing, led to 5 fewer reinfarctions and 5 fewer ventricular fibrillations per 1000 treated.[18] The cost was increased cardiogenic shock, heart failure, persistent hypotension, and bradycardia (in total, 88 serious adverse events). In the United States, metoprolol and atenolol are the only β-blockers licensed for intravenous use in AMI. Overall, however, no convincing data emerge for routine early intravenous β-blockade.[19] With selected and carefully monitored exceptions, it is simpler to introduce oral β-blockade later when the hemodynamic situation has stabilized. The current American College of Cardiology (ACC)–American Heart Association (AHA) guidelines recommend starting half-dose oral β-blockade on day 2 (assuming hemodynamic stability) followed by dose increase to the full or the maximum tolerated dose, followed by long-term postinfarct β-blockade.[20]

Postinfarction secondary prevention. (1) Administer β-blockade for all postinfarct patients with an ejection fraction (EF) of 40% or less unless contraindicated, with use limited to carvedilol, metoprolol succinate, or bisoprolol, which reduce mortality *(Class 1, Level of Evidence A);* (2) administer β-blockade for 3 years in patients with normal LV function after AMI or ACS; *(Class I, Level B).* It is also reasonable to continue β-blockade beyond 3 years *(Class IIa, Level B).*[21]

Benefits of postinfarct β-blockade. In the postinfarct phase, β-blockade reduces mortality by 23% according to trial data[22] and by 35% to 40% in an observational study on a spectrum of patients including diabetics.[23] Timolol, propranolol, metoprolol, and atenolol are all effective and licensed for this purpose. Metoprolol has excellent long-term data.[24] Carvedilol is the only β-blocker studied in the reperfusion era and in a population also receiving ACE inhibitors.[25] As the LV dysfunction was an entry point, the carvedilol dose was gradually uptitrated, and all-cause mortality was reduced. The mechanisms concerned are multiple and include decreased ventricular arrhythmias[26] and decreased reinfarction.[27] β-Blockers with partial agonist activity are relatively ineffective, perhaps because of the higher heart rates.

The only outstanding questions are (1) whether low-risk patients really benefit from β-blockade (there is an increasing trend to omit β-blockade especially in patients with borderline hyperglycemic values); (2) when to start (this is flexible and, as data for early β-blockade are not strong,[22] oral β-blocker may be started when the patient's condition allows, for example from 3 days onward[25] or even later at about 1 to 3 weeks); and (3) how long β-blockade should be continued. Bearing in mind the risk of β-blockade withdrawal in patients with angina, many clinicians continue β-blockade administration for the long term once a seemingly successful result has been obtained. The benefit in high-risk groups such as older adults or those with low EFs increases progressively over 24 months.[23]

The *high-risk patients* who should benefit most are those often thought to have contraindications to β-blockade.[23] Although CHF was previously regarded as a contraindication to β-blockade, post-infarct patients with heart failure benefited more than others from β-blockade.[23] Today this category of patient would be given a β-blocker after treatment of fluid retention cautiously with gradually increasing doses of carvedilol, metoprolol, or bisoprolol. The SAVE trial[27] showed that ACE inhibitors and β-blockade are additive reducing postinfarct mortality, at least in patients with reduced EFs. The benefit of β-blockade when added to combination therapy with ACE inhibitors reduces mortality by 23% to 40%.[23,25] Concurrent therapy of CCBs or aspirin does not diminish the benefits of postinfarct β-blockade.

Despite all these strong arguments and numerous recommendations, β-blockers are *still underused in postinfarct patients* at the expense of many lives lost. In the long term, 42 patients have to be treated for 2 years to avoid one death, which compares favorably with other treatments.[22]

Lack of Outcome Studies in Angina

Solid evidence for a decrease in mortality in postinfarct follow-up achieved by β-blockade has led to the assumption that this type of treatment must also improve the outcome in effort angina or unstable angina. Regretfully, there are no convincing outcome studies to support this belief. In unstable angina, the short-term benefits of metoprolol were borderline.[14] In effort angina, a meta-analysis of 90 studies showed that β-blockers and CCBs had equal efficacy and safety, but that β-blockers were better tolerated[28] probably because of short-acting nifedipine capsules, which were then often used. In angina plus hypertension, direct comparison has favored the CCB verapamil (see next section).

Other Cardiac Indications for β-Blockers

While this chapter addresses the specific role of β-blockers in patients with ischemic heart disease only, there are other established uses for β-blocker therapy, which include *hypertrophic obstructive cardiomyopathy*, the treatment of *catecholaminergic polymorphic ventricular tachycardia* (VT) with high-dose β-blockers to prevent exercise-induced VT; in *mitral stenosis with sinus rhythm*, where β-blockade benefits patients by decreasing resting and exercise heart rates; *in mitral valve prolapse,* where β-blockade is the standard procedure for control of associated arrhythmias, and in both *dissecting aortic aneurysms;* and in *Marfan syndrome* with aortic root involvement, where β-blockade has an important role in reducing the rate of pressure rise within the left ventricle (dp/dt) and the shear stress imposed on the proximal aortic wall.

These conditions will be referenced and discussed in other sections of this book.

Noncardiac Indications for β-Blockade

Stroke. In an early trial the nonselective blocker propranolol was only modestly beneficial in reducing stroke (although ineffective in reducing coronary artery disease [CAD]).[29] The β_1 selective agents are more effective in stroke reduction.[30]

Vascular and noncardiac surgery. β-blockade exerts an important protective effect in selected patients. Perioperative death from cardiac causes and MI were reduced by bisoprolol in high-risk patients undergoing vascular surgery.[31] A risk-based approach to noncardiac surgery is proposed by a very large observational study on 782,969 patients. In those at no or very low cardiac risk, β-blockers were without benefit and in fact were associated with more adverse events, including mortality. In those at very high cardiac risk, mortality decreased by 42%, with a number needed to treat of only 33.[32] Thus risk factor assessment is vital (see original article for revised cardiac risk index). In patients undergoing vascular surgery but otherwise not at very high risk, perioperative metoprolol gave no benefit yet increased intraoperative bradycardia and hypotension.[33]

Impact of POISE study. In the major prospective PeriOperative ISchemic Evaluation (POISE) study on a total of 8351 patients, perioperative slow-release metoprolol decreased the incidence of nonfatal MI from 5.1% to 3.6% ($P < 0.001$), yet increased total perioperative mortality from 2.3% to 3.1% ($P < 0.05$), with increased stroke rates and markedly increased significant hypotension and bradycardia. *Thus, routine perioperative inception of metoprolol therapy is not justified.* As metoprolol exerts markedly heterogenous cardiovascular effects according to metabolic genotype, involving subtypes of CYP450 2D6,[5] genetic differences may have accounted for part of the adverse cardiovascular findings in POISE and another study.[33]

In an important focused update given by ACC-AHA,[34] the major recommendations are the following: (1) Class I indication for perioperative β-blocker use in patients already taking the drug; (2) Class IIa recommendations for patients with inducible ischemia, coronary artery disease, or multiple clinical risk factors who are undergoing vascular (i.e. high-risk) surgery and for patients with CAD or multiple clinical risk factors who are undergoing intermediate-risk surgery; (3) Initiation of therapy, particularly in lower-risk groups, requires careful consideration of the risk/benefit ratio; (4) If initiation is selected, it should be started well before the planned procedure with careful perioperative titration to achieve adequate heart rate control while avoiding frank bradycardia or hypotension. In light of the POISE results, routine administration of perioperative β-blockers, particularly in higher fixed-dose regimens begun on the day of surgery, cannot be advocated.

Thyrotoxicosis. Together with antithyroid drugs or radioiodine, or as the sole agent before surgery, β-blockade is commonly used in thyrotoxicosis to control symptoms, although the hypermetabolic state is not decreased. β-blockade controls tachycardia, palpitations, tremor, and nervousness and reduces the vascularity of the thyroid gland, thereby facilitating operation. In thyroid storm, intravenous propranolol IV in slow 1–2 mg boluses may be repeated every 10–15 min until the desired effect is achieved. Alternatively, esmolol, 500 micrograms/Kg IV bolus, followed by 50–200 micrograms/Kg/min for maintenance may be administered; circulatory collapse is a risk, so that β-blockade should only be used in thyroid storm if LV function is normal as shown by conventional noninvasive tests.

Anxiety states. Although propranolol is most widely used in anxiety (and is licensed for this purpose in several countries, including the United States), probably all β-blockers are effective, acting not centrally but by a reduction of peripheral manifestations of anxiety such as tremor and tachycardia.

Glaucoma. The use of local β-blocker eye solutions is now established for open-angle glaucoma; care needs to be exerted with occasional systemic side effects such as sexual dysfunction, bronchospasm, and cardiac depression. Among the agents approved for treatment of glaucoma in the United States are the nonselective agents timolol (Timoptic), carteolol, levobunolol, and metipranolol. The cardioselective betaxolol may be an advantage in avoiding side effects in patients with bronchospasm.

Migraine. Propranolol (80 to 240 mg daily, licensed in the United States) acts prophylactically to reduce the incidence of migraine attacks in 60% of patients. The mechanism is presumably by beneficial vasoconstriction. The antimigraine effect is prophylactic and not for attacks once they have occurred. If there is no benefit within 4 to 6 weeks, the drug should be discontinued.

Esophageal varices. β-blockade has been thought to prevent bleeding by reducing portal pressure. No benefit was found in a randomized study.[35]

Pharmacologic Properties of Various β-Blockers

β-blocker "generations." *First-generation nonselective agents,* such as propranolol, block all the β-receptors (both β_1 and β_2). *Second-generation cardioselective agents,* such as atenolol, metoprolol, acebutolol, bisoprolol, and others, have relative selectivity for the β_1 (largely cardiac) receptors when given in low doses (Fig. 1.10). *Third-generation vasodilatory* agents have added properties (Fig. 1.2), acting chiefly through two mechanisms: first, direct vasodilation, possibly mediated by release of nitric oxide as for carvedilol (see Fig. 1.2) and nebivolol[3]; and, second, added

β_1 *VS* β_2 *SELECTIVITY*

β_1-SELECTIVE

- Bradycardia
- Negative inotropy
- BP ↓
- Less bronchospasm
- Fewer peripheral effects
  - Metabolic effects
  - Circulatory

NON-SELECTIVE (β_1 β_2)

- Similar cardiac and antihypertensive effects
- More marked pulmonary and peripheral effects

Fig. 1.10 β_1- versus β_2-cardioselectivity. In general, note several advantages of cardioselective β-blockers (exception: heart failure). Cardioselectivity is greatest at low drug doses. (Figure © L. H. Opie, 2012.)

α-adrenergic blockade, as in labetalol and carvedilol. A third vaso-dilatory mechanism, as in pindolol and acebutolol, acts via β_2-ISA, which stimulates arterioles to relax. Acebutolol is a cardioselective agent with less ISA than pindolol that was very well tolerated in a 4-year antihypertensive study.[36]

Nonselective agents (combined β_1-β_2-blockers). The prototype β-blocker is propranolol, which is still often used worldwide and is a World Health Organization essential drug. By blocking β_1-recep-tors, it affects heart rate, conduction, and contractility, yet by blocking β_2-receptors, it tends to cause smooth muscle contrac-tion with risk of bronchospasm in predisposed individuals. This same quality might, however, explain the benefit in migraine when vasoconstriction could inhibit the attack. Among the nonse-lective blockers, nadolol and sotalol are much longer acting and lipid insoluble.

Combined β_1-β_2-α-blockers. Carvedilol is very well supported for preferential use in heart failure, in which this combination of receptor blockade should theoretically be ideal, as shown by better outcomes than with metoprolol in the COMET study.[37]

Cardioselective agents (β_1-selectivity). Cardioselective agents (acebutolol, atenolol, betaxolol, bisoprolol, celiprolol, and meto-prolol) exert antihypertensive effects equally to the nonselective ones (see Fig. 1.10). Selective agents are preferable in patients with chronic lung disease or chronic smoking, insulin-requiring diabetes mellitus, and in stroke prevention.[30] Cardioselectivity varies among agents but is always greater at lower doses. Bisoprolol is among the most selective. Cardioselectivity declines or is lost at high doses. No β-blocker is completely safe in the presence of asthma; low-dose cardioselective agents can be used with care in patients with bron-chospasm or chronic lung disease or chronic smoking. In angina and hypertension, cardioselective agents are just as effective as noncardioselective agents. In acute MI complicated by stress-induced hypokalemia, nonselective blockers theoretically should be better antiarrhythmics than β_1-selective blockers.

Vasodilating β-blockers. Carvedilol and nebivolol are the proto-types (see Fig. 1.2). These agents could have added value in the therapy of hypertension by achieving vasodilation and, in the case of nebivolol, better reduction of LVH is claimed.[38]

Antiarrhythmic β-blockers. All β-blockers are potentially antiarrhythmic by virtue of Class II activity (see Fig. 1.11). Sotalol is a unique β-blocker with prominent added Class III antiarrhyth-mic activity (see Fig. 1.11; Chapter 9) and will be discussed in greater detail elsewhere.

EXCESS β-ADRENERGIC SIGNALS IN HF

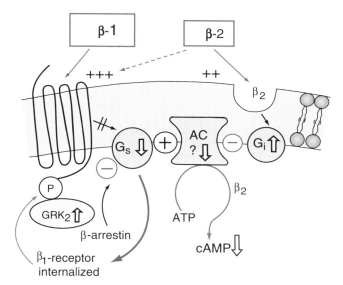

β₁-**down regulated**
CONTRACTION ⇩

β₂-**mediated effects**
CONTRACTION ⇩
Apoptosis ⇩

Fig. 1.11 β-adrenergic receptors in advanced heart failure. Downregulation and uncoupling of β-adrenergic receptor signal systems results in depressed levels of cyclic adenosine monophosphate *(cAMP)* and decreased contractility, which may be viewed as an autoprotective from the adverse effects of cAMP. Note: (1) β-receptor downregulation starts as a result of inhibitory phosphorylation of the receptor mediated by G protein–coupled receptor kinase *(GRK₂;* previously β₁ adrenergic receptor kinase [β₁ARK]), GRK₂ increases in response to excess β-adrenergic stimulation of the receptor, (2) β-receptor uncoupling from G-protein, *Gₛ* results from β-arrestin activity, (3) β-receptor downregulation is a result of internalization, (4) increased inhibitory G-protein *(Gᵢ)* is a result of increased messenger ribonucleic acid activity, (5) β₂ receptors are relatively upregulated and appear to exert an inhibitory effect on contractile via enhanced Gᵢ. *AC,* Adenyl cyclase; *ATP,* adenosine triphophate. (Figure © L. H. Opie, 2012. For details, see Opie LH, *Heart Physiology from Cell to Circulation.* Philadelphia: Lippincott Williams and Wilkins; 2004:508.)

Specific β-Blockers Used in Clinical Practice

Of the large number of β-blockers, the ideal agent for hypertension or angina might have (1) advantageous pharmacokinetics (simplicity, agents not metabolized in liver); (2) a high degree of cardioselectivity (bisoprolol); (3) long duration of action (several); and (4) a favorable metabolic profile, especially when associated with vasodilatory properties (carvedilol and nebivolol).

Propranolol. *(Inderal)* is the historical gold standard because it is approved for so many different indications, including angina, acute MI, postinfarction secondary prevention, hypertension, arrhythmias, migraine prophylaxis, anxiety states, and essential tremor. However, propranolol is not β_1-selective. Being lipid soluble, it has a high brain penetration and undergoes extensive hepatic first-pass metabolism. Central side effects may explain its poor performance in quality-of-life studies. Propranolol also has a short half-life so that it must be given twice daily unless long-acting preparations are used. The other β-blockers agents are described below alphabetically:

Acebutolol. *(Sectral)* is the cardioselective agent with ISA that gave a good quality of life in the 4-year TOMH study in mild hypertension. In particular, the incidence of impotence was not increased.[39]

Atenolol. *(Tenormin)* was one of the first of the cardioselective agents and now in generic form is one of the most widely used drugs in angina, in postinfarction secondary prevention, and in hypertension. However, its use as first-line agent in hypertension is falling into disfavor,[40] with poor outcomes, including increased all-cause mortality when compared with the CCB amlodipine in ASCOT.[41] There are very few trials with outcome data for atenolol in other conditions, with two exceptions: the ASIST study in silent ischemia[11] and INVEST in hypertensives with coronary artery disease. Here atenolol had equality of major clinical outcomes with verapamil at the cost of more episodes of angina, more new diabetes, and more psychological depression.[42,43] Note that atenolol was often combined with a diuretic and verapamil with an ACE inhibitor. In the British Medical Research Council trial of hypertension in older adults, atenolol did not reduce coronary events.[29] More recently, in the LIFE Trial, atenolol was inferior to the ARB losartan in the therapy of hypertensives with LVH.[44]

Bisoprolol. *(Zebeta in the United States, Cardicor or Emcor in the United Kingdom)* is a highly β_1-selective agent, more so than atenolol, licensed for hypertension, angina heart failure in the United Kingdom, but only for hypertension in the United States. It was the drug used in the large and successful CIBIS-2 study in heart failure, in which there was a large reduction not only in total mortality but also in sudden death.[45] In CIBIS-3, bisoprolol compared well with enalapril as first-line agent in heart failure.[46] A combination of low-dose bisoprolol and low-dose hydrochlorothiazide (Ziac) is available in the United States (see Combination Therapy, p. 13).

Carvedilol. (*Coreg in the United States, Eucardic in the United Kingdom*) is a nonselective vasodilator α-β-blocker with multimechanism vasodilatory properties mediated by antioxidant activity, formation of nitric oxide, stimulation β-arrestin-MAP-kinase[47] and α-receptors, that has been extensively studied in CHF[48] and in postinfarct LV dysfunction.[25] Metabolically, carvedilol may increase insulin sensitivity.[49] In the United States, it is registered for hypertension, for CHF (mild to severe), and for post-MI LV dysfunction (EF ≤40%), but not for angina.

Labetalol. (*Trandate, Normodyne*) is a combined α- and β-blocking antihypertensive agent that has now largely been supplanted by carvedilol except for acute intravenous use as in hypertensive crises (see Table 1.4).

Metoprolol. (*Toprol-XL*) is cardioselective and particularly well studied in AMI and in postinfarct protection. Toprol-XL is approved in the United States for stable symptomatic Class 2 or 3 heart failure.[50] It is also registered for hypertension and angina. *Lopressor, shorter acting,* is licensed for angina and MI.

Nadolol. (*Corgard*) is very long acting and water soluble, although it is nonselective. It is particularly useful when prolonged antianginal activity is required.

Nebivolol. (*Nebilet in the United Kingdom, Bystolic in the United States*) is a highly cardioselective agent with peripheral vasodilating properties mediated by nitric oxide.[38] Hepatic metabolites probably account for the vasodilation[51] and the long biological half-life.[52] Nebivolol reverses endothelial dysfunction in hypertension, which may explain its use for erectile dysfunction in hypertensives.[53] There are also metabolic benefits. In a 6-month study, nebivolol, in contrast to atenolol and at equal BP levels, increased insulin sensitivity and adiponectin levels in hypertensives.[54] Nebivolol given in the SENIORS trial to older adult patients with a history of heart failure or an EF of 35% or less reduced the primary composite end-point of all-cause mortality and cardiovascular hospitalizations, also increasing the EF and reducing heart size.[55]

Penbutolol. (*Levatol*) has a modest ISA, similar to acebutolol, but is nonselective. It is highly lipid soluble and is metabolized by the liver.

Table 1.4

Drugs used in hypertensive urgencies and emergencies

Clinical requirement	Mechanism of antihypertensive effect	Drug choice	Dose
Urgent reduction of severe acute hypertension	NO donor	Sodium nitroprusside infusion (care: cyanide toxicity)	0.3–2 µg/kg/min (careful monitoring)
Hypertension plus ischemia (± poor LV)	NO donor	Infusion of nitroglycerin 20–200 µg/min or isosorbide dinitrate 1–10 mg/h	Titrate against BP
Hypertension plus ischemia plus tachycardia	β-blocker (especially if good LV)	Esmolol bolus or infusion	50–250 µg/kg/min
Hypertension plus ischemia plus tachycardia	α-β-blocker	Labetalol bolus or infusion	2–10 mg 2.5-30 µg/kg/min
Hypertension plus heart failure	ACE inhibitor (avoid negative inotropic rugs)	Enalaprilat (IV) Captopril (sl)	0.5–5 mg bolus 12.5–25 mg sl
Hypertension without cardiac complications	Vasodilators, including those that increase heart rate	Hydralazine Nifedipine (see text)[a] Nicardipine : bolus : infusion	5–10 mg boluses 1–4 mg boluses 5–10 mg sl (care) 5–10 µg/kg/min 1–3 µg/kg/min
Severe or malignant hypertension, also with poor renal function	Dopamine (DA-1) agonist; avoid with β-blockers	Fenoldopam[b]	0.2–0.5 µg/kg/min
Hypertension plus pheochromocytoma	α-β-or combined α-β-blocker (avoid pure β-blocker)	Phentolamine Labetalol: bolus: infusion	1–4 mg boluses 2–10 mg 2.5–30 µg/kg/min

[a]Not licensed in the United States; oral nifedipine capsules contraindicated.
[b]Licensed as *Corlopam* for use in severe or malignant hypertension in the United States; for detailed infusion rates, see package insert. Note tachycardia as side effect must not be treated by β-blockade (package insert).
ACE, Angiotensin-converting enzyme; *BP,* blood pressure; *IV,* intravenous; *LV,* left ventricular; *NO,* nitric oxide; *sl,* sublingual.

Modified from Foex, et al. *Cardiovascular Drugs in the Perioperative Period.* New York: Authors' Publishing House; 1999, with permission. Nitrate doses from Table 6, Niemenen MS, et al. *Eur Heart J.* 2005;266:384.

Sotalol. *(Betapace, Betapace AF)* is a unique nonselective β-blocker that has Class 3 antiarrhythmic activity. It is licensed for life-threatening ventricular arrhythmias as Betapace, and now also as Betapace AF for maintenance of sinus rhythm in patients with symptomatic atrial fibrillation or atrial flutter. Sotalol is a water-soluble drug, excreted only by the kidneys, so that Betapace AF is contraindicated in patients with a creatinine clearance of less than 40 mL/min.

Timolol. *(Blocarden)* was the first β-blocker shown to give postinfarct protection and it is one of the few licensed for this purpose in the United States. Other approved uses are for hypertension and in migraine prophylaxis.

Ultrashort-Acting Intravenous β-Blockade

Esmolol. *(Brevibloc)* is an ultrashort-acting β_1-blocker with a half-life of 9 minutes, rapidly converting to inactive metabolites by blood esterases. Full recovery from β-blockade occurs within 30 minutes in patients with a normal cardiovascular system. *Indications* are situations in which on-off control of β-blockade is desired, as in SVT in the perioperative period, or sinus tachycardia (noncompensatory), or emergency hypertension in the perioperative period (all registered uses in the United States). Other logical indications are emergency hypertension (pheochromocytoma excluded) or in unstable angina.[56] *Doses* are as follows: For *SVT,* loading by 500 µg/kg/min over 1 minute, followed by a 4-minute infusion of 50 µg/kg/min (US package insert). If this fails, repeat loading dose and increase infusion to 100 µg/kg/min (over 4 minutes). If this fails, repeat loading dose and then infuse at rates up to 300 µg/kg/min. Thereafter, to maintain control, infuse at adjusted rate for up to 24 hours. For *urgent perioperative hypertension,* give 80 mg (approximately 1 mg/kg) over 30 seconds and infuse at 150 to 300 µg/kg/min if needed. For more gradual control of BP, follow routine for SVT. Higher doses are usually required for BP control than for arrhythmias. After the emergency, replace with conventional antiarrhythmic or antihypertensive drugs. For *older adult patients with non–ST-elevation MI* requiring acute β-blockade despite symptoms of heart failure, a cautious infusion of 50–200 µg/kg/min may be tried.[57] *Cautions* include extravasation of the acid solution with risk of skin necrosis.

Concomitant Diseases and Choice of β-Blocker

Respiratory disease. Cardioselective β_1-blockers in low doses are best for patients with reversible bronchospasm. In patients with a history of asthma, no β-blocker can be considered safe.

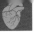

Associated cardiovascular disease. For *hypertension plus effort angina,* see "β-blockers for hypertension" earlier in this chapter. In patients with *sick sinus syndrome,* pure β-blockade can be dangerous. β-blockers with ISA may be best. In patients with *Raynaud phenomenon,* propranolol with its peripheral vasoconstrictive effects is best avoided. In active *peripheral vascular disease,* β-blockers are generally contraindicated, although the evidence is not firm.

Renal disease. The logical choice should be a β-blocker eliminated by the liver rather than the kidney (see Fig. 1.7). Of those, the vasodilating β-blocker nebivolol conserved the estimated glomerular filtration rate in patients with heart failure better than did metoprolol.[58]

Diabetes mellitus. In diabetes mellitus, the risk of β-blockade in insulin-requiring diabetics is that the premonitory symptoms of hypoglycemia might be masked. There is a lesser risk with the cardioselective agents. In type 2 diabetics with hypertension, initial β-blocker therapy by atenolol was as effective as the ACE inhibitor, captopril, in reducing macrovascular endpoints at the cost of weight gain and more antidiabetic medication.[59] Whether *diabetic nephropathy* benefits as much from treatment with β-blockade is not clear. ARBs and ACE inhibitors have now established themselves as agents of first choice in diabetic nephropathy. Carvedilol combined with renin angiotensin system (RAS) blocker therapy in diabetic patients with hypertension results in better glycemic control and less insulin resistance than combination therapy that includes metoprolol.[60] Although better glycemic control should theoretically translate into fewer cardiovascular events and other adverse outcomes, the short-term nature of this study does not allow conclusions on outcomes.

Those at risk of new diabetes. The use of β-blockers and diuretics poses a risk of new diabetes,[61] which should be lessened by a truly low dose of the diuretic or by using another combination. Regular blood glucose checks are desirable.

Side Effects of β-Blockers

The *four major mechanisms for β-blocker side effects* are (1) smooth muscle spasm (bronchospasm and cold extremities), (2) exaggeration of the cardiac therapeutic actions (bradycardia, heart block, excess negative inotropic effect), (3) central nervous system penetration (insomnia, depression), and (4) adverse metabolic side effects. The *mechanism of fatigue* is not clear. When compared with propranolol, however, it is reduced by use of either a cardioselective β-blocker or a vasodilatory agent, so that both central and peripheral hemodynamic effects may be involved. When patients are appropriately selected, double-blind studies show no differences between a cardioselective agent such as atenolol and placebo. This may be because atenolol is not lipid soluble and should have lesser effects on bronchial and vascular smooth muscle than propranolol. When *propranolol* is given for hypertension, the rate of serious side effects (bronchospasm, cold extremities, worsening of claudication) leading to withdrawal of therapy is approximately 10%.[62] The rate of withdrawal with atenolol is considerably lower (approximately 2%), but when it comes to dose-limiting side effects, both agents can cause cold extremities, fatigue, dreams, worsening claudication, and bronchospasm. Increasing heart failure remains a potential hazard when β-blockade therapy is abruptly started at normal doses in a susceptible patient and not tailored in.

Central side effects. An attractive hypothesis is that the lipid-soluble β-blockers (epitomized by propranolol) with their high brain penetration are more likely to cause central side effects. An extremely detailed comparison of propranolol and atenolol showed that the latter, which is not lipid soluble, causes far fewer central side effects than does propranolol.[63] However, depression remains an atenolol risk.[64] The lipid-solubility hypothesis also does not explain why metoprolol, which is moderately lipid soluble, appears to interfere less with some complex psychological functions than does atenolol and may even enhance certain aspects of psychological performance.[65]

Quality of life and libido. In the first quality-of-life study reported in patients with hypertension, propranolol induced considerably more central effects than did the ACE inhibitor captopril.[66] More modern β-blockers, with different fundamental properties, all leave the quality of life largely intact in hypertensives. However, there are a number of negatives. First, *weight gain* is undesirable and contrary to the lifestyle pattern required to limit cardiovascular diseases, including the metabolic syndrome and hypertension. Second, β-blockade may precipitate *diabetes*,[67] a disease that severely limits the quality of life. Third, during *exercise*, β-blockade reduces the total work possible by approximately 15% and increases the sense of fatigue. Vasodilatory β-blockers may be exceptions but lack outcome studies in hypertension. *Erectile dysfunction* is an age-dependent complication of β-blockade. In a large group with mean age 48 years, erectile problems took place in 11% given a β-blocker, compared with 26% with a diuretic and 3% with placebo.[68] β-blockers have consistently impaired sexual intercourse more than an ACE inhibitor or ARB, the latter improving sexual output.[69] Changing to nebivolol may improve erections.[53] Sildenafil (Viagra) or similar agents should also help, but are relatively contraindicated if the β-blocker is used for angina (because of the adverse interaction with nitrates, almost always used in those with angina).

Adverse metabolic side effects and new-onset diabetes. The capacity of β-blockers to increase new diabetes, whether given for hypertension or postinfarct,[61] comes at a time when diabetes is increasingly recognized as major cardiovascular hazard (see Chapter 4). A wise precaution is to obtain fasting blood glucose levels and, if indicated, a glucose tolerance curve before the onset of chronic β-blockade and at annual intervals during therapy. Note that the vasodilatory β-blockers carvedilol and nebivolol both promote formation of nitric oxide and both have a better metabolic profile than comparator cardioselective agents, without, however, long-term outcome data in hypertension (see "Specific β-Blockers" later in this chapter, see also Fig. 1.2).

β-blockade withdrawal. Chronic β-blockade increases β-receptor density. When β-blockers are suddenly withdrawn, angina may be exacerbated, sometimes resulting in MI. Treatment of the withdrawal syndrome is by reintroduction of β-blockade. Best therapy is to avoid this condition by gradual withdrawal.

Contraindications to β-Blockade

The absolute contraindications to β-blockade can be deduced from the profile of pharmacologic effects and side effects (Table 1.5). Cardiac absolute contraindications include severe bradycardia, preexisting high-degree heart block, sick sinus syndrome, and overt LV failure unless already conventionally treated and stable (Fig. 1.12). Pulmonary contraindications are overt asthma or severe bronchospasm; depending on the severity of the disease and the cardioselectivity of the β-blocker used, these may be absolute or relative contraindications. The central nervous system contraindication is severe depression (especially for propranolol). Active peripheral vascular disease with rest ischemia is another contraindication. The metabolic syndrome suggests caution.

Overdose of β-Blockers

Bradycardia may be countered by intravenous atropine 1 to 2 mg; if serious, temporary transvenous pacing may be required. When an infusion is required, glucagon (2.5 to 7.5 mg/h) is logical because it stimulates formation of cAMP by bypassing the occupied β-receptor. However, evidence is only anecdotal.[70] Logically an infusion of a phosphodiesterase inhibitor, such as amrinone or milrinone, should

Table 1.5

β-Blockade: contraindications and cautions

(Note: cautions may be overridden by the imperative to treat, as in
  postinfarct patients)

Cardiac

**Absolute: Severe bradycardia, high-degree heart block, cardiogenic
  shock, overt untreated left ventricular failure** (versus major use in
  early or stabilized heart failure).
Relative: Prinzmetal's angina (unopposed α-spasm), high doses of other
  agents depressing SA or AV nodes (verapamil, diltiazem, digoxin,
  antiarrhythmic agents); in angina, *avoid sudden withdrawal.*

Pulmonary

Absolute: Severe asthma or bronchospasm. Must question for past or
  present asthma. Risk of fatalities.
Relative: Mild asthma or bronchospasm or chronic airways disease. Use
  agents with cardioselectivity plus β_2-stimulants (by inhalation).

Central Nervous

Absolute: Severe depression (especially avoid propranolol).
Relative: Vivid dreams: avoid highly lipid-soluble agents (see Fig. 1.7) and
  pindolol; avoid evening dose. Visual hallucinations: change from
  propranolol. Fatigue (all agents). If low cardiac output is cause of
  fatigue, try vasodilatory β-blockers. Erectile dysfunction may occur
  (check for diuretic use; consider change to nebivolol and/or ACE
  inhibitor/ARB). Psychotropic drugs (with adrenergic augmentation) may
  adversely interact.

Peripheral Vascular, Raynaud Phenomenon

Absolute: Active disease: gangrene, skin necrosis, severe or worsening
  claudication, rest pain.
Relative: Cold extremities, absent pulses, Raynaud phenomenon. Avoid
  nonselective agents (propranolol, sotalol, nadolol); prefer vasodilatory
  agents.

Diabetes Mellitus

Relative: Insulin-requiring diabetes: nonselective agents decrease
  reaction to hypoglycemia; use selective agents. Note successful use of
  atenolol in type 2 diabetes in prolonged UK trial at cost of weight gain
  and more antidiabetic drug usage.

Metabolic Syndrome or Prediabetes

β-blockers may increase blood sugar by 1–1.5 mmol/L and impair insulin
  sensitivity especially with diuretic cotherapy; consider use of carvedilol
  or nebivolol.

Continued on following page

Table 1.5

β-Blockade: contraindications and cautions (Continued)

Renal Failure

Relative: As renal blood flow falls, reduce doses of agents eliminated by kidney (see Fig. 1.7).

Liver Disease

Relative: Avoid agents with high hepatic clearance (propranolol, carvedilol, timolol, acebutolol, metoprolol). Use agents with low clearance (atenolol, nadolol, sotalol). See Fig 1.7. If plasma proteins low, reduce dose of highly bound agents (propranolol, pindolol, bisoprolol).

Pregnancy Hypertension

β-blockade increasingly used but may depress vital signs in neonate and cause uterine vasoconstriction. Labetalol and atenolol best tested. Preferred drug: methyldopa.

Surgical Operations

β-blockade may be maintained throughout, provided indication is not trivial; otherwise stop 24 to 48 hours beforehand. May protect against anesthetic arrhythmias and perioperative ischemia. Preferred intravenous drug: esmolol. Use atropine for bradycardia, β-agonist for severe hypotension.

Age

β-blockade often helps to reduce BP but lacks positive outcome data. Watch pharmacokinetics and side effects in all older adult patients.

Smoking

In hypertension, β-blockade is less effective in reducing coronary events in smoking men.

Hyperlipidemia

β-blockers may have unfavorable effects on the blood lipid profile, especially nonselective agents. Triglycerides increase and HDL-cholesterol falls. Clinical significance unknown but may worsen metabolic syndrome. Vasodilatory agents, with intrinsic sympathomimetic activity or α-blocking activity, may have mildly favorable effects.

ACE, Angiotensin-converting enzyme; *AV,* atrioventricular; *ARB,* angiotensin receptor blocker; *BP,* blood pressure; *HDL,* high-density lipoprotein; *SA,* sinoatrial. Adapted from Kjeldssen, LIFE elderly substudy. *JAMA.* 2002;288:1491.

help cAMP to accumulate. Alternatively, dobutamine is given in doses high enough to overcome the competitive β-blockade (15 μg/kg/min). In patients without ischemic heart disease, an infusion (up to 0.10 μg/kg/min) of isoproterenol may be used.

β-BLOCKER CONTRAINDICATIONS

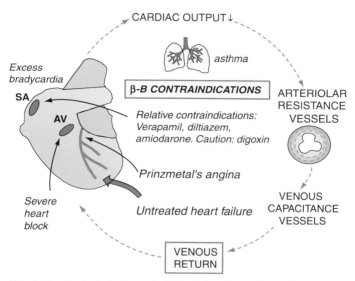

Fig. 1.12 Contraindications to β-blockade. Metabolic syndrome (not shown) is a relative contraindication to β-blockade for hypertension. *AV,* Atrioventricular, *SA,* sinoatrial. (Figure © L. H. Opie, 2012.)

Summary

1. *Clinical conditions for which β-blockers are beneficial.* β-blockers still come closest to providing all-purpose cardiovascular therapy with the conspicuous absence of any benefit for lipid problems. Approved indications include angina, hypertension, AMI, postinfarct follow-up, arrhythmias, and now heart failure. Data for postinfarct protection and for mortality reduction in CHF are particularly impressive. Other data are less compelling (Table 1.6).

2. *In heart failure,* solid data support the essential and earlier use of β-blockers in stable systolic heart failure, to counter the excessive adrenergic drive. Only three agents have been studied in detail, namely carvedilol, metoprolol, and bisoprolol, of which only the first two are approved for heart failure in the United States. In older adults, nebivolol improved EF in systolic but not diastolic heart failure. Following the recommended protocol with slow, incremental doses of the chosen agent is essential.

Table 1.6

Summary of use of β-blockers in cardiovascular disease.

Conditions	Must use[a] (Level A)	May use (Level B)	Do not use (Data Poor)
Heart failure	✓✓		
Post-MI	✓✓		
Arrhythmias (ventricular, post-MI)	✓✓		
Arrhythmias (others)		✓	
ACS, unstable angina (NSTE)		✓	
ACS, acute-phase MI		✓	
Stable angina without MI		✓	
Hypertension (initial choice)			Selective
Hypertension (selected)		✓	
Metabolic syndrome			Careful

[a]Unless contraindicated.
Note: "Must use" can override "Do not use." ✓✓ = strongly indicated; ✓ = indicated.
ACS, Acute coronary syndrome; *MI*, myocardial infarction; *NSTE*, non-ST elevation.
For concepts, see reference 40.

3. ***For coronary heart disease,*** β-blockade is very effective symptomatic treatment, alone or combined with other drugs, in 70% to 80% of patients with classic effort angina. However, atenolol-based therapy was no better at lessening major outcomes than verapamil-based therapy, and worse for some minor outcomes. β-blockers are part of the essential postinfarct protection armamentarium. For ACSs, indirect evidence suggests a quadruple follow-up regime of aspirin, statin, ACE inhibitor, and β-blockade, but there are no compelling outcome trials. Overall, there is no clinical evidence that β-blockers slow the development of coronary artery disease.

4. ***In hypertension*** β-blockers have lost their prime position, although they reduce the BP effectively in 50% to 70% of those with mild to moderate hypertension. The crucial study showed that for equal brachial pressures, the aortic pressure was less reduced with atenolol than with the CCB amlodipine, which could explain why β-blockers reduce stroke less than several other agents. Older adults with hypertension, especially those of the black ethnic group, respond less well to β-blocker monotherapy. The previously recommended combination of β-blockers and diuretics may provoke new diabetes, with lesser risk if the diuretic dose is truly low.

5. ***In arrhythmias*** β-blockers are among the more effective ventricular antiarrhythmics.

6. ***Metabolic side effects,*** including new diabetes, may be important to monitor. β-blockers can be diabetogenic even without

diuretics. The vasodilatory β-blockers carvedilol and nebivolol appear to be exceptions and have outcome studies only in heart failure.

7. ***Is there still a role for propranolol?*** There is no particular advantage for this original "gold standard" drug, with its poor quality-of-life outcomes, unless hypertension or angina with some other condition in which experience with propranolol is greater than with other β-blockers (e.g., POTS, hypertrophic cardiomyopathy, migraine prophylaxis, anxiety, or essential tremor).

8. ***Other β-blockers*** are increasingly used because of specific attractive properties: cardioselectivity (acebutolol, atenolol, bisoprolol, metoprolol), vasodilatory capacity and possible metabolic superiority (carvedilol and nebivolol), positive data in heart failure (carvedilol, metoprolol, bisoprolol, nebivolol), or postinfarct protection (metoprolol, carvedilol, timolol), lipid insolubility and no hepatic metabolism (atenolol, nadolol, sotalol), long action (nadolol) or long-acting formulations, ISA in selected patients to help avoid bradycardia (pindolol, acebutolol), and well-studied antiarrhythmic properties (sotalol). Esmolol is the best agent for intravenous use in the perioperative period because of its extremely short half-life.

9. ***Evidence-based use*** supports the use of those agents established in large randomized trials because of the known doses and clearly expected clinical benefits. For example, for postinfarct protection propranolol, metoprolol, carvedilol, and timolol are the best studied, of which only carvedilol has been studied in the reperfusion era. For stabilized heart failure, carvedilol, metoprolol, and bisoprolol have impressive data from large trials. Carvedilol especially merits attention, being licensed for a wide clinical range, from hypertension to LV dysfunction to severe heart failure, and having best trial data in heart failure. For arrhythmias, sotalol with its class 3 properties stands out.

Nitrates and Newer (or Nontraditional) Antianginals

Introduction

This section focuses on the antianginal effects of nitrates, one of *three major classes of traditional antianginal agents*, including β-blockers and CCBs (Fig. 1.13), as well as an expanding fourth

ACTION OF ANTIANGINALS

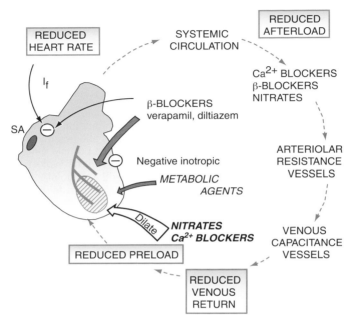

Fig. 1.13 Proposed antianginal mechanisms for the major four classes of antianginal agents: nitrates, β-blockers, calcium channel blockers, and metabolic agents (for details of metabolic agents, see Fig. 2.7). *SA,* Sinoatrial. (Figure © L. H. Opie, 2012.)

class of novel antianginals that act principally by reducing late inward sodium current (ranolazine), by metabolic modulation without major hemodynamic effects (trimetazidine), or by inhibition of the sinus node (ivabradine). Mechanistically, nitrates and CCBs are coronary vasodilators, with nitrates also reducing preload and CCBs afterload while β-blockers reduce oxygen demand by slowing heart and imparting a negative inotropic effect.

This section reviews (1) the organic nitrates, including both their antianginals effects and other hemodynamic effects, and (2) more novel agents with diverse antianginal properties, which include ranolazine, ivabradine, and trimetazidine. It is important to emphasize that the treatment and prophylaxis of angina to ameliorate symptoms is but one component of a more encompassing overall management strategy that includes proven "disease-modifying" therapies such as aspirin, P2Y$_{12}$ inhibitors, statins, inhibitors of the renin-angiotensin system (angiotensin-converting enzyme [ACE] inhibitors and ARBs), statins, and other dyslipidemic agents (ezetimibe, icosapent ethyl) in addition to treatment of symptomatic myocardial ischemia.

Mechanisms of Action of Nitrates in Angina and Heart Failure

Nitrates provide an exogenous source of vasodilator nitric oxide (NO˙, usually given as NO), a very short-lived free radical, thereby inducing coronary vasodilation even when endogenous production of NO˙ is impaired by CAD. Thus, nitrates act differently from the other classes of antianginals (see Fig. 1.13). Chronic nitrate use may produce tolerance, which can be a significant clinical problem. The main treatment strategy is to minimize or prevent the development of tolerance, with the major emphasis on the adverse role of excess NO˙ that produces harmful peroxynitrite.[71] The thrust of basic work has shifted to endogenously produced NO˙ as a ubiquitous physiologic messenger, as described by Ignarro, Furchgott, and Murad,[72] the winners of the 1998 Nobel Prize for Medicine. Although endogenously produced NO˙ has many functions (such as a role in vagal neurotransmission) quite different from the NO˙ derived from exogenous nitrates, there are important shared vasodilatory effects.

Coronary and peripheral vasodilatory effects. A distinction must be made between antianginal and coronary vasodilator properties. Nitrates preferentially dilate large coronary arteries and arterioles greater than 100 mm in diameter[73] to (1) redistribute blood flow along collateral channels and from epicardial to endocardial regions and (2) relieve coronary vasospasm and dynamic epicardial stenosis, including the coronary arterial constriction that may be induced by exercise and thereby relieving exercise-induced myocardial ischemia. Thus, nitrates are effective in dilating epicardial coronary arteries and reducing coronary vascular resistance, which, in turn, promotes augmented coronary flow to ischemic myocardium, in contrast to more potent arterial dilators such as dipyridamole and other vasodilators (such as nifedipine) that act more distally in the arterial tree and which pose the risk of diverting nutritive coronary blood away from ischemic myocardium to nonischemic myocardium, which may induce a "coronary steal" phenomenon.

The additional peripheral hemodynamic effects of nitrates, originally observed by Lauder Brunton,[74] also cannot be ignored in that nitrates do reduce both afterload and preload of the heart (Fig. 1.14).

ACTION OF NITRATES ON CIRCULATION

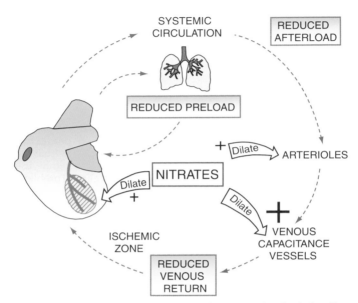

Fig. 1.14 Schematic diagram of effects of nitrate on the circulation. The major effect is on the venous capacitance vessels with additional coronary and peripheral arteriolar vasodilatory benefits. (Figure © L. H. Opie, 2012.)

Reduction in myocardial oxygen demand. Nitrates increase the venous capacitance, causing pooling of blood in the peripheral veins and thereby a reduction in venous return and in ventricular volume. There is less mechanical stress on the myocardium and this corresponding reduction in LV wall tension decreases myocardial oxygen demand. In addition, a modest fall in the aortic systolic pressure also reduces the oxygen demand.

Endothelium and vascular mechanisms. The fundamental mechanism of nitrate biological effect is the enzyme-mediated release of highly unstable NO' from the nitrate molecule (Fig. 1.15).[75] An intact vascular endothelium is required for the vasodilatory effects of some vascular active agents (thus acetylcholine physiologically vasodilates but constricts when the endothelium is damaged). Nitrates vasodilate whether or not the endothelium is physically intact or functional. Prolonged nitrate therapy with formation of peroxynitrite may, however, inhibit endothelial nitric oxide synthase (NOS), which is one of several postulated

NITRATE MECHANISMS

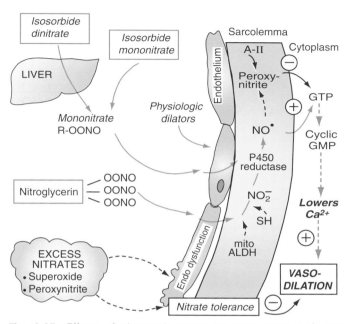

Fig. 1.15 Effects of nitrates in generating nitric oxide (NO˙) and stimulating guanylate cyclase to cause vasodilation. Nitrate tolerance is multifactorial in origin, including the endothelial effects of peroxynitrite and superoxide that ultimately inhibit the conversion of guanosine triphosphate *(GTP)* to cyclic guanosine monophosphate *(GMP)*. Note that mononitrates bypass hepatic metabolism and the mitochondrial aldehyde dehydrogenase-2 *(mito ALDH)* step required for bioactivation of nitroglycerin. Hence reduced or genetic lack of ALDH-2 may also be a cause of nitrate tolerance.[8] *Endo*, endothelial; *OONO*, peroxynitrite, *SH,* sulfhydryl. (Figure © L. H. Opie, 2008.)

mechanisms of nitrate tolerance. Similarly, long-term use of long-acting nitrates may cause endothelial dysfunction mediated by free radicals (see later, Fig. 1.16).[71,76] Whether this problem extends to aggravation of preexisting endothelial dysfunction is uncertain. Thus, nitrate tolerance and endothelial dysfunction have partially shared pathogenetic mechanisms.

Nitrates, after entering the vessel wall, are bioconverted to release NO˙, which stimulates guanylate cyclase to produce cyclic guanosine monophosphate (GMP; see Fig. 1.15). In addition, NO˙ acts potentially via direct S-nitrosylation of a number of proteins,

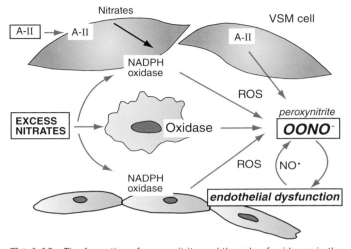

Fig. 1.16 The formation of peroxynitrite and the role of oxidases in the process. Excess nitrate administration leads to stimulation of the oxidase system. The end result is increased endothelial dysfunction. Angiotensin II stimulates the vascular smooth muscle *(VSM)* cells to form peroxynitrite. Some of the procedures that diminish these processes, leading to endothelial dysfunction, include administration of carvedilol (strong data), high doses of atorvastatin (human volunteer data), and the angiotensin receptor blocker telmisartan (experimental data). *NADPH,* Nicotinamide adenine dinucleotide phosphate; *NO·,* Nitric oxide; *OONO,* peroxynitrite; *ROS,* reactive oxygen species. (Figure © L. H. Opie, 2012.)

altering their physiologic properties via a posttranslational modification step. NO· may also be "scavenged" by the superoxide (O_2^-) radical, generating peroxynitrate ($ONOO^-$), which in high concentrations contributes to nitrate toxicity (Fig. 1.16) and the induction of nitrate tolerance. Conversely, low concentrations enhance the vasodilator effects of NO·.

Overall the best-known mechanism linked to clinical practice is that calcium in the vascular myocyte falls, and vasodilation results (see Fig. 1.15). Sulfhydryl (SH) groups are required for such formation of NO· and the stimulation of guanylate cyclase. Nitroglycerin powerfully dilates when injected into an artery, an effect that is probably limited in humans by reflex adrenergic-mediated vasoconstriction. Hence (1) nitrates are better venous than arteriolar dilators, and (2) there is an associated adrenergic reflex tachycardia[77] that can be attenuated by concurrent β-blockade.

Effects of NO' on myocardial relaxation and contractile proteins. NO' has a fundamental role as a modulator of myocardial relaxation, mediated at least in part by cyclic GMP (see Fig. 1.15).[78] This effect is independent of the restoration of coronary blood flow that in turn can reverse ischemic diastolic dysfunction. Furthermore, NO' improves diastolic function in human heart muscle where it acts on the contractile proteins by increasing troponin I phosphorylation of the springlike cytoskeletal protein titin.[79] In long-term therapy, NO' donors may limit or reverse LV hypertrophy (LVH).[80] These studies raise the possibility that organic nitrates may exert a role in the management of systemic hypertension, in which LVH is a marker and modulator of long-term cardiovascular risk.

Pharmacokinetics of Nitrates

Bioavailability and half-lives. Because the various nitrate preparations differ so appreciably, each needs to be considered separately. As a group, nitrates are absorbed from the mucous membranes, the skin, and the gastrointestinal (GI) tract. The prototype agent, nitroglycerin, has pharmacokinetics that are not well understood. It rapidly disappears from the blood with a half-life of only a few minutes, largely by extrahepatic mechanisms that convert the parent molecule to longer-acting and active dinitrates.[81] Isosorbide dinitrate, on the other hand, must first be converted in the liver to active mononitrates (see Fig. 1.15) that have half-lives of approximately 4 to 6 hours with ultimate renal excretion. The mononitrates are completely bioavailable without any hepatic metabolism, with half-lives of 4–6 hours. Of the many nitrate preparations (Table 1.7), sublingual nitroglycerin remains the gold standard for acute anginal attacks.[82] In practice, patients are often also given long-acting nitrates, except that in order to avoid or minimize the likelihood of nitrate tolerance, it is important that physicians should prescribe a 6–10-hour nitrate free interval each day, though this approach does pose the possible risk of precipitating angina during the nitrate-free interval, which is often at night.[82]

Data for Use: Clinical Indications for Nitroglycerin Preparations

Short-Acting Nitrates for Acute Exertional Angina

Sublingual nitroglycerin is very well established in the initial therapy of exertional angina, yet may be ineffective, frequently because the patient has not received proper instruction or because of severe headaches. When angina starts, the patient should rest in

---

Table 1.7

Nitrates: doses, preparations, and duration of effects

Compound	Route	Preparation and dose	Duration of effects and comments
Amyl nitrite	Inhalation	2–5 mg	10 sec–10 min; for diagnosis of LV outflow obstruction in hypertrophic cardiomyopathy.
Nitroglycerin (trinitrin, GTN)	(a) Sublingual tablets	0.3–0.6 mg up to 1.5 mg	Peak blood levels at 2 min; $t_{\frac{1}{2}}$ approximately 7 min; for acute therapy of effort or rest angina. Keep tightly capped.
	(b) Spray	0.4 mg/metered dose	Similar to tablets at same dose.
	(c) Ointment	2%; 6 × 6 ins or 15 × 15 cm or 7.5–40 mg	Apply 2 × daily; 6-h intervals; effect up to 7 h after first dose. No efficacy data for chronic use.
	(d) Transdermal patches	0.2–0.8 mg/h patch on for 12 h, patch off for 12 h	Effects start within minutes and last 3–5 h. No efficacy data for second or third doses during chronic therapy.
	(e) Oral; sustained release	2.5–13 mg 1–2 tablets 3 × daily	4–8 h after first dose; no efficacy data for chronic therapy.
	(f) Buccal	1–3 mg tablets 3 × daily	Effects start within minutes and last 3–5 h. No efficacy data for second or third doses during chronic therapy.
	(g) Intravenous infusion (discontinued in US)	5–200 µg/min (care with PVC); Tridil 0.5 mg/mL or 5 mg/mL; Nitro BID IV 5 mg/mL	In unstable angina, increasing doses are often needed to overcome tolerance. High-concentration solutions contain propylene glycol; crossreacts with heparin.

Drug		Dose	Notes
Isosorbide dinitrate (sorbide nitrate) Isordil	(a) Sublingual	2.5–15 mg	Onset 5–10 min, effect up to 60 min or longer.
	(b) Oral tablets	5–80 mg 2–3 × daily	Up to 8 h (first dose; then tolerance) with 3 × or 4 × daily doses; 2 × daily 7 h apart may be effective but data inadequate.
	(c) Spray	1.25 mg on tongue	Rapid action 2–3 min.
	(d) Chewable	5 mg as single dose	Exercise time increased for 2 min–2.5 h.
	(e) Oral; slow-release	40 mg once or 2 × daily	Up to 8 h (first dose; 2 × daily not superior to placebo).
	(f) Intravenous infusion	1.25–5 mg/h (care with PVC)	May need increasing doses for unstable angina at rest.
	(g) Ointment	100 mg/24 h	Not effective during continuous therapy.
Isosorbide 5-mononitrate	Oral tablets	20 mg 2 × day (7 h apart); 120–240 mg 1 × daily (slow release)	12–14 h after chronic dosing for 2 weeks. Efficacy up to 12 h after 6 weeks.
Pentaerythritol tetranitrate (not in US)	Sublingual	10 mg as needed	No efficacy data.

Long acting ([(b), (e), and (g)], available in the United States: Nitroglycerin Extended Release, nitroglycerin transdermal patch. (a), (c), and (d) are short-acting, and (f) is intravenous.
Available in the United States: Extended Release Isosorbide dinitrate, Isosorbide mononitrate.
GTN, glyceryl trinitrate; IV, Intravenous; LV, left ventricular; PVC, polyvinylchloride tubing; $t_{1/2}$; half-life.

the sitting position (standing may promote syncope, while a recumbent position enhances venous return and increased work of the heart) and take sublingual nitroglycerin (0.3 to 0.6 mg) every 5 minutes until the discomfort abates. In general, it is not advised that patients consume more than three sublingual nitroglycerin tablets over 15 minutes; persistent rest angina unresponsive to multiple nitroglycerin tablets may presage an ACS or AMI, and should be regarded as a medical emergency. *Nitroglycerin spray* is an alternative mode of oral administration, which is more acceptable to some patients. It vasodilates sooner than does the tablet, which might be of special importance in those with dryness of the mouth.[83]

Isosorbide dinitrate may be given *sublingually* (5 mg) to abort an anginal attack and then exerts antianginal effects for approximately 1 hour. Because the dinitrate requires hepatic conversion to the mononitrate, the onset of antianginal action (mean time: 3.4 minutes) is slower than with nitroglycerin (mean time: 1.9 minutes), so that the manufacturers of the dinitrate compound recommend sublingual administration of this drug only if the patient is unresponsive to or intolerant of sublingual nitroglycerin. After oral ingestion, hemodynamic and antianginal effects persist for several hours. Single doses of isosorbide dinitrate confer longer protection against angina than can single doses of sublingual nitroglycerin (see Table 1.7).

Short-Acting Nitrates for Angina Prophylaxis

While most physicians and patients regard sublingual nitroglycerin as an acute treatment intervention to abort an angina attack, it is important to emphasize that sublingual nitroglycerin or nitrolingual spray can also be used prophylactically to prevent an angina attack when there is a regular, predictable pattern of exertional angina that is elicited with a particular precipitant such as brisk walking up an incline or climbing a hill, exposure to cold, eating a large meal, etc. Patients can be encouraged to take a short-acting nitrate preparation several minutes prior to the onset of the expected offending activity in order to obtain a potentially therapeutic coronary vasodilatory effect.

Long-Acting Nitrates for Angina Prophylaxis

As noted, long-acting nitrates are not continuously effective if regularly taken over a prolonged period, unless allowance is made for a nitrate-free or nitrate-low interval (Table 1.8).[84-87] Worsening of endothelial dysfunction is a potential complication of long-acting nitrates that should be avoided,[88] and the common practice of routine use of long-acting nitrates for exertional angina[7] may have to be reevaluated.

Table 1.8

Interval therapy for effort angina by eccentric nitrate dosage schedules designed to avoid tolerance		
Preparation	**Dose**	**Reference**
Isosorbide dinitrate	30 mg at 7 am, 1 pm[a]	Thadani and Lipicky, 1994[84]
Isosorbide mononitrate (Robins-Boehringer-Wyeth-Ayerst; Pharma-Schwartz)	20 mg at 8 am and 3 pm	Parker, 1993[85]
Isosorbide mononitrate, Extended-release (Key-Astra)	120–240 mg daily	Chrysant, 1993[86]
Transdermal nitrate patches	7.5–10 mg per 12 h; patches removed after 12 h	DeMots, 1989[87]
Phasic release nitroglycerin patch	15 mg, most released in first 12 h[b]	Parker, 1989[c]

[a]Efficacy of second dose not established; no data for other doses.
[b]No data for other doses.
[c]*Eur Heart J.* 1989;10(Suppl. A):43–49.

Isosorbide dinitrate (oral preparation) is frequently given for the prophylaxis of angina. An important question is whether regular therapy with isosorbide dinitrate gives long-lasting protection (3–5 hours) against angina. In a crucial placebo-controlled study, exercise duration improved significantly for 6 to 8 hours after single oral doses of 15 to 120 mg isosorbide dinitrate, but for only 2 hours when the same doses were given repetitively four times daily.[89] Marked tolerance develops during sustained therapy, despite much higher plasma isosorbide dinitrate concentrations during sustained than during acute therapy.[89] While eccentric twice-daily treatment with extended-release isosorbide dinitrate (*Tembids*) 40 mg administered in the morning and 7 hours later was not superior to placebo in a large multicenter study,[84] such dosing schedules of isosorbide dinitrate are still often used in an effort to avoid tolerance.

Mononitrates have similar dosage and effects to those of isosorbide dinitrate. Nitrate tolerance, likewise a potential problem, can be prevented or minimized when rapid-release preparations (*Monoket, Ismo*) are given twice daily in an eccentric pattern with doses spaced by 7 hours.[85] Using the slow-release preparation (*Imdur*), the dose range 30–240 mg once daily was tested for antianginal activity. Only higher dose 120 and 240 mg daily improved exercise times at 4 and 12 hours after administration, even after

42 days of daily use.[86] These high doses were reached by titration over 7 days. A daily dose of 60 mg, still often used, was ineffective.

Transdermal nitroglycerin patches are designed to permit the timed release of nitroglycerin over a 24-hour period. Despite initial claims of 24-hour efficacy, major studies have failed to show prolonged improvement, and nitrate tolerance is an issue with more continuous dosing.

Nitrates for Acute Coronary Syndromes

Large trials have failed to show a consistent reduction in mortality in either unstable angina and non-ST elevation MI or in ST-elevation MI. Therefore, the goal of nitrate therapy is pain relief or management of associated acute heart failure[90] or severe hypertension.

Intravenous nitroglycerin is widely regarded as being effective in the management of pain in patients with ACS, although without properly controlled trials. Nitroglycerin should be infused at an initial rate of 5 μg/min (or even 2.5 μg/min in patients with borderline hypotension), using nonadsorptive delivery systems. Although earlier studies used progressive uptitration of infusion rates to relief of pain (with eventual rates of >1000 μg/min in some patients), this strategy should be limited in general because of the risks of tolerance induction and subsequent "rebound." Given that even 10 μg/min nitroglycerin induces some degree of tolerance within 24 hours,[91] an infusion rate of 10–50 μg/min is recommended in most cases.[92] Nitrate patches and nitroglycerin ointment should not be used. Intravenous therapy, which can be titrated upward as needed, is far better for control of pain, and because of the short half-live of intravenous nitroglycerin, rapid downtitration is usually effective if BP decreases.

Percutaneous coronary intervention. Intracoronary nitroglycerin is often used to minimize ischemia, for example, caused by coronary spasm, either with or without oral CCBs.

Acute Heart Failure and Acute Pulmonary Edema

No clear guidelines exist regarding management of *acute decompensated heart failure*. In an observational study of more than 65,000 patients, intravenous nitroglycerin gave similar outcomes to what was achieved previously with intravenous nesiritide and better results than dobutamine, though randomized trail data are largely lacking.[93]

In *acute pulmonary edema* from various causes, including acute MI, nitroglycerin can be strikingly effective, with some risk of precipitous falls in BP and of tachycardia or bradycardia. Sublingual nitroglycerin in repeated doses of 0.8 to 2.4 mg every 5 to 10 minutes can relieve dyspnea within 15 to 20 minutes, with a fall of LV filling pressure and a rise in cardiac output.[94] Intravenous nitroglycerin, however, is usually a better method to administer nitroglycerin because the dose can be rapidly adjusted upward or downward depending on the clinical and hemodynamic response. Infusion rates required may be higher than the maximal use for acute MI (i.e., above 200 μg/min), but this is premised on the need for only a brief infusion when pulmonary edema is present without systemic hypotension. A similar approach has been validated with intravenously infused isosorbide dinitrate.[95]

Heart Failure With Reduced Ejection Fraction

Both short- and long-acting nitrates are used as unloading agents in the relief of symptoms in acute and chronic heart failure. Their dilating effects are more pronounced on veins than on arterioles, so they are best suited to patients with raised pulmonary wedge pressure and clinical features of pulmonary congestion. There is a beneficial, synergistic interaction between nitrates and hydralazine whereby the latter helps to lessen nitrate tolerance,[96] probably acting through inhibition of free radical formation. This may explain why the combination of nitrates and hydralazine is effective in heart failure.[97] The combination of high-dose isosorbide dinitrate (60 mg four times daily) plus hydralazine was better than placebo in decreasing mortality, yet nonetheless inferior to an ACE inhibitor in severe heart failure.[98] However, heart failure patients treated with the hydralazine-isosorbide dinitrate combination had more significant improvements in both EF and NYHA functional class compared to enalapril. Thus, there is a firm therapeutic rationale for using additive, or combination, vasodilator therapy in heart failure patients.[98]

As in treating exertional angina, *nitrate tolerance* remains a problem. Intermittent dosing designed to counter periods of expected dyspnea (at night, or during anticipated exercise) is one approach.[99] Escalating doses of nitrates provide only a short-term solution and should, in general, be avoided.

Beneficial Combination of Isosorbide Dinitrate and Hydralazine in African American Patients With Heart Failure

The combination of hydralazine and isosorbide dinitrate is approved for use in the United States as BiDil (Nitromed, Inc) for patients with heart failure who self-identify as black. Approval was based in part on results of the African American Heart Failure Trial (A-HeFT) showing that BiDil use was associated with a 43% reduction in death and a 39% reduction in hospitalizations.[100] The combination used was isosorbide dinitrate 20 mg and hydralazine 37.5 mg, both given three times daily.

Despite the proven efficacy of this additive vasodilator combination in African Americans, it remains unclear whether there could be a potentially incremental role of such combination therapy in other ethnic groups of patients with severe heart failure or in whom other forms of pharmacotherapy are relatively contra-indicated, for example, on the basis of renal dysfunction.

Side Effects, Contraindications, and Drug Interactions

Side Effects

Hypotension is the most serious and headache the most common side effect (Table 1.9). Headache characteristically occurs with sublingual nitroglycerin, and at the start of therapy with long-acting nitrates.[82] Often the headaches pass over while antianginal efficacy is maintained; yet headaches may lead to loss of treatment adherence. Concomitant aspirin reduces the occurrence of headaches. In chronic lung disease, arterial hypoxemia may result from vaso-dilation and increased venous admixture.

Nitrate Contraindications

With right ventricular involvement in AMI, a nitrate-induced fall in LV filling pressure may aggravate hypotension. A systolic BP of less than 90 mmHg is a contraindication. Recent ingestion of sildenafil or its equivalent means that nitrate therapy must be delayed or avoided (see "Nitrate Interactions with Other Drugs," pp. 43–44).

Nitrate Interactions With Other Drugs

Many of the proposed interactions of nitrates are pharmacody-namic, involving potentiation of vasodilatory effects, as with the CCBs. However, the chief example of vasodilator interactions is with the selective phosphodiesterase-5 (PDE-5) inhibitors such as sildenafil and similar agents used for erectile dysfunction. In addi-tion, PDE-5 inhibitors are used increasingly for the therapy of pul-monary hypertension (see Chapter 11), and their potential benefits in heart failure are likewise being explored. As a group, these agents can cause serious hypotensive reactions when com-bined with nitrates (see Fig. 1.16). Hence the package insert of each agent forbids coadministration to patients taking nitrates in any form either regularly or intermittently. For example, sildenafil decreases the BP by approximately 8.4/5.5 mmHg, and by much more in those taking nitrates. The exertion of sexual intercourse also stresses the cardiovascular system further. As a group, these drugs should also not be given with α-adrenergic blockers. In case of inadvertent *PDE-5-nitrate combinations*, administration of an α-adrenergic agonist or even of norepinephrine may be needed.

Table 1.9

Nitrate precautions and side effects

Precautions

Need airtight containers.
Nitrate sprays are inflammable.

Common side effects

Headaches *initially* frequently limit dose; often respond to aspirin.
Facial flushing may occur.
Sublingual nitrates may cause halitosis.

Serious side effects

Syncope and hypotension may occur.
Hypotension risks cerebral ischemia.
Alcohol or other vasodilators may augment hypotension.
Tachycardia frequent.
Methemoglobinemia: with prolonged high doses. Give IV methylene blue
(1–2 mg/kg)

Contraindications

In ***hypertrophic obstructive cardiomyopathy***, nitrates may exaggerate
outflow obstruction.
Sildenafil (or similar agents): risk of hypotension or even acute MI.

Relative contraindications

Cor pulmonale: decreased arterial pO_2.
Reduced venous return risky in constrictive pericarditis, tight mitral
stenosis.

Tolerance

Continuous high doses lead to tolerance that eccentric dosage may avoid.
Cross-tolerance between formulations.

Withdrawal symptoms

Gradually discontinue long-term nitrates.

IV, Intravenous; *MI,* myocardial infarction.

Additionally, whenever a male patient presents with an anginal attack or ACS, whether or not precipitated by sexual intercourse, one essential question that must be considered or probed is whether the patient has recently taken sildenafil (Viagra), vardenafil (Levitra), or tadalafil (Cialis) (Fig. 1.17)? If so, an important corollary question is how soon thereafter can a nitrate be safely administered. In clinical practice, nitrates may be started 24 hours

SERIOUS NITRATE INTERACTION

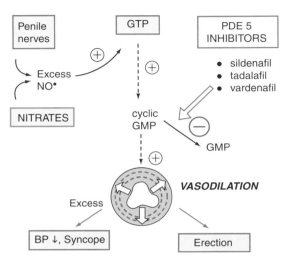

Fig. 1.17 A serious nitrate-drug interaction. The mechanism of normal erection involves penile vasodilation mediated by guanosine triphosphate *(GTP)* and cyclic guanosine monophosphate *(GMP)*. The phosphodiesterase-5 inhibitors *(PDE 5)* such as sildenafil (Viagra) act by inhibiting the enzymatic breakdown of penile cyclic GMP to GMP with increased vasodilation. This is not confined to the penis, and peripheral vasodilation added to that caused by nitrates gives rise to an excess fall of blood pressure *(BP)* and possible syncope. Hence the use of PDE 5 inhibitors in any patient taking nitrates is contraindicated. *NO˙*, Nitric oxide. (Figure © L. H. Opie, 2012.)

after sildenafil[82] and for vardenafil, while for the longer-acting tadalafil, the corresponding interval is 48 hours.[101]

Nitrate Tolerance and Nitric Oxide Resistance

Nitrate Tolerance

Nitrate tolerance often limits nitrate efficacy. Thus longer-acting nitrates, although providing higher and better-sustained blood nitrate levels, paradoxically often seem to lose their efficacy with time. This is the phenomenon of nitrate tolerance (see Fig. 1.15).

Strategies to Prevent or Minimize Nitrate Tolerance

In effort angina, many studies now show that symptomatic tolerance can be lessened by interval dosing. Eccentric twice-daily doses of isosorbide mononitrate (Monoket, Ismo) or once-daily treatment with 120 or 240 mg of the extended-release formulation of mononitrate (Imdur) maintain clinical activity but may nonetheless lead to endothelial dysfunction.[76] There is considerable evidence that nitrate effects on blood vessels and platelets are SH-dependent.[102-104] Concomitant therapy with SH donors such as N-acetylcysteine (NAC) potentiates nitroglycerin effects, both hemodynamically[105] and on platelet aggregation.[106] Concomitant nitroglycerin-NAC therapy may also limit tolerance induction clinically[107] while improving outcomes in unstable angina pectoris.[108] Additional simple procedures that might be tried are folic acid supplementation, supplemental L-arginine,[109] and vitamin C.[76]

Nitrate Rebound and Pseudotolerance

Rebound is the abrupt increase in anginal frequency during accidental nitrate withdrawal (e.g., displacement of an intravenous infusion) or during nitrate-free periods.[110,111] Nitrate pseudotolerance probably accounts for the "zero hour phenomenon," whereby patients receiving long-acting nitrate therapy experience worsening of angina just prior to routine administration of medication.[87] The purported underlying mechanisms are unopposed vasoconstriction (angiotensin II, catecholamines, and endothelin) during nitrate withdrawal with attenuation of net vasodilator effect of NO˙.[112]

Nitric Oxide Resistance

NO˙ resistance may be defined as *de novo* hyporesponsiveness to NO˙ effects, whether vascular or antiaggregatory. It also occurs with other "direct" donors of NO˙, such as sodium nitroprusside. The occurrence of NO˙ resistance accounts for the finding that some patients with heart failure respond poorly to infused NO˙ donors, irrespective of prior nitrate exposure.[113] The mechanisms of NO˙ resistance in platelets relate primarily to incremental redox stress mediated by superoxide anion release.[114] There is a close association between NO˙ resistance and endothelial dysfunction as in ACS.[115] Platelet resistance to NO˙ is an adverse prognostic marker.[116]

Combination Therapy for Angina

Existing data are inadequate to evaluate the overall efficacy of combinations of nitrates plus β-blockers and CCBs when compared with optimal therapy by each other or by any one agent alone.

The previous landmark COURAGE Trial continues to reflect current American practice, and these findings have been largely validated and reinforced by the recent large international ISCHEMIA Trial published in April 2020.[117a-c] Almost all received a statin and aspirin, 86% to 89% a β-blocker, and 65% to 78% an ACE inhibitor or ARB. Nitrate use declined from 72% at the start to 57% at 5 years. However, only 43% to 49% were given a CCB.[117d]

β-blockade and long-acting nitrates are often combined in the therapy of angina (see Table 1.10). Both β-blockers and nitrates decrease the oxygen demand, and nitrates increase the oxygen supply; β-blockers block the tachycardia caused by

Table 1.10

Proposed step-care for angina of effort

1. **General:** History and physical examination to exclude valvular disease, anemia, hypertension, thromboembolic disease, thyrotoxicosis, and heart failure. Check risk factors for coronary artery disease (smoking, hypertension, blood lipids, diabetes, obesity). Must stop smoking. Check diet.
2. **Prophylactic drugs.** Give aspirin, statins and ACE inhibitors. Control BP.
3. **Start-up.** *First-line therapy.* Short-acting nitrates are regarded as the basis of therapy, to which is added either a β-blocker or CCB (heart-rate lowering or DHP) β-blocker if prior infarct or heart failure. Otherwise level of evidence only C.[a] May use CCB (preferably verapamil as in INVEST[42] or diltiazem or long-acting dihydropyridine).
4. **Second-line therapy** is the combination of a short-acting nitrate with a β-blocker plus a CCB (DHP).
5. **Third-line therapy.** The add-on choice is between long-acting nitrates, ivabradine, nicorandil, ranolazine, perhexiline (Australia and New Zealand), or trimetazidine (Europe).
6. **PCI with stenting** may be attempted at any stage in selected patients, especially for highly symptomatic single vessel disease.
7. **Consider bypass surgery** after failure to respond to medical therapy or for left main stem lesion or for triple vessel disease, especially if reduced LV function. Even response to medical therapy does not eliminate need for investigation.
8. **Nitrate failure** may occur at any of these steps. Consider nitrate tolerance or worsening disease or poor compliance.

[a]Gibbons RJ, et al. ACC/AHA 2002 guideline update for the management of patients with chronic stable angina—summary article: a report of the American College of Cardiology/American Heart Association Task Force on practice guidelines (Committee on the Management of Patients with Chronic Stable Angina). *J Am Coll Cardiol.* 2003;41:159–168.
ACE, Angiotensin-converting enzyme; *BP,* blood pressure; *CCB,* Calcium channel blocker; *DHP,* dihydropyridine; *LV,* left ventricular; *PCI,* percutaneous coronary intervention.

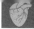

nitrates. β-blockade tends to increase heart size and nitrates to decrease it.

CCBs and short-acting nitroglycerin are often combined. In a double-blind trial of 47 patients with effort angina, verapamil 80 mg three times daily decreased the use of nitroglycerin tablets by 25% and prolonged exercise time by 20%.[118] No outcome data have been reported. *CCBs and long-acting nitrates* are also often given together, however, again without support from outcome trial data.

Nitrates, β-blockers, and CCBs may also be combined as triple therapy. The ACTION study was a very large outcome study in which long-acting nifedipine GI therapeutic system (GITS; Procardia XL, Adalat CC) was added to preexisting antianginal therapy, mostly β-blockers (80%) and nitrates (57% nitrates as needed, and 38% daily nitrates).[7] The CCB reduced the need for coronary angiography or bypass surgery, and reduced new heart failure. In hypertensive patients added nifedipine gave similar but more marked benefits plus stroke reduction.[119] There are two lessons: first, dual medical therapy by β-blockers and nitrates is inferior to triple therapy (added DHP CCBs); and second, hypertension in stable angina needs vigorous antihypertensive therapy as in triple therapy. However, we argue that "optimal medical therapy" should consider a metabolically active agent.

Calcium Channel Blockers

Introduction

CCBs (calcium antagonists) act chiefly by vasodilation and reduction of the peripheral vascular resistance. They remain among the most commonly used agents for hypertension and angina. Their major role in these conditions is now well established, based on the results of a series of large trials. CCBs are a heterogeneous group of drugs that can chemically be classified into the DHPs and the non-DHPs (Table 1.11), their common pharmacologic property being selective inhibition of L-type channel opening in vascular smooth muscle and in the myocardium (Fig. 1.18). Distinctions between the DHPs and non-DHPs are reflected in different binding sites on the calcium channel pores, and in the greater vascular selectivity of the DHP agents.[120] In addition, the non-DHPs, by virtue of nodal inhibition, reduce the heart rate (heart rate–lowering [HRL] agents). Thus, verapamil and diltiazem more closely resemble the β-blockers in their therapeutic spectrum, with one major difference: CCBs should be used cautiously in heart failure, particularly in the setting of a recent Q-wave MI or ST-segment elevation myocardial infarction (STEMI).[121]

Table 1.11

Binding sites for CCBs, tissue specificity, clinical uses, and safety concerns				
Site	Tissue specificity	Clinical uses	Contraindications	Safety concerns
DHP binding				
Prototype: nifedipine Site 1	Vessels > myocardium > nodes Vascular selectivity $10 \times$ N, A $100 \times$ Nic, I, F $1000 \times$ Nis	Effort angina (N, A) Hypertension (N,[a] A, Nic, I, F, Nis) Vasospastic angina (N, A) Raynaud phenomenon	Unstable angina, early-phase AMI, systolic heart failure (possible exception: amlodipine)	Nifedipine capsules: excess BP fall especially in older adults; adrenergic activation in ACS Longer-acting forms: safe in hypertension, no studies on ACS
Non-DHP binding				
"Heart rate lowering" Site 1B, D Site 1C, V	SA and AV nodes > myocardium = vessels	Angina: effort (V, D), unstable (V), vasospastic (V, D) Hypertension (D,[a]V) Arrhythmias, supraventricular (D,[b] V) Verapamil: postinfarct patients (no US license)	Systolic heart failure; sinus bradycardia or SSS; AV nodal block; WPW syndrome; AMI (early phase)	Systolic heart failure, especially diltiazem. Safety record of verapamil may equal that of β-blockade in older adult patients with hypertension

[a]Long-acting forms only.

[b]Intravenous forms only.

FDA-approved drugs for listed indications in parentheses. *A*, Amlodipine; *ACS*, acute coronary syndrome; *AMI*, acute myocardial infarction; *AV*, atrioventricular; *BP*, blood pressure; *CCB*, calcium channel blocker; *D*, diltiazem; *DHP*, dihydropyridine; *F*, felodipine; *FDA*, Food and Drug Administration; *I*, isradipine; *N*, nifedipine; *Nic*, nicardipine; *Nis*, nisoldipine; *SA*, sinoatrial; *SSS*, sick sinus syndrome; *V*, verapamil; *WPW*, Wolff-Parkinson-White syndrome.

Ca^{2+} MOVEMENTS

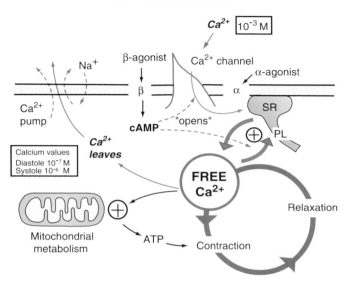

Fig. 1.18 Role of calcium channel in regulating myocardial cytosolic calcium ion movements. α, Alpha-adrenergic receptor; β, beta-adrenergic receptor; *cAMP,* cyclic adenosine monophosphate; *PL,* phospholamban; *SR,* sarcoplasmic reticulum. (Figure © L.H. Opie, 2012.)

Mechanisms of Action and Pharmacologic Properties

Calcium Channels: L and T Types

The most important property of all CCBs is selectively to inhibit the inward flow of charge-bearing calcium ions when the calcium channel becomes permeable or is "open." Previously, the term *slow channel* was used, but now it is realized that the calcium current travels much faster than originally thought, and that there are at least two types of calcium channels, the L and T. The conventional long-lasting opening calcium channel is termed the *L-type channel,* which is blocked by CCBs and increased in activity by catecholamines. The function of the L-type is to permit the influx of the requisite amount of calcium ions needed for initiation of contraction via the release of stored calcium ions from the SR (see Fig. 1.18). The T-type (*T* for transient) channel opens at more negative potentials than the L-type. It plays an important role in the initial depolarization of sinus and AV nodal tissue and is relatively upregulated in the failing myocardium. Currently there are no specific T-type blockers clinically available.

In smooth muscle (see Fig. 1.6), calcium ions regulate the contractile mechanism independently of troponin C. Interaction of calcium with calmodulin forms calcium-calmodulin, which then stimulates myosin light chain kinase (MLCK) to phosphorylate the myosin light chains to allow actin-myosin interaction and, hence, contraction. cAMP inhibits the MLCK. By contrast, β-blockade, by lessening the formation of cAMP, removes the inhibition on MLCK activity, and therefore promotes contraction in smooth muscle, which explains why asthma may be precipitated, and why the peripheral vascular resistance often rises at the start of β-blocker therapy (Fig. 1.19).

HEMODYNAMICS: β-BLOCKERS vs CCBs

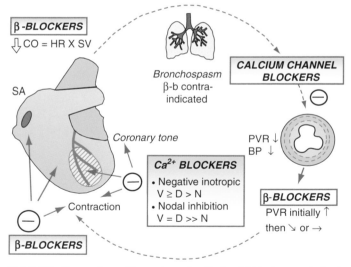

Fig. 1.19 Comparison of hemodynamic effects of β-blockers and of calcium channel blockers *(CCBs)*, showing possibilities for combination therapy. *BP,* Blood pressure; *CO,* cardiac output; *D,* diltiazem; *HR,* heart rate; *N,* nifedipine as an example of dihydropyridines; *PVR,* peripheral vascular resistance; *SA,* sinoatrial node; *SV,* stroke volume; *V,* verapamil. (Figure © L.H. Opie, 2012.)

Cellular Mechanisms: β-Blockade Versus CCBs

Both these categories of agents are used primarily for angina and hypertension, yet there are important differences in their subcellular mode of action. Both have a negative inotropic effect, whereas only CCBs relax vascular and (to a much lesser extent) other smooth muscle (Fig. 1.6). CCBs "block" the entry of calcium through the calcium channel in both smooth muscle and myocardium, so that less calcium is available to the contractile apparatus. The result is vasodilation and a negative inotropic effect, which in the case of the DHPs is usually modest because of the unloading effect of peripheral artery vasodilation.

CCBs versus β-blockers. CCBs and β-blockers have hemodynamic and neurohumoral differences. Hemodynamic differences are well defined (see Fig. 1.19). Whereas β-blockers inhibit the renin-angiotensin system by decreasing renin release and oppose the hyperadrenergic state in heart failure, CCBs as a group have no such inhibitory effects.[122] This difference could explain why β-blockers but not CCBs are an important component for treating heart failure.

Classification of CCBs and Differences Among Drugs in Class

Dihydropyridines (DHPs)

The DHPs all bind to the same sites on the α_1-subunit (the N sites), thereby establishing their common property of calcium channel antagonism (Fig. 1.20). To a different degree, they exert a greater inhibitory effect on vascular smooth muscle than on the myocardium, conferring the property of vascular selectivity (see Table 1.11, Fig. 1.21). There is nonetheless still the potential for myocardial depression, particularly in the case of agents with less selectivity and in the presence of prior myocardial disease (particularly extensive MI)[123] or β-blockade. For practical purposes, effects of DHPs on the SA and AV nodes can be ignored.

Nondihydropyridine (non-DHP) or Heart Rate-Lowering (HRL) CCBs

Both verapamil and diltiazem bind to two different sites on the α_1-subunit of the calcium channel (see Fig. 1.20) yet have many properties in common with each other. The first and most obvious distinction from the DHPs is that verapamil and diltiazem both act on nodal tissue, being therapeutically effective in SVTs. Both tend to decrease impulse formation from the sinus node and slow heart rate. Both

CALCIUM CHANNEL MODEL

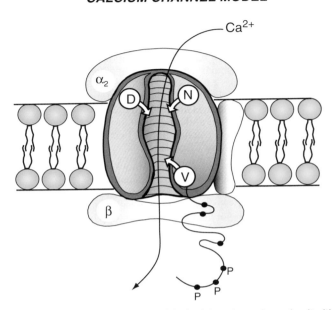

Fig. 1.20 Proposed molecular model of calcium channel α_1-subunit with binding sites for nifedipine *(N)*, diltiazem *(D)*, and verapamil *(V)*. It is thought that all dihydropyridines bind to the same site as nifedipine. Amlodipine has additional subsidiary binding to the V and D sites. *P* indicates sites of phosphorylation in response to cyclic adenosine monophosphate (see Fig. 1.18), which acts to increase the opening probability of the calcium channel. (Figure © L.H. Opie, 2012.)

inhibit myocardial contraction more than the DHPs or, put differently, are less vascular selective (see Fig. 1.21). These properties, added to peripheral vasodilation, lead to substantial reduction in the myocardial oxygen demand. Such "oxygen conservation" makes the HRL agents much closer than the DHPs to the β-blockers, with which they share some similarities of therapeutic activity.

Specific CCB Agents

Verapamil

Verapamil (Isoptin, Calan, Verelan), the prototype non-DHP agent, remains the CCB with the most licensed indications. Both verapamil and diltiazem have multiple cardiovascular effects (see Fig. 1.22).

CARDIAC VS VASCULAR SELECTIVITY

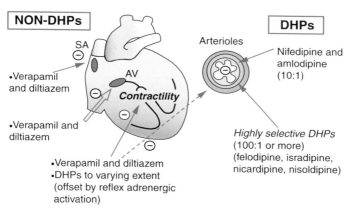

Fig. 1.21 As a group, the dihydropyridines *(DHPs)* are more vascular selective, whereas the non-DHPs verapamil and diltiazem act equally on the heart and on the arterioles. *AV,* Atrioventricular; *SA,* sinoatrial. (Figure © L.H. Opie, 2012.)

Electrophysiology. Verapamil inhibits the action potential of the upper and middle regions of the AV node where depolarization is calcium mediated. Verapamil thus inhibits one limb of the reentry circuit, believed to underlie most paroxysmal SVTs (see Fig. 1.23). Increased AV block and the increase in effective refractory period of the AV node explain the reduction of the ventricular rate in atrial flutter and fibrillation. Hemodynamically, verapamil combines arteriolar dilation with a direct negative inotropic effect (see Table 1.12).

Pharmacokinetics. Oral verapamil takes 2 hours to act and peaks at 3 hours. Therapeutic blood levels (80 to 400 ng/mL) are seldom measured. The elimination half-life is usually 3 to 7 hours but increases significantly during chronic administration and in patients with liver or advanced renal insufficiency. Despite nearly complete absorption of oral doses, bioavailability is only 10% to 20%. There is a high first-pass liver metabolism by multiple components of the P-450 system, including CYP3A4, the latter explaining why verapamil increases blood levels of several statins such as atorvastatin, simvastatin, and lovastatin, as well as ketoconazole. Because of the hepatic CYP3A4 interaction, the US Food and Drug Administration (FDA) warns that the 10-mg dose of simvastatin should not be exceeded in patients taking verapamil. Ultimate

VERAPAMIL OR DILTIAZEM, MULTIPLE EFFECTS

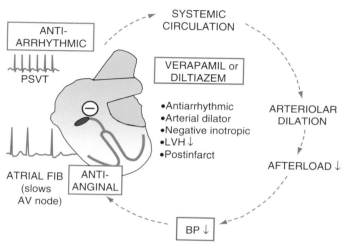

Fig. 1.22 Verapamil and diltiazem have a broad spectrum of therapeutic effects. *Atrial fib,* Atrial fibrillation; *AV,* atrioventricular; *BP,* blood pressure; *LVH,* left ventricular hypertrophy; *PSVT,* paroxysmal supraventricular tachycardia. (Figure © L.H. Opie, 2012.)

BETA & I*f* EFFECTS ON SA NODE

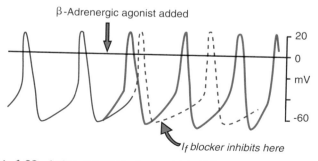

Fig. 1.23 Action potential of sinoatrial *(SA)* node, with effect of β-adrenergic stimulation and of inhibition of current I$_f$, relevant to recent development of a specific I$_f$ blocker. (Figure © L.H. Opie, 2012.)

excretion of the parent compound, as well as the active hepatic metabolite norverapamil, is 75% by the kidneys and 25% by the GI tract. Verapamil is 87% to 93% protein bound, but no interaction with warfarin has been reported. When both verapamil and digoxin are given together, their interaction causes digoxin levels to rise, probably as a result of a reduction in the renal clearance of digoxin.

Verapamil doses. The usual total oral dose is 180–360 mg daily, but no more than 480 mg given once or twice daily (long-acting formulations) or three times daily for standard short-acting preparations should be administered (see Table 1.12). Large differences in pharmacokinetics among individuals indicates that careful dose titration is required, so that 120 mg daily may be adequate for those with hepatic impairment or for older adults. During chronic oral dosing, the formation of norverapamil metabolites and altered rates of hepatic metabolism suggest that less frequent or smaller daily doses of short-acting verapamil may be used.[124] For example, if verapamil has been given at a dose of 80 mg three times daily, then 120 mg twice daily should be equipotent and well tolerated. Lower doses are required in older adult patients or those with advanced renal or hepatic disease or when there is concurrent β-blockade. Intravenous verapamil is much less used for supraventricular arrhythmias since the advent of adenosine and the ultra–short acting β-blocker, esmolol.

Slow-release preparations. Calan SR or Isoptin SR releases the drug from a matrix at a rate that responds to food, whereas Verelan releases the drug from a rate-controlling polymer at a rate not sensitive to food intake. The usual doses are 240–480 mg daily. The SR preparations are given once or twice daily and Verelan once daily. A controlled-onset, extended-release tablet (Covera-HS; COER-24; 180 or 240 mg tablets) is also taken once daily at bedtime.

Data for Clinical Use: Indications for Verapamil

Angina and myocardial ischemia. In chronic stable exertional angina, verapamil acts by a combination of afterload reduction and a mild negative inotropic effect, plus reduction of exercise-induced tachycardia and coronary vasoconstriction. The heart rate usually stays the same or falls modestly. In a major outcome study in patients with CAD with hypertension, INVEST, verapamil-based therapy was compared with atenolol-based therapy, the former supplemented by the ACE inhibitor trandolapril and the latter by a thiazide, if required, to achieve the BP goal.[42] Major outcomes were very similar, but verapamil-based therapy resulted in less angina and new diabetes. Verapamil doses of 240–360 mg daily were the

Table 1.12

Oral heart rate-lowering CCBs: salient features for cardiovascular use

Agent	Dose	Pharmacokinetics and metabolism	Side effects and contraindications	Kinetic and dynamic interactions
Verapamil				
Tablets (for IV use, see p. 78)	180–480 mg daily in two or three doses (titrated)	Peak plasma levels with 1–2 h. Low bioavailability (10%–20%), high first-pass metabolism to long-acting norverapamil Excretion: 75% renal; 25% GI; t1/2 3–7 h	Constipation; depression of SA, AV nodes, and LV; CI sick sinus syndrome, digoxin toxicity, excess β-blockade, LV failure; obstructive cardiomyopathy	Levels ↑ in liver or renal disease Hepatic interactions; inhibits CYP3A4, thus decreases breakdown of atorvastatin, simvastatin, lovastatin/St. John's wort reduces plasma verapamil Digoxin levels increased
Slow release (SR) Verelan (Ver) Covera-HS (timed)	As above, two doses (SR) Single dose (Ver) Single bedtime dose	Peak effects: SR 1–2 h, Ver 7–9h, t½ 5–12 h Codelayed 4- to 6-h release	As above	As above

Diltiazem				
Tablets (for IV use see p. 79)	120–360 mg daily in three or four doses	Onset: 15–30 min. Peak: 1–2 h; $t_{1/2}$ 5 h. Bioavailable 45% (hepatic). Active metabolites. 65% GI loss.	As for verapamil, but no constipation	As for verapamil, except little or no effect on digoxin levels, liver interactions less prominent Cimetidine and liver disease increase blood levels Propranolol levels increased
Prolonged SR, CD, XR Tiazac	As above, 1 (XR, CD, Tiazac) or 2 doses	Slower onset, longer $t_{1/2}$, otherwise similar	As above	As above

AV, Atrioventricular; *CCB*, calcium channel blocker; *CI*, confidence intervals; *GI*, gastrointestinal; *IV*, intravenous; *LV*, left ventricular; *SA*, sinoatrial; *SR*, slow release; $t_{1/2}$, plasma elimination half-life; *Ver*, Verelan.

69 «

approximate equivalent of atenolol 50–100 mg daily. For patients with Prinzmetal's variant angina, therapy is based on CCBs, including verapamil, and high does may be needed.[125] Abrupt withdrawal of verapamil may precipitate rebound angina.

Hypertension. Verapamil is approved for mild to moderate hypertension in the United States. Besides the outcome study in CAD with hypertension (preceding section), in a long-term, double-blind comparative trial, mild to moderate hypertension was adequately controlled in 45% of patients who received verapamil 240 mg daily,[126] versus 25% control for hydrochlorothiazide 25 mg daily, versus 60% for the combination. Verapamil combinations can include diuretics, β-blockers, ACE inhibitors, angiotensin receptor blockers (ARBs), or centrally acting agents. During combination with α-blockers, a hepatic interaction may lead to excess hypotension.

Supraventricular arrhythmias. Verapamil is licensed for the prophylaxis of repetitive SVTs and for rate control in chronic atrial fibrillation. For acute attacks of SVTs, when there is no myocardial depression, a bolus dose of 5 mg to 10 mg (0.1 to 0.15 mg/kg) given over 2 minutes restores sinus rhythm within 10 minutes in 60% of cases (package insert). However, this use is now largely supplanted by intravenous adenosine (see Fig. 1.24). When used for uncontrolled atrial fibrillation (but with caution if there is LV failure), verapamil may safely be given (0.005 mg/kg/min, increasing) or as an intravenous bolus of 5 mg (0.075 mg/kg) followed by double the dose if needed. The maximal total dose of intravenous verapamil is 20–30mg when used as repetitive boluses. In atrial flutter, AV block is increased. In all SVTs, including atrial flutter and fibrillation, the presence of a bypass tract (Wolff-Parkinson-White [WPW] syndrome) contraindicates verapamil.

Hypertrophic cardiomyopathy. In hypertrophic cardiomyopathy, verapamil has been the CCB best evaluated. It is licensed for this purpose in Canada. When given acutely, it lessens symptoms, reduces the outflow tract gradient, improves diastolic function, and enhances exercise performance by 20% to 25%. Verapamil should not be given to patients with resting outflow tract obstruction. No long-term, placebo-controlled studies with verapamil are available. In retrospective comparisons with propranolol, verapamil appeared to decrease sudden death and gave better 10-year survival.[127] The best results were obtained by a combination of septal myectomy and verapamil. A significant number of patients on long-term verapamil develop severe side effects, including SA and AV nodal dysfunction, and occasionally overt heart failure.

Postinfarction secondary prevention. For postinfarct protection, verapamil is approved in the United Kingdom and in

ADENOSINE INHIBITION OF AV NODE

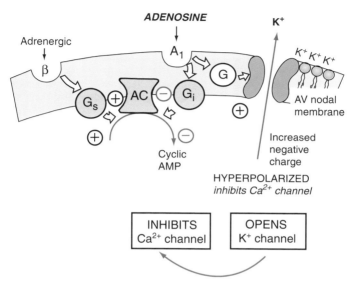

Fig. 1.24 Adenosine inhibits the atrioventricular *(AV)* node by effects on ion channels. Adenosine acting on the adenosine 1 *(A$_1$)* surface receptor opens the adenosine-sensitive potassium channel to hyperpolarize and inhibit the AV node and also indirectly to inhibit calcium channel opening. *AC,* Adenylate cyclase; *AMP,* adenosine monophosphate; β, β-adrenoreceptor; *G,* G protein, nonspecific; *G$_i$,* inhibitory G protein; *G$_s$,* stimulatory G protein. (Figure © L.H. Opie, 2012.)

Scandinavian countries when β-blockade is contraindicated. Verapamil 120 mg three times daily, started 7 to 15 days after the acute phase in patients without a history of heart failure and no signs of CHF (but with digoxin and diuretic therapy allowed), was protective and decreased reinfarction and mortality by approximately 25% over 18 months.[128] As noted above, both verapamil and diltiazem may have clinical utility for reducing recurrent cardiac events in selected patients (principally those with non-Q-wave MI or NSTEMI) where there is no evidence of LV systolic dysfunction, generally defined as an EF <40%.[129-131]

Side effects. Verapamil has a less active effect on vascular smooth muscle and thus less vasodilatory side effects than the DHPs, with less flushing or headaches or pedal edema (Table 1.13). Reflex

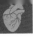
Table 1.13

Reported side effects of the three prototypical CCBs and long-acting dihydropyridines

	Verapamil covera-HS (%)	Diltiazem short-acting (%)	Diltiazem XR or CD (%)	Nifedipine capsules[a] (%)	Nifedipine XL, CC, GITS (%)	Amlodipine 10 mg (%)	Felodipine ER 10 mg (%)
Facial flushing	<1	0–3	0–1	6–25	0-4	3	5
Headaches	< placebo	4–9	< placebo	3–34	6	< placebo	4
Palpitation	0	0	0	Low-25	0	4	1
Light-headedness, dizziness	5	6–7	0	12	2–4	2	4
Constipation	12	4	1–2	0	1	0	0
Ankle edema, swelling	0	6–10	2–3	6	10–30	10	14
Provocation of angina	0	0	0	Low-14	0	0	0

[a]No longer used in the United States.

Side effects are dose related; no strict direct comparisons between the CCBs. Percentages are placebo-corrected. *CCB*, Calcium channel blocker.

Data from Opie LH. *Clinical Use of Calcium Antagonist Drugs*. Boston: Kluwer; 1990. p. 197, and from package inserts.

tachycardia is uncommon because of the inhibitory effects on the SA node. LV depression remains the major potential side effect, especially in patients with preexisting congestive heart failure (CHF) due to largely extensive MI. Why constipation occurs only with verapamil of all the CCBs is not known.

Contraindications to verapamil. (Fig. 1.25, Table 1.14). Contraindications, especially in the intravenous therapy of SVTs, are sick sinus syndrome; preexisting AV nodal disease; and excess therapy with β-blockade, digitalis, quinidine, or disopyramide. In the WPW syndrome complicated by atrial fibrillation, intravenous verapamil is contraindicated because of the risk of anterograde conduction through the bypass tract (see Fig. 1.26). Verapamil is also contraindicated in VT (wide QRS-complex) because of excess myocardial depression, which may be lethal. Myocardial depression, if secondary to the SVT, is not a contraindication, whereas preexisting LV systolic failure warrants cautious use.

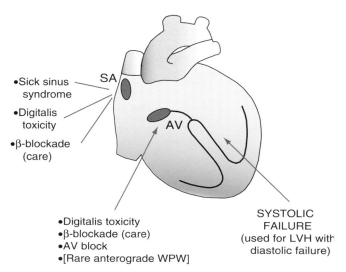

NON-DHP CONTRAINDICATIONS

- •Sick sinus syndrome
- •Digitalis toxicity
- •β-blockade (care)

SA

AV

- •Digitalis toxicity
- •β-blockade (care)
- •AV block
- •[Rare anterograde WPW]

SYSTOLIC FAILURE
(used for LVH with diastolic failure)

Fig. 1.25 Contraindications to verapamil or diltiazem. For use of verapamil and diltiazem in patients already receiving β-blockers, see text. *AV,* Atrioventricular; *LVH,* left ventricular hypertrophy; *SA,* sinoatrial; *WPW,* Wolff-Parkinson-White preexcitation syndrome. (Figure © L.H. Opie, 2012.)

Table 1.14

Comparative contraindications of verapamil, diltiazem, dihydropyridines, and β-adrenergic blocking agents

Contraindications	Verapamil	Diltiazem	DHPs	β-blockade
Absolute				
Severe sinus bradycardia	0/+	0/+	0	++
Sick sinus syndrome	++	++	0	++
AV conduction defects	++	++	0	++
WPW syndrome	++	++	0	++
Digoxin toxicity, AV block[a]	++	++	0	++
Asthma	0	0	0	+++
Bronchospasm	0	0	0	0/++
Heart failure	+++	+++	++	Indicated
Hypotension	+	+	++	+
Coronary artery spasm	0	0	0	+
Raynaud and active peripheral vascular disease	0	0	0	+
Severe mental depression	0	0	0	+
Severe aortic stenosis	+	+	++	+
Obstructive cardiomyopathy	0/+	0/+	++	Indicated
Relative				
Insulin resistance	0	0	0	Care
Adverse blood lipid profile	0	0	0	Care
Digoxin nodal effects	Care	Care	0	Care
β-blockade	Care	Care	0	0
Disopyramide therapy	Care	Care	0	Care
Unstable angina	Care	Care	++	0
Postinfarct protection	May protect	0 (+ if no LVF)	++	Indicated

[a]Contraindication to rapid intravenous administration
+++ = Absolutely contraindicated; ++ = strongly contraindicated; + = relative contraindication; 0 = not contraindicated. "Indicated" means judged suitable for use by author (L.H. Opie), not necessarily FDA approved. *AV,* Atrioventricular; *DHP,* dihydropyridine; *FDA,* Food and Drug Administration; *LVF,* left ventricular failure; *WPW,* Wolff-Parkinson-White syndrome.

Drug Interactions With Verapamil

β-blockers. Depending on the dose and the state of the sinus node and the myocardium, the combination of oral verapamil with a β-blocker may be well tolerated or not. In practice, clinicians can often safely combine verapamil with β-blockade

AV NODAL RE-ENTRY VERSUS WPW

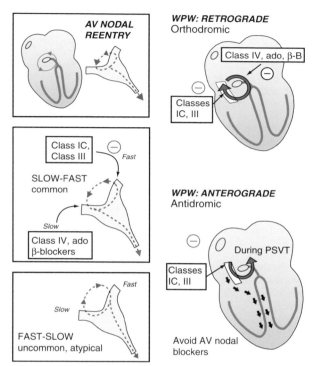

Fig. 1.26 Atrioventricular *(AV)* nodal reentry and Wolff-Parkinson-White *(WPW)* or preexcitation syndrome. The *top left panel* shows AV nodal reentry without WPW. The common pattern is slow-fast *(middle panel)*, whereas fast-slow conduction *(bottom left panel)* is uncommon. The slow and fast fibers of the AV node are artificially separated for diagrammatic purposes. The right panel shows WPW with the bypass tract as a white band. During paroxysmal supraventricular tachycardia *(PSVT)*, when anterograde conduction occurs over the AV node and retrograde conduction most commonly through the accessory pathway, the QRS pattern should be normal (orthodromic supraventricular tachycardia [SVT], *top right panel*). Less commonly, the accessory pathway is used as the anterograde limb and the AV node (or a second accessory pathway) is the retrograde limb (antidromic SVT, *bottom right panel*). The QRS pattern shows the pattern of full preexcitation. In such preexcited atrial tachycardias, agents that block the AV node may enhance conduction over the accessory pathway to the ventricles *(red downward arrows)*, leading to rapid ventricular rates that predispose to ventricular fibrillation. Sites of action of various classes of antiarrhythmics are indicated. *Ado,* Adenosine; *β-B,* β-blocker. (Figure © L.H. Opie, 2012.)

in the therapy of angina pectoris or hypertension, provided that due care is taken (monitoring for heart rate and heart block). In older adults, prior SA and AV nodal disease must be excluded. For hypertension, a combination of a β-blocker plus verapamil is therapeutically effective, although heart rate, AV conduction, and LV function may sometimes be adversely affected. To avoid any hepatic pharmacokinetic interactions, verapamil is best combined with a hydrophilic β-blocker such as atenolol or nadolol, rather than one that is metabolized in the liver, such as metoprolol, propranolol, or carvedilol.

Digoxin. Verapamil inhibits the digoxin transporter, P-glycoprotein, to increase blood digoxin levels, which is of special relevance when both are used chronically to inhibit AV nodal conduction. In digitalis toxicity, rapid intravenous verapamil is absolutely contraindicated because it can lethally exaggerate AV block. In the absence of digitalis toxicity or AV block, oral verapamil and digoxin should be used very cautiously, and digoxin levels needs to be checked. Whereas digoxin can be used for heart failure with atrial fibrillation, verapamil is negatively inotropic and should be avoided.

Antiarrhythmics. The combined negative inotropic potential of verapamil and disopyramide is considerable. Cotherapy with flecainide may also produce additive negative inotropic and dromotropic effects.

Statins and other agents. Verapamil inhibits the hepatic CYP3A isoenzyme, and therefore potentially increases the blood levels of atorvastatin, simvastatin, and lovastatin, which are all metabolized by this isoenzyme.[132] It also increases blood levels of cyclosporin, carbamazepine (Tegretol), and theophylline, and this CYP3A inhibition is also expected to increase blood levels of ketoconazole and sildenafil. Conversely, phenobarbital, phenytoin, and rifampin are CYP3A4 inducers in metabolizing verapamil so that its blood levels fall.

Therapy of verapamil toxicity. There are few clinical reports on management of verapamil toxicity. Intravenous calcium gluconate (1 to 2 g) or half that dose of calcium chloride, given over 5 minutes, helps when heart failure or excess hypotension is present. If there is an inadequate response, positive inotropic or vasoconstrictory catecholamines are administered or, alternatively, glucagon or hyperinsulinemic-euglycemic therapy is given.[133] Intravenous atropine (0.5 to 1 mg) or isoproterenol is used to shorten AV conduction. A pacemaker may be needed.

Diltiazem

Although molecular studies show different channel binding sites for diltiazem and verapamil (see Fig. 1.20), in clinical practice they have somewhat similar therapeutic spectra and contraindications, so that they are often classified as the non-DHPs or HRL agents (see Fig. 1.21). Clinically, diltiazem is used for the same spectrum of disease as is verapamil: angina pectoris, hypertension, supraventricular arrhythmias, and rate control in atrial fibrillation or flutter (see Fig. 1.22). Diltiazem has a low side-effect profile, similar to or possibly better than that of verapamil; specifically the incidence of constipation is much lower (Table 1.13). On the other hand, verapamil is registered for more indications.

Pharmacokinetics. Following oral administration of diltiazem, more than 90% is absorbed, but bioavailability is approximately 45% (first-pass hepatic metabolism). The onset of action of short-acting diltiazem is within 15–30 minutes (oral), with a peak at 1–2 hours. The elimination half-life is 4–7 hours; hence, dosage every 6–8 hours of the short-acting preparation is required for sustained therapeutic effect. The therapeutic plasma concentration range is 50–300 ng/mL. Protein binding is 80–86%. Diltiazem is acetylated in the liver to deacyldiltiazem (40% of the activity of the parent compound), which accumulates with chronic therapy. Unlike verapamil and nifedipine, only 35% of diltiazem is excreted by the kidneys (65% by the GI tract). Because of the hepatic CYP3A4 interaction, the FDA warns that dosage of simvastatin should not exceed 10 mg when used with diltiazem.

Diltiazem doses. The dose of diltiazem is 120–360 mg, given in four daily doses of the short-acting formulation or once or twice a day with slow-release preparations. Cardizem SR permits twice-daily doses. For once-daily use, Dilacor XR is licensed in the United States for hypertension and Cardizem CD and Tiazac for hypertension and angina.

Data for Use: Clinical Indications for Diltiazem

Exertional angina and myocardial ischemia. The efficacy of diltiazem in chronic stable angina is at least as good as propranolol or other β-blockers, and the dose is titrated from 120–360 mg daily (see Table 1.12). In vasospastic angina, diltiazem 240–360 mg/day reduces the number of episodes of ischemic chest discomfort.

Diltiazem for supraventricular arrhythmia. Intravenous diltiazem (Cardizem injectable) is approved for arrhythmias but not for acute hypertension. The main electrophysiologic effect is a negative chronotropic and dromotropic effect on the AV node; the functional and effective refractory periods are prolonged by diltiazem, so that diltiazem is approved for termination of an attack of supraventricular tachyarrhythmia and for the rapid decrease of the ventricular response rate in atrial flutter or fibrillation. For acute conversion of paroxysmal SVT, after exclusion of WPW syndrome (see Fig. 1.26) or for slowing the ventricular response rate in atrial fibrillation or flutter, it is given as 0.25 mg/kg over 2 minutes with electrocardiogram and BP monitoring. If the response is inadequate, the dose is repeated as 0.35 mg/kg over 2 minutes. Acute therapy is usually followed by an infusion of 5–15 mg/h for up to 24 hours. Diltiazem overdose is treated as for verapamil. Oral diltiazem can be used for the elective as well as prophylactic control (90 mg three times daily) of most supraventricular tachyarrhythmias.

Diltiazem for hypertension. In the major long-term outcome study, the Nordic Diltiazem (NORDIL) trial, which included more than 10,000 patients, diltiazem followed by an ACE inhibitor if needed to reach BP goals was as effective in preventing the primary combined cardiovascular endpoint as treatment based on a diuretic, a β-blocker, or both.[134] In the multicenter VA study of antihypertensive monotherapy, diltiazem was shown to be the most effective among five agents (atenolol, thiazide, doxazosin, and captopril) in reducing BP, and was especially effective in older adult white patients and in black patients.[135] Nonetheless, reduction of LV hypertrophy was limited/inconclusive at 1 year of follow-up, possibly because a short-acting diltiazem formulation was used.[136]

Postinfarction secondary prevention. While β-blockers have been used extensively as secondary prevention in post-MI patients for decades, there has been a paucity of data to support the benefits of β-blockers in patients with prior MI. HRL CCBs have been viewed historically as being contraindicated in post-MI secondary prevention. This concern about the presumed "negative inotropic effects" of HRL CCBs was fueled primarily by the negative results of the Multicenter Diltiazem Post-Infarction Trial (MDPIT) more than 30 years ago. While there was clearly an increased rate of death or MI in the 20% of MDPIT patients with clinical or radiographic pulmonary congestion and among subjects with an EF <40%, these deleterious findings were observed principally in the ~30% of participants who had presented clinically with extensive anterior Q-wave MI associated with LV systolic dysfunction. In the MI patients without pulmonary congestion or LV systolic dysfunction, there was no evidence for an excess in death and/or MI rate.

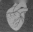

By contrast, and importantly, among the 27% of enrolled subjects in MDPIT with non-Q-wave MI (NSTEMI), the first recurrent cardiac event rate (death or MI) was reduced by approximately 40% during a mean 2-year follow-up from 15% in the placebo group to 9% in the diltiazem group (HR 0.66, 96% CI 0.44, 0.98). It is relevant to cite, however, that these findings were observed only in a subset of the overall study population, though these were prespecified analyses. Despite these findings of a salutary benefit of diltiazem in this group of patients, this has become a virtually forgotten therapeutic agent for postinfarction secondary prevention.

Side effects. Normally side effects of the standard preparation are few and limited to headaches, dizziness, and ankle edema in approximately 6–10% of patients (see Table 1.13). With high-dose diltiazem (360 mg daily), constipation may also occur. Bradycardia and first-degree AV block may occur with all diltiazem preparations. In the case of intravenous diltiazem, side effects resemble those of intravenous verapamil, including hypotension and the possible risk of asystole and high-degree AV block when there is preexisting nodal disease. In postinfarction patients with preexisting poor LV function, most notably among the subset of patients with recent, extensive anterior Q-wave MI or post-STEMI, mortality was shown to be increased by diltiazem, not decreased. Occasionally, severe skin rashes such as exfoliative dermatitis are found.

Contraindications. Contraindications resemble those of verapamil (see Fig. 1.25, Table 1.14): preexisting marked depression of the sinus or AV node, hypotension, myocardial failure, and WPW syndrome. Postinfarction LV failure, as described above, with an EF of less than 40% is a contraindication to diltiazem administration (based on the results of the older MDPIT trial).[137]

Drug interactions and combinations. Unlike verapamil, the effect of diltiazem on the blood digoxin level is often slight or negligible.[138] In fact, one carefully performed study failed to show any increase in serum digoxin levels despite the graded increase in oral diltiazem dosing in normal subject volunteers.[138] As in the case of verapamil, there are the expected hemodynamic interactions with β-blockers. Nonetheless, diltiazem plus a β-blocker may be an effective combination when used with care for angina pectoris management, taking precaution for excess bradycardia or AV block or hypotension. Occasionally diltiazem plus a DHP CCB is used for refractory coronary artery spasm, the rationale being that two different binding sites on the calcium channel are involved (see Fig. 1.20). Diltiazem plus long-acting nitrates may lead to excess hypotension. As in the case of verapamil, but probably less so,

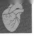
diltiazem may inhibit CYP3A cytochrome, which is expected to increase blood levels of cyclosporin, ketoconazole, carbamazepine (Tegretol), and sildenafil.[132] Conversely, cimetidine inhibits the hepatic cytochrome system breaking down diltiazem to increase circulating levels.

Nifedipine: The Prototypic and First DHP CCB

The major actions of the DHPs can be simplified to one: arteriolar dilation (see Fig. 1.21). The direct negative inotropic effect is usually outweighed by arteriolar unloading effects and by reflex adrenergic stimulation (see Fig. 1.27), except in patients with heart failure. Nifedipine was the first of the DHPs. In the short-acting capsule form, originally available, it rapidly vasodilates to relieve severe hypertension and to terminate attacks of coronary vasospasm. The peripheral vasodilation and a rapid drop in BP led to rapid reflex adrenergic activation with tachycardia (Fig. 1.27). Such

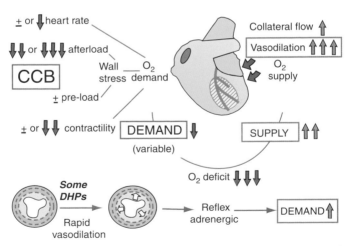

Fig. 1.27 Mechanisms of antiischemic effects of calcium channel blockers. Note that the rapid arteriolar vasodilation resulting from the action of some short-acting dihydropyridines (DHPs) may increase myocardial oxygen demand by reflex adrenergic stimulation. *CCB,* Calcium channel blocker; *O_2,* oxygen. (Figure © L.H. Opie, 2012.)

proischemic effects probably explain why the short-acting DHPs in high doses have precipitated serious adverse events in unstable angina.[123,139] The inappropriate use of short-acting nifedipine can explain much of the adverse publicity that once surrounded the CCBs as a group,[140] so that the focus has now changed to the long-acting DHPs, which are free of such dangers.[141] The subsequent introduction of truly long-acting compounds, such as amlodipine or the extended-release formulations of nifedipine (GITS, XL, CC), and of others such as felodipine and isradipine, has led to much greater usage of the DHPs

Long-Acting Nifedipine Formulations

The long-acting nifedipine formulations (Procardia XL in the United States, Adalat LA elsewhere; Adalat CC) are now widely used in the treatment of hypertension, in exertional angina, and in vasospastic angina.

Pharmacokinetics. Almost all circulating nifedipine is broken down by hepatic metabolism by the cytochrome P-450 system to inactive metabolites (high first-pass metabolism) that are largely excreted in the urine. The long-acting, osmotically sensitive tablet (nifedipine GITS, marketed as Procardia XL or Adalat LA) releases nifedipine from the inner core as water enters the tablet from the GI tract (see Table 1.12). This process results in stable blood therapeutic levels of approximately 20 to 30 ng/mL over 24 hours. With a core-coat system (Adalat CC), the blood levels over 24 hours are more variable, with the trough-peak ratios of 41% to 91%.

Doses of nifedipine. In exertional angina, the usual daily dose 30–90 mg of Procardia XL or Adalat LA (Adalat CC is not licensed in the United States for angina). Dose titration is important to avoid precipitation of ischemic pain in some patients. In cold-induced angina or in coronary spasm, the doses are similar and capsules (in similar total daily doses) allow the most rapid onset of action. In hypertension, standard doses are 30–90 mg once daily of Procardia XL or Adalat CC. In older adults or in patients with severe liver disease, doses should be reduced.

Data for Use: Clinical Indications for Nifedipine

Exertional angina. In the United States only Procardia XL and not Adalat CC is licensed for exertional angina, when β-blockade and nitrates are ineffective or not tolerated. Whereas capsular nifedipine modestly increases the heart rate (that may aggravate angina), the extended-release preparations leave the heart rate unchanged.[142] Their antianginal activity and safety approximate that of the β-blockers, albeit at the cost of more subjective symptoms.[143] In the ACTION study on patients with stable coronary disease, one of the largest studies on effort angina (n ≈ 7800), 80% already receiving β-blockade, the major benefits of added long-acting nifedipine were less new heart failure, less coronary angiography, and less bypass surgery.[144] In the retrospective substudy on hypertensives (mean initial 151/85 mmHg falling to 136/78 mmHg) new heart failure decreased by 38% and major stroke by 32%, without altering cardiovascular death.[145]

Vasospastic angina. Long-acting nifedipine is widely used as a powerful arterial vasodilator with few serious side effects and is now part of the accepted therapy for vasospastic angina, although its use as a DHP CCB has been largely supplanted by amlodipine. However, in unstable angina at rest and in ACSs not felt to be vasospastic in origin, nifedipine in any formulation should not be used as monotherapy, as it may be associated with hypotension, reflex tachycardia, a coronary steal phenomenon, and worsening myocardial ischemia.[123,139]

Systemic hypertension. Long-acting nifedipine and other DHPs are increasingly used with excellent efficacy and tolerability. The major outcome study with nifedipine GITS, the INSIGHT study, showed equivalence in mortality and other major outcomes to the diuretic, with less new diabetes or gout or peripheral vascular disease and more heart failure.[146] Capsular forms are not licensed for hypertension in the United States because of intermittent vasodilation and reflex adrenergic discharge, as well as the short duration of action. Procardia XL and Adalat CC are, however, approved and the dose is initially 30 mg once daily up to 90 mg daily.

Contraindications and cautions. (Fig. 1.28, Table 1.15). These include hemodynamically significant severe valvular aortic stenosis or obstructive hypertrophic cardiomyopathy (danger of exaggerated pressure gradient), clinically evident heart failure or LV dysfunction (added negative inotropic effect), unstable angina with threat of infarction (in the absence of concurrent β-blockade), and preexisting hypotension.

Minor side effects. Two residual side effects of note are headache, as for all arteriolar dilators, and ankle edema, caused by precapillary dilation. The bilateral ankle edema caused by nifedipine is distressing to patients but is not due to cardiac failure; if required, it can be treated by dose reduction, by conventional diuretics, or by an ACE inhibitor. Nifedipine itself has a mild diuretic effect. The low incidence of acute vasodilatory side effects, such as flushing and tachycardia, is because of the slow rate of rise of blood DHP levels.

DHP CONTRAINDICATIONS

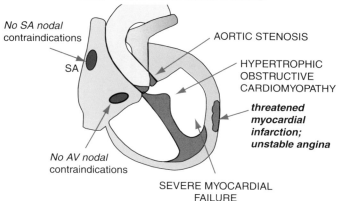

Fig. 1.28 Contraindications to dihydropyridines *(DHPs)* are chiefly obstructive lesions such as aortic stenosis or hypertrophic obstructive cardiomyopathy, and heart failure. Unstable angina (threatened infarction) is a contraindication unless combined nifedipine plus β-blockade therapy is used or unless (rarely) coronary spasm is suspected. *AV,* Atrioventricular; *SA,* sinoatrial. (Figure © L.H. Opie, 2012.)

Drug interactions. Cimetidine and grapefruit juice (e.g., large amounts >1–2 quarts) inhibit the hepatic CYP3A4 P-450 enzyme system breaking down nifedipine, thereby substantially increasing its blood levels. Phenobarbital, phenytoin, and rifampin induce this system metabolizing so that nifedipine blood levels should fall (not mentioned in package insert). In some reports, blood digoxin levels rise. Volatile anesthetics interfere with the myocardial calcium regulation and have inhibitory effects additional to those of nifedipine.

Rebound angina/ischemia after cessation of nifedipine therapy. In patients with vasospastic angina, the manufacturers recommend that the dose be tapered to discontinuation and not abruptly discontinued.

Combination with β-blockers and other drugs. In patients with largely preserved LV function (EF ≥40%), nifedipine may be freely combined with β-blockade (Fig. 1.29), provided that excess hypotension is avoided. In significant LV systolic dysfunction (e.g., EF <40%), the added negative inotropic effects may precipitate overt heart failure. In the therapy of exertional or vasospastic angina, nifedipine is often combined with nitrates. In the therapy of hypertension, nifedipine may be combined with diuretics, β-blockers,

Table 1.15

Long-acting dihydropyridines for oral use

Agent	Dose and major trials	Pharmacokinetics and metabolism	Side effects and contraindications	Interactions and precautions
Amlodipine (Norvasc, Istin)	5–10 mg once daily (ALLHAT, VALUE, ASCOT)	t_{max} 6–12 h. Extensive but slow hepatic metabolism, 90% inactive metabolites; 60% renal; $t_½$ 35–50 h. Steady state in 7–8 days.	Edema, dizziness, flushing, palpitation. CI: severe aortic stenosis, obstructive cardiomyopathy, LVF, unstable angina AMI. May use amlodipine in CHF class 2 or 3, but best avoided.	Prolonged $t_½$ up to 56 h in liver failure. Reduce dose, also in older adults and in patients with heart failure. Hepatic metabolism via CYP3A4, interaction with simvastatin (do not exceed 20 mg simvastatin, FDA recommendation), atorvastatin and lovastatin. Grapefruit juice: caution, interaction not established.
Nifedipine prolonged release XL, LA, GITS, Adalat CC; Procardia XL	30–90 mg once daily (INSIGHT, ACTION)	Stable 24-h blood levels. Slow onset, approximately 6 h.	S/E: headache, ankle edema. CI: severe aortic stenosis, obstructive cardiomyopathy, LVF. Unstable angina if no β-blockade.	Added LV depression with β-blockade. Avoid in unstable angina without β-blockade. Nifedipine via CYP 3A4 interacts with simvastatin (limit simvastatin to 20 mg) and probably atorvastatin, lovastatin. Cimetidine and liver disease increase blood levels.

Felodipine ER (Plendil)	5–10 mg once daily (HOT)	t_{max}, 3–5 h. Complete hepatic metabolism (P-450) to inactive metabolites 75% renal loss, $t_{1/2}$ 22-27 h.	Edema, headache, flushing. CI as above except for CHF class 2 and 3 (mortality neutral).	Reduce dose with cimetidine, age, liver disease. Anticonvulsants enhance hepatic metabolism; grapefruit juice decreases CYP3A4 and markedly increases blood felodipine.

AMI, Acute myocardial infarction; *CHF*, congestive heart failure; *CI*, confidence intervals; *FDA*, Food and Drug Administration; *LV*, left ventricular; *LVF*, left ventricular failure; *S/E*, side effect; $t_{1/2}$, plasma elimination half-life; t_{max}, time to peak blood level.

CCBs VERSUS β-BLOCKADE, CV EFFECTS

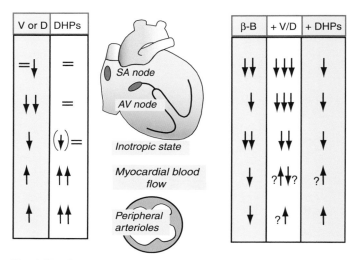

Fig. 1.29 Proposed hemodynamic effects of calcium channel blockers *(CCB)*, singly or in combination with β-blockade *(β-B)*. Note that some of these effects are based on animal data, and extrapolation to humans needs to be made with caution. *AV,* Atrioventricular; *D,* diltiazem; *DHP,* dihydropyridines; *SA,* sinoatrial; *V,* verapamil. (Figure © L.H. Opie, 2012.)

methyldopa, ACE inhibitors, or ARBs. Combination with prazosin or (by extrapolation) other α-blockers may lead to adverse hypotensive interactions.

Amlodipine: The First of the Second-Generation DHPs

The major specific advantages of amlodipine (Norvasc; Istin in the United Kingdom) are (1) the slow onset of action and the long duration of activity (see Table 1.15) and (2) the vast experience with this drug in hypertension. It was the first of the longer acting "second-generation" CCBs. It binds to the same site as other DHPs (labeled *N* in Fig. 1.20). The charged nature of the molecule means that its binding is not entirely typical, with very slow association and dissociation, so that the channel block is slow in onset and offset. Additionally, it also binds to the same sites as verapamil and diltiazem, albeit to a lesser degree, so that with justification its binding properties are regarded as unique.[147]

Pharmacokinetics. Peak blood levels are reached after 6–12 hours, followed by extensive hepatic metabolism to inactive metabolites. The plasma levels increase during chronic dosage probably because of the very long half-life. The elimination half-life is 35–48 hours, increasing slightly with chronic dosage. In older adults, the clearance is reduced and the dose may need reduction. Regarding drug interactions, no effect on digoxin levels has been found, nor is there any interaction with cimetidine (in contrast to verapamil and nifedipine). Because of the hepatic CYP3A4 interaction, the FDA warns that the 20-mg dose of simvastatin should not be exceeded in patients taking amlodipine. There is no known adverse effect with grapefruit juice ingestion.

Data for Use: Clinical Indications for Amlodipine

Hypertension. Amlodipine has an outstanding record in major BP trials (Table 1.16).[148] As initial monotherapy, a common starting dose is 5 mg daily going up to 10 mg. In a large trial on mild hypertension in a middle-aged group over 4 years, amlodipine 5 mg daily was the best tolerated of the agents compared with an α-blocker, β-blocker, diuretic, and ACE inhibitor.[149] In the largest outcome study, ALLHAT, amlodipine had the same primary outcome (fatal and nonfatal coronary heart disease) as the diuretic and ACE-inhibitor groups, but with modestly increased heart failure while decreasing new diabetes.[150] In another mega-trial, ASCOT-BP Lowering Arm, amlodipine usually in combination with the ACE inhibitor perindopril gave much better outcomes than a β-blocker usually combined with a diuretic.[151] Specifically, all cardiovascular events were decreased, including heart failure; new diabetes was less; and decreased mortality led to premature termination of the trial.

The important *ACCOMPLISH* trial, comparing initial antihypertensive treatment with benazepril plus amlodipine versus benazepril plus hydrochlorothiazide, was terminated early as the CCB–ACE inhibitor combination was clearly demonstrated as superior to the ACE inhibitor-diuretic combination.[152] Both primary and secondary endpoints were reduced by approximately 20%. For cardiovascular deaths, nonfatal MI, and nonfatal stroke, the hazard ratio was 0.79 (95% CI 0.67–0.92, $P = 0.002$).[152] When matching the reductions in BP exactly, the benefits were the same.[153] The progression of nephropathy was slowed to a greater extent with this combination.[154]

In hypertensive type 2 diabetics, ALLHAT showed that amlodipine was as effective as the diuretic in the relative risk of cardiovascular disease.[155] In advanced diabetic nephropathy, amlodipine

Table 1.16

Amlodipine: major outcome trials in hypertension

Acronym	Numbers and duration	Comparison	End points
ALLHAT[150]	9048 in amlodipine arm	Amlodipine vs others (diuretic, ACE inhibitor, α-blocker)	Equal CHD, stroke, all-cause mortality, at same BP target; more HF, less new diabetes
ASCOT[151]	18,000 patients, 5 years, BP > 160/100 or 140/90 on drug; age 40–80; 3+ risk factors for CHD	Amlodipine vs atenolol 2nd: A + perindopril vs. atenolol + thiazide	Mortality reduced, major fall in all CV events
VALUE, Amlodipine[148]	15,245 patients, age 50+, initial BP 155/87 mm Hg	Amlodipine vs. valsartan ± thiazide	Equal cardiac and mortality outcomes
ACCOMPLISH[152,153]	11,506 patients, at high risk for events	Benazepril + amlodipine vs. benazepril + hydrochlorothiazide	Hazard ratio 0.79 for CV death, nonfatal MI, and nonfatal stroke (CI, 0.67–0.92; $P = 0.002$)

ACCOMPLISH, Avoiding Cardiovascular Events through Combination Therapy in Patients Living with Systolic Hypertension; *ACE,* angiotensin-converting enzyme; *ALLHAT,* Antihypertensive and Lipid-Lowering treatment to prevent Heart Attack Trial; *ASCOT,* Anglo Scandinavian Cardiac Outcomes Trial; *BP,* blood pressure; *CHD,* coronary heart disease; *CI,* confidence intervals; *CV,* cardiovascular; *HF,* heart failure; *MI,* myocardial infarction; *VALUE,* Valsartan Antihypertensive Long-term Use Evaluation Trial.

compared with irbesartan protected from MI, whereas irbesartan decreased the heart failure and the progression of nephropathy.[156]

Exertional angina and coronary artery disease. Amlodipine is well tested in effort angina, with an antianginal effect for 24 hours, and often better tolerated than β-blockers. In CAMELOT, amlodipine was given for 2 years to 663 patients with angiographic CAD; amlodipine decreased cardiovascular events by 31% versus enalapril despite similar BP reduction.[157,158] Although atheroma volume fell in this trial, arterial lumen dimensions were unchanged. In PREVENT, amlodipine given to patients with coronary angiographic disease had reduced outcome measures after 3 years.[159] Exercise-induced ischemia was more effectively reduced by amlodipine than by the β-blocker atenolol, whereas ambulatory ischemia was better reduced by atenolol, and for both settings the combination was the best.[160] However, the CCB–β-blocker combination is often underused, though this largely reflects clinicians' concerns of using simultaneously two pharmacologic agents that possess negative chronotropic and negative inotropic effects. While the previous COURAGE Trial in stable ischemic heart disease patients found high rates of usage for aspirin, statins, and inhibitors of the renin-angiotensin system as part of what the authors termed "optimal medical therapy," there were lower overall rates of usage of antianginal agents, particularly nitrates and CCBs.[161] Exercise-induced ischemia is at the basis of effort angina. After the anginal pain is relieved by nitrates, the EF takes approximately 30 minutes to recover, a manifestation of postischemic stunning. Amlodipine markedly attenuates such stunning,[162] hypothetically because cellular calcium overload underlies stunning. In Prinzmetal's vasospastic angina, another approved indication, amlodipine 5 mg daily lessens symptoms and ST changes. For cardiovascular protection in hypertension, amlodipine was the major drug in the important ASCOT study reducing strokes, total major events, and mortality.[151]

Contraindications, cautions, and side effects. Amlodipine has the same contraindications as other DHPs (see Fig. 1.28). It is untested in unstable angina, AMI, and during long-term follow-up in patients with ischemic heart disease. First principles strongly suggest that it should not be used in the absence of concurrent β-blockade. In heart failure, CCBs as a group are best avoided, but amlodipine may be added, for example, for better control of angina. In liver disease, the dose should be reduced. Of the side effects, peripheral edema is most troublesome, occurring in approximately 10% of patients at 10 mg daily (see Table 1.13). In women there is more edema (15%) than in men (6%). Next in significance are dizziness (3–4%) and flushing (2–3%). Compared with verapamil, edema is more common, while headache and constipation are less common. Compared with placebo, headache is not increased (package insert). Amlodipine gave an excellent quality of life compared with other agents in the TOMH study.[149]

Felodipine

Felodipine (Plendil ER) shares many of the standard properties of other long-acting DHPs. In the United States, it is only approved for hypertension in a starting dose of 5 mg once daily, then increasing to 10 mg or decreasing to 2.5 mg as needed. As monotherapy, it is approximately as effective as nifedipine. Initial felodipine monotherapy was the basis of a very large outcome study (Height of Hypertension [HOT]) in Scandinavia in which the aim was to compare BP reduction to different diastolic levels, 90, 85, or 80 mmHg.[163] Combination with other agents such as ACE inhibitors and β-blockers was often required to attain BP treatment goals. Best results were found with the lowest BP group in diabetics, in whom hard endpoints such as cardiovascular mortality was reduced. Felodipine, like other DHPs, combines well with β-blockers.[164] There are two drug interactions of note: cimetidine, which increases blood felodipine levels, and anticonvulsants, which markedly decrease levels, both probably acting at the level of the hepatic enzymes. Grapefruit juice markedly inhibits the metabolism. The high vascular selectivity of felodipine led to extensive testing in heart failure, yet achieved no sustained clinical benefit in the large Ve-HeFT-III trial in which it was added to conventional vasodilator therapy.[165]

Third-Generation Dihydropyridines

Third-generation DHP CCBs inhibit T-type calcium channels on vascular muscular cells such as those localized on postglomerular arterioles. The first of these agents, mibefradil, had to be withdrawn after a series of initially successful studies because of hepatic side effects. Now there is interest in a newer agent, *manidipine*.[166] In the DEMAND study on 380 subjects for a mean of 3.8 years, combined manidipine and ACE-inhibitor therapy reduced both macrovascular events and albuminuria in hypertensive patients with type 2 diabetes mellitus, whereas the ACE inhibitor did not. The proposed mechanism was reduced postglomerular resistance and decreased intraglomerular pressure. Cardioprotective effects extended beyond improved BP and metabolic control. Worsening of insulin resistance was almost fully prevented in those on combination therapy, which suggested additional effects possibly manidipine-mediated activation of adipocyte peroxisome proliferator-activated receptor-γ. The authors estimated that approximately 16 subjects had to be treated with the combined therapy to prevent one major cardiovascular event. Much larger trials are required to place the third-generation CCBs firmly on the therapeutic map.

Summary

1. **Spectrum of Use.** CCBs are widely used in the therapy of hypertension and vasospastic angina, but are often underused in exertional angina, particularly in combination with β-blockers. The major mechanism of action is via calcium channel blockade in the arterioles, with peripheral or coronary vasodilation thereby explaining the major effects in hypertension and in effort angina. The HRL CCBs have a prominent negative inotropic effect, and inhibit the sinus and the AV nodes, which imparts also a negative chronotropic effect. These inhibitory cardiac effects are absent or muted in the DHPs, of which nifedipine is the prototype, now joined by amlodipine, felodipine, and others. Of these, amlodipine is very widely used in hypertension with proven outcome benefit. As a group, the DHPs are more vascular selective and more often used in hypertension than the HRL agents, also called the non-DHPs. Only the non-DHPs, verapamil and diltiazem, have antiarrhythmic properties by inhibiting the AV node. Both DHPs and non-DHPs are useful in the management of exertional angina and myocardial ischemia, albeit acting through different mechanisms and often underused especially in the United States.

2. **Safety and Efficacy.** Previous serious concerns about the long-term safety of the CCBs as a group have been annulled by seven large outcome studies in hypertension, with one in angina pectoris. Nonetheless, as with all drugs, cautions and contraindications as noted in the preceding sections need to be considered.

3. **Ischemic Heart Disease.** All the CCBs are effective in ameliorating both rest and exertional angina, particularly if the etiology is vasospastic in origin, and these agents are also effective in blunting myocardial ischemia with efficacy and safety rather similar to β-blockers. The largest angina outcome study, ACTION, showed the benefits of adding a long acting DHP to prior β-blockade. In unstable angina the DHPs are specifically contraindicated in the absence of β-blockade because of their tendency to vasodilation-induced reflex adrenergic activation. Although the use of the HRL non-DHPs in unstable angina is relatively well supported by data, they have in practice been supplanted by β-blockers—though, as noted previously, a vasospastic etiology would strongly favor the use of HRL CCBs

such as diltiazem or verapamil. In postinfarction patients, verapamil or diltiazem may be used if β-blockade is not tolerated or contraindicated, provided that there is no heart failure, although it is not approved for this purpose in the United States. Diltiazem has been shown to reduce first recurrent cardiac events in selected postinfarction patients, notably those with non-Q-wave MI or NSTEMI. There are insufficient trials data to support the use of DHP CCBs in postinfarction patients.

4. *Hypertension.* Strong overall evidence from a series of large outcome studies favors the safety and efficacy on hard endpoints, including coronary heart disease, of longer-acting DHPs. One large outcome study in coronary heart disease patients shows that the non-DHP verapamil gives overall results as effective as atenolol, with less new incident diabetes cases.

5. *Diabetic Hypertension.* ALLHAT showed that amlodipine was as effective as the diuretic or the ACE inhibitor in the relative risk of cardiovascular disease. Other data suggest that initial antihypertensive therapy in diabetics should be based on an ACE inhibitor or ARB, especially in those with nephropathy. To achieve current BP goals in diabetics, it is almost always necessary to use combination therapy, which would usually include an ACE inhibitor or ARB, and a CCB besides a diuretic or β-blocker.

6. *Heart Failure.* Heart failure remains a general contraindication to the use of all CCBs, with two exceptions: diastolic dysfunction based on LV hypertrophy, and otherwise well-treated systolic heart failure when amlodipine may be cautiously added if needed, for example, for additional symptomatic control of angina. Diltiazem and verapamil should be avoided in patients with significantly LV systolic dysfunction (generally an EF <40% in the setting of recent, extensive Q-wave MI or STEMI), or in the setting of clinical or radiographic pulmonary congestion.

Newer (Nontraditional) Antianginal Agents (or Metabolic and Other Nontraditional Antianginal Agents)

In addition to the standard pharmacotherapy drug classes that include beta-blockers, calcium channel blockers, and nitrates, several newer antianginal therapies are now available for the symptomatic treatment of both angina and myocardial ischemia. These include ranolazine, trimetazidine, ivabradine, and nicorandil, which are detailed in the following section.

Ranolazine

Ranolazine is an inhibitor of late sodium channel influx (late I_{Na}) during repolarization (Fig. 1.30). This reduces intracellular sodium concentrations, which, in turn, lowers intracellular calcium concentrations, which results in lower ventricular diastolic wall tension, a reduction in oxygen consumption, and improvement in angina symptoms. In addition, ranolazine is believed to be a partial fatty acid oxidation inhibitor with a resultant attenuation of oxidative stress.[108] Ranolazine reduces angina without any significant reductions in heart rate, BP, or rate-pressure product during exercise and is hemodynamically neutral, thus making it a useful therapeutic option in patients who are at risk of hypotension or bradycardia with the use or uptitration of traditional antianginals. Ranolazine also prolongs the ventricular action potential and QTc interval through inhibition of the rapid delayed rectifier potassium current (I_{Kr}) in a dose-dependent manner. Ranolazine alone,

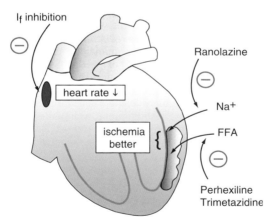

NOVEL ANTIANGINALS

Fig. 1.30 Novel antianginal agents work in different ways. I_f inhibition by ivabradine increases myocardial oxygen demand by decreasing the heart rate. Ranolazine decreases the inflow of sodium by the slow sodium current during ischemia and thereby lessens the intracellular sodium and calcium load. Perhexiline inhibits free fatty acid *(FFA)* oxidation at the level of the enzyme CPT-1. Trimetazidine inhibits fatty acid oxidation at the level of the mitochondrial long-chain oxidation and, in addition, improves whole-body insulin sensitivity. (Figure © L. H. Opie, 2012.)

or as combination therapy with β-blockers or CCBs, significantly decreases the frequency of angina and NTG use, improves exercise duration and delays the onset of ST depression during exercise (MARISA, CARISA, and ERICA).

In a randomized, double-blind trial of 6566 patients with non-ST elevation MI who were managed with either ranolazine or placebo in addition to the background therapy,[167] ranolazine was not associated with a significant decrease in the primary composite end-point of cardiovascular death, MI between the two groups (21.8% ranolazine versus 23.5% placebo, $P = 0.11$).[168] However, recurrent ischemia was significantly reduced in the ranolazine group (13.9% versus 16.1% for placebo, $P = 0.03$).[168] Furthermore, despite a small increase in QTc, there was no significant increase in documented arrhythmia (3.0% versus 3.1%, $P = 0.84$), supporting the safety of this medication.[168] In a prespecified analysis, the authors of the MERLIN-TIMI 36 trial evaluated the antianginal efficacy of ranolazine in a large subgroup of over 5500 patients with chronic angina who presented with ACS, and showed that ranolazine compared to placebo was associated with significant reduction in the primary composite end-point of cardiovascular death, MI, or recurrent ischemia.[169] These findings from MERLIN-TIMI 36 trial demonstrate that ranolazine is an effective antianginal agent but does not reduce mortality.[169] In patients with diabetes mellitus, ranolazine has demonstrated significant reductions in HbA1c, thus making it an appealing option for managing angina in these patients.[110,111] In a *post hoc* analysis of the CARISA trial, there was a 0.48% ± 0.18% ($P = 0.008$) reduction in HbA1c with 750 mg twice-daily dosing and a 0.70% ± 0.18% ($P = 0.0002$) reduction in HbA1c with 1000 mg twice-daily dosing when compared to placebo after 12 weeks of therapy.[110] Additionally, as a part of the MERLIN-TIMI 36 trial, the patients with diabetes treated with ranolazine had a significant reduction in HbA1c, had a greater likelihood of having an HbA1c <7% at 4 months, and were less likely to have a ≥1% increase in HbA1c at 1 year.[111] A recent randomized controlled trial, the Type 2 Diabetes Evaluation of Ranolazine in Subjects with Chronic Stable Angina (TERISA), enrolled 949 patients with diabetes, CAD, and stable angina who were being treated with one to two antianginals at baseline to treatment with ranolazine or placebo.[170] Ranolazine was found to significantly lower weekly angina frequency and weekly sublingual nitroglycerin use.[170]

Trimetazidine. Widely used as an antianginal drug in Europe but not in the United States or United Kingdom. It is a partial inhibitor of fatty acid oxidation without hemodynamic effects. Short-term clinical studies have demonstrated significant benefits including a reduction in weekly angina episodes and improved exercise time, but large, long-term trials are needed.[171] In diabetic patients with

CAD, trimetazidine decreased blood glucose, increased forearm glucose uptake, and improved endothelial function.[172] An interesting proposal is that, because it acts independently of any BP reduction, it could be used as an antianginal in those with erectile dysfunction in place of nitrates to allow free use of sildenafil and similar agents.

There is increasingly strong evidence that trimetazidine may also be useful in the treatment of chronic systolic heart failure[173] secondary to improvements in myocardial energetics. In heart failure, added trimetazidine gives benefit to conventional therapy including β-blockades and RAS inhibition.[174] In a small series of neurologic patients, treatment with trimetazidine worsened previously diagnosed Parkinson disease,[175] which should become a contraindication to its use.

Ivabradine. *(Procoralan)* is a blocker of the pacemaker current I_f, and hence does not act directly on the metabolism but indirectly by decreasing the heart rate and thus the metabolic demand of the heart. Its antianginal potency is similar to that of β-blockade[176] and amlodipine.[177] There is no negative inotropic effect or BP reduction as with β-blockers, nor is there any rebound on cessation of therapy.[178] Ivabradine is licensed in the United Kingdom and other European countries for use in angina when β-blockers are not tolerated or are contradicted. In practice, it may be combined with β-blockade with clinical benefit,[179] but in this study the β-blocker was not upwardly titrated to achieve maximal heart rate reduction. Theoretically there is less risk of severe sinus node depression than with β-blockade because only one of several pacemaker currents is blocked, whereas β-blockade affects all. The downside is that the current I_f is also found in the retina, so that there may be disturbance of nocturnal vision with flashing lights (phosphenes)[180] that could impair driving at night and is often transient. In heart failure patients, the SHIFT study established the clinical benefits of ivabradine in a group of patients with moderate systolic heart failure whose heart rates remained elevated despite β-blockade,[181] though here is some controversy as to whether adequate β-blocker doses had been used during the conduct of the trial.[182] Only 23% of the patients were at trial-established target doses and only half were receiving 50% or more of the targeted β-blocker dose.

Nicorandil. (not approved for use in the United States) Has a double cellular mechanism of action, acting both as a potassium channel activator and having a nitrate-like effect, which may explain why experimentally it causes less tolerance than nitrates. It is a nicotinamide nitrate, acting chiefly by dilation of the large coronary arteries, as well as by reduction of pre- and afterload. It is widely used as an antianginal agent in Japan. In the IONA study, 5126 patients with stable angina were followed for a mean of 1.6 years. Major coronary events including ACS were reduced.[183]

Summary

A. Nitrates:

1. ***Mechanisms of action.*** Nitrates act by venodilation and relief of coronary vasoconstriction (including that induced by exercise) to ameliorate anginal attacks. They are also arterial dilators and reduce aortic systolic pressure. Their unloading effects also benefit patients with heart failure with high LV filling pressures.

2. ***Intermittent nitrates for exertional angina.*** Sublingual nitroglycerin remains the basic therapy, usually combined with a β-blocker, a CCB, or both with careful assessment of lifestyle, BP, and blood lipid profile. As the duration of action lasts for minutes, nitrate tolerance is unusual because of the relatively long nitrate-free intervals between attacks. Intermittent isosorbide dinitrate has a delayed onset of action because of the need for hepatic transformation to active metabolites, while the duration of action is longer than with nitroglycerin.

3. ***For angina prophylaxis.*** Both short-acting and long-acting nitrates can be used effectively in advance of exertional angina precipitants and can play important roles in angina prophylaxis. Short-acting sublingual nitroglycerin or nitrolingual spray administered several minutes in advance of a known angina trigger may prevent exertional attacks.

4. ***For unstable angina at rest or early-phase acute MI.*** A nitrate-free interval is not possible, and short-term treatment for 24 to 48 hours with intravenous nitroglycerin is frequently effective; however, escalating doses are often required to overcome tolerance. Intravenous nitroglycerin in acute MI may be beneficial in enhancing coronary collateral flow, and in the setting of heart failure or increased LV filling pressures (or pulmonary capillary wedge pressure), intravenous nitroglycerin may increase venous capacitance and decrease preload.

5. ***Treatment of heart failure.*** Nitrates may effectively lower preload and reduce pulmonary congestion, though tolerance may also develop with chronic use. Isosorbide dinitrate combined with hydralazine may be of benefit in heart failure with or without ACE inhibitor therapy. A proprietary combination (BiDil) is approved for heart failure in patients who self-identify as African-American.

6. ***Nitrate tolerance.*** The current understanding of the mechanism tolerance focuses on free radical formation (superoxide and peroxy nitrite) with impaired bioconversion of nitrate to active NO˙. During the treatment of effort angina

by isosorbide dinitrate or mononitrate, substantial evidence suggests that eccentric doses with a nitrate-free interval largely avoid clinical tolerance, but endothelial dysfunction remains a long-term hazard. Besides addition of hydralazine (see previous discussion), other, less well-tested measures include administration of antioxidants, statins, ACE inhibitors, and folic acid. Increasing data show that endothelial dysfunction, in which aldehyde formation plays a role, is incriminated in nitrate tolerance. Coadministration with carvedilol or possibly nebivolol as the β-blockers of choice should help to prevent or delay tolerance, yet prospective clinical trials are lacking.

7. ***Interaction with PDE-5 inhibitors.*** Nitrates can interact very adversely with such agents, which are now often used to alleviate erectile dysfunction. The latter is common in those with cardiovascular disease, being a manifestation of endothelial dysfunction. The coadministration of these PDE-5 inhibitors with nitrates is therefore contraindicated. If any of these agents has been used, there has to be an interval of 24–48 hours (the longer interval for tadalafil) before nitrates can be given therapeutically with reasonable safety but still with great care.

References

Complete reference list available at www.expertconsult.com.

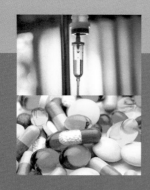

第2章
高血压的药物治疗

　　虽然对生活方式的干预是所有高血压治疗指南推荐的基石，但大多数患者仍然需要降血压药物来治疗。

　　目前已有十类不同的药物可用于降血压，包括利尿药、钙通道阻滞剂、血管紧张素转化酶抑制剂、血管紧张素Ⅱ受体拮抗剂、醛固酮受体拮抗剂、β受体拮抗剂、交感神经抑制剂、α1肾上腺素能受体拮抗剂、直接血管扩张剂、直接肾素抑制剂。其中，每类药物都针对高血压的发展和维持、心血管或肾脏并发症相关的一个或多个病理生理过程。例如，卡维地洛同时具有β受体和α受体的阻断特性；螺内酯是一种盐皮质激素受体拮抗剂，但在较高剂量时也能起到利尿药的作用。这些药物被归入高血压药物治疗最常使用的类别。

　　在降血压药物的总体使用原则方面，虽然指南倾向于在特定的患者群体中推荐某些药物类别，但目前已有的证据表明，比药物类别更重要的是所实现的降压幅度，或者说"降压才是硬道理"。另外，多项研究表明，联合治疗的降压效果更明显、不良反应更少。医师在用药时，要根据患者的临床表现进行个体化用药；并发症的存在也有可能影响用药的倾向性；需注意对不良反应的控制，因为不良反应的存在可能会导致药物依从性降低。此外，必须强调的是，对患者生活方式的教育比个性化用药选择更重要。

在高血压的药物治疗各论方面，本章对每类药物的作用机制、同类不同种药物的区别、临床应用、不良反应、药物相互作用都进行了详细介绍，主要为以下几点。

（1）噻嗪类利尿药仍然被推荐作为高血压治疗的一线药物，并显示出广泛的心血管获益优势。袢利尿药被用于治疗出现严重容量负荷或严重肾功能不全的患者。在使用利尿药过程中，还需注意监测血钾、血镁等电解质情况。

（2）钙通道阻滞剂因其显著且广谱的降压效果，也是原发性高血压治疗的一线药物，尤其适用于老年人及有其他钙通道阻滞剂适应证的情况，如心绞痛、微血管功能障碍、雷诺现象等。需要注意的是，由于β受体阻滞剂和维拉帕米对心率和心肌收缩能力有共同的负性作用，此两种药物不能同时使用。

（3）血管紧张素转化酶抑制剂除降血压外，有证据表明其与血管紧张素Ⅱ受体拮抗剂均可对血管有额外的保护作用，尤其是在糖尿病和慢性肾脏病患者中。血管紧张素转化酶抑制剂在使用过程中，还需注意咳嗽、高钾血症、血肌酐升高等可能出现的不良反应。血管紧张素转化酶抑制剂禁用于怀孕或可能怀孕的女性。

（4）β受体阻滞剂不再被推荐用于原发性高血压的初始治疗。

舟　君

2

Antihypertensive Therapies

LUKE J. LAFFIN · GEORGE L. BAKRIS

Introduction

The formal classification and blood pressure (BP) threshold to define an individual as having hypertension continues to vary based on available evidence. The appraisal of such evidence by professional associations and societies has led to different BP thresholds adopted in guidelines worldwide.[1,2] Given that the thresholds by which we define hypertension can and will continue to evolve, it is less helpful to think of hypertension in a binary sense, but more helpful to view increasing BP as a risk factor with a continuous linear-log relationship with coronary artery disease, stroke, heart failure (HF), and cardiovascular (CV) mortality. Ultimately, most clinicians would be operationally well served to consider defining hypertension as a BP level above which investigation and treatment does more good than harm.[3]

While lifestyle intervention is the cornerstone of therapy by all guidelines, most people will also require antihypertensive medications. There are ten different medication classes available to lower BP. Each class addresses one or more of the multiple pathophysiological processes that are associated with development and maintenance of hypertension (Fig. 2.1) and subsequent CV and renal complications (Fig. 2.2). Although guidelines tend to favor certain drug classes in specific patient populations, it is critical to remember that the current available evidence suggests that more important than a specific class of medication used, is the magnitude of BP lowering achieved.[4]

Individualizing the choice of medication based on the clinical presentation,[5] keeping in mind the presence of other comorbid conditions and desire to limit adverse effects that may lead to medication nonadherence is critical. Additionally, it must be emphasized that more important than individualizing medication choice while treating hypertension, is appropriate patient education about lifestyle modifications.[4]

HYPERTENSION MECHANISMS

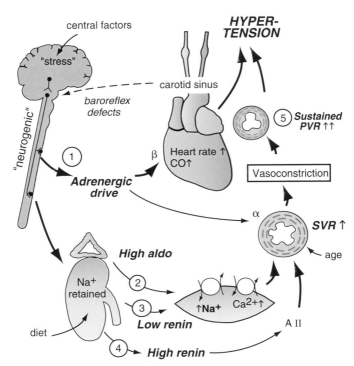

Fig. 2.1 Predominant mechanisms in the development and maintenance of hypertension. (1) Increased adrenergic drive as found especially in younger patients with hypertension. (2 and 3) Renal-angiotensin-aldosterone mediated mechanisms, including low renin hypertension as in those with inherently higher aldosterone levels or renal sodium retention (sodium epithelial channel). (4) High-renin hypertension, as seen in renal dysfunction. (5) Increased systemic vascular resistance *(SVR)*. *aldo*, Aldosterone; *CO*, cardiac output; *PVR*, peripheral vascular resistance. (Figure © L.H. Opie, 2012)

An overview of the major drug classes and contemporary hypertension guidelines is initially discussed in the chapter. This is followed by a discussion of each pharmacologic class available for the treatment of hypertension, and the associated mechanism of action, data for use, side effects, and drug interactions for each drug class.

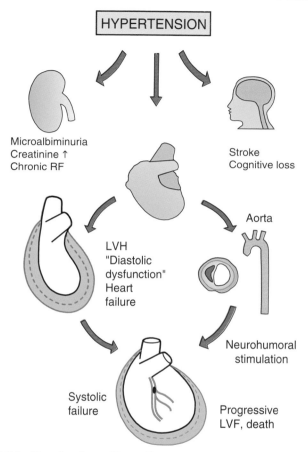

Fig. 2.2 Hypertension and its cardiovascular complications. Cardiovascular complications are the most common cause of death. Uncontrolled hypertension also leads to renal failure *(RF)* and cerebrovascular complications such as stroke. The two major cardiovascular events are heart failure and development of aortic and coronary artery disease. Left ventricular hypertrophy *(LVH)* can be the first manifestation of hypertensive heart disease and result in subsequent diastolic dysfunction or left ventricular systolic dysfunction. These complications can ultimately lead to heart failure with preserved or reduced ejection fraction. *LVF,* Left ventricle failure. (Figure © L.H. Opie, 2012)

Drug Class Overview and Guidelines

Blood pressure–lowering medications can be grouped into ten major categories, with some subcategories within the group (Table 2.1). These categories act by different mechanisms and at different sites in the body to address alterations in BP (Fig. 2.3). Certain antihypertensive medications may lower BP by more than a single mechanism. For example, carvedilol has both β- and α-blocking properties, and spironolactone is a mineralocorticoid receptor antagonist, but also acts as a diuretic at higher doses. Care was taken to classify such drugs in the category that they are most commonly encountered. Table 2.2 provides a broad overview of the more commonly used drug categories for the outpatient managements of hypertension, including compelling indications and contraindications. Table 2.3 provides an overview of the medications used in the treatment of hypertensive emergency.[6]

The most contemporary guidelines for the treatment of elevated BP in the United States were published in 2017 and endorsed by the American College of Cardiology and the American Heart

Table 2.1

Medication classes for the treatment of hypertension

Diuretics
- Thiazide-type
- Loop

Calcium channel blockers "CCBs"
- Dihydropyridine
- Nondihydropyridine

Angiotensin converting enzyme inhibitors "ACE inhibitors"
Angiotensin II receptor blockers "ARBs"
Mineralocorticoid receptor antagonists
β-blockers
- Nonselective
- Cardio selective
- Vasodilating
- Intrinsic sympathomimetic

Central sympatholytic agents
α_1-adrenoreceptor antagonists
Direct vasodilators
Direct renin inhibitors – only aliskiren

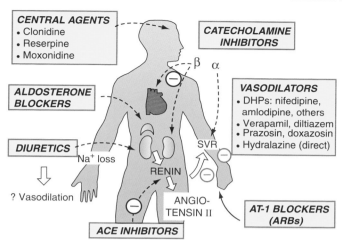

Fig. 2.3 Sites of action for antihypertensive agents. Because hypertension is frequently multifactorial in origin, it may be difficult to find the ideal drug for a given patient and drug combinations are often used at low to moderate doses, which often produce better blood pressure lowering than a single agent at a maximum dose. *ACE*, Angiotensin-converting enzyme; *ARBs*, angiotensin receptor blockers; *AT-1*, angiotensin II subtype 1; *DHP*, dihydropyridine; *SVR*, systemic vascular resistance. (Figure © L.H. Opie, 2012)

Association among other professional organizations.[4] Additional American guidelines for the treatment of resistant hypertension were published in the fall of 2018.[7] The European Society of Hypertension/European Society of Cardiology (ESH/ESC) BP guidelines were also published in the fall of 2018.[2] A comparison of these guidelines demonstrates more similarities than differences.[8] Highlighted in both is a stronger push toward use of combination therapy (i.e., multiple medications in a single tablet or pill). The ESH/ESC guidelines recommend this strategy as initial therapy in all hypertensive patients, while United States guidelines recommend such a strategy for patients that are greater than 20/10 mmHg above systolic and/or diastolic BP goals. Multiple studies demonstrate the value of combination therapy as more effective with fewer side effects.

Table 2.2

General guidelines for selecting drug treatment for hypertension

Class of drug	Favored indications	Possible indications	Compelling contraindications	Possible contraindications
Diuretics (thiazide-type)	Heart failure Older adults with hypertension Systolic hypertension Black patients	Obesity	Gout	Pregnancy Dyslipidemia Metabolic syndrome
Diuretics (loop)	Heart failure Renal failure		Hypokalemia	
Mineralocorticoid receptor antagonists	Heart failure Post-MI Primary Aldosteronism	Resistant hypertension	Hyperkalemia Renal failure	Diabetic renal disease
Calcium channel blockers	Angina Older adults Systolic hypertension	Peripheral vascular disease Diabetes African origin	Heart block[a] Clinical heart failure (exception amlodipine)	Preexisting lower extremity edema
ACE inhibitors	Left ventricular systolic dysfunction or failure Proteinuria	CV protection Type 2 nephropathy	Pregnancy Hyperkalemia Bilateral renal artery stenosis	Severe cough

Angiotensin-II antagonists (ARBs)	ACE inhibitor cough LVH Heart failure	Post MI	Pregnancy Bilateral renal artery stenosis Hyperkalemia	Severe aortic stenosis
β-blockers	Angina Tachyarrhythmias Post-MI Heart failure	Pregnancy Diabetes	Asthma, severe COPD Heart block[b]	Obesity Metabolic syndrome Athletes and exercising patients Erectile dysfunction

[a]Grade 2 or 3 atrioventricular block with verapamil or diltiazem.
[b]Grade 2 or 3 atrioventricular block.

ACE, Angiotensin-converting enzyme; *Aldo*, aldosterone; *ARB*, angiotensin receptor blocker; *BP*, blood pressure; *CCB*, calcium channel blocker; *COPD*, chronic obstructive pulmonary disease; *CV*, cardiovascular; *LVH*, left ventricular hypertrophy; *MI*, myocardial infarction.

Table 2.3

Drugs for the management of hypertensive emergencies

Agent	Dose	Onset/duration of action (after discontinuation)	Precautions/contraindications
Parenteral vasodilators			
Nitroprusside	0.25–10.0 µg/kg/min as IV infusion maximal dose for 10 min only	1–2 min after infusion	Nausea, vomiting, muscle twitching; with prolonged use may cause thiocyanate intoxication, methemoglobinemia acidosis, cyanide poisoning
Fenoldopam	0.1–0.3 µg/kg/min IV infusion, increase every 15 min until BP goal is reached	5–15 min/30–60 min	Headache, tachycardia, flushing, local phlebitis
Nitroglycerin	5–200 µg/min as IV infusion, 5 µg/min increase every 5 minutes	1–5 min/3–5 min	Headache, reflex tachycardia, vomiting, flushing, methemoglobinemia
Nicardipine	5–15 mg/h infusion	1–5 min/30–40 min, but may exceed 12 h after prolonged infusion	Reflex tachycardia, nausea, vomiting, headache, increased intracranial pressure; hypotension may be protracted after prolonged infusions
Clevidipine	2 mg/h IV infusion, increase every 2 min with 2 mg/h as IV bolus, repeated, or 15–30 mg/min by IV infusion	2–3 min/5–15 min	Headache and reflex tachycardia
Hydralazine	10–20 mg as IV bolus or 10–40 mg IM, repeat every 4–6 h	10 min IV/>1 h IV; 20–30 min IM/4–6 h IM	Tachycardia, headache, vomiting
Enalaprilat	0.625–1.250 mg every 6 h IV	15–15 min/4–6 h	Renal failure in patients with bilateral renal artery stenosis, hypotension, history of angioedema

Parenteral adrenergic inhibitors

Labetalol	0.25–0.5 mg/kg IV bolus; 2–4 mg/min as IV infusion until BP goal is reached, 5–20 mg/h subsequently	5–10 min/3–6 h	History of 2nd- or 3rd-degree AV block, HFrEF, asthma, bradycardia
Metoprolol	2.5–5 mg IV bolus over 2 min, repeat every 5 min to maximum of 15 mg	1–2 min/5–8 h	History of 2nd- or 3rd-degree AV block, HFrEF, asthma, bradycardia
Esmolol	0.5–1 mg/kg IV bolus or 50–300 µg/kg/min by infusion	1–2/10–30 min	Greater than first-degree heart block, bradycardia, HFrEF, asthma
Phentolamine	0.5–1 mg/kg as IV bolus OR 50–300 µg/kg/min by infusion	1–2/10–30 min	Tachyarrhythmias, orthostatic hypotension
Clonidine	150–300 µg IV bolus in 5–10 min	30 min/4–6 h	Sedation and rebound hypertension

AV, atrioventricular; BP, blood pressure; HFrEF, heart failure with reduced ejection fraction; IV, intravenous.
Adapted from Van den Born BH, Lip GYH, Brguljan-Hitij J, et al. ESC Council on hypertension position document on the management of hypertensive emergencies. Eur Heart J Cardiovasc Pharmacother. 2019;5(1):37-46.

Diuretics

Mechanism of Action

Diuretics alter physiologic renal mechanisms to increase the flow of urine with greater excretion of sodium or natriuresis. This results in a wide range of effects on BP. Moreover, thiazide type diuretics also result in mild vasodilation and, hence, provide an additional mechanism for BP lowering.[9]

Thiazide-type diuretics inhibit the reabsorption of sodium and chloride in the more distal part of the nephron. This distal cotransporter is insensitive to loop diuretics. Increased sodium reaches the distal tubules to stimulate exchange with potassium, particularly in the presence of an activated renin-angiotensin-aldosterone system. Thiazides may also increase the active excretion of potassium in the distal renal tubule. Oral formulations are rapidly absorbed from the gastrointestinal tract to produce a diuresis within 1 to 2 hours, although the overall longevity of this effect varies significantly between the most commonly used thiazide-type diuretics in the United States, hydrochlorothiazide (HCTZ) and chlorthalidone.

Loop diuretics, including the most commonly used furosemide and torsemide, inhibit the $Na^+/K^+/2Cl-$ cotransporter associated with the transport of chloride across the lining cells of the ascending limb of the loop of Henle. This site of action is reached intraluminally, after the drug has been excreted by the proximal tubule. The effect of the cotransport inhibition is that chloride, sodium, potassium, and hydrogen ions all remain intraluminally and are lost in the urine with the possible side effects of hyponatremia, hypochloremia, hypokalemia, and an alkalosis. In comparison with thiazide-type diuretics, there is a relatively greater urine volume and relatively less loss of sodium.

Thiazide-type diuretics as a class differ from the loop diuretics in that they have a longer duration and site of action. Additionally, thiazides are so-called low-ceiling diuretics, because the maximal response is reached at a relatively low dose and they demonstrate a decreased capacity to exert a predictable in the presence of renal failure.[10] The fact that thiazides and loop diuretics act at different tubular sites explains their additive effects, termed sequential nephron block.

Potassium-sparing diuretics such as amiloride and triamterene are occasionally used in combination with thiazide-type diuretics to reduce hypokalemia and lessen the incidence of serious ventricular arrhythmias in hypertension.[11] Amiloride acts on the renal epithelial sodium channel[12] and triamterene inhibits the sodium-proton exchanger, so that both lessen sodium reabsorption in the distal tubules and collecting tubules. Unto themselves they are comparatively weak diuretics.

Differences Within Class

Among thiazide-type diuretics, HCTZ is the most widely used. It has a bioavailability ranging from 60% to 80%. Its absorption may be decreased in HF and/or chronic kidney disease (CKD.) Chlorthalidone and indapamide differ from HCTZ, and hence are called thiazide-like (leading to the terminology of thiazide-type encompassing both thiazide and thiazide-like diuretics.) Both chlorthalidone and indapamide are preferentially recommended for the treatment of resistant hypertension.[7] Indapamide is widely used in Europe and is available in the United States, but much less commonly used. Head-to-head comparisons among thiazide-type diuretics do not demonstrate significant differences for BP reduction when equivalent doses are used. However, comparisons between thiazide and thiazide-type diuretics have clear differences regarding magnitude and duration of BP reduction.[9,13] Moreover, chlorthalidone at a dose of 25 mg is comparatively effective to 50 mg of HCTZ, particularly with respect to the treatment of nocturnal hypertension.[13]

Thiazide-like and thiazide diuretics can be very different pharmacokinetically.[14] Chlorthalidone compared to HCTZ has both a considerably longer half-life, approximately 40–60 hours, and a larger volume of distribution. Metolazone is a powerful thiazide, diuretic with a quinazoline structure. An important advantage of metolazone is efficacy even despite decreased kidney function and is usually used in concert with loop diuretics for edema management. The duration of action is up to 24 hours. In combination with furosemide, metolazone may provoke a profound diuresis, with known risk of excessive volume and potassium depletion. Tables 2.4 and 2.5 highlight important pharmacokinetic differences between loop and thiazide diuretics.

Among loop diuretics, furosemide is the most widely used. However, its use can be complicated by erratic absorption, with wide bioavailability ranges and a half-life of <6 hours.[15] Also complicating the use of furosemide is that the coefficient of variation for absorption varies for different generic products. As such, substituting one furosemide formulation for another will not standardize patient absorption and thus response. Bumetanide and torsemide are more predictable for oral absorption.

The short duration of action of loop diuretics means that frequent doses are needed when sustained diuresis is required in patients with hypertension. Twice-daily doses of furosemide should

Table 2.4

Commonly encountered loop diuretics: doses and kinetics		
Drug	**Dose**	**Pharmacokinetics**

Furosemide	10–40 mg oral, 2 × for BP
	Up to 250–2000 mg
	oral or IV
		Diuresis within 10–20 min
		  Peak diuresis at 1.5 h
		  Total duration of action 4–5 h
		  Renal excretion
		  Variable absorption
		  10%–100%

Bumetanide	0.5–2 mg oral 1–2 × daily
	(not licensed for BP
	treatment)
		Peak diuresis 75–90 min
		  Total duration of action 4–5 h
		  Renal excretion
		  Absorption 80%–100%

Torsemide	5–20 mg oral 1 × daily
	for BP
		Diuresis within 10 min of IV
		  dose; peak at 60 min
		  Oral peak effect 1–2 h
		  Oral duration of diuresis
		  6–8 h
		  Absorption 80%–100%

BP, Blood pressure control; *IV*, intravenous.

Table 2.5

Commonly encountered thiazide-type diuretics: doses and duration of action		
	Dose	**Duration of action (h)**
Hydrochlorothiazide	12.5–25 mg, 12.5 mg preferred	16–24
Chlorthalidone	12.5–50 mg, 12.5 to 15 preferred (BP)	≈40–60
Metolazone	2.5–5 mg (BP); 5–20 mg (HF)	24
Chlorothiazide	250[a]–1000 mg	6–12
Indapamide	1.25–2.5 mg, 1.25 mg preferred (BP); 2.5–5 mg (HF)	24

[a]Lowest effective antihypertensive dose not known; may prefer to use other agents for blood pressure control.
BP, Blood pressure; *HF*, heart failure.

be given in the early morning and midafternoon to avoid nocturia. Furosemide causes a greater and earlier (0 to 6 hours) absolute loss of sodium than HCTZ. However, because of its short duration of action, the total 24-hour sodium loss may be insufficient to maintain the slight volume contraction needed for sustained antihypertensive action.[16] In *oliguria* (not induced by volume depletion), as the glomerular filtration rate (GFR) drops to less than 20 mL/min, very high dose of furosemide may be required because of decreasing luminal excretion. In *hypertension*, twice-daily low-dose furosemide can be effective even as monotherapy or combined with other agents and is increasingly needed as renal function deteriorates[17]; however, torsemide, because of its longer half-life, is preferred among those who require a loop diuretic for hypertension management.

With respect to bumetanide and torsemide, their clinical effects and side effects are very similar to furosemide. As in the case of furosemide, a combined diuretic effect is obtained by addition of a thiazide diuretic. In contrast to furosemide, oral absorption of both agents is predictable at 80% or more.[10] In the United States, bumetanide use for hypertension is an off-label indication, but if used should be given three times a day because of its short half-life.[4] It is much more effective for diuresis, intravenously, in low-albumin states. Torsemide demonstrates a longer duration of action than furosemide and bumetanide. The consistency of torsemide's absorption and its longer duration of action are distinguishing pharmacologic features among loop diuretics.

Clinical Application

Thiazide diuretics remain among the medication classes recommended for first-line therapy for hypertension.[4] Thiazide-type diuretics demonstrate wide-ranging CV benefits. Diuretics were key components of an additive regimen used by the Veterans Administration (VA) Cooperative Study Group started in the 1960s, a study that convincingly proved the benefits of BP control. Both the severe (diastolic, 115–129 mmHg) and mild to moderate (diastolic, 90–104 mmHg) subgroups demonstrated reduced CV morbidity and mortality with BP reduction.[18,19] Only 2.7 patients needed to be treated to prevent a major CVD event in either BP group. There are outcome trials with doses of 100 and 200 mg of HCTZ, however, had very high adverse event profiles.[18]

Chlorthalidone is effective in both BP reduction and improving CV outcomes. Chlorthalidone is preferred for hypertension the major reason being that HCTZ has no outcome studies in hypertension at the doses commonly used, i.e., 12.5 and 25 mg/day.[20] Low-dose diuretics are often the initial agent of choice in low-renin groups such as older adults and in black patients.[21] By contrast, in younger white patients (mean age 51 years) only one-third responded to escalating doses of HCTZ over 1 year.[22] Thus the BP response rate in hypertension to thiazide-type monotherapy is variable and may be underwhelming, depending in part on the age and race of the patient, and also on the patient's oral sodium intake.

Chlorthalidone was the sole agent used in three seminal BP trials: The Systolic Hypertension in the Elderly Program (SHEP),[23] the Antihypertensive and Lipid-Lowering Treatment to Prevent Heart Attack Trial (ALLHAT)[24] and the Systolic Blood Pressure Intervention Trial (SPRINT).[25]

SHEP examined the impact of first-line chlorthalidone based antihypertensive therapy compared with placebo on the incidence of stroke and other CV events in 4736 participants over the age of 60, with isolated systolic hypertension for an average of 4.5 years. The chlorthalidone-based regimen decreased the incidence of stroke by 36%, myocardial infarction (MI) by 27%, HF by 54%, and overall CV morbidity by 32%.[26]

ALLHAT randomized 42,000 participants with hypertension and known CV disease or at least one other coronary artery disease risk factor to initial BP-lowering therapy with chlorthalidone, doxazosin, lisinopril, or amlodipine. There was no difference among these four agents for the primary outcome or mortality. However, secondary outcomes were similar except for a 38% higher rate of HF with amlodipine; a 10% higher rate of combined CVD, a 15% higher rate of stroke, and a 19% higher rate of HF with lisinopril; and a 20% higher rate of CVD, a 20% higher rate of stroke, and an 80% higher rate of HF with doxazosin, compared with chlorthalidone.[24] For stroke, there was a statistically significant race-by-treatment interaction. Chlorthalidone was superior to lisinopril in preventing incident stroke only in blacks.

Most recently, the primary diuretic used in the SPRINT was chlorthalidone.[25] Published in 2015, it was the major impetus for guideline recommendations for more aggressive BP lowering. The enrolled population was non-diabetics at elevated CV risk. The trial was stopped early due to a significant reduction of the primary composite endpoint of major adverse CV events in the lower BP target group. Interestingly the same BP targets were studied in the Action to Control Cardiovascular Risk in Diabetes (ACCORD) BP trial published in 2010 and did not demonstrate a significant reduction in major adverse CV events.[27] There are many theories about why a significant difference in adverse events was seen in SPRINT and not in ACCORD. Commonly cited reasons include the addition of acute decompensated HF as a component of the composite primary endpoint in SPRINT and was likely impacted by the use of chlorthalidone rather than HCTZ in ACCORD-BP.[28] In a meta-analysis of 108 trials, chlorthalidone was better in lowering systolic BP, at the cost of more hypokalemia.[29]

The major outcome trial for indapamide is the Hypertension in the Very Elderly Trial (HYVET) study.[30] Patients 80 years of age or older with a systolic BP of 160 mmHg or higher received indapamide 1.5 mg with the angiotensin-converting enzyme (ACE) inhibitor perindopril (2 or 4 mg) added if necessary, to achieve the target BP of 150/80 mmHg. Benefits were a significant reduction of 21% in death from any cause, with 39% reduction in stroke deaths as well as a 64% reduction in HF.

One trial that suggests combination therapy with an ACE-inhibitor and HCTZ may not be preferable to an ACE-inhibitor and calcium channel antagonist combination is The Avoiding Cardiovascular Events Through Combination Therapy in Patients Living With Systolic Hypertension trial (ACCOMPLISH). It investigated the ideal initial combination therapy by comparing an ACE-inhibitor and diuretic or ACE-inhibitor and calcium channel blocker (CCB) combination. The trial randomized 11,506 patients to benazepril/amlodipine or benazepril/HCTZ. During a mean follow-up of 2.5 years, benazepril/amlodipine was associated with reduced CV events (9.6% versus 11.8%).[31] The most significant criticism of the trial was the use of a short-acting HCTZ, rather than the long-acting chlorthalidone. However, a 2010 follow-up 24-hour ambulatory BP monitoring study from the ACCOMPLISH authors studied 573 patients on the HCTZ formulation and found no significant difference in BPs throughout a 24-hour period.[32]

Loop diuretics should not be used as first-line therapy in hypertension, since there are no outcome data with them. They should be reserved for conditions of clinically significant fluid overload (i.e., HF and significant fluid retention with vasodilator drugs, such as minoxidil) or in the presence of advanced renal failure.

Side Effects

Many side effects of thiazides are like those of the loop diuretics and are dose dependent. These side effects include those with established mechanisms (electrolyte and metabolic derangements) and other side effects that are not as well understood mechanistically (such as erectile dysfunction.) Thiazide-related biochemical side effects are more common with longer-acting formulation at increasing doses. Lower doses of thiazide-type diuretics produce fewer biochemical alterations and provide full antihypertensive as shown in several large trials. In the SHEP study, chlorthalidone 12.5 mg was initially used and after 5 years 30% of the subjects were still on the lower dose.[23]

Volume depletion. The possibility of excessive diuresis exists, thus resulting in reduced intravascular volume and ventricular filling so that the cardiac output drops and tissues become under-perfused. The renin-angiotensin system (RAS) and the sympathetic nervous system are further activated in a volume depleted state. Patients can manage their therapy well by tailoring a flexible diuretic schedule to their own needs. This can also include every other day dosing of chlorthalidone that has a very long duration of action.

Hypokalemia and Hypomagnesemia

Hypokalemia is likely an over-feared complication, especially when low doses of thiazides are used.[33] Nevertheless, the frequent combination of thiazide-type diuretics with the potassium-retaining agents including the ACE inhibitors, angiotensin II receptor blockers (ARBs), or mineralocorticoid receptor antagonists is appropriate, with the alternative, but lesser, risk of *hyperkalemia,* particularly in the presence of renal impairment.

Dietary potassium increases are the simplest recommendation to provide patients that experience hypokalemia. High-potassium and low-sodium intake may be achieved by fresh foods and salt substitutes. If unable to achieve via one's diet, a potassium-sparing agent, coadministration with an ACE-inhibitor, ARB, or a mineralocorticoid receptor antagonist is preferable to oral potassium supplementation, especially because the supplements do not correct hypomagnesemia.

Conventional doses of diuretics rarely cause magnesium deficiency,[34] but hypomagnesemia, like hypokalemia, is blamed for arrhythmias of QT-prolongation during diuretic therapy.

Hyponatremia

Thiazides and thiazide-like diuretics can cause hyponatremia, especially in older patients (more so in women) in whom free water excretion is impaired. In SHEP, hyponatremia occurred in 4% of patients treated with chlorthalidone versus 1% in the placebo group. Occurring rapidly (within 2 weeks), mild thiazide-induced hyponatremia can cause a vague constellation of symptoms including fatigue and nausea. When severe hyponatremia occurs, it may result in confusion, seizures, coma, and death. Hyponatremia occurs more so with thiazide-type diuretics than loop diuretics because thiazide-type diuretics do not interfere with the ability of the kidney to maximally concentrate urine

Diabetes

Diuretic therapy for hypertension increases the risk of new diabetes by approximately one-third, versus placebo.[14] The thiazides are more likely to provoke diabetes if combined with a β-blocker.[35-39] This risk depends on the thiazide dose and possibly on the type of β-blocker, in that carvedilol or nebivolol are exceptions. Patients with a familial tendency to diabetes or those with the metabolic syndrome are probably more prone to the diabetogenic side effects. Although there are no large prospective studies on the effects of loop diuretics on insulin insensitivity or glucose tolerance in hypertensive patients, it is clearly prudent to avoid hypokalemia and to monitor both serum potassium and blood glucose values.

Hyperuricemia and Gout

Thiazide-induced hyperuricemia can occur as a result of volume contraction and competition of thiazides with uric acid for renal tubular secretion. Most diuretics decrease renal urate excretion with the risk of increasing blood uric acid, causing gout in a subset of patients. In 5789 persons with hypertension, 37% were treated with a diuretic. Use of any diuretic (HR 1.48; CI 1.11–1.98), a thiazide diuretic (HR 1.44; CI 1.00–2.10), or a loop diuretic (HR 2.31; CI 1.36–3.91) increased the risk of gout.[40] Cotherapy with losartan lessens the rise in uric acid.[41] Use of loop diuretics more than doubles the risk of gout.

Changes in blood lipids. Thiazides may increase the total blood cholesterol in a dose-related fashion.[42] Low-density lipoproteins (LDL) cholesterol and triglycerides increase after 4 months with HCTZ (40-mg daily mean dose).[43] In the TOMH study, low-dose chlorthalidone (15 mg daily) increased cholesterol levels at 1 year but not at 4 years.[44] Atherogenic blood lipid changes, like those found with thiazides, may also be found with loop diuretics.

Hypercalcemia

Thiazide diuretics tend to retain calcium by increasing proximal tubular reabsorption (along with sodium). The benefit is a decreased risk of hip fractures in older adults.[45] Conversely, especially in hyperparathyroidism, hypercalcemia may be precipitated.

Erectile Dysfunction

In the TOMH study, low-dose chlorthalidone (15 mg daily given over 4 years) was the only one of several antihypertensive agents that doubled impotence.[46]

Sulfonamide Sensitivity

In addition to the metabolic side effects seen with previously used high doses, thiazide diuretics rarely cause sulfonamide-type immune side effects including intrahepatic jaundice, pancreatitis, blood dyscrasias, pneumonitis, interstitial nephritis, and photosensitive dermatitis. Ethacrynic acid is the only nonsulfonamide diuretic and is used generally only in patients allergic to other diuretics. It closely resembles furosemide in dose (25 and 50 mg tablet), duration of diuresis, and side effects. If ethacrynic acid is not available for a sulfonamide-sensitive patient, a gradual challenge with furosemide or, even better, torsemide may overcome sensitivity.[47]

Drug Interactions

Adverse interactions include the blunting of thiazide effects by nonsteroidal antiinflammatory drugs (NSAIDs) and coadministration of corticosteroids, which may cause salt retention to disrupt the action of thiazide-type diuretics. Lithium levels should be monitored closely in lithium-treated patients because thiazide diuretics can reduce lithium excretion and precipitate lithium toxicity.[48] Antiarrhythmic that prolong the QT-interval, such as Class IA or III agents including sotalol, may precipitate torsades de pointes in the presence of diuretic-induced hypokalemia. Cotherapy with certain aminoglycosides can precipitate ototoxicity. Nonsteroidal antiinflammatory drugs lessen the renal response to loop diuretics, presumably by interfering with formation of vasodilatory prostaglandins.[49] High doses of furosemide may competitively inhibit the excretion of salicylates to predispose to salicylate poisoning with tinnitus. Steroid or adrenocorticotropic hormone (ACTH) therapy may predispose to hypokalemia.

Calcium Channel Blockers

Mechanism of Action

Calcium channel blockers (CCBs) impede the movement of extracellular calcium through ion-specific channels within the cell wall (Fig. 2.4). This ultimately reduces calcium flux inward, which results in arterial dilation via smooth muscle relaxation and subsequent BP lowering. They may also cause a decrease in cardiac contractility and a slowing of AV conduction velocities.[50] Calcium channel blockers act primarily to reduce peripheral vascular resistance and, within the renal vasculature, produce natriuresis by increasing renal blood flow, dilating afferent arterioles, and increasing glomerular filtration pressure. Nondihydropyridine CCBs also importantly reduce albuminuria by improving glomerular permselectivity and lowering the perfusion pressure of the kidney (Fig. 2.5).[51,52]

Differences Among Drugs in Class

A major differentiating point amongst CCBs is the classification of dihydropyridine and nondihydropyridine CCBs. Commonly used

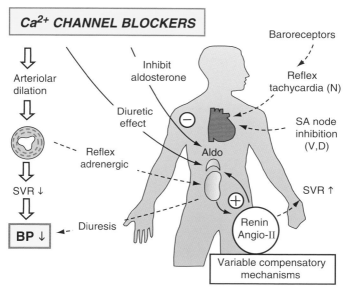

Fig. 2.4 Calcium channel blocker mechanism of action. Calcium channel blockers (CCBs) act largely by peripheral artery dilation. They also evoke counterregulatory mechanisms that depend on stimulation of renin and formation of angiotensin, as well as on reflex release of norepinephrine. Currently only long-acting CCBs are used in the treatment of hypertension because this effect is not seen to an appreciable extent with longer acting preparations. The inhibition of aldosterone release obviates overall fluid retention. *Aldo*, Aldosterone; *BP*, blood pressure; *D*, diltiazem; *N*, nifedipine; *SA*, sinoatrial; *SVR*, systemic vascular resistance; *V*, verapamil. (Figure © L.H. Opie, 2012)

dihydropyridine CCBs include amlodipine and nifedipine. Commonly encountered nondihydropyridine CCBs include verapamil and diltiazem.

Dihydropyridines with short elimination half-lives typically cause reflex tachycardia and sympathetic activation.[53] This effect has been mitigated with the advent of longer-acting and extended-release preparations.

Nondihydropyridine CCBs produce more negative chronotropic and inotropic effects than dihydropyridines, which is important for patients with cardiac arrythmias or who require concomitant administration of β-blockade.

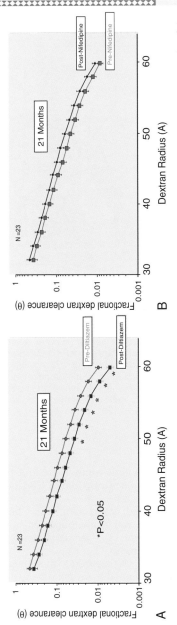

Fig. 2.5 Effects of diltiazem and nifedipine on glomerular permselectivity to dextran after 2 years of either agent in patients with diabetes. Patients in the study were >50 years old and had >5 years of type 2 diabetes and >10 years of hypertension all with >300 mg/day albuminuria. Data showed a significant reduction in glomerular permeability by diltiazem and worsening by nifedipine.

Among nondihydropyridine CCBs, verapamil has more negative chronotropic effects than diltiazem, an effect that makes each useful for acute intravenous treatment and chronic prevention of atrial tachyarrhythmias.

Clinical Application

CCBs demonstrate significant BP reduction across all patient groups, irrespective of sex, race, ethnicity, age, and dietary sodium intake. Thus, they are among the medication classes noted to be first-line therapy for the treatment of primary hypertension.[4]

There are several long-term CV outcome studies with CCBs in hypertension, and the overwhelming result is that CCBs are safe and effective, particularly for prevention of stroke.[54]

CCBs compared with placebo reduced stroke, coronary heart disease, major CV events, and CV death with, however, a trend to increased HF.[55] When compared to BP treatment with diuretics or β-blockers, CCBs had the same effect on CV death and total mortality, increased HF, with a trend toward decreased stroke. Additionally, there were fewer cases of new-onset diabetes with CCBs than with β-blockers or diuretics.[24,56]

Amlodipine is often used in combination with an ACE inhibitor and provided greater antihypertensive efficacy and better protection against CV events, mortality, and the development of new diabetes than did atenolol-based therapy in the ASCOT trial.[57]

ACCOMPLISH suggests that a combination of ACE inhibitor and CCB, rather than ACE inhibitor–thiazide diuretic, should be the preferred initial therapy in a high-risk hypertensive population.[31] Significantly, initial antihypertensive treatment with benazepril plus amlodipine slowed progression of nephropathy to a greater extent than did benazepril plus HCTZ.[58]

CCBs are particularly effective in older adult patients and do not have more prominent effects in one race or another. They are an ideal choice for the treatment of hypertension if there exist other compelling indications for a CCB such as angina pectoris, microvascular dysfunction, Raynaud phenomenon, or supraventricular tachycardia (use of nondihydropyridine).

The totality of data for the use of CCBs in the treatment of hypertension suggest that an initial strategy of CCB therapy can prevent all major types of CV disease, aside from HF. Initial dihydropyridine CCBs do not reduce the rate of progression of renal disease to the extent as inhibitors of the RAS; however, nondihydropyridine CCBs, such as diltiazem, can reduce albuminuria.

Side Effects

CCBs, unlike many other classes of antihypertensive therapy, do not lead to metabolic disturbances in potassium, glucose, uric acid, or lipid metabolism. However, they are not free from side effects. Higher doses of dihydropyridine CCBs often result in some degree of edema, and can additionally cause flushing, headache, and tachycardia. Lower extremity edema is the most commonly observed of these side effects and is particularly manifest in patients that display indiscretion in dietary sodium intake. Interestingly, a combination with an ACE-inhibitor or ARB is the best way to reduce dihydropyridine CCB–associated edema.[59]

Nondihydropyridine CCBs are contraindicated in patients with bradycardia, sick sinus syndrome, or more advanced heart block (in the absence of a pacemaker.) Additionally, caution must be used in patients with atrial tachyarrhythmias and an accessory bypass tract. Nondihydropyridine CCBs are generally contraindicated in left ventricular systolic dysfunction, acute myocardial infarction, and individuals at high risk of HF with reduced ejection fraction. As an example, use of a diuretic initially in the treatment of hypertension was significantly more effective in preventing HF than any other drug class, including a CCB.[60,61] Amlodipine's effects in HFrEF was studied with two significant clinical trials, PRAISE 1 and PRAISE 2, given that is does not have negative inotropic effects. PRAISE 1 suggested a trend toward CV benefit of amlodipine in individuals with nonischemic cardiomyopathy, but PRAISE 2 demonstrated no significant effect on CV outcomes compared with placebo.[62] Thus, use of amlodipine is not contraindicated in HFrEF, but it is often used in those individuals with HFrEF and hypertension.

In patients with CKD, it is uncommon to use CCBs as monotherapy while treating hypertension. Findings from the African American Study of Kidney Disease (AASK)[63] demonstrated that amlodipine was inferior to an ACE-inhibitor in preventing a reduction renal function in nondiabetic patients. Amlodipine was also shown to be inferior to irbesartan in in patients with hypertension, nephropathy and type 2 diabetes.[64]

Drug Interactions

CCBs have many important drug interactions. Chief among them are that diltiazem and verapamil interact with digoxin and cyclosporine, among others. They increase digoxin levels and increase plasma levels of cyclosporine, thus decreasing the dosing requirement for cyclosporine.

Verapamil and diltiazem are metabolized by CYP3A4 pathway; therefore, inducers and inhibitors are likely to result in decreased and increased plasma levels of these two CCBs, respectively. Because of their shared negative effects on heart rate and myocardial contractility, β-blockers and verapamil are not used simultaneously. Pharmacokinetic data show small increases in statin exposure with coadministration of amlodipine and lovastatin or simvastatin. There is no evidence of significant interaction when amlodipine is given with atorvastatin, pitavastatin, rosuvastatin, fluvastatin, and pravastatin.[65]

Angiotensin-Converting Enzyme Inhibitors

Mechanism of Action

Frequent reference is made to the role of the RAS in CV pathologic conditions. The effect of excess angiotensin II and aldosterone contribute to adverse maladaptive vascular processes. Major effects of renin-angiotensin blockade are due to reduced circulating and local concentrations of angiotensin II, and subsequent effect on systemic arterioles, renovascular hemodynamics, the adrenal zona glomerulosa, and the sympathetic nervous system.

ACE inhibitors act on the ACE enzyme that generates angiotensin II from angiotensin I and inactivates the breakdown of bradykinin. Angiotensin I originates in the liver from angiotensinogen under the influence of the enzyme renin, a protease that is made in the juxtaglomerular cells of the kidney. Renin release is stimulated by impaired renal blood flow as seen in ischemia or hypotension, salt depletion or sodium diuresis, and β-adrenergic stimulation.

Understandably, ACE inhibition should work by lessening the complex and widespread effects of angiotensin II. Angiotensin II has essential structural as well as functional effects. A degree of the antihypertensive effect of ACE inhibition may be attributable to withdrawal of angiotensin II's effect on vascular smooth muscle, which increases arteriolar wall thickness and maintains increased systemic vascular resistance. Additionally, angiotensin II affects matrix protein composition in the heart and blood vessels by promoting the synthesis and deposition of collagen and other structural proteins (Table 2.6). Angiotensin II also stimulates that release of aldosterone from the adrenal cortex. Thus, ACE inhibition is also associated with aldosterone reduction and has potential

Table 2.6

Potential pathogenic properties of angiotensin II

Heart

- Myocardial hypertrophy
- Interstitial fibrosis

Coronary arteries

- Endothelial dysfunction with deceased release of nitric oxide
- Coronary constriction via release of norepinephrine
- Increased oxidative stress; oxygen-derived free radicals formed via NADH oxidase
- Promotion of inflammatory response and atheroma
- Promotion of LDL cholesterol uptake

Kidneys

- Increased intraglomerular pressure
- Increased protein leak
- Glomerular growth and fibrosis
- Increased sodium reabsorption

Adrenals

- Increased formation of aldosterone

Coagulation system

- Increased fibrinogen
- Increased PAI-1 relative to tissue plasminogen factor

LDL, Low-density lipoprotein; *NADH*, nicotine adenine dinucleotide, reduced; *PAI*, plasminogen activator inhibitor.

indirect natriuretic and potassium-retaining effects. Aldosterone formation does not, however, stay fully blocked during prolonged ACE inhibitor therapy. ACE inhibitors also demonstrate indirect antiadrenergic effects because angiotensin II promotes the release of norepinephrine and enhances adrenergic tone. Furthermore, angiotensin II amplifies the vasoconstriction achieved by α_1-receptor stimulation.

ACE activity is prominent in the vascular endothelium of the lungs, but occurs in all vascular beds, including the coronary arteries. Ultimately, ACE inhibition produces vasodilatory effects. The contribution of ACE inhibitors leading to increased local formation of bradykinin is because bradykinin is inactivated by two kininases, kininase I and II. ACE is a kininase II. Bradykinin acts on its receptors in the vascular endothelium to promote the release nitric oxide and vasodilatory prostaglandins. High bradykinin levels are likely ACE-inhibitor related, although high bradykinin levels may also provide additional vasodilation and other benefits not observed with ARBs.

Differences Among Drugs in Class

A major factor in the overall efficacy of ACE inhibitor therapy is the wide heterogeneity in activity of the renin-angiotensin-aldosterone (RAAS) among patients. Activation of the RAS is linked with the sympathetic nervous system and participates in complex stress responses and in early development of hypertension.[66] Similarly, activation of the RAS and sympathetic nervous system are seen in obese and CKD patients.[67] Dietary sodium loading can suppress the BP-lowering effect of an ACE inhibitor, while it is enhanced by salt restriction and concomitant diuretic therapy. Dose-response curves with ACE inhibitors are particularly flat, but their peak effects vary. Overall, there are few advantages and differences between the different ACE inhibitors. Table 2.7 outlines some of the major differences among agents in this class of BP-lowering medications.

Clinical Application

ACE inhibitors are among the four agents that are recommended as first-line therapy for the treatment of primary hypertension by the American College of Cardiology and American Heart Association.[4] In addition to hypertension, ACE inhibitors are indicated for treatment of patients with proteinuric CKD and HF with reduced ejection fraction. Aside from BP lowering, evidence suggests ACE

Table 2.7

Summary of pharmacologic properties and doses of commonly used ACE inhibitors		
Drug	**Elim T$_{1/2}$ (hours)**	**Hypertension (usual daily dose)**
Captopril	4–6 (total captopril)	25–50 mg 2 × or 3 ×
Benazepril	11	10–80 mg in 1–2 doses
Enalapril	6; 11 (accum)	5–20 mg in 1–2 doses
Fosinopril	12	10–40 mg 1 × (or 2 ×
Perindopril	3–10	4–8 mg 1 ×
Quinapril	1.8	10–40 mg in 1–2 doses
Ramipril	13–17	2.5–10 mg in 1–2 doses
Trandolapril	10	0.5–4 mg 1 × then 4 mg 2 ×
Lisinopril	7; 12 (accum)	10–40 mg 1 × (may need high dose if given 1 ×)

accum, Accumulation half-life, *ACE*, Angiotensin-converting enzyme; *T$_{1/2}$*, half-life.

inhibitors and ARBs also confer some added vascular protection, especially in diabetic patients and in CKD.

ACE inhibitors can be used as monotherapy in patients with mild to moderate hypertension, even in low-renin patients, or in combination with other standard agents. For monotherapy, moderate dietary salt restriction is especially important.[68] Differences in sodium intake and the relative activity of the renin-angiotensin mechanism explain why not all mild to moderate hypertensive patients respond to monotherapy with ACE inhibition.

The largest outcome trial that included ACE inhibitors (in the form of lisinopril) is the Antihypertensive Lipid-Lowering Heart Attack Trial (ALLHAT). The lisinopril-based therapy was slightly inferior to chlorthalidone or amlodipine but the reduction in the primary end point (fatal and nonfatal myocardial infarction) was not different from thiazide-type diuretic or amlodipine.[24]

ACE inhibitors tend to be effective as monotherapy in BP reduction in most patient groups except older black patients, in whom higher doses or combination therapy may be needed. For example, in ALLHAT, lisinopril resulted in less stroke protection than chlorthalidone or amlodipine for black patients (which accounted for approximately one-third of the study population), likely because the trial design did not allow combination with either a diuretic or a dihydropyridine CCB. There is a very wide overlap in the range of plasma renin activity between black and white individuals, but mean plasma renin activity tends to be lower in black cohorts,[69] and the antihypertensive efficacy of ACE inhibitor monotherapy is generally reduced in blacks compared with whites. Lesser BP efficacy in black patients, especially in older adults, can be overcome by addition of low-dose diuretics or higher doses of the ACE inhibitor. A particularly useful combination is ACE inhibitors with thiazide diuretics to enhance BP-lowering effects and to lessen metabolic side effects, because diuretics increase circulating renin activity and angiotensin II levels, which ACE inhibitors counter by inhibiting the conversion of angiotensin I to angiotensin II.

Although mechanistically a diuretic and ACE inhibitor combination makes sense, an even more attractive combination may be an ACE inhibitor and CCB. In the ACCOMPLISH trial, the ACE inhibitor benazepril plus amlodipine gave better reduction in morbidity and mortality than did amlodipine plus HCTZ. It must be noted that this superiority was only found when the estimated glomerular filtration rate (eGFR) was more than 60 mL/min.[58]

In the HOPE trial of patients at high risk of coronary heart disease, the addition of ramipril provided substantial cardioprotection in the form of a 22% risk reduction when compared to placebo.[70] Although initially attributed to an unspecified protective effect of ACE inhibitor that was independent of BP because the reported difference in office BPs between treatment arms was only about 3 / 2 mmHg, uncertainty exists as to whether this was related to the extra antihypertensive effect provided by the ACE inhibitor, especially with respect to nocturnal BPs, because the ramipril was given as 10 mg at night with substantial BP differences in an ABPM substudy. In that study, Ramipril reduced 24-hour ambulatory BP by about 10 / 4 mmHg, a difference of sufficient magnitude to explain the benefits of ACE inhibitor compared with placebo.[71] In the EUROPA study, perindopril given in a high dose of 8 mg to patients with established coronary disease but with other otherwise relatively low risk gave substantial CV protection especially by reducing the occurrence of MI.[72] Ultimately a large body of experimental evidence supports the notion that there are direct vascular protective effects, and in three trials of HF, an additional BP-independent effect of ACE inhibitors has been shown.[73]

In patients with hypertension and diabetes, with nephropathy and proteinuria, ACE inhibitors and ARBs provide preferential dilation of the renal efferent arterioles, immediately reducing intraglomerular pressure and thereby protecting against progressive glomerulosclerosis.

In the AASK, nondiabetic patients with presumed hypertensive nephrosclerosis were randomized into a 3x2 factorial study that tested three drugs (ramipril, metoprolol, and amlodipine) and two BP targets (<140 / 90 mmHg or <125 / 75 mmHg) for 5 years.[63] Ramipril demonstrated superiority in protecting against the composite renal end point (>50% or >25 mL/ min loss of GFR from baseline, end-stage renal disease occurrence, or death.)

In renovascular hypertension, in which circulating renin is high and a critical part of the hypertensive mechanism, ACE inhibition is logical first-line therapy. A low-test dose is recommended because the hypotensive response may be dramatic. With standard doses of ACE inhibitors, the GFR falls acutely to largely recover in cases of unilateral, but not bilateral, disease. Careful follow-up of renal blood flow and function is required. The primary goal of therapy for patients with hemodynamically significant renal arterial disease (RAD) is control of hypertension and preservation of kidney function. The risks versus benefits of medical and interventional therapies in treating patients with RAD have been under debate for many years.

The three current therapeutic options available to treat patients with RAD include (a) medical management, (b) surgical revascularization, and (c) percutaneous angioplasty (PTRA) with or without stent placement. The largest clinical trial of renal artery revascularization versus medical therapy alone was the

Cardiovascular Outcomes in Renal Atherosclerotic Lesions (CORAL) trial.[74] It enrolled 947 participants with systolic hypertension and atherosclerotic renal artery stenosis despite the use of two or more BP medications. All patients were given candesartan in addition to randomization percutaneous revascularization or no revascularization. Revascularization had similar outcomes to medical therapy alone, thus again calling into question the benefit of revascularization. This trial has been criticized for selection bias, because patients enrolled were not among those likely to benefit and high-risk patients were not enrolled. In summary, those patients like the participants in CORAL are unlikely to derive benefit from revascularization and should be treated with RAS blockade initially.

Side Effects

Despite the fact that ACE inhibitors do not alter glucose tolerance, blood uric acid, or cholesterol levels, they remain a popular drug choice among patients with metabolic syndrome and another pre-existing CV disease. Side effects are typically class specific and not drug specific. Cough remains one of these common side effects. The incidence was 5.5% of HOPE participants. Increased formation of bradykinin and prostaglandins may play a role, because ARBs have a much lower incidence of cough.

ACE inhibitors are the leading cause of drug-induced angioedema in the United States because they are widely used. However, the overall incidence is low, with many estimates suggesting a less than 0.5% risk.[75] Most commonly angioedema is encountered in the lips, tongue, and face, although intestinal angioedema can be seen. Switching therapy to an ARB should be considered if there are compelling indications for RAS blockade given its lower incidence[76]; however, there are also isolated instances of ARB-associated angioedema.

Hyperkalemia is only really a problem in patients with reduced kidney function or low renal blood flow, as seen in advanced HF. Concomitant use of multiple RAS blockers, aldosterone antagonists, and high-potassium diets can increase the incidence of hyperkalemia.

A critically important possible effect with ACE inhibitor use is an increase in serum creatinine, and thus a decreased glomerular filtration rate. This is due to a preferential relaxing of the renal efferent arterioles and subsequent reduction of the intraglomerular pressure. If such a decline in renal function is seen during acute or chronic use of an ACE inhibitor, this identifies individuals likely to experience long-term renal protective benefits. Unfortunately, there is a clinical trend to discontinue ACE inhibitors after small increases in serum creatinine. Overreacting to small changes in GFR can lead to inappropriate withdrawal of ACE inhibitors from patients who could benefit from these therapies. Increases in serum creatinine up to approximately 30% are tolerable and common during the initiation of ACE inhibition.[77] As noted above, such changes do not usually represent true renal injury, and the failure of serum creatinine to increase acutely and chronically with ACE inhibition is an undesirable sign, particularly in diabetic patients, because it strongly suggests that the drugs have not reduced glomerular filtration pressure and thus are unlikely to slow the progression to end-stage renal disease.[78]

ACE inhibitors are contraindicated in women who are pregnant or likely to become pregnant because of the possibility of fetal defects or death.

Drug Interactions

Indomethacin, which inhibits prostaglandin synthesis, partially reduces the hypotensive effect of ACE inhibitors. They may precipitate hyperkalemia when combined with potassium-retaining agents such as spironolactone. Although in the past ACE inhibitors and ARBs had been used together for extra renal protection in proteinuric patients, coadministration of an ACE inhibitor and an ARB is contraindicated based on the results of ONTARGET,[76,79] which demonstrated increased serious renal adverse events and hyperkalemia when compared with monotherapy with either agent. Similarly, elevated risk is seen when an ACE inhibitor or ARB is combined with the direct-renin inhibitor.[80,81]

Angiotensin II Receptor Blockers

Mechanism of Action

Clinically used ARBs should be more formally considered as angiotensin II receptor subtype 1 (AT-1) blockers. Angiotensin-II stimulates AT-1 which ARBs specifically act on. As described above when discussing the mechanism of ACE inhibitors, angiotensin-II promotes CV pathologic effects including vasoconstriction, mitogenic activity, cytokine production, reactive oxygen species formation, and aldosterone production. Because ACE inhibitors exert their major effects by inhibiting the formation of angiotensin II, it follows that direct antagonism of the receptors for angiotensin II

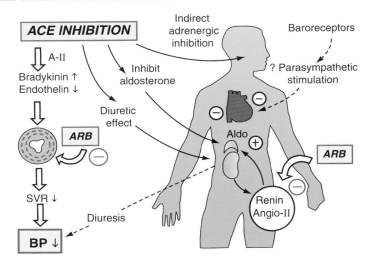

Fig. 2.6 **Angiotensin-converting enzyme *(ACE)* inhibitor and angiotensin receptor blockers *(ARBs)*.** Proposed mechanisms whereby these agents may have their antihypertensive effects. Note that the major effect is on the peripheral arterioles causing vasodilation and a fall in the systemic vascular resistance *(SVR)*. Indirect inhibition of adrenergic activity also promotes arteriolar dilation. Several ancillary mechanisms are at work, including renal and indirect adrenal effects, as well as possible central inhibition. Parasympathetic activity may also be stimulated. *AII & Angio-II*, Angiotensin II; *Aldo*, aldosterone; *BP*, blood pressure. (Figure © L.H. Opie, 2012.)

should duplicate many or most of the effects of ACE inhibition. These are illustrated in Fig. 2.6. ARBs largely avoid the bradykinin-related side effects of ACE inhibitors, such as cough and angioedema. A brief comparison is provided in Table 2.8.

Differences Among Drugs in Class

There are no significant differences in efficacy or other clinical characteristics among older ARBs. However, the last two ARBs approved, olmesartan and azilsartan, have greater BP-lowering efficacy, with slightly great effect of azilsartan than older agents.[82-84] Newer ARBs such as azilsartan more effectively reduce BP than older agents, particularly over 24 hours. For example, losartan and valsartan, when given once daily, do not control BP to the same magnitude as other ARBs.[85]

Table 2.8

Comparison of certain properties of ARBs and ACE inhibitors relevant to use in hypertension		
Property	**ARB**	**ACE Inhibitor**
Major site of block	AT-1 receptor	Converting enzyme
Major claims, basic science	More complete AT-1 block, AT-2 activity increased; latter may be beneficial (not certain)	Block of two receptors: AT-1, AT-2. Inhibition of breakdown of protective bradykinin
Side effects	Generally similar to placebo; cough unusual; angioedema very rare but reported	Dry cough; angioedema higher in black (1.6%) than nonblack patients (0.6%)
Licensed for hypertension?	Yes	Yes
Major clinical claims in hypertension	Equal BP reduction to ACE-inhibitors, little or no cough, excellent tolerability, well tested in LVH and in diabetic nephropathy	Well tolerated, years of experience especially in HF, good quality of life; used in coronary prevention trials (HOPE, EUROPA, PEACE)

ACE, angiotensin-converting enzyme; *ARBs*, angiotensin II receptor blockers; *AT-1*, angiotensin II receptor subtype 1; *AT-2*, angiotensin II receptor subtype 1I; *BP*, blood pressure; *HF*, congestive heart failure; *LDL*, low-density lipoprotein.

To this end, azilsartan was granted approval of a superiority claim by the United States Food and Drug Administration (FDA) based on the results of a pivotal clinical trial comparing the mean change in 24-hour ambulatory systolic BP of azilsartan, olmesartan, and valsartan in 1291 patients with stages 1 and 2 hypertension.[83] Azilsartan at a dose of 80 mg daily lowered systolic BP by 14 mmHg compared to 11.7 mmHg with olmesartan at 40 mg daily and 320 mg of valsartan daily lowered by only 10 mmHg.

Elevated levels of uric acid are reduced by losartan administration. Elevated levels are linked to the incidence and progression of CV disease.[86,87] Telmisartan was found to have some mild peroxisome proliferator-activated receptor activity at standard doses[88]; however, in unpublished clinical studies, it failed to show a metabolic benefit.

ARBs vary widely in their volume of distribution. Bioavailability also varies widely. However, the excellent tolerability of all the drugs in this class provides a wide therapeutic window that allows most of these drugs to be given once daily with 24-hour efficacy in BP reduction. However, based on their short plasma elimination half-lives, losartan, valsartan, and eprosartan require twice-daily dosing to maintain 24 hours of effective BP lowering in some patients.

Clinical Application

The ARBs are highly effective antihypertensive agents that are also particularly well tolerated. Some have argued that ARBs should entirely supplant ACE inhibitors in the treatment of hypertension, stating that the risk-to-benefit analysis indicates that there is little, if any, reason to use ACE inhibitors for the treatment of hypertension.[89]

There have been clinically meaningful differences in antihypertensive efficacy demonstrated between the classes of RAS blockers.[90] In a meta-analysis of 354 randomized trials, dose-response analysis among antihypertensive drug classes showed that ARBs had numerically higher reductions in office systolic BP compared with ACE inhibitors.[91]

When looking solely at hypertension treatment, there are no prospective randomized controlled trials that show a morbidity or mortality reduction with ACE inhibitors or ARBs against placebo. Years ago, the major argument against using ARBs ubiquitously was that they were not available in a generic formulation. Most if not all ACE inhibitors and ARBs are available as generic formulations, and cost to the patient becomes less relevant. Furthermore, many fixed drug combinations of both ACE inhibitors and ARBs with thiazides and amlodipine are available, thus allowing simplification of the therapeutic regimen with synergistic effects of the two BP-lowering medications.

Telmisartan is the only ARB truly indicated for the reduction of CV morbidity in patients with atherosclerotic CV disease, based on the results of the ONTARGET trial. A large study on more than 25,000 persons at high CV risk, ONTARGET demonstrated that the ACE inhibitor ramipril and the ARB telmisartan are equally good in reducing CV outcomes, including stroke.[79]

In the Losartan Intervention for Endpoint reduction in hypertension study (LIFE), the primary hypothesis was that losartan would be more effective than atenolol in reducing CV morbidity and mortality in patients with primary hypertension and signs of left ventricular hypertrophy (LVH).[37] With similar reduction in BP, losartan prevented more CV morbidity and death than did atenolol, and there was greater regression of LVH with losartan than with atenolol.[92] Similarly, losartan lowered the risk of stroke more than atenolol did.[93]

Some data suggest ARBs, like ACE inhibitors, are less effective in reducing both clinic and ambulatory BP among African Americans than among Caucasians, although addition of a thiazide diuretic to the regimen results in equivalent BP reductions in the two ethnic groups.[94]

Clearly BP reduction is linked to a slowing of the progression of kidney disease and to a reduction in albuminuria, and most prominently in diabetics, ARBs and other RAS blockers are significantly more effective other classes of antihypertensive drugs.[95] Importantly there are data establishing the role of losartan and irbesartan in, respectively, delaying or preventing the decline in renal function in diabetic patients with hypertension who had modest renal impairment upon trial enrollment. The results of the RENAAL[64] and IDNT[96] demonstrate this effect.

The Effects of Losartan on Renal and Cardiovascular Outcomes in Patients with Type 2 Diabetes and Nephropathy (RENAAL) trial was a randomized double-blind study comparing losartan with placebo, on top of standard antihypertensive treatment. The primary outcome of RENAAL was a composite of a doubling of the baseline serum creatinine, progression to end-stage renal disease, or death. Prespecified secondary end points evaluated a composite of morbidity and mortality from CV causes, proteinuria, and the rate of progression of renal disease. Losartan reduced the incidence of a doubling of the serum creatinine concentration and end-stage renal disease but had no effect on the rate of death. The composite of morbidity and mortality from CV causes was statistically no different between placebo and intervention.

The Irbesartan in Diabetic Nephropathy Trial (IDNT) was a prospective, randomized, double-blind clinical trial that compared irbesartan, amlodipine, and placebo in the treatment of hypertensive patients with nephropathy caused by type 2 diabetes mellitus. The primary composite end point was the same as RENAAL and included a doubling of the baseline serum creatinine concentration, the development of end-stage renal disease, or death from any cause. A lower risk of the primary composite end point was seen with irbesartan. There were no significant differences in the rates of death from any cause or in the CV composite end point.

Side Effects

The ARBs have excellent tolerability and a low side effect profile. These effects are compared with ACE inhibitors in Table 2.9. Although there has recently been concern about production of generic versions of certain ARBs (losartan, valsartan, and irbesartan) that are contaminated with carcinogens, the impurities arose during manufacture of the ingredients in factories located in China

Table 2.9

ACE inhibitors and ARBs: side effects and contraindications

ACE inhibitors: side effects, class

- Cough—common
- Hypotension—variable (care with renal artery stenosis; severe heart failure)
- Deterioration of renal function (related in part to hypotension)
- Angioedema (rare, but potentially fatal)
- Renal failure (rare, risk with bilateral renal artery stenosis)
- Hyperkalemia (in renal failure, especially with K-retaining diuretics)
- Skin reactions (especially with captopril)

ACE inhibitors: Side effects first described for high-dose captopril

- Loss of taste
- Neutropenia especially with collagen vascular renal disease
- Proteinuria
- Oral lesions; scalded-mouth syndrome (rare)

ACE inhibitors and ARBs: shared contraindications and cautions

- Pregnancy all trimesters (NB: prominent FDA warning)
- Severe renal failure (caution if creatinine >2.5–3 mg/dL, 220–265 μmol/L)
- Hyperkalemia requires caution or cessation
- Bilateral renal artery stenosis or equivalent lesions
- Preexisting hypotension
- Severe aortic stenosis or obstructive cardiomyopathy
- Often less effective in black subjects without added diuretic

ACE, Angiotensin-converting enzyme; *ARB,* angiotensin receptor blocker; *FDA,* Food and Drug Administration; *K,* potassium.

and India, and this does not include all medications or manufacturers in this class.[97]

The adverse effect profiles of the first ARBs were often comparable to or less than those seen with placebo administration. We do not see the same degree of cough as with ACE inhibitors, and angioedema rates are lower.[98]

There are several caveats common to ACE inhibitors and ARBs, including a need to reduce the dose in volume-depleted states, monitoring for acute kidney injury and/or hyperkalemia, and absolutely avoiding use in pregnancy. Care is required in liver or renal disease because most ARBs are either metabolized by the liver or directly excreted by the bile or the kidneys. A similar mechanism to ACE inhibitors results in an increase in serum creatinine, often observed as BP is lowered in patients with modest renal impairment.

With respect to metabolic complications of ARB therapy, losartan was associated with fewer cases of new diabetes than atenolol.[99] Candesartan was associated with less insulin resistance than HCTZ,[100] and valsartan was associated with fewer cases than amlodipine.[101] The meta-analysis of LIFE, SCOPE, and VALUE trials has shown that losartan, candesartan, as well as valsartan can cause a clinically significant decrease in the incidence of new-onset diabetes, with a combined estimated relative risk of 0.80 for all the three ARBs.[102]

Drug Interactions

Losartan has the highest potential for drug interactions due to its involvement with the hepatic cytochrome P450 enzyme system. Olmesartan is not metabolized by the cytochrome P450 enzyme system, reducing the risk of interactions with drugs metabolized by these enzymes. No significant drug interactions involving valsartan, irbesartan, or candesartan have been reported. Coadministration of telmisartan and digoxin may increase digoxin concentrations, but to a small degree, the clinical significance of which is questionable.[103]

Mineralocorticoid Receptor Antagonists

Mechanism of Action

Although once described as aldosterone blockers, pharmacotherapies such as eplerenone and spironolactone are more appropriately termed mineralocorticoid receptor antagonists. Originally aldosterone was thought to be the sole physiologic ligand for the mineralocorticoid receptor, and that aldosterone increased BP via its sodium retention and subsequent volume effect. More contemporary data demonstrate that other ligands exist for the mineralocorticoid receptor (in addition to aldosterone); cortisol can significantly activate the mineralocorticoid receptor (particularly in HF with reduced ejection fraction and hypertension). Additionally, although the sodium-retaining effects of aldosterone are relevant for BP elevations, recent data demonstrate that aldosterone and MR activation raises BP predominantly via its effects on the vasculature and central nervous system. Aldosterone exerts multiple physiologic actions that raise BP, including mediation of increased extracellular fluid volume and promotion of vasoconstriction. Aldosterone specifically acts on mineralocorticoid receptors in epithelial cells in the distal renal tubule and collecting duct to promote sodium reabsorption and potassium excretion.

Differences Among Drugs in Class

Eplerenone is a newer, more selective mineralocorticoid receptor antagonist with significantly fewer antiandrogenic effects than spironolactone. This greatly enhances its tolerability and likely patient adherence to pharmacotherapy. Preclinical studies with eplerenone have demonstrated a >100-fold lower affinity for androgen and progesterone receptors than is the case for spironolactone. Spironolactone is moderately more potent than eplerenone in competing for mineralocorticoid receptors.[104]

Clinical Application

Clearly if primary aldosteronism is identified as the cause of a patient's elevated BPs, then use of a mineralocorticoid antagonist is indicated, particularly if unable to address with surgical treatment. Medical therapy with eplerenone or spironolactone can be used in patients with bilateral adrenal adenomas, adenomas that cannot be excised surgically, in individuals with bilateral adrenal hyperplasia, and in those with significant responses to mineralocorticoid receptor antagonists who do not desire surgery. Of note, surgical removal of an aldosterone-producing adenoma (unilateral disease) can improve BP and normalizes a patient's biochemical profile; however, a significant percentage of patients are not cured of hypertension even with adrenalectomy.[105] The persistence of hypertension is usually owing to underlying primary hypertension or development of nephrosclerosis given a long history of elevated BP.

There also exist a subset of patients who, although they do not meet the strict criteria for primary aldosteronism, still display an inappropriately elevated serum aldosterone and have robust BP lowering with the addition of spironolactone or eplerenone.[5] Perhaps this partially explains the seminal results of the PATHWAY-2 trial published in 2015.[106]

This study is the most comprehensive study of pharmacotherapy for resistant hypertension to date and demonstrates that spironolactone is the most effective add-on drug for the treatment of resistant hypertension, when compared with bisoprolol and doxazosin. As such, guidelines now recommend the addition of a mineralocorticoid receptor antagonist (spironolactone or eplerenone) as fourth-line therapy for uncontrolled hypertension.[7] Subsequent additional pharmacotherapies are based on expert opinion, lacking large-scale clinical trials, and should be individualized for the patient.

In general, the combined use of spironolactone and adequate doses of a thiazide-type diuretic is recommended for the treatment of resistant hypertension in order to maximize efficacy and reduce risk of spironolactone-induced hyperkalemia. It should be noted however, that hyperkalemia is seen predominantly in people with reduced kidney function, i.e., eGFR $<45\,mL/min/1.73\,m^2$ and/or those with a baseline potassium of $>4.5\,mEq/L$.[107]

Given the side effects associated with spironolactone, eplerenone use is increasing given its efficacy and decreased antiandrogenic effects. There are also significant data on its benefits in patients with hypertensive heart disease demonstrating a similar degree of efficacy in the regression of LVH and BP lowering, eplerenone was as effective as enalapril in regressing LVH and lowering BP and was equally effective in lowering BP in black and white patients with hypertension.[108]

Side Effects

Major adverse effects of mineralocorticoid receptor blockers include sexual dysfunction.

A major reason for spironolactone treatment discontinuation is its tendency to produce undesirable sexual adverse effects including erectile dysfunction, gynecomastia, and breast tenderness. These adverse effects are due to the binding of spironolactone to progesterone and androgen receptors. The Randomized Aldactone Evaluation Study (RALES) of spironolactone in HF with reduced ejection fraction reported a 10% incidence of gynecomastia or breast pain in its male patients receiving 25–50 mg per day of spironolactone versus 1% on placebo.[109] The Eplerenone Post–Acute Myocardial Infarction Heart Failure Efficacy and Survival Study (EPHESUS) demonstrated that the more selective mineralocorticoid receptor antagonist eplerenone provides a reduced incidence of gynecomastia that was no different than placebo.[110]

Hyperkalemia especially in setting of coexisting renal dysfunction or HF is clearly a concern when adding spironolactone or eplerenone to a medication regimen.

Judicious monitoring of serum potassium with clear attention and education regarding dietary potassium restriction, and consideration for concomitant use of appropriate diuretics, are paramount.

Drug Interactions

When aldosterone antagonists are used in combination with ACE inhibitors or ARBs, particularly in patients who have renal insufficiency, there is an increased risk of hyperkalemia. Often concomitant treatment for hypertension includes a diuretic appropriate for renal function, thus lessening the risk of excess serum potassium. The metabolism of eplerenone is via the is CYP3A4 pathway and it should be used judiciously with inhibitors of CYP3A4 activity.

Although not a true "drug" per se, excess sodium intake facilitates the deleterious effects of mineralocorticoid receptor activation.[111,112] This is even true in a normotensive state where high sodium intake aldosterone produces blood-pressure–independent target organ damage acting through inflammatory and profibrotic pathways. Thus, a low-sodium diet enhances the effect of mineralocorticoid receptor antagonism.

β-Blockers

Mechanism of Action

There are multiple mechanisms by which β-blockers lower BP. Among the likely mechanisms are reducing heart rate and cardiac output, inhibiting the release of renin (the release of which is partly regulated by β_1-adrenoceptors in the renal juxtaglomerular apparatus), inhibiting the central nervous system, improving vascular compliance, reducing norepinephrine release, and attenuating of the pressor response to catecholamines. β-adrenoceptors bind norepinephrine and epinephrine. β-blockers prevent binding to the β-adrenoceptor by competing for the binding site (Fig. 2.7).

Differences Among Drugs in Class

The pharmacologic effect of β-blockers are heterogeneous based on certain factors such as the degree of β_1-selectivity, presence of intrinsic sympathomimetic activity, α_1-blocking effect, lipid solubility, degree of first-pass hepatic metabolism, penetration into the central nervous system, endothelial nitric oxide production and vasodilation in the case of nebivolol, as well as the potency of medication effect and duration of action.

β-Blockers tend to have similar pharmacotherapeutic effects, despite these differences, but alterations in these properties may make certain drugs more attractive choices for individual patients. Broadly β-blockers may be grouped or termed as nonselective or

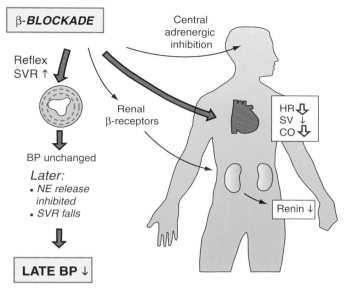

Fig. 2.7 Proposed antihypertensive mechanisms of β-blockers. An early fall in heart rate *(HR)*, stroke volume *(SV)*, and cardiac output *(CO)* does not lead to a corresponding fall in blood pressure *(BP)* because of baroreflex-mediated increased peripheral alpha-adrenergic vasoconstriction, with a rise in systemic vascular resistance *(SVR)*. Within a few days β-blockade of prejunctional receptors on the terminal neuron, with consequent inhibition of release of norepinephrine *(NE)*, may explain why the SVR reverts to normal. The BP then decreases. In the case of vasodilatory β-blockers there is an early decrease in SVR and a more rapid fall in BP. (Figure © L.H. Opie, 2012)

selective. Nonselective β-blockers bind both β$_1$- and β$_2$-adrenoreceptors, whereas the "cardio-selective" β-blockers have significantly higher affinity for the β$_1$-receptors.

Carvedilol and labetalol are β-blockers that not only block β-adrenoreceptors but also antagonize α-adrenoreceptors.[113] Unlike most β-blocking drugs, these additional α-blocking properties result in vasodilating activity and can lead to a reduction in peripheral vascular resistance that acts to maintain higher levels of cardiac output. Nebivolol also has additional vasodilator actions, unrelated to its β$_1$-selective antagonism. This is related to an enhancement of nitric oxide activity.[114]

β-Blockers may also be sorted based on their pharmacokinetic properties and grouped as those primarily eliminated by hepatic metabolism, and those drugs excreted unchanged by the kidney. The former is lipid soluble and include propranolol and metoprolol. They can have a significant effect on the central nervous system, short half-lives, wider variations in plasma concentration, and cause an increased incidence of side effects compared to the latter group: water-soluble agents. Water-soluble β-blockers such as atenolol are eliminated unchanged by the kidney and do not have the same degree of central nervous system penetration. They also tend to show less variance in bioavailability and have longer serum half-lives.

Given the high incidence of hypertension and end-stage renal disease (ESRD), an often-times underappreciated issue in patients is the dialyzability of certain β-blockers.[115] Atenolol and metoprolol are extensively cleared by hemodialysis compared with the negligible dialytic clearance of carvedilol.

Clinical Application

β-Blockers are no longer recommended for initial therapy in the treatment of primary hypertension and are now often relegated to fourth- or fifth-line therapy in the absence of other compelling indications.[7]

Propranolol was the first β-blocker approved as an oral antihypertensive agent. Since that time, many publications have demonstrated that β-blockers do not protect against heart attack better than other classes and suggest an increased risk of stroke.[116-118] A Cochrane Review published in 2012, which assessed the role of β-blockade as first-line therapy for hypertension, found that initiating treatment of hypertension with β-blockers leads to modest reductions in CV disease and no significant effects on mortality. As such, the effects of β-blockers are inferior to those of other antihypertensive drugs.[119]

The Anglo-Scandinavian Cardiac Outcomes Trial (ASCOT) conducted between 1998 and 2000 recruited patients with high BP and three or more additional risk factors for CV disease. In its BP lowering arm, it demonstrated that amlodipine and perindopril did not reduce CV morbidity and mortality compared to atenolol and bendroflumethiazide. However, the trial was underpowered and was stopped early due to a significant reduction in all-cause mortality in the amlodipine/perindopril arm (11%). Secondary outcomes suggest a possible reduction in CV morbidity and mortality using amlodipine and perindopril, although this has been ascribed to differences in BP between the two study arms. The primary composite outcome of nonfatal MI and fatal coronary artery disease demonstrated a nonstatistically significant reduction of 10% in the amlodipine/perindopril treatment arm. The lack of statistical significance may have been due to early trial termination. The amlodipine-based arm had a significantly lower BP than the atenolol-based arm throughout the entire study, which may explain the differences in outcomes.[57] Of note, the amlodipine-based arm also demonstrated a significant reduction in new-onset diabetes mellitus and decreased risk of developing peripheral artery disease or renal impairment.

The ASCOT Legacy study is a long-term follow-up of 8580 patients. It demonstrated long-term beneficial effects on mortality of antihypertensive treatment with a CCB-based treatment regimen and lipid lowering with a statin. Patients on amlodipine-based treatment had fewer stroke deaths and patients on atorvastatin had fewer CV deaths more than 10 years after trial closure.[120]

The relative ineffectiveness of β-blockade for primary prevention may be attributed to multiple effects including loss of insulin sensitivity with resultant increased risk of diabetes; increase in plasma triglyceride and lowering of high-density lipoprotein (HDL) cholesterol; increase in body weight; and, as noted in a substudy of the ASCOT trial, a lesser reduction in central as opposed to peripheral BP[121] and an increase in BP variability.[122]

However, we must recognize that, based on an analysis of more than 200,000 persons with more than 20,000 outcome events in the BP Trialists' Collaboration, there were no differences in the proportionate risk reductions achieved with different BP-reducing regimens.[123] The major determinant of CV outcomes is overall degree of BP lowering.

First-line therapy with β-blockers is recommended for patients with recent myocardial infarction, left ventricular systolic dysfunction, hypertrophic cardiomyopathy, and tachyarrhythmias. β-blockers may be useful in patients with BP driven particularly by excess adrenergic activation,[5] or with concomitant palpitations, tachycardia, and anxiety. Sufferers from migraine headache and essential tremor may also benefit. β-blockers tend to be less effective in older patients.[116]

Ideally in the treatment of hypertension, a β-blocker would be long acting, cardio-selective, and has metabolically favorable effects. β-blockers can be used in combination with other antihypertensive drugs to achieve. Combinations of β-blockers with one or another agent from all other classes have been successful in the therapy of hypertension. Nonetheless, combination with another drug suppressing the RAS, such as an ACE inhibitor or an ARB, is not logical. Labetalol can be used in hypertensive emergencies (Table 2.3).

Side Effects

Asthma and reactive airway disease may worsen while administering β-blockers. β-blockers that are β_1-selective (i.e., atenolol, metoprolol, and nebivolol) inhibit cardiac β_1-receptors but have less influence on bronchial smooth muscles theoretically resulting in less symptoms. However, higher doses of β_1-selective agents will also block β_2-receptors. Caution must be used in acute decompensated HF, higher degrees of heart block, and baseline bradycardia.

There is concern about use of β-blockers in diabetic patients, because they may worsen glucose tolerance, as well as masking the symptoms of, and prolong recovery from, hypoglycemia. They may also cause weight gain.[124] Although the risk of metabolic effects differs among the types of β-blocker used,[125] the Glycemic Effects in the Diabetes Mellitus: Carvedilol-Metoprolol Comparison in Hypertensives (GEMINI) study compared the effects of carvedilol versus metoprolol tartrate on glycemic and metabolic control. Participants had hypertension, diabetes, and were already receiving therapy with a blocker of the RAS. Use of carvedilol resulted in equivalent BP-lowering relative to metoprolol but did not affect glycemic control and improved some components of the metabolic syndrome, including improved insulin sensitivity and glycemic control. Additionally, carvedilol demonstrated less progression to microalbuminuria.[126] GEMINI also found that weight gain was less with carvedilol compared to metoprolol.[127] Combinations of β-blockers and diuretics should be applied thoughtfully in patients with diabetes whenever possible to avoid worsening of glycemic control given that they both may have negative metabolic effects.

Caution must be used when discontinuing a β-blocker. This is particularly true at higher doses. Withdrawal may be followed by adrenergically mediated symptoms. Therefore, a stepwise reduction in patient receiving higher doses is advised, particularly in high-risk patients.

β-Blockers have the potential to increase serum triglyceride levels and reduce HDL cholesterol levels by interfering with lipid metabolism, although this is less prevalent with newer vasodilating β-blockers and β-blockers with intrinsic sympathomimetic activity.[42]

Drug Interactions

Combining β-blockers with nondihydropyridine CCBs can synergistically depress the sinoatrial and atrioventricular nodes and lead to negative chronotropy and inotropy. This is also true of their use with other antiarrhythmic drugs that have negative inotropic effects.

Central Sympatholytic Agents

Mechanisms of Action

Central sympatholytic agents lower BP by decreasing sympathetic outflow to the heart and peripheral circulation. More specifically, they stimulate central α_2-adrenergic receptors in the rostral ventro-lateral medulla (i.e., brainstem), thereby reducing sympathetic nerve activity, and by inhibition of presynaptic release of norepinephrine from peripheral sympathetic nerve terminals.[128,129] Activation of imidazoline-1 receptors in the brainstem also contributes to a sympatholytic effect and BP-lowering effects that are independent of central α_2-adrenergic receptors.[130] Clonidine activates both imidazoline and α_2-adrenergic receptors. Guanfacine and guanabenz are more selective α_2-adrenergic receptors. Methyldopa does not activate imidazoline-1 receptors.

Differences Among Drugs in Class

Methyldopa, reserpine (no longer available), clonidine, guanabenz, and guanfacine are the most notable drugs in this class. Methyldopa, or α-methyldopa, was the first of the class to be commonly used and is a prodrug. It is still used in certain instances despite adverse central nervous system symptoms and potentially serious hepatic and blood side effects. α-Methyldopa does not directly reduce BP; it first requires conversion to α-methyl norepinephrine in the central nervous system, which leads to activation of central α_2-adrenergic receptors and inhibition of sympathetic outflow. In hypertensive patients, methyldopa reduces BP mainly by reducing systemic vascular resistance with minimal effects on heart rate or cardiac output.[131]

Clonidine, guanabenz, and guanfacine provide the BP-lowering effects of methyldopa with none of the rare but serious auto-immune reactions. A transdermal form of clonidine may be applied weekly and minimizes the risks of rebound hypertension seen with oral clonidine. Guanabenz resembles clonidine but may cause less fluid retention. It is predominantly eliminated via hepatic biotrans-formation, so dose adjustment is required in those with chronic liver diseases. Guanfacine is a similar agent that can be given once daily (and typically at bedtime to decrease the occurrence of day-time somnolence), with less risk of rebound hypertension if abruptly discontinued. Guanfacine demonstrates 12 to 25 times higher selectivity than clonidine for the α_2-adrenergic receptors when compared to the α_1-adrenergic receptors and reduces BP mainly by reducing total vascular resistance rather than cardiac output.[132-134] Guanfacine reduces resting heart rate both at rest and during exercise with minimal effects on cardiac output.

In contrast to the above-mentioned agents, reserpine reduces BP by depleting norepinephrine stores in the peripheral postganglionic sympathetic nerve terminals without reducing central sympathetic discharge.[135] It is easiest to use in a low dose, which carries most of the BP-lowering effect with fewer side effects than higher doses. Reserpine has been extensively used in the past as an effective antihypertensive agent particularly when combined with thiazide-type diuretics.[136]

Clinical Application

Although it was once the backbone of antihypertensive therapy, α-methyldopa is generally only used in pregnant women with hypertension because of its established safety profile in pregnancy,[137] owing to a lack of teratogenicity or fetal side effects. Maternal cardiac output, uterine blood flow, and renal blood flow are also unaffected by α-methyldopa.

In patients who are adherent to treatment, central sympatholytic drugs remain an important adjunct therapy for hypertension, particularly if it may be classified as "refractory hypertension" with overactivation of the sympathetic nervous system (as is usually characterized by elevated heart rate or cardiac output).[138,139]

In the VA Cooperative study, clonidine was among the more effective of the agents tested. It worked equally well in younger and older age groups, and in black and white patients. The major disadvantage in that trial was that clonidine demonstrated the highest incidence of drug intolerance, which was present in 14% of participants.[140]

Guanabenz has been shown to be effective in reducing LVH in hypertensive patients[129] and may help attenuate morning hypertension when administered at night-time.[141]

Side Effects and Drug Interactions

Side effects of α-methyldopa that ultimate require drug discontinuation are infrequent. However, there are numerous potential side effects including positive Coombs test, drug-induced fever, pancreatitis, hemolytic anemia, hepatic dysfunction, nasal congestion, exacerbation of parkinsonism, hyperprolactinemia, and gynecomastia.

Rebound hypertension is another major concern in certain drugs with a short half-life, such as oral clonidine. Abrupt cessation is known to precipitate symptoms of sympathetic over activity, and result in anxiety, tremor, headache, palpitation, and rebound hypertension within 1–3 days of discontinuation.[142,143] The rebound phenomenon may be amplified in patients under concurrent treatment with β-adrenergic blockers due to unopposed α-adrenergic vasoconstriction, and β-adrenergic blockers should not be initiated as single agents in withdrawing patients. Therapy for rebound includes treatment with α-blockers (or with combined α- and β-blockers if tachycardia is severe).

Higher doses of reserpine have been associated with significant side effects, including nasal stuffiness, peptic ulcer disease, and depression.

α_1-Adrenoreceptor Antagonists

Mechanisms of Action

It is important to understand that what are commonly referred to as "α-blockers" in today's medical parlance lower BP by selective inhibition of postsynaptic α_1-adrenoreceptors. They dilate both the resistance and capacitance sides of the vasculature, because blocking α_1-adrenoreceptors antagonizes catecholamine-induced constriction of both arterial and venous vascular beds. Initial study of α-receptor antagonists led to the development of phentolamine and phenoxybenzamine. These are nonselective agents and essentially cause a biochemical sympathectomy by blocking both pre- and postsynaptic α_1-adrenoreceptors. In contemporary practice, these are reserved for the pretreatment of patients with known pheochromocytoma undergoing surgery. Labetalol and carvedilol, discussed above, both have α_1-blocking properties that contribute to their antihypertensive effect.

Differences Among Drugs in Class

Postsynaptic α_1-adrenoreceptors in use today include prazosin, terazosin, and doxazosin. These agents differ predominantly in their pharmacokinetic profiles. Prazosin was originally approved for use in the United States. Although useful when initially developed, is not commonly used today. This is because of its relatively short duration of action resulting in compulsory multiple daily doses to provide sustained BP lowering. Use of prazosin over a longer time frame was also associated with waning antihypertensive effectiveness because of the expansion of extracellular and plasma volumes in patients with hypertension consuming typical levels of dietary sodium. Terazosin and, subsequently, doxazosin are later-generation selective postsynaptic α_1-adrenoreceptors that have much longer half-lives and durations of action than prazosin, which allow for once-daily dosing.

Clinical Application

α_1-Adrenoreceptors antagonists are not recommended as first-line BP-lowering therapy. This was made clear during the Antihypertensive and Lipid-Lowering Treatment to Prevent Heart Attack Trial.[24]

Before ALLHAT, encouraging data for α-blockers was demonstrated in the Treatment of Mild Hypertension Study (TOMHS). With 2 mg per day of doxazosin, BP decreases were compared with placebo, lisinopril, amlodipine, and acebutolol.[144] In the background of lifestyle modification including weight loss, dietary sodium reduction, alcohol restriction, and increased physical activity, doxazosin lowered systolic BP by almost 16 mmHg in nonblack participants and 9 mmHg in black participants, which was similar to that seen with lisinopril but not as much as with chlorthalidone, amlodipine, and acebutolol.[145] Blood cholesterol decreased with doxazosin, and the incidence of impotence was lowest in the doxazosin group.[146]

ALLHAT randomized more than 42,000 North American participants with stage 1 or 2 hypertension and an additional CV risk factor to amlodipine, chlorthalidone, lisinopril, or doxazosin. The doxazosin arm of the ALLHAT study was terminated early by the data safety and monitoring board and National Heart Lung and Blood Institute only 3.3 years into the trial. Two reasons exist for the early termination decision. The first was futility in the primary end point event rates between the chlorthalidone and doxazosin arms. Notably the primary end point was fatal coronary artery disease or nonfatal myocardial infarction. The other, more important reason was that ALLHAT participants randomized to doxazosin experienced more combined CV disease, stroke, and HF than participants in the chlorthalidone study arm.[147,148]

At annual study visits, systolic BP was between 2 and 3 mmHg higher in the doxazosin compared with the chlorthalidone treatment arm. In ALLHAT participants with glucose disorders, doxazosin was equally as effective as chlorthalidone in preventing the occurrence of the primary study end point; however, there were higher rates of combined CV disease and HF despite lower glucose levels in the doxazosin group.[149] One major caveat that must be stated with respect to ALLHAT is that in-study use of diuretics was not allowed as either second- or third-line therapy in any of the ALLHAT randomized treatment groups as would optimally be done in contemporary medical practice (i.e., combination of an α-blocker and diuretic). Given the known fluid retention seen with doxazosin, this may explain why the doxazosin arm of the ALLHAT study was terminated because of an excess of HF, compared with the reference diuretic, chlorthalidone.[148]

α_1-Adrenoreceptors antagonists are also not indicated as therapy for the initial treatment of resistant hypertension. This was demonstrated in the PATHWAY-2 trial of spironolactone versus placebo, bisoprolol, and doxazosin to determine the optimal treatment for drug-resistant hypertension.[106]

Among 335 participants with uncontrolled BP already taking an antihypertensive regimen of an ACE or ARB, CCB, and diuretic, add-on of once-daily oral spironolactone 25 mg, doxazosin modified release 4 mg, bisoprolol 5 mg, or placebo was studied with respect to systolic BP lowering. The average reduction in home systolic BP by spironolactone i.e., -8.7 mmHg was superior to placebo ($P < 0.0001$), and superior to doxazosin (-4.03; $P < 0.0001$) and to bisoprolol (-4.48; $P < 0.0001$).

In addition to their BP-lowering effect, α_1-adrenoreceptors antagonists demonstrate favorable effects on metabolic and lipid profiles. In TOMHS, doxazosin reduced total cholesterol by 6%, LDL cholesterol by 7%, and increased HDL cholesterol by 5%. Doxazosin was the only pharmacotherapy in TOMHS that lowered fasting blood glucose as well as fasting insulin levels.[150] These beneficial effects are due to antagonism of the α_1-adrenoreceptors that results in an increase in LDL receptor number, down-regulation of hydroxymethylglutaryl-coenzyme A (HMG-CoA) reductase, reduced synthesis of very-low-density lipoprotein (VLDL), and up-regulation of lipoprotein lipase activity.[151]

Despite the results of ALLHAT, α_1-adrenoreceptors antagonists may be used as adjunct therapy to other antihypertensive drug classes, preferably in combination with diuretic antihypertensive pharmacotherapy regimens. A well-established niche for α_1-adrenoreceptors antagonists is in older men with benign prostatic hypertrophy and hypertension. This is because α_1-blockers also increase mean and peak urinary flow rates, as well as reduce lower urinary tract symptoms.

Side Effects

When used over a prolonged period, α_1-blockers cause expansion of the extracellular fluid and plasma volumes, which leads to weight gain and an attenuation of the BP-lowering efficacy in persons who are consuming moderate or greater levels of dietary sodium. Use of diuretics in combination with α_1-blockers is beneficial because these agents minimize the expansion of the extracellular and plasma volumes while providing additional reductions in

BP. Given this known volume expansion effect, α_1-adrenoreceptors antagonists should be used very judiciously in patients with HF. Fluid retention is the likely explanation why the doxazosin arm of the ALLHAT study was terminated because of an excess of HF, compared with reference diuretic.[148]

Although minimal adverse metabolic and lipid effects are seen when prescribing α-blockers, side effects can include drowsiness, diarrhea, and postural hypotension. Tolerance of α-blockers, related to retaining fluid, may develop during chronic therapy requiring increasingly aggressive diuretic regimens.

Drug Interactions

In elderly individuals, particularly when taken in combination with diuretics or central sympatholytic agents, such clonidine, orthostatic hypotension is a concern, particularly because it results in only modest incremental BP lowering.

Direct Vasodilators

Mechanisms of Action

Hydralazine, nitrates, nitroprusside, and minoxidil are the most commonly encountered direct vasodilators in clinical practice. Hydralazine exerts its BP-lowering effect by dilating resistance arterioles, therefore reducing peripheral resistance. As there is no dilating effect of the venous circulation, oftentimes a baroreflex-mediated venoconstriction occurs, resulting in an increase in venous return to the heart.[152] Additionally, a direct catecholamine-mediated positive inotropic and chronotropic stimulation of the heart leads to increased cardiac output, which runs antithetical to its BP-lowering effect. Hydralazine therapy should be combined with medications that are sympathetic inhibitors to prevent expression of this reflex, and often patients will benefit from combining with a diuretic agent to prevent sodium retention caused by reduced renal perfusion pressure.

Similarly, minoxidil dilates resistance vessels with minimal effect on the venous bed.[153] Minoxidil activates adenosine triphosphate-sensitive potassium channels in arterial smooth muscle leading to a hyperpolarized smooth muscle membrane with calcium influx through voltage-gated calcium channels being inhibited, and cytosolic calcium concentration is reduced.[154]

Nitrates and sodium nitroprusside are nitric oxide donors. The resultant vascular consequences are in part related to the generation of nitric oxide gas as a consequence of their metabolic breakdown.[155] However, the ultimate vascular effect is different depending on the specific drug and its concentration at the site of action. Oral nitrates cause veins, conduit arteries, and small arteries to relax, but they are not powerful arteriolar dilators. Nitroprusside does act on arterioles and lowers systemic vascular resistance when administered intravenously.

Differences Among Drugs in Class

Hydralazine is metabolized in the liver, primarily by N-acetylation. The plasma half-life is short, but the clinical effect appears to be longer, and studies have demonstrated efficacy even when given as a twice-a-day regimen.[156] Dosing in clinical hypertension varies from 25 mg twice a day to 100 mg three times a day. Minoxidil is also metabolized in the liver, and its oral absorption is 100%. Its use is limited to men with severe hypertension and/or renal insufficiency due to the numerous side effects noted below. Minoxidil is often prescribed as a twice-daily pill, starting at 2.5 mg to 5 mg. Much higher doses have been studied, but they increase the potential for adverse effects.

Long-term nitrates include oral isosorbide dinitrate, isosorbide mononitrate, or transcutaneous nitroglycerin preparations. These are more widely used to treat angina or HFrEF than to provide sustained BP lowering in hypertension.

Clinical Application

Although still used as a fifth- or sixth-line agent in patients with resistant hypertension,[7] use of hydralazine has been supplanted with the introduction of CCBs, which exert similar vasodilation effects without nearly the degree of side effects. Hydralazine is still used widely in the developing countries because it is inexpensive. Hydralazine is most commonly used in the United States when it is combined with nitrates in patients with HF with reduced ejection fraction. This is particularly effective in black patients.[157] Regrettably, as needed, hydralazine has been adopted, for unknown reasons, as a drug of choice for asymptomatic hospitalized patients with elevated BPs. This practice should be discouraged and may cause more harm than good.

No long-term outcome trials of oral nitrates for the treatment of hypertension exist. Small, short-term studies display effective BP lowering in isolated systolic hypertension in the elderly.[158] Longer-acting nitrate formulations are effective in lowering systolic BP without the development of nitrate tolerance, particularly when used with an antioxidant, such as hydralazine.[159]

In the treatment of severe left ventricular failure or hypertensive emergency, sodium nitroprusside is an effective continuous intravenous agent that acutely reduces impedance to left ventricular emptying.[160,161] It may be increased from low initial starting doses until the desired hemodynamic parameters are achieved.

Side Effects and Drug Interactions

Adverse effects of direct vasodilators include predictable tachycardia, fluid retention, and headache, caused by the vasodilation, especially soon after beginning therapy. These can be reduced with use of β-blockade and diuretics.

Use of long-acting nitrates may cause headache, but can be prevented by slow increases in doses, and resolves with continuous administration. Similar to long-acting nitrates, headache and nausea are common side effects with nitroprusside. However, the major concern during prolonged infusion is the development of cyanide toxicity. Blood levels of thiocyanate may be monitored as a guide to prevent the development of cyanide toxicity.

Hydralazine, because it is N-acetylated, puts patients at risk of drug-induced lupus with high doses and long-term use.[162] It is more likely to be seen in patients that are slow acetylators and is less often seen in African American patients.

Minoxidil causes severe renal sodium retention that requires large doses of loop diuretics to counteract. Pulmonary and lower extremity edema may be the result of fluid retention and increased capillary pressure from arteriolar dilation without venous dilation. Particularly in patients with CKD, pericardial effusions may develop.[163] Tachycardia due to reflex sympathetic activation may account for electrocardiographic changes, which present during the first days of minoxidil treatment. Additionally, angina may be heightened in patients with coronary artery disease. Hirsutism is also a quite common side effect of minoxidil, and reverses after a few months after discontinuation. Other side effects may include nasal congestion, nausea, breast tenderness, and dermatological complications.

References

Complete reference list available at www.expertconsult.com.

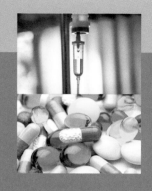

第3章
心力衰竭的药物治疗

　　心力衰竭是一大类临床综合征的总称，包括多种不同表型及临床表现，如急性心力衰竭、慢性心力衰竭。根据射血分数，慢性心力衰竭又可分为射血分数减低型、射血分数轻度减低型、射血分数改善型、射血分数保留型。不同的表型和临床表现有不同的用药及治疗目标。

　　对于急性心力衰竭，治疗主要基于低灌注和（或）淤血的临床证据，利尿药和扩血管药常用于缓解淤血症状。在低心输出量导致低灌注和低血压、组织缺血缺氧性损伤的患者中，应考虑使用正性肌力药物。

　　对于心源性休克，若患者持续低血压，尤其是在优化扩容升压治疗后仍持续性低灌注的患者，应使用血管升压药，如去甲肾上腺素、大剂量多巴胺、大剂量肾上腺素等。

　　对于慢性心力衰竭的治疗，自该版图书出版以后，陆续有新的大型临床试验结果公布，至2021年，欧洲心脏病学会（European Society of Cardiology，ESC）、美国心脏病学会（American College of Cardiology，ACC）、美国心脏协会（American Heart Association，AHA）等主流心血管学会都对心力衰竭的治疗发布了许多更新的指南。其中对于慢性射血分数减低型心力衰竭，β受体阻滞剂、血管紧张素转化酶抑制剂或血管紧张素受体−脑啡肽酶抑制剂、盐皮质激素受体拮抗剂、钠−葡萄糖协同转运蛋白2抑制剂是目前治疗的基石，即"新四联"。针对射血分数减低型心力衰竭的一些相关情况，还应按需使用抗凝药物、抗心律失常、静脉补铁、ω-3脂肪酸等多种治疗。对于射血分数保留型心力衰竭，钠−葡萄糖协同转运蛋白2抑制剂和血管紧张素受体−脑啡肽酶抑制剂分别获得了2a和2b类的推荐。并且，2021年的指南新增了射血分数轻度减低型心力衰竭和射血分数改善型心力衰竭这两个分类概念，更加强调动态监测心力衰竭发展的"纵向"过程及治疗的连续性。

心力衰竭的药物治疗除针对心力衰竭本身外，还需针对造成心力衰竭的心血管基础疾病（如冠状动脉粥样硬化性心脏病、心肌病、心脏瓣膜病、心肌炎等）进行治疗。

舟　君

Heart Failure

JEFFERSON L. VIEIRA · MANDEEP R. MEHRA

Introduction

Drug therapies for heart failure (HF) differ depending on the phenotype of presentation.[1-3] Distinctive phenotypes of presentation have different management targets, ranging from acute decompensated HF (ADHF) to chronic HF with reduced ejection fraction (HFrEF) or preserved ejection fraction (HFpEF).[4-6] For the purposes of this discussion, we shall focus on drug therapy for specific phenotypic syndromes including ADHF, HFrEF, and HFpEF. Preventive care, self-management, cardiac rehabilitation, device-based therapies, and surgical management of HF are discussed elsewhere.

Acute Decompensated Heart Failure

Introduction

Acute decompensated HF is a life-threatening condition generally defined as a first occurrence (*de novo*) or, more frequently a presentation of acute worsening of preexisting chronic HF with prior reported admissions for decompensation.[7-9] It affects primarily the elderly and often requires urgent evaluation and hospitalization (Table 3.1).[4,10,11]

Patients with *de novo* ADHF usually have a sudden presentation, with pulmonary edema or cardiogenic shock, while those with acute decompensation of chronic HF tend to show progressive signs and symptoms before acute presentation. These differences are explained by compensatory mechanisms, the capacity of the pulmonary lymphatic system and preexisting use of diuretic therapy.[12-14] Also, although acute decompensation of chronic HF can happen without known precipitants, most patients have identifiable triggers such as infection, arrhythmia, anemia, pulmonary embolism, acute coronary syndrome (ACS), and nonadherence.[15-17]

Table 3.1

New York Heart Association (NYHA) functional classification and American College of Cardiology/American Heart Association (ACC/AHA) stages of heart failure

NYHA functional classification

Class I—Patients with heart disease without resulting limitation of physical activity. Ordinary physical activity does not cause heart failure symptoms such as fatigue or dyspnea.

Class II—Patients with heart disease resulting in slight limitation of physical activity. Symptoms of heart failure develop with ordinary activity but there are no symptoms at rest.

Class III—Patients with heart disease resulting in marked limitation of physical activity. Symptoms of heart failure develop with less than ordinary physical activity but there are no symptoms at rest.

Class IV—Patients with heart disease resulting in inability to carry on any physical activity without discomfort. Symptoms of heart failure may occur even at rest.

ACC/AHA stages of heart failure

Stage A—At high risk for heart failure but without structural heart disease or symptoms of heart failure.

Stage B—Structural heart disease but without signs or symptoms of heart failure. This stage includes patients in NYHA class I with no prior or current symptoms or signs of heart failure.

Stage C—Structural heart disease with prior or current symptoms of heart failure. This stage includes patients in any NYHA class with prior or current symptoms of heart failure.

Stage D—Refractory heart failure requiring specialized interventions. This stage includes patients in NYHA class IV with refractory heart failure.

Although prehospital management is recommended, it should not delay transfer to an appropriate medical environment.[18] The assessment includes discrimination of severity and adjudication of the relative contribution of either congestion or perfusion to the bedside clinical profile. In the absence of cardiogenic shock, immediate echocardiography is not mandatory, since initial treatment of ADHF is similar for patients with HFrEF or HFpEF, which centers around decongestion with diuretic therapy and maintenance of adequate peripheral perfusion using either vasodilators or in selected situations, inotropic support.[17] There is some controversy as to whether chronic therapies for HF should be reduced or stopped during acute decompensations. Current guidelines suggest that patients should continue long-term HF therapies in the setting of ADHF, except in the presence of hemodynamic instability, hyperkalemia or severely impaired renal function. The clinical supposition in such cases is that the neurohormonal activation may be necessary during acute decompensation to maintain cardiorenal hemodynamics. In these cases, daily dosages of neurohormonal antagonists may be down-titrated or withheld temporarily until stabilization, with rapid reexposure once the acute state abates.[1] The choice of drug therapy will need to take prognostic variables into account and parameters such as an elevated blood urea nitrogen (BUN) level ≥ 43 mg/dL, low systolic blood pressure (BP) <115 mmHg, high serum creatinine level ≥ 2.75 mg/dL, and increased troponin I level signify elevated risk.[15,16,19] Permanent signs of congestion and renal dysfunction have been shown to be among the most important prognostic variables.[20-23] The routine use of a pulmonary artery catheter is not recommended and should be restricted to hemodynamically unstable patients with an unknown mechanism of deterioration and influences the therapy which in such cases tends to be targeted towards the hemodynamic aberration.[20,24] A clinical approach that may act as a surrogate to invasive hemodynamic parameters has been widely used to classify patients into therapeutic categories (Fig. 3.1).[25,26] Patients with a "wet" profile have correlated higher pulmonary capillary wedge pressure (PCWP ≥ 18 mmHg) while those with a "cold" profile have lower cardiac indexes (CI ≤ 2.2 L/min/m^2).[25,27] Fig. 3.2 summarizes the 2016 European Society of Cardiology (ESC) algorithm for management of patients admitted with ADHF based on clinical profiles.

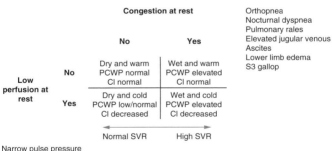

Fig. 3.1 Clinical profiles based on the presence of symptoms and signs of congestion and peripheral hypoperfusion. *CI*, Cardiac index; *PCWP*, pulmonary capillary wedge pressure; *S3*, third heart sound; *SVR*, systemic vascular resistance. (Based on data from Nohria A, Tsang SW, Fang JC, et al. Clinical assessment identifies hemodynamic profiles that predict outcomes in patients admitted with heart failure. *J Am Coll Cardiol* 2003;41(10):1797–1804.)

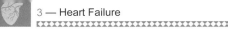

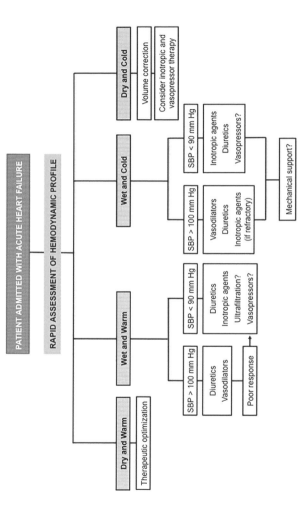

Fig. 3.2 Algorithm for management of patients admitted with acute heart failure *(AHF)* based on clinical profiles. (Data from Poni-kowski P, Voors AA, Anker SD, et al. 2016 ESC guidelines for the diagnosis and treatment of acute and chronic heart failure: The task force for the diagnosis and treatment of acute and chronic heart failure of the European Society of Cardiology (ESC). Developed with the special contribution of the Heart Failure Association (HFA) of the ESC. *Eur Heart J* 2016.)

Pharmacotherapy

Diuretics

Congestion is the leading cause of hospitalization in patients with ADHF.[28,29] Although robust evidence is lacking, clinical experience has demonstrated that diuretics effectively improve hemodynamics and congestive symptoms, even in the setting of *de novo* ADHF, in which pulmonary edema may occur without significant volume overload.[30] During ADHF hospitalization, net changes in weight and fluid balance are commonly used to assess response to decongestive therapies.[31]

Diuretics are classified according to their major site of action, chemical structure, or type of diuresis. Table 3.2 summarizes the doses and site of action of most diuretics commonly used in patients with acute and chronic HF. The optimal regimen is often influenced by renal function, preexisting diuretic therapy and urgency of decongestion. Loop diuretics, such as furosemide, torsemide, and bumetanide, have the most potent diuretic effect and remain the diuretic of choice for treating ADHF.[30,32] These agents act by directly inhibiting the sodium–potassium–chloride cotransporter (NKCC) at the thick ascending limb of the loop of Henle. They also inhibit a second cotransporter isoform that is widely expressed throughout the body, including the ear, which probably explains the side effect of ototoxicity associated with their use.

Loop diuretics are organic anions that are heavily bound to proteins as they circulate, reaching the tubular lumen predominantly by active secretion rather than glomerular filtration and thus maintain efficacy unless renal function is severely impaired. While structurally similar as a class, these agents have substantial differences in pharmacokinetics. The oral bioavailability of furosemide ranges from 10% to 90% and is determined by absorption from the gastrointestinal tract into the bloodstream, which is decreased in patients with severe ADHF-associated bowel edema. In contrast, the oral bioavailability of torsemide and bumetanide remain high (>90%), making oral and intravenous (IV) doses similar.[33] In addition, torsemide has a longer half-life when compared to furosemide or bumetanide. In healthy individuals, an oral dose of a loop diuretic may be as effective as an IV dose because the diuretic bioavailability that is above the natriuretic threshold is approximately equal. However, the natriuretic threshold increases in patients with HF and the oral dose may not provide a high enough serum level to elicit a significant natriuresis.[34] Therefore, IV therapy is recommended in patients with ADHF to achieve a higher and consistent bioavailability, allowing rapid onset of action within few minutes.

Table 3.2

Doses of diuretics commonly used in patients with heart failure

Diuretic class	Site	Starting dose	Maintenance dose	Half-life
Carbonic anhydrase inhibitors*				
Acetazolamide	Proximal tubule	250–375 mg orally/IV once a day	One dose every other day or once daily for 2 days alternating with a day of rest	2.4–5.4 hours
Loop diuretics [a]				
Bumetanide[b]	Ascending loop of Henle	Oral: 0.5–2 mg once or twice IV or IM: 0.5–1 mg once or twice	Oral doses may be titrated every 4 hours IV doses may be titrated every 2–3 hours Maximum recommended dose is 10 mg/day	1–1.5 hours
Furosemide[b]		Oral: 20–80 mg once or twice IV or IM: 20–40 mg once or twice	Maximum dose: 600 mg/day	30–120 min (normal renal function) 9 hr (end-stage renal disease)
Torsemide[b]		Oral or IV: 10–20 mg once	200 mg	3.5 hours

3 — Heart Failure

Thiazide-like diuretics [c]				
Chlorothiazide	Distal convoluted tubule	Oral or IV: 500–1000 mg once or twice	1000 mg once or twice	45–120 minutes
Chlorthalidone		12.5–50 mg once	100 mg	45–60 hours
Hydrochlorothiazide		12.5–50 mg once or twice	200 mg	6–15 hours
Metolazone		2.5–10 mg once	20 mg	6–20 hours
Potassium-sparing diuretics				
Amiloride	Collecting duct	5–10 mg once or twice	20 mg	6–9 hours
Mineralocorticoid-receptor antagonists [c,d]				
Spironolactone	Collecting duct	12.5–25 mg once	50–100 mg [e]	1–2 hours
Eplerenone		25–50 mg once	50–100 mg [e]	3–6 hours
Sequential nephron blockade				

Metolazone 2.5–10.0 mg once + loop diuretic
Hydrochlorothiazide 25–100 mg once or twice + loop diuretic
Chlorothiazide (IV) 500–1000 mg once + loop diuretic

IV, Intravenous.

*Carbonic anhydrase inhibitors can be used to treat the edema of congestive heart failure but are not commonly used for this purpose.

[a] Dose of intravenous and oral loop diuretics are similar

[b] Equivalent doses: 40 mg furosemide = 1 mg bumetanide = 20 mg torsemide

[c] Do not use if estimated glomerular filtration rate is <30 mL/min/1.73 m^2

[d] Minimal diuretic effect

[e] Doses up to 400 mg may be used in hepatology

Modified from Mullens W, Damman K, Harjola VP, Mebazaa A, Brunner-La Rocca HP, Martens P, et al. The use of diuretics in heart failure with congestion - a position statement from the Heart Failure Association of the European Society of Cardiology. *Eur J Heart Fail* 2019;21(2):137–155.

Diuretic dosing should be individualized and titrated according to hemodynamic response. Patients on chronic loop diuretic therapy may need higher doses in the setting of acute decompensation of chronic HF. The DOSE trial prospectively compared diuretic strategies in patients with ADHF and suggested that 2.5 times the usual home dose is associated with better symptom improvement than low dose, at the cost of some renal impairment.[35] The DOSE trial also showed no difference in outcomes between continuous IV infusion and intermittent bolus strategies, suggesting that both approaches could be considered when managing significant volume overload or diuretic resistance. Clinical experience, however, has demonstrated that when the effect of high-dose loop diuretic is suboptimal, a continuous infusion may be superior to reduce toxicity and maintain stable serum drug levels. Given the steep dose-response curve of loop diuretics, prompt doubling of dose at 2-hour intervals might allow the attainment of a ceiling dose earlier. Increasing the dose above the ceiling can lead to additional natriuresis by extending the time during which serum drug levels exceeds the natriuretic threshold, which makes it appear as if a ceiling does not exist.[30]

Impaired diuretic response is a common complication in patients with ADHF and is associated with increased rehospitalization and mortality. Although not fully understood, diuretic resistance is thought to result from a complex interplay between cardiac and renal dysfunction, specific renal adaptation, and escape mechanisms.[30,33,36] In fact, the magnitude of natriuresis following a given dose of diuretics declines over time as a result of the braking phenomenon, an appropriate homeostatic response that prevents excessive volume depletion during continued diuretic therapy. However, in patients with secondary hyperaldosteronism, such as those with HF, this phenomenon can be pronounced, leading to an increased reabsorption of sodium and contributing to diuretic resistance.[37] Furthermore, chronic treatment with a loop diuretic results in compensatory hypertrophy of the distal tubular cells, which bypasses the proximal effect of the loop diuretic.[38]

The coexistence of HF and impaired renal function is another common cause of diuretic resistance, as decreased renal blood flow and impaired tubular secretion may lead to insufficient therapeutic urinary drug concentrations. Among these patients, it is important to distinguish between underlying kidney disease and cardiorenal syndrome, which is being increasingly recognized as a complication of ADHF. The pathways to these distinct conditions involve not only hemodynamic deterioration but also neurohormonal, inflammatory, and intrinsic renal mechanisms.[39] It is hypothesized that the cardiorenal syndrome may represent a backward failure, with elevated right-sided filling pressures contributing more to renal dysfunction than low cardiac output (CO).[40] Traditional therapy with diuretics can contribute to cardiorenal syndrome, probably by further neurohormonal activation and worsening intrarenal hemodynamics, while vasodilator or inotropic therapy has not been shown to help.[39] In most cases, however, worsening of renal function in the setting of aggressive diuresis may reflect hemodynamic or functional changes in glomerular filtration rather than actual renal tubular injury.[41] Because residual clinical congestion is a predictor of poor outcomes in HF, a small to moderate increase in the BUN/creatinine ratio should not prevent further diuretic therapy if clinical evidence of congestion is still present in patients with ADHF.[42-44]

A useful approach for overcoming diuretic resistance is by sequential nephron blockade, which is the concurrent use of diuretics acting upon different segments of the nephron to produce an additive or synergistic diuretic response.[32] There is some evidence that a stepped pharmacologic strategy with early assessment of urinary output and sequential nephron blockade might result in equal decongestion when compared to mechanical ultrafiltration (UF), without significant renal impairment.[45-47] A post hoc analysis of the CARRESS-HF, DOSE, and ROSE-ADHF trials compared the efficacy of a urine-output guided diuretic adjustment versus standard high-dose loop diuretics therapy for the management of cardiorenal syndrome in patients with ADHF.[46] Compared with standard therapy, the stepped pharmacologic algorithm dosed to maintain urine output between 3 and 5 L/day resulted in greater weight change and more net fluid loss after 24 hours with slight improvement in renal function. A practical stepped pharmacologic algorithm to diuretic assessment in ADHF is reflected in Fig. 3.3.

Combined diuretic therapy using any of several thiazide-type diuretics can more than double daily natriuresis, although care must be taken for symptomatic hypotension, renal dysfunction, and electrolyte abnormalities.[32,48,49] Both IV chlorothiazide and oral metolazone have been shown to provide significant increases in urine-output when added to furosemide monotherapy, with chlorothiazide inducing a larger diuretic effect but at higher costs and greater need for potassium replacement.[48] There are no randomized controlled trials to establish whether a preferable thiazide exists in the treatment of ADHF.

Potassium-sparing diuretics, such as spironolactone, eplerenone, amiloride, and triamterene, should be considered to prevent hypokalemia associated with loop and thiazide diuretics use. Spironolactone and eplerenone are synthetic mineralocorticoid-receptor antagonists (MRAs) with a strong recommendation for patients with symptomatic chronic HFrEF, while amiloride and triamterene are epithelial sodium channel blockers that do not affect the mineralocorticoid receptor.[1,2,50]

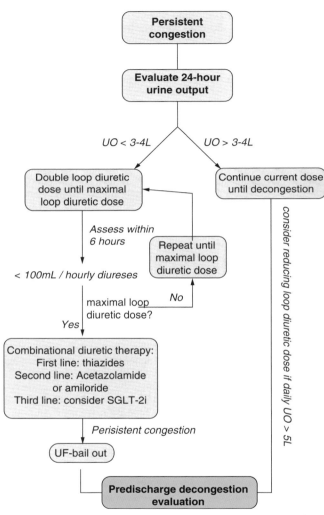

Fig. 3.3 A practical stepped pharmacologic algorithm to diuretic assessment in acute heart failure. Total loop diuretic dose can be administered either as continuous infusion or bolus infusion. *SGLT-2i*, Sodium-glucose cotransporter 2 inhibitor; *UF*, ultrafiltration; *UO*, urine output. (Modified from Mullens W, Damman K, Harjola VP, et al. The use of diuretics in heart failure with congestion—a position statement from the Heart Failure Association of the European Society of Cardiology. *Eur J Heart Fail* 2019;21(2):137–155.)

Carbonic anhydrase inhibitors, such as acetazolamide, potently inhibit sodium bicarbonate reabsorption in the proximal tubules, resulting in increased sodium levels in the loop of Henle where loop diuretics may exert their natriuretic action. These agents may be particularly useful during concomitant metabolic alkalosis, but, when used repeatedly, can lead to metabolic acidosis and hypokalemia. Other potential drugs for further decongestion, such as the arginine vasopressin (AVP) antagonists, have been investigated as adjuncts to standard HF therapies and will be addressed in other sections.

Other approaches that may also be helpful in patients with diuretic resistance are UF or hypertonic saline solution (HSS 3%) administration. The potential benefit of veno-venous UF is the removal of isotonic fluid without neurohormonal activation seen with diuretics. A trial comparing UF to diuretic therapy in patients with ADHF showed that UF was associated with greater weight loss by 48 hours but no difference in dyspnea score when compared to the control group. UF was associated with a reduction in rehospitalization and unscheduled office visits.[51] By contrast, other trials have observed a higher frequency of adverse events in patients treated with UF, including worsening of renal function in the CARRESS-HF and venous access complications in the AVOID-HF, which was not completed by the sponsor.[45,52] Based on these concerns, current HF guidelines do not recommend routine use of UF, which should be restricted to patients with congestion not responding to a stepped-care diuretic strategy. HSS 3% administration along with high-dose furosemide in selected hyponatremic patients with systemic congestion and renal dysfunction may be associated with greater clinical response and renal function preservation.[53,54] However, routine use of HSS 3% is controversial and further studies are needed before use can be endorsed.

Vasodilators

Although there is no robust evidence to support their routine use, IV vasodilators are the second most commonly used agents to relieve congestive symptoms in patients with ADHF.[55-57] Some vasodilators may act primarily on arterial resistance, leading to a decrease in afterload, while others act predominantly on venous capacitance with consequent reduction in preload. Most vasodilators, however, have balanced action on both afterload and preload.

Vasodilators are indicated in situations of pulmonary and systemic edema with or without hypoperfusion and are particularly helpful during hypertensive ADHF. However, they must be used with caution in patients who are preload or afterload dependent, such as those with severe diastolic dysfunction or aortic stenosis, since these agents can cause significant hypotension. Moreover, the use of vasodilators requires intensive BP monitoring and dose titration, and they should be avoided in patients with hypotension, hypovolemia, and recent use of phosphodiesterase (PDE)-5 inhibitors such as sildenafil, vardenafil, and tadalafil.

As a class, traditional direct-acting vasodilators, such as organic nitrates, sodium nitroprusside, and nesiritide (Table 3.3), act as an exogenous source of nitric oxide (NO) to activate soluble guanylate cyclase (sGC), producing cyclic guanosine monophosphate (cGMP) and consequent vascular smooth muscle relaxation (Fig. 3.4).[55] Conversely, novel vasodilator agents targeting new pathways have been developed, including serelaxin, natriuretic peptides, neurohormonal antagonists, and sGC stimulators and sGC activators.

Organic Nitrates

Organic nitrates, such as nitroglycerin, isosorbide dinitrate, and isosorbide mononitrate, reduce ventricular preload primarily via venodilation. At higher doses, especially in the presence of

Table 3.3

Intravenous vasodilators used to treat acute heart failure				
Vasodilator	Initial dose	Dose range	Main side effects	Other
Nitroglycerin	10–20 µg/min	40–400 µg/min	Hypotension, headache	Tolerance on continuous use
Isosorbide dinitrate	1 mg/h	2–10 mg/h	Hypotension, headache	Tolerance on continuous use
Sodium nitroprusside	0.3 µg/kg/min	0.3–5 µg/kg/min	Hypotension, isocyanate toxicity	Light sensitive
Nesiritide	Bolus 2 µg/kg Infusion 0.01 µg/kg/min	0.01–0.03 µg/kg/min	Hypotension	

Modified from Ponikowski P, Voors AA, Anker SD, et al. 2016 ESC guidelines for the diagnosis and treatment of acute and chronic heart failure: the task force for the diagnosis and treatment of acute and chronic heart failure of the European Society of Cardiology (ESC). Developed with the special contribution of the Heart Failure Association (HFA) of the ESC. *Eur Heart J* 2016;18(8):891–975.

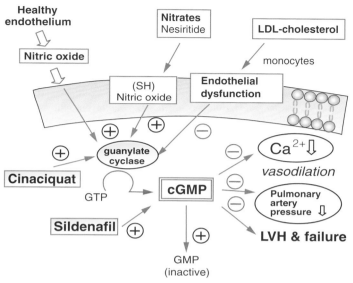

Fig. 3.4 Nitric oxide, nitroprusside, and nesiritide stimulate guanylate cyclase to form cyclic guanosine monophosphate *(cGMP)* with vasodilatory properties. *GTP,* guanosine-5′-triphosphate; *LDL,* low-density lipoprotein; *LVH,* left ventricular hypertrophy; *SH,* Sulfhydryl. (Figure © L.H. Opie, 2012.)

vasoconstriction, these agents can decrease systemic vascular resistance (SVR) and left ventricular (LV) afterload, consequently increasing stroke volume (SV) and CO.[55] Nitrates are also partially selective for epicardial coronary arteries, thus justifying use in ADHF associated with ACS. [57]

Nitrate indication is largely based upon hemodynamic response and expert opinion, as evidence is scarce and has relatively limited methodological quality.[58,59] Intravenous administration is recommended for greater bioavailability and ease of titration. Low initial doses of nitroglycerin (NTG) are recommended, with rapid up-titration increments every 5 minutes as required and tolerated. Aggressive early up-titration of NTG is associated with a significant reduction in pulmonary capillary wedge pressure (PCWP) that reaches a maximum effect at 2 to 3 hours and declines subsequently within the following 24 hours due to tachyphylaxis.[60] Tachyphylaxis is described as a rapid and significant attenuation of hemodynamic effects, limiting NTG usefulness in the treatment of patients with ADHF. The most common side effects of NTG are hypotension, headache, and nausea.

Sodium Nitroprusside

In contrast to NTG, sodium nitroprusside (SNP) causes balanced arterial and venous dilation, therefore reducing both the preload and the afterload. The use of SNP in patients with ADHF results in a significant decrease in systemic BP, right atrial pressure (RAP), pulmonary arterial pressure (PAP), PCWP, SVR, and pulmonary vascular resistance (PVR). SNP has a very short half-life, of seconds to a few minutes, and is particularly effective in the setting of ADHF secondary to elevated afterload such as acute aortic or mitral regurgitation, ventricular septal rupture, or hypertensive emergency.[61]

Administration of SNP requires close hemodynamic monitoring due to its potent hemodynamic effects. Although severe hypotension is rare and resolves quickly, significant vasodilation of the intramyocardial vasculature may cause a "coronary steal" phenomenon. Therefore, SNP is not recommended in the setting of ACS. Also, sudden withdrawal may cause a "rebound hypertension" effect and gradual tapering is advised, ideally transitioning to oral vasodilators.

The major limitation to the use of SNP is its metabolism to cyanide. When doses >400 μg/min are used for long periods of time, especially in patients with renal and/or hepatic dysfunction, the accumulation of SNP metabolites can lead to the development of cyanide, or rarely thiocyanate, toxicity, which may be fatal. The first sign of cyanide toxicity is lactic acidosis, and the most common side effects of thiocyanate toxicity are mental status changes, nausea, and abdominal pain. Thiocyanate can be removed with dialysis, and cyanide toxicity has been successfully managed with infusions of thiosulfate, sodium nitrate, and hydroxycobalamin.[57] There are no randomized clinical trials of SNP in patients with ADHF and, as with NTG, their indication is based upon hemodynamic response and expert opinion.

Nesiritide

Nesiritide is a synthetic analogue form of the human B-type natriuretic peptide (BNP), manufactured from *Escherichia coli* with recombinant DNA technology. It causes balanced arterial and venous dilation, resulting in significant reductions in filling pressures and mild increases in CO.

In patients with ADHF, the administration of nesiritide has been investigated more extensively than both NTG and SNP. The VMAC trial tested the safety and efficacy of nesiritide in patients with ADHF and reported a significantly greater decrease in PCWP compared to both NTG and placebo, with no evidence of tachyphylaxis.[60] Nesiritide, but not NTG, was also associated with significant improvements in patient-reported dyspnea at 3 hours. The ASCEND-HF trial tested nesiritide in a broad population of patients with ADHF and demonstrated a modest improvement in dyspnea when compared to placebo, but no difference in the composite outcome of death or HF hospitalization at 30 days.[62] While there was no increase in renal failure with nesiritide, the incidence of symptomatic hypotension was higher with nesiritide. Those findings were consistent with the latter ROSE-ADHF trial, which assessed the effects of low-dose nesiritide in patients with ADHF and showed no benefits on urine output, congestion, renal function, or clinical outcomes, but more symptomatic hypotension.[63]

Because of its high cost and lack of clear clinical benefit beyond other vasodilator therapies, such as NTG or SNP, nesiritide is not recommended as a first-line drug for patients with ADHF. Neither should it be used for the indication of replacing diuretic therapy, enhancing natriuresis, preventing cardiorenal syndrome, or improving survival. However, in selected patients who remain symptomatic despite standard therapy, a trial of nesiritide may be helpful.

Novel Vasodilators

Given the central role of vasodilator therapy in ADHF, there has been considerable enthusiasm for developing other types of vasodilator therapies. Serelaxin is a recombinant form of the human peptide relaxin-2, a hormone that regulates CV and renal adaptation to improve arterial compliance during pregnancy in humans.[64] It acts primarily via receptor-based increase of intracellular NO, with additional activation of matrix metalloproteinases, upregulation of endothelin type-B receptors, and expression of vascular endothelial growth factor (VEGF). Low-dose serelaxin decreases RAP and PCWP, while high-dose increases CO.[65] The RELAX-ADHF trial tested the efficacy of serelaxin by randomizing patients with ADHF to a 48-hour infusion of either serelaxin or placebo within 16 hours of hospital presentation.[66] Serelaxin improved short-term dyspnea and was associated with reduced worsening signs or symptoms of HF, shorter hospital length of stay (LOS), and improved biomarkers of end-organ dysfunction including troponin, N-terminal pro-BNP (NT-proBNP), creatinine, and transaminases. Following a similar protocol, RELAX-ADHF-2 trial aimed to confirm the beneficial effects of serelaxin on CV mortality and worsening HF, but failed to meet either of its primary outcomes.[64] These seemingly contradictory results suggest that serelaxin decongests the system rapidly, but with no improvement in CV outcomes.

Ularitide is a synthetic form of urodilatin, another natriuretic peptide, which is produced in the distal renal tubules with vasodilating, natriuretic, and diuretic effects. The TRUE-ADHF trial randomized patients with ADHF to continuous infusion of ularitide or placebo for 48 hours and found no difference in the risk of long-term CV mortality between the groups despite ularitide improving PCWP, SVR, CI, and dyspnea.[67] Additionally, ularitide increased creatinine associated with a doubling of hypotension.

Neurohormonal antagonism started aggressively during ADHF hospitalization and on top of more established therapy has been tested in large-scale trials, with mostly disappointing results. The ASTRONAUT trial found that the addition of aliskiren, a direct renin inhibitor (DRI), to standard ADHF therapy did not reduce mortality or hospitalization outcomes and was associated with higher rates of hyperkalemia, renal dysfunction, and hypotension.[68] Likewise, there was no benefit with tezosentan, a nonselective endothelin antagonist, or TRV027, an angiotensin type-1 (AT-1) receptor antagonist, over matching placebo in the VERITAS and BLAST-ADHF trials, respectively.[69,70] In contrast, the PIONEER-HF trial showed that sacubitril–valsartan, an angiotensin receptor-neprilysin inhibitor (ARNI), reduced NT-proBNP to a greater degree than enalapril among eligible patients admitted with acute decompensated HF.[71] Of note, side effects including hyperkalemia and hypotension were similar between the two drugs. Nevertheless, because reduction in biomarkers is a surrogate outcome, a larger trial powered for clinical outcomes is warranted.

The sGC stimulators and the sGC activators have a mechanism of action similar to that of organic nitrates, since both classes of drugs activate the sGC in smooth muscle cells, thus leading to the synthesis of cGMP and subsequent vasodilation. However, unlike traditional nitrates, sGC stimulators and sGC activators can induce sGC in its NO-insensitive state. Intravenous cinaciguat showed dose-dependent improvement in hemodynamic parameters but failed to demonstrate effectiveness in clinical trials for ADHF due to a high incidence of treatment induced hypotensive events requiring emergency intervention.[72] Subsequently, oral vericiguat was evaluated in two dose-finding studies within the SOCRATES program. In the SOCRATES-REDUCED trial, vericiguat showed a significant reduction in NT-proBNP and a trend toward fewer hospitalizations in patients with HFrEF.[73] In the SOCRATES-PRESERVED trial, it did not change NT-proBNP but was associated with better quality-of-life assessments in patients with HFpEF.[74] Recently, the oral sGC stimulator vericiguat was tested in the VICTORIA trial, which randomized patients with NYHA class II-IV HF, LVEF $\leq$ 45%, and a recent decompensation event to receive vericiguat or placebo. Over a median follow-up of 10.8 months, the incidence of CV death or HF hospitalization was significantly lower among patients receiving vericiguat, but there was no difference in all-cause mortality. Verici-guat was safe and well tolerated and did not require monitoring of renal function or electrolytes.[75]

Several other agents can reduce afterload and improve hemo-dynamic parameters, such as nitroxyl donors, short-acting calcium channel blockers, and potassium channel activators. However, robust randomized clinical trials for such agents are lacking.

Inotropes

Inotropic agents should be considered selectively in patients with advanced HF and low CO syndrome resulting in hypoperfusion, hypotension (relative and absolute), and end-organ dysfunction to prevent hemodynamic collapse and stabilize the clinical situa-tion. They are also a reasonable pharmacologic bridge to cardiac transplantation in patients with end-stage HF.

The mechanism of action for most inotropes involves their abil-ity to increase intracellular calcium, either by increasing influx into the cell or stimulating release from the sarcoplasmic reticulum. How-ever, there is long-standing concern that even short-term use of IV inotropes might lead to hypotension, atrial or ventricular arrhyth-mias, and death.[76-79] In particular, patients with ischemic heart dis-ease (IHD) may be at higher risk of further myocardial ischemia due to reduced coronary perfusion and increased oxygen consumption. In any case, inotropic therapy should be started at very low doses, up-titrated under close monitoring, and discontinued as soon as appro-priate organ perfusion is reestablished (Table 3.4). Inotropes are not indicated in patients with HFPEF, and there is limited evidence to suggest that one particular agent is better than another.

β-Adrenergic Agonists

Dobutamine

Dobutamine is the most widely used β-adrenergic agent for inotro-pic support. It is a synthetic analog of dopamine, with strong β_1 ago-nist activity as well as minor effects on β_2- and α_1-receptors. It has been suggested that the inotropic activity of dobutamine results from combined β_1 and α_1 stimulation in the myocardium. β_1-stimulation enhances cardiac contractility through increases in intracellular cyclic adenosine monophosphate (cAMP) and cal-cium. At low doses, β2-stimulation generally offsets α1-adrenergic activity, resulting in peripheral artery vasodilation that occasionally may lead to symptomatic hypotension. At higher doses, though, peripheral vasoconstriction predominates through vascular

Table 3.4

Positive inotropes and/or vasopressors used to treat acute heart failure

Agents	Adrenergic receptors agonists				Calcium sensitizer	PDE III inhibitor
	Dopamine	Dobutamine	Norepinephrine	Epinephrine	Levosimendan	Milrinone
Mechanism of action	Dopa > β HD, α	β1 > β2 > α	α > β1 > β2	β1 = β2 > α	Calcium sensitization HD, PDE III inhibition	PDE III inhibition
Inotropic effect	↑↑	↑↑	(↑)	↑↑	↑	↑
Arterial vasodilatation	↑↑ (renal, LD)	↑ (HD)	0	↑	↑↑	↑↑
Vasoconstriction	↑↑ (HD)	↑ or 0	↑↑	↑ (HD)	0	0
Pulmonary vasodilatation			↓ or 0 (at high PVR)	↓ or 0 (at high PVR)	↑↑	↑↑
Elimination t1/2	2 min	2.4 min	3 min	2 min	1.3h (active metabolite, 80h)	2.5 h
Infusion dose	<3 μg/kg/min: renal vasodilation 3–5 μg/kg/min: inotropic >5 μg/kg/min: vasoconstrictor	1–20 μg/kg/min	0.02–10 μg/kg/min	0.05–0.5 μg/kg/min	0.05–0.2 μg/kg/min	0.375–0.75 μg/kg/min
Bolus dose	No	No	No	1 mg during CPR every 3–5 min	6–12 μg/kg over 10 min (optional)	25–75 μg/kg over 10–20 min

CPR, Cardiopulmonary resuscitation; Dopa, dopaminergic receptors; HD, high dose; LD, low dose; PDE, phospodiesterase; PVR, pulmonary vascular resistances. From Farmakis D, Agostoni P, Baholli L, et al. A pragmatic approach to the use of inotropes for the management of acute and advanced heart failure: An expert panel consensus. Int J Cardiol. 2019;297:83–90. https://doi.org/10.1016/j.ijcard.2019.09.005.

α_1-receptor stimulation. Since it has no dopaminergic effects, dobutamine is less prone to induce hypertension than is dopamine.

Dobutamine provides hemodynamic support with a dose-dependent increase in SV and CO and modest decreases in SVR and PCWP, referred to as an inodilatory effect. Lower doses might improve perfusion in patients with cardiogenic shock, but higher doses are generally recommended for more profound hypoperfusion states.

Dobutamine may induce serious atrial and ventricular arrhythmias at any infusion dose, particularly in the context of myocarditis and electrolyte imbalance. It also increases heart rate (HR) and myocardial oxygen demand and should be used cautiously in patients with recent myocardial ischemia. Hypersensitivity to dobutamine is a rare and unrecognized cause of eosinophilic myocarditis after prolonged infusion. Also, β-receptors may be downgraded or therapeutically blocked in patients with advanced HF so that intolerance to dobutamine may ensue. In the absence of cardiogenic shock, either levosimendan or milrinone could be alternatives for treating ADHF when β-blockade is thought to be contributing to hypoperfusion.[80]

Clinical trials and HF registries have documented excess mortality in patients receiving intermittent or continuous dobutamine infusion, despite its beneficial hemodynamic effects.[81-83] Thus, dobutamine should be restricted to HF patients with pulmonary congestion and low CO syndrome. In this setting, dobutamine appears to be as effective as milrinone.[84]

Dopamine

Dopamine is a catecholamine-like agent, with complex effects that vary greatly with dose. At low doses, dopamine acts primarily on dopamine-1 receptors to dilate renal, splanchnic, and cerebral arteries. Although it has been proposed that dopamine might improve renal blood flow promoting natriuresis through direct distal tubular effects, data supporting such a potential benefit are limited. The DAD-HF study suggested that a combination of low-dose furosemide and low-dose dopamine as a continuous infusion for 8 hours was equally effective as high-dose furosemide but associated with improved potassium homeostasis and preservation of renal function.[85] The follow-up DAD-HF II trial, however, found no differences in mortality rates, HF hospitalization, or overall dyspnea relief with the combined therapy.[86] These findings are consistent with the ROSE-ADHF trial, which found that neither low-dose dopamine nor low-dose nesiritide enhanced decongestion or improved renal function in patients with ADHF.[63] Notably, both DAD-HF II and ROSE-ADHF studies showed a higher incidence of tachycardia in the dopamine group.

At intermediate doses, dopamine acts as a precursor in the synthesis of norepinephrine (NE), an agonist of both adrenergic and dopaminergic receptors, and an inhibitor of NE reuptake, increasing SV and CO with variable effects on HR. Both the β_1-stimulation and the rapid release of NE can precipitate tachycardia as well as atrial and ventricular arrhythmias. Tachyphylaxis to the inotropic effects of dopamine may develop, in part, because myocardial NE stores often become depleted in patients with advanced HF.

At higher doses, dopamine also stimulates α-receptors leading to pulmonary and peripheral artery vasoconstriction. In the treatment of shock, dopamine compares similarly to NE as the first-line vasopressor agent with respect to 28-day mortality but is associated with an increased risk of arrhythmias.[87] Also, vasoconstriction dosages carry significant risk of precipitating limb and end-organ ischemia and should be used with caution. Discontinuation from high infusion rates should be done gradually to no less than 3 μg/kg/min, to minimize potential hypotensive response of low-dose dopamine.

Epinephrine

Epinephrine is the first-line vasopressor for cardiac arrest and anaphylactic shock. It acts as a complete β-receptor agonist, with dose-dependent α-agonism effect at higher doses. At lower doses, epinephrine acts predominantly on β_1-receptors, with less prominent effects on β_2 and α_1, resulting in an overall increase in CO with balanced vasodilator and vasoconstrictor effects. At higher doses, it increases SVR and BP, with combined inotropic and vasopressor effect. Common side effects, particularly at high doses, include tachycardia, arrhythmias, poor peripheral perfusion, headaches, anxiety, cerebral hemorrhage, and pulmonary edema. There is also a risk of local tissue necrosis with extravasation.

Isoproterenol

This relatively pure β-stimulant should be considered in cardiogenic shock secondary to bradycardia or when excessive β-blockade is thought to be contributing to hypoperfusion. It increases inotropy and chronotropy through β_1-stimulation, with a variable response on BP, depending upon the degree of concomitant β_2-vasodilator stimulation. The cardiac effects of isoproterenol may lead to palpitations, sinus tachycardia, and more serious arrhythmias. Other common side effects are hypotension, angina pectoris, flushing, headache, restlessness, and sweating. Patients with IHD may be at higher risk of further myocardial ischemia due to increased oxygen consumption. Also, there are some concerns regarding cost effectiveness of isoproterenol when compared to significantly cheaper alternative chronotropic agents.

Phosphodiesterase Inhibitors

Intravenous PDE-3 inhibitors, such as milrinone and enoximone (also available for oral use), decrease the rate of cAMP degradation, leading to enhanced inotropy, chronotropy, and lusitropy in cardiomyocytes. They also cause significant peripheral and pulmonary vasodilation via inhibition of vascular PDE, reducing preload and afterload while increasing contractility (Fig. 3.5).

Since PDE-3 inhibitors do not act via β-receptor stimulation, their effects are not offset by concomitant β-blocker therapy as are those of dobutamine or dopamine. Additionally, this independence of adrenergic pathways also allows for synergistic effects with the β-agonist inotropes. Nevertheless, while the hemodynamic effects of PDE-3 inhibitors can be helpful for short-term support, the increased levels of myocardial cAMP predispose to life-threatening arrhythmias, and the routine use of these agents for periods longer than 48 hours is not recommended. Milrinone is widely available for clinical use. Intravenous infusions may be started with a slow bolus over 10–20 minutes, which is often omitted due to hypotensive effects. The dose requires adjustments in the presence of renal dysfunction.

Major side effects include hypotension and atrial and ventricular arrhythmias. The OPTIME-CHF trial compared the effects of short-term IV milrinone versus placebo in patients with acute decompensation of chronic HF not requiring inotropic support. It showed that routine use of IV milrinone for ADHF was not associated with a reduction in hospital-based resource utilization at 60 days but increased the risk of sustained hypotension and atrial arrhythmias.[77] In addition, a later subanalysis revealed increased mortality and rehospitalization in patients with IHD receiving milrinone when compared to placebo.[88] Retrospective analysis of the ADHERE registry also found an increased in-hospital mortality associated with dobutamine or milrinone when compared to NTG or nesiritide.[83] However, given that sicker patients were treated with inotropes, it is difficult to know if the adjustments were sufficient.

Calcium Sensitizers

Calcium sensitizers increase the sensitivity of troponin C fibers to ionic calcium that is already available in the cytoplasm, improving myocardial contractility with no additional calcium overload and

INOTROPIC DILATORS

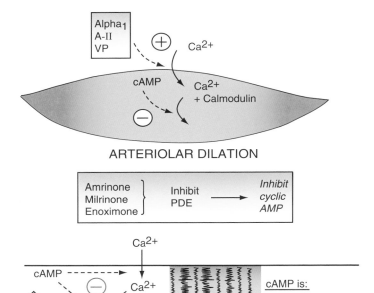

Fig. 3.5 **Inotropic dilators ("inodilators").** Increase of cyclic adenosine monophosphate in vascular smooth muscle *(top)* and in myocardium *(bottom)*. α_1, α_1-Adrenergic stimulation; *A-II*, Angiotensin-II; *cAMP,* cyclic adenosine monophosphate; *PDE,* phosphodiesterase; *SR,* Sarcoplasmic reticulum; *VP,* vasopressin. (Figure © L.H. Opie, 2012.)

minimal increase in oxygen demand. The most widely studied calcium sensitizer is levosimendan, while pimobendan is primarily used as a veterinary medication.[89] Neither levosimendan nor pimobendan, however, are pure calcium sensitizers, as both share some PDE-3 inhibitor activity that may be partially responsible for their inotropic and vasodilator properties. Levosimendan exerts additional pleiotropic effects through the opening of potassium-dependent adenosine triphosphate (ATP) channels in vascular smooth muscle cells and mitochondria.[90]

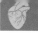

Although not approved for any use in the United States, levosimendan is currently available worldwide, including some countries in Europe and South America. It is indicated as short-term therapy for patients with ADHF who need inotropic support in the absence of severe hypotension. Intravenous infusions may be given with a bolus over 10 minutes, which is usually omitted due to the risk of significant hypotension. Due to an active long-acting metabolite, the hemodynamic effects of levosimendan can last for up to at least a week after stopping the infusion.[91]

Despite a dose-dependent improvement in indices of cardiac performance, including a reduction in PCWP and afterload and an increase in CO, there is limited evidence of clinical benefit from levosimendan therapy. Initial clinical studies, such as LIDO and RUSSLAN, suggested a survival advantage from levosimendan when compared to dobutamine or placebo, respectively.[81,92] The sequential more definitive trials REVIVE I and REVIVE II demonstrated a significant improvement in symptoms, BNP level, and hospital LOS with levosimendan therapy. However, there were more episodes of hypotension and cardiac arrhythmias in the levosimendan group, as well as a nonsignificant increase in early mortality when compared to placebo.[93] The SURVIVE trial demonstrated no survival difference between levosimendan and dobutamine during long-term follow-up of patients with ADHF despite evidence for an early reduction of plasma BNP level with levosimendan. Levosimendan therapy was also associated with more episodes of atrial fibrillation (AFib) and hypokalemia.[80]

Novel Inotropes

Omecamtiv Mecarbil

Omecamtiv mecarbil is a direct cardiac myosin activator that enhances effective actin-myosin cross-bridge formation and creates a force-producing state that is not associated with cytosolic calcium accumulation. Thus, omecamtiv mecarbil is believed to act as a calcium-sensitizer with pure inotropy action and no pleiotropic effects. Earlier studies have shown that it is safe, well tolerated, and produces dose-dependent increases in systolic ejection time, SV, EF, and fractional shortening.[94] In the ATOMIC-AHF trial, IV omecamtiv mecarbil did not meet the primary outcome of dyspnea improvement in patients with ADHF compared to placebo, except in the higher-dose group. It did, however, increase systolic ejection time and decrease LV end-systolic diameter.[95]

Istaroxime

Istaroxime is an investigational drug that mediates lusitropism through inhibition of sodium-potassium ATPase and stimulation of the sarcoendoplasmic reticulum calcium ATPase type 2a (SER-CA2a). In the phase 2 HORIZON-HF trial, the addition of istaroxime to standard therapy lowered PCWP and HR and increased systolic BP in patients with ADHF. Also, higher doses of istaroxime appeared to be associated with more improvement in diastolic function.[96] The role of this agent remains uncertain at this time.

Vasopressors

Vasopressor therapy should be reserved for patients with persistent hypotension, especially in the management of cardiogenic shock when hypoperfusion is evident despite optimization of filling pressures. Vasopressors increase vasoconstriction, which leads to increased SVR and mean arterial pressure (MAP), improving end-organ perfusion at the cost of peripheral perfusion and increased afterload. Among patients without preexisting cardiac dysfunction under vasopressor therapy, CO is either maintained or actually increased. However, the impact on CO in HF patients will depend on the balance between contractility improvement and afterload increase. Therefore, it is generally recommended to begin vasopressor therapy at very low doses, often in combination with inotropes.

The most often used vasopressors are NE, high-dose dopamine, high-dose epinephrine, vasopressin, and phenylephrine (Table 3.4). NE has a high affinity for α_1-receptors and moderate affinity for β-adrenergic receptors (Fig. 3.6), resulting in marked vasoconstriction with mild to modest increase in HR, CO, and myocardial oxygen demand. In general, NE is the vasopressor of choice for generalized shock. The SOAP II trial evaluated first-line vasopressor selection in patients with generalized shock and showed that, among the pre-specified cardiogenic shock subgroup, dopamine was associated with a higher risk of death and arrhythmia when compared to NE.[87] Although the SOAP II trial was the largest study in patients with generalized shock, a scientific statement from the American Heart Association (AHA) raised questions about the external validity and applicability of the findings in the subgroup with cardiogenic shock.[97] Therefore, NE might be the vasopressor of choice in many patients with shock, especially those presenting with arrhythmias, but whether it the optimal first-line vasoactive medication to treat cardiogenic shock remains unclear. Side effects include tachycardia, reflex bradycardia, anxiety, pulmonary edema, headache,

ADRENERGIC TERMINAL NEURON

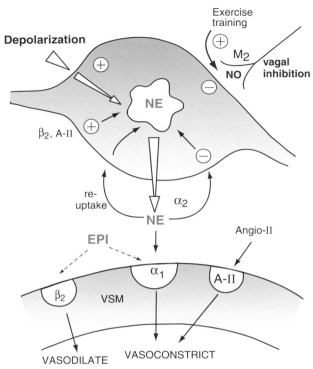

Fig. 3.6 Neuromodulation of vascular tone. *Upper panel,* terminal neuron; *lower panel,* vascular smooth muscle *(VSM).* Adrenergic sympathetic depolarization *(top left)* leads to release of norepinephrine *(NE)* from the storage granules of the terminal neurons into the synaptic cleft that separates the terminals from the arterial wall to act on postsynaptic vasoconstrictive β_1-receptors. NE also stimulates presynaptic β_2-receptors to invoke feedback inhibition of its own release, to modulate excess release of NE. Vagal cholinergic stimulation releases nitric oxide *(NO),* which acts on muscarinic receptors (subtype two, *M2*) to inhibit the release of NE, thereby indirectly causing vasodilation. Circulating epinephrine *(EPI)* stimulates vascular vasodilatory β_2-receptors but also presynaptic receptors on the nerve terminal that promote release of NE. Angiotensin-II *(A-II)* formed in response to renin released from the kidneys in shock-like states is also powerfully vasoconstrictive, acting both by inhibition of NE release (presynaptic receptors, schematically shown to the left of the terminal neuron) and also directly on arteriolar receptors. (Figure © L.H. Opie, 2012.)

and hypertension. As with all catecholamines and vasodilators, there is risk of local tissue necrosis with extravasation.

Phenylephrine is a selective α_1-receptor agonist with potent arterial vasoconstrictor effect and minimal cardiac inotropy or chronotropy. It is particularly useful in patients with severe hypotension related to systemic vasodilation, such as septic shock, rather than to a decrease in CO. Thus, it should be reserved for patients in whom NE is contraindicated due to arrhythmias or who have failed other vasopressors.

As noted above, both dopamine and epinephrine may also be used for their vasoconstrictor properties. Dopamine is a precursor of NE and epinephrine, which acts in a dose-dependent fashion on dopaminergic receptors as well as α- and β-receptors. Epinephrine has essentially α_1- and β- activity, increasing SVR, HR, CO, and BP (Fig. 3.6).

Angiotensin II is a naturally occurring hormone secreted as part of the renin-angiotensin system that results in systemic vasoconstriction. In the ATHOS-3 trial, IV angiotensin II at a rate of 20 ng/kg/min adjusted to increase the mean arterial BP to at least 75 mmHg effectively increased BP and reduced vasopressor needs in patients with refractory vasodilatory shock.[98] Although angiotensin II has been better studied in vasodilatory shock, it may be beneficial in both cardiogenic shock and cardiac arrest as well.[99]

Vasopressin is an endogenous vasopressor stored mainly in the posterior lobe of the pituitary gland and myocardium.[100] In a retrospective study of 36 patients who developed cardiogenic shock after myocardial infarction (MI), IV vasopressin therapy increased mean arterial BP without adversely affecting PCWP, CI, urine output, or other inotropic requirements.[101] In a prospective randomized clinical trial of 48 patients, the combined infusion of vasopressin and NE proved to be superior to infusion of NE alone in the treatment of cardiocirculatory failure in catecholamine-resistant vasodilatory shock.[102] A meta-analysis of randomized clinical trials compared vasopressin or terlipressin, which is a vasopressin analog not available in the United States, with supportive care in vasodilatory shock and showed no difference in short-term mortality.[103] Currently, vasopressin is used as a second-line agent in refractory vasodilatory shock, particularly septic shock or anaphylaxis that is unresponsive to epinephrine.

Special Situations

Acute Coronary Syndromes

The acute onset of severe myocardial ischemia, with or without infarction, can result in decreased CO and/or elevated filling pressures.[104] The coexistence of ADHF within ACS identifies a high-risk cohort, for whom aggressive therapy aiming at reperfusion should be rapidly instituted. Primary angioplasty is the strategy of choice for patients with ST-elevation MI.[105-107] Inopressor therapy can offer pharmacological support to improve hemodynamics during cardiogenic shock but should be administered at the lowest possible doses to avoid further ischemia. Inodilator agents are not recommended in the absence of shock.[108]

Hypertensive Emergency

Hypertensive ADHF accounts for approximately 10% of all ADHF cases, being most common in patients with HFpEF.[7] ADHF precipitates in the setting of markedly elevated afterload, and typically manifests as acute pulmonary edema. Aggressive BP reduction with IV vasodilators and diuretics is recommended. Calcium channel blockers (CCBs) without significant myocardial depressant effects, such as nicardipine and clevidipine, may be helpful in patients presenting with hypertensive ADHF.[109] Intravenous clevidipine has a rapid onset of action, high clearance, and no effect on ventricular contractility or central venous pressure (CVP), and is currently approved for the acute management of severe hypertension. Intravenous esmolol, a β-blocker, may be also used, but it is contraindicated in severe bradycardia heart block, cardiogenic shock, and overt HF.

Right Ventricular Heart Failure

Isolated right-sided or right ventricular (RV) HF is generally caused by acute RV infarction, severe pulmonary hypertension, or acute pulmonary embolism. Acute RV infarction should be approached as any other ACS, including early reperfusion and primary angioplasty when indicated. However, patients with RV infarction are very preload-dependent and can develop severe hypotension in response to nitrates or other preload-reducing agents. Hemodynamic stabilization with careful volume loading to a goal CVP of 10–12 mmHg can be beneficial, especially in patients with MAP <60 mmHg.[110] After ensuring adequate filling pressures, inotropic support can further augment RV CO. However, these principals do not apply to chronic right-sided HF.

The RV is also sensitive to increases in afterload, which is affected by the PVR. Selective pulmonary artery vasodilation includes treatment with NO, prostacyclin analogues, endothelin receptor antagonists, or, less frequently, certain CCBs. Hemodynamically unstable patients due to acute pulmonary embolism should be treated with immediate reperfusion either with thrombolysis, catheter-based approach, or surgical embolectomy.

Cardiogenic Shock

Cardiogenic shock is defined as a state of sustained hypotension (systolic BP <90 mmHg for ≥30 min) and a reduced CI (<2.2 L/min/m^2) in the presence of normal or elevated PCWP (>15 mmHg) and inadequate tissue perfusion (e.g., elevation in lactate levels).[97,111] Acute MI with LV dysfunction is the most frequent cause of cardiogenic shock.[7] In patients with a recent ACS, mechanical complications such as papillary muscle rupture, ventricular septal defect, and free wall rupture may present as cardiogenic shock within 24 hours of hospitalization.[112] Also, around 2%–6% patients may develop postcardiotomy cardiogenic shock following cardiac surgery. Therefore, immediate echocardiography is mandatory in all individuals presenting with cardiogenic shock. Other, less common etiologies include advanced valvular heart disease, arrhythmias, cardiac tamponade, cardiac constriction, pulmonary embolism, peripartum cardiomyopathy, acute coronary dissection, acute myocarditis, and drug poisoning.[97]

Fluid challenge for up to 30 minutes, either with saline or ringer lactate, is recommended as the first-line treatment if there is no sign of overt fluid overload. Pharmacological therapy with inotropic and vasopressor agents aims to improve organ perfusion by increasing CO and BP. Despite their frequent use, few clinical outcome data are available to guide the initial selection of such therapies in patients with cardiogenic shock. Dobutamine is the most used inotrope, while levosimendan may be an alternative to patients already on oral β-blockade.[113,114] Norepinephrine is recommended as the first-line vasopressor agent in the treatment of shock, as the use of dopamine is associated with a greater number of adverse events, such as arrhythmia.[87] Short-term MCS, including extracorporeal membrane oxygenation (ECMO), may be considered as a bridge to heart transplantation or to other mechanical intervention in refractory cases. Currently, the intra-aortic balloon pump (IABP) is still the most widely used MCS device in cardiogenic shock. However, among patients with MI and cardiogenic shock, the use of an IABP did not improve mortality or any long-term secondary outcome in the IABP-SHOCK II trial.[115] Therefore, routine use of an IABP cannot be recommended.

Heart Failure Patients With Reduced Ejection Fraction

Introduction

There has been substantial progress in the pharmacological management of chronic HF over the past three decades. The positive results of successive landmark clinical trials are reflected in clinical practice guidelines, which, in turn, have become standard of HF care. In general, the goals of treatment are to improve symptoms, functional capacity, and general quality of life, prevent disease progression and recurrent admissions, and prolong survival. To accomplish these goals, HFrEF should be viewed as a continuum that comprises four interrelated stages with incremental therapy at each stage aimed at modifying risk factors (A), treating structural heart disease (B-D), and reducing morbidity and mortality.[3,34]

Currently, the recommendation for patients with stage A HF is largely preventive and should focus on risk factor modification and treatment of atherosclerotic vascular disease. There is robust evidence showing that the onset of HF may be delayed or prevented through interventions aimed at modifying risk factors or treating asymptomatic LV systolic dysfunction. The SPRINT trial showed that intensive BP control in subjects with a high CV risk was associated with a 38% relative risk reduction in the development of overt HF.[116] In patients with stable coronary artery disease (CAD) without LV dysfunction, meta-analyses of randomized clinical trials have shown a modest benefit of angiotensin converting–enzyme (ACE) inhibitors, with a reduction in major CV outcomes, including HF.[117] The antidiabetic sodium-glucose cotransporter 2 (SGLT-2) inhibitors reduced the composite risk of CV death or HF hospitalization in patients with type 2 diabetes mellitus (T2DM), regardless of established CV disease or HF.[118-120] There is also reasonable evidence that intensive statin therapy, but not aspirin or other antiplatelet agents, may prevent or delay the onset of HF after ACS, with the most gain in patients with elevated levels of BNP.[121,122]

Several mechanisms contribute to the progression of HF, such as neurohormonal activation, endothelial dysfunction, venous congestion, and myocardial remodeling. Once patients have established structural heart disease, the choice of pharmacotherapy will depend on their NYHA functional class. For patients with structural heart disease but without signs or symptoms of HF (stage B), the therapeutic goal should be the prevention of further cardiac remodeling. In asymptomatic patients with chronically reduced LV ejection fraction (LVEF), an ACE inhibitor should be used to prevent the risk of HF hospitalization.[123,124] In all patients with a recent or remote history of MI or ACS, β-blockers and ACE inhibitors should be used, regardless of LVEF. It is noteworthy that β-blocker therapy should only be initiated after acute MI has resolved to avoid the risk of cardiogenic shock.[125,126]

Symptomatic patients (stages C and D) have a worse prognosis, particularly after hospital admission for ADHF. The major goals of treatment in patients with structural heart disease and previous or current symptoms (stage C) are to alleviate symptoms and reduce morbidity by reversing or slowing the cardiac and peripheral dysfunction. Neurohormonal antagonists, such as ACE inhibitors, angiotensin receptor blockers (ARBs), β-blockers, MRAs, and ARNIs, have been shown to improve outcomes in HFrEF and are recommended, unless contraindicated or not tolerated. More recently, the SGLT-2 inhibitor dapagliflozin was also associated with improved clinical outcomes among patients with symptomatic HFrEF, irrespective of T2DM status, signaling a new approach in the treatment of HF.

Additional pharmacological agents, such as hydralazine plus nitrate, ivabradine, and digoxin, should be considered in selected patients. Patients with refractory end-stage HF (stage D) may be eligible for specialized, advanced treatments, such as LV assist devices (LVADs) and heart transplantation.

Neurohormonal Activation

HFrEF classically develops after an index event that could be an acute injury to the heart, a long-standing hemodynamic overload, or a response to genetic variations that disrupt contractile function or lead to myocyte death. The circulatory changes that arise from impaired cardiac pumping and/or filling trigger a series of compensatory mechanisms referred to as neurohormonal activation. This historical term reflects early observations that many of the molecules that are elaborated in response to HFrEF are produced by the neuroendocrine system. However, most neurohormones such as NE and angiotensin II are now known to be synthesized directly within the myocardium and, therefore, act in an autocrine or paracrine manner.[127]

The sympathetic nervous system (SNS) and the renin–angiotensin–aldosterone system (RAAS) are the major neurohormonal systems, working collectively to maintain CO through increased retention of salt and water, peripheral vasoconstriction, and increased contractility.[128] The activation of inflammatory mediators also contributes to maintain early CV homeostasis through cardiac repair and remodeling.[129] However, sustained and chronic neurohormonal activation has deleterious effects and leads to progressive ventricular remodeling and worsening HF.[130] Further activation of the natriuretic peptide (NP) system briefly offsets these harmful effects but is unable to sustain compensation for chronic neurohormonal activation over time.[131]

Neuroendocrine modulation with β-blockers targeting the SNS and ACE inhibitors, ARBs, and MRAs targeting the RAAS have become the cornerstone of medical therapy to reduce morbidity and mortality in patients with chronic HFrEF. Most recently, the ARNIs further improved clinical outcomes by targeting both the RAAS and the NP system.

Pharmacotherapy

β-Blockers

SNS activation is one of the earliest responses to a decrease in CO, resulting in both increased release and decreased reuptake of catecholamines at adrenergic nerve endings.[132,133] It plays a complex role in HF, with both beneficial and adverse effects. In the short term, catecholamine-mediated chronotropic and inotropic responses help to maintain CO while increased SVR and venous tone preserve BP and preload. NE and angiotensin II also mediate constriction of the efferent arterioles, allowing for stable glomerular filtration rate (GFR) despite a low renal perfusion, and stimulate sodium retention and volume expansion, improving SV via the Frank–Starling law.[133]

Over time, however, these responses become detrimental, resulting in disruptions of β-adrenergic signaling and impaired mobilization of intracellular calcium.[128] As a consequence, increased SNS activation has been implicated in the development and progression of HF through multiple mechanisms, involving cardiac, renal, and vascular function. In the heart, it may lead to downregulation and functional desensitization of β-adrenergic receptors, cardiomyocyte hypertrophy, necrosis, apoptosis, and fibrosis. In the kidneys, SNS activation stimulates salt and water retention, attenuates response to natriuretic factors, and activates the RAAS, which in turn promotes a positive feedback loop that adversely affects hemodynamic and cardiac remodeling. In the peripheral vessels, it also mediates neurogenic vasoconstriction and vascular hypertrophy.[132,134]

The association between SNS activation, reflected by an increase in the plasma NE concentration, and mortality in patients with HFrEF raised the possibility of therapeutic efficacy for sympathetic inhibition. The potential mechanisms by which β-blockers improve outcomes in HFrEF are likely related to reducing the detrimental effects of sustained SNS activation by competitively antagonizing β-adrenergic receptors. Particular benefits might include decreased myocyte death from catecholamine-induced necrosis, antiarrhythmic and HR-lowering effects, upregulation of β_1-receptors, and inhibition of renin secretion. In addition, β-blockers directly reduce myocardial oxygen consumption and BP, revert production of fetal protein isoforms, and prevent proapoptotic and cardiotoxic effects of cAMP-mediated calcium overload.[135-137]

β-Blockers also strongly modulate cardiac remodeling, improve symptoms, reduce hospitalizations, and prolong survival in patients with HFrEF. Recommendations for their use are mainly based on the outcomes of large randomized placebo-controlled trials.

The three β-blockers that have been shown to reduce the risk of death in patients with chronic HFrEF are carvedilol, bisoprolol, and extended-release metoprolol succinate (CR/XL). Nebivolol was also associated with a reduction in the composite outcome of mortality or CV hospitalizations, but it did not reduce mortality alone and is not approved by the US Food a Drug Administration (FDA) for the treatment of HFrEF.

The MDC was the first randomized clinical trial testing a β-blocker, the short-acting metoprolol tartrate, in subjects with idiopathic dilated cardiomyopathy (DCM) and NYHA class II-III.[138] At 12 months, the metoprolol group had significant improvement in quality-of-life assessments, LVEF, and exercise capacity. There was also a nonsignificant 34% relative risk reduction in the combined outcome of death or need for cardiac transplantation, which was driven entirely by the reduction in transplantation, since there was no difference in all-cause mortality. The following MERIT-HF trial also investigated the impact of metoprolol on mortality in subjects with symptomatic HFrEF. However, it was larger, included patients with IHD as well as idiopathic DCM, and used the metoprolol succinate, which has a better pharmacological profile than metoprolol tartrate because of its extended-release formulation (CR/XL) and longer half-life.[139] The MERIT-HF trial was stopped early at a mean follow-up of 12 months after an interim analysis demonstrated a 34% relative risk reduction in all-cause mortality in subjects with NYHA class II–IV HF and LVEF $\leq$40% with metoprolol CR/XL compared to placebo. Additional secondary outcomes showed a reduction in all-cause hospitalization and CV events. Of note, metoprolol CR/XL reduced mortality from both sudden cardiac death and progressive pump failure while nearly 95% of the study population was already taking a concomitant ACE inhibitor or ARB at baseline.

The first study performed with bisoprolol in HFrEF was the CIBIS trial, which showed a nonsignificant trend toward 20% lower mortality and 30% fewer HF hospitalizations at a mean follow-up of 1.9 years in the bisoprolol group.[140] The subsequent follow-up CIBIS-II trial had greater statistical power to detect a mortality benefit and included approximately four times as many subjects as did CIBIS.[141] The CIBIS-II was stopped early, at about 16 months, after the second interim analysis demonstrated a 34% relative risk reduction in all-cause mortality in patients with NYHA class III–IV HF and LVEF $\leq$35% with bisoprolol compared to placebo. At the time of CIBIS-II publishing, standard HFrEF therapy included diuretics, ACE inhibitors, nitrates, and digoxin. Other benefits of bisoprolol therapy, such as a reduction in the risk of sudden cardiac death, HF hospitalizations, and all-cause hospitalizations, were observed regardless of the HF etiology.

Of the three FDA-approved β-blockers for the treatment of HFrEF, carvedilol has been the most studied. The US Carvedilol Heart Failure Program was designed as a stratified clinical program consisting of four component trials to evaluate nonfatal outcomes in subjects with mild to severe HF and LVEF ≤35%.[142] Although mortality was not a predefined primary outcome for the combined trials, it was prospectively measured by a safety committee, which prematurely stopped the program at a mean follow-up of 6.5 months due to a highly significant 65% relative risk reduction in mortality associated with the use of carvedilol across all four trials. The following ANZ-Carvedilol trial was conducted primarily to determine the effect of carvedilol therapy on LVEF and exercise tolerance in subjects with HF due to ischemic heart disease. The study concluded that carvedilol therapy for 12 months reduced LV volumes and preserved exercise performance at a lower rate-pressure product.[143] At 19 months, there was also a significant 26% relative risk reduction in the clinical composite of death or hospitalization with carvedilol compared to placebo. However, the ANZ-Carvedilol trial was not powered to determine statistically significant effects on mortality, and therefore, the 24% relative risk reduction in mortality alone did not achieve statistical significance.

Taken together, the outcomes of the US Carvedilol HF Program and the ANZ-Carvedilol trial provided a strong rationale for other large, randomized mortality studies, such as the COPERNICUS and the CAPRICORN trials. The COPERNICUS trial was specifically designed to evaluate the impact of carvedilol in a population with more advanced HF than was studied in previous trials, including subjects with NYHA class III–IV and severely reduced LVEF <25%.[144] After a mean follow-up of 10.4 months, carvedilol was associated with a 34% relative risk reduction in annual mortality rates, as well as reductions in rehospitalizations, hospital length of stay, and cardiogenic shock when compared to placebo. In addition, subjects in the carvedilol group felt better and were less likely to develop any serious adverse event. The CAPRICORN trial tested the effects of carvedilol in patients with acute MI and LV dysfunction with LVEF ≤40% and showed no difference in the prespecified primary composite outcome of mortality and CV hospitalization when compared to placebo.[145] However, all-cause mortality was reduced by 23% in the carvedilol group, a magnitude nearly identical to the results of the BHAT trial, which tested propranolol in patients with acute MI and was published two decades before.[146] Importantly, almost all subjects in CAPRICORN were taking an ACE inhibitor, while approximately one-half had received thrombolysis and/or primary angioplasty.

Differences in β-blockers clinically used in HFrEF are associated to β$_1$-receptor selectivity, presence of α$_1$-receptor antagonism, antioxidant properties, and vasodilating effects.[136] Both metoprolol and bisoprolol are second-generation agents that block β_1-receptors to a much greater extent than β_2-receptors, without antioxidant properties or vasodilating effects. Metoprolol is 75-fold selective, whereas bisoprolol has approximately 120-fold higher affinity for human β_1-versus β_2-receptors. This is important because their effects are mainly restricted to areas containing β_1 receptors, especially the heart and part of the kidney. Also, side effects linked to β_2-blockade, such as bronchospasm, peripheral vasoconstriction, and abnormalities of glucose and lipid metabolism, are less common with β_1-selective agents, although receptor selectivity weakens at higher doses. Conversely, carvedilol is a third-generation nonselective β-blocker that competitively blocks β_1-, β_2-, and α-receptors with some antioxidant properties. Approximately 80% of adrenergic receptors in the normal myocardium are β_1-receptors. However, due to β_1 downregulation in HF, β_2 may rise up to 40% of the total adrenergic receptors.[135,147] Interestingly, β_2 also mediates the effects of catecholamines in the heart, and as a result, it becomes a relatively important mediator of inotropic support and arrhythmogenic effects of sympathetic stimulation in patients with HF.[148] The human heart also expresses α_1-receptors, although at much lower levels than β-receptors. The importance of cardiac α_1-receptors in the pathophysiology of HF is still controversial, but their role in the vasoconstriction of major arteries, such as the aorta, pulmonary arteries, mesenteric vessels, and coronary arteries, is well known. Consequently, carvedilol blockade of α_1-receptors causes vasodilation of blood vessels and might help to improve afterload while posing a higher risk for hypotension.

The hypothesis that multiple adrenergic blockade is more effective than selective β_1-adrenergic blockade was tested in the COMET trial, which remains the largest and most well-designed head-to-head trial of β-blockers in HF.[149] The COMET trial randomized subjects with NYHA class II–IV HF and LVEF $\leq$35% to carvedilol or short-acting metoprolol tartrate in addition to other standard therapies and showed that carvedilol was more effective in reducing all-cause mortality. The generalizability of these findings is limited given that the degree of β-blockade may not have been equivalent in the two arms of COMET. The mean dose of metoprolol achieved in COMET was lower than the ones given in the MDC and MERIT-HF trials, which resulted in significantly lesser HR reductions when compared to carvedilol. Another potential concern is that metoprolol tartrate differs from the extended-release metoprolol succinate (CR/XL) used in MERIT-HF, the main trial showing a survival benefit of metoprolol compared with placebo in HFrEF patients. Metoprolol tartrate produces a less sustained β_1-blockade because of its shorter half-life and has not been shown to reduce mortality in the MDC trial. There have been no trials directly comparing outcomes on carvedilol and extended-release metoprolol succinate (CR/XL).

The COMET trial supports the hypothesis that meaningful differences exist in the clinical effects of different β-blockers, suggesting that their beneficial effects in HFrEF may not necessarily be a class effect. For instance, some β-blockers with intrinsic sympathomimetic activity, such as xamoterol, have been shown to increase, rather than reduce, mortality in patients with HFrEF.[150] Other β-blockers, such as bucindolol and nebivolol, had a neutral effect on overall mortality rates in the BEST and SENIORS trials. Bucindolol is a third-generation nonselective β-blocker, with additional weak α-blocking properties and some intrinsic sympathomimetic activity. Although it failed to reduce total mortality in the BEST trial, a prespecified subanalysis suggested a survival benefit restricted to white participants that might be secondary to a polymorphism in β₁-receptors in that population.[151] Nebivolol is a selective β_1-receptor antagonist with some vasodilatory effects that are partially mediated by NO production via activation of β_3-adrenergic receptors. It is approximately 3.5 times more β_1-selective than bisoprolol and, along with carvedilol, is one of the few β-blockers to cause vasodilation. The SENIORS trial tested the effects of nebivolol on mortality and morbidity in patients ≥70 years old with stable HF.[152] At a mean follow-up of 21 months, nebivolol therapy resulted in a significant 14% relative risk reduction in the primary composite outcome of all-cause mortality or CV hospitalizations compared to placebo but did not reduce all-cause mortality. In the United States, nebivolol is only approved for the treatment of hypertension, while in Europe it is registered for use in hypertension and HF as well.

Overall, the results of the COMET, BEST, and SENIORS trials highlight the importance of using doses and formulations of β-blockers with proven benefit in clinical trials. In accordance with clinical practice guidelines recommendations, β-blockers should be up-titrated to reach maximally tolerated doses whenever possible. Evidence-based doses for recommended β-blockers are listed in Table 3.5. However, the abrupt withdrawal of adrenergic support may lead to exacerbation of congestive HF and significant negative chronotropy. Thus, therapy with β-blockers is recommended for clinically stable patients and should be initiated at very low doses and up-titrated gradually, with dose doubling no earlier than every 2 weeks as tolerated. Nevertheless, patients may experience some fluid retention within the first 3–5 days of treatment and should be advised to weigh themselves on a daily basis. Fluid retention can be managed by increasing the diuretic dose until weight returns to baseline and should not prevent future up-titration of the β-blocker.

Table 3.5

Drugs for the prevention and treatment of chronic heart failure with reduced ejection fraction		
Drug	**Starting dose**	**Target dose**
β-Blockers		
Bisoprolol	1.25 mg once	10 mg once
Carvedilol	3.125 mg twice	25 mg twice[a]
Metoprolol succinate	12.5–25 mg once	200 mg once
Angiotensin-converting enzyme inhibitors		
Captopril	6.25 mg 3 times	50 mg 3 times
Enalapril	2.5 mg twice	10–20 mg twice
Lisinopril	2.5–5.0 mg once	20–35 mg once
Ramipril	1.25–2.5 mg once	10 mg once
Trandolapril	0.5 mg once	4 mg once
Angiotensin receptor blocker		
Candesartan	4–8 mg once	32 mg once
Losartan	25 mg once	150 mg once
Valsartan	40 mg twice	160 mg twice
Angiotensin receptor neprilysin inhibitor		
Sacubitril–valsartan	24 mg/26 mg twice	97 mg/103 mg twice
Mineralocorticoid receptor antagonist		
Eplerenone	25 mg once	50–100 mg once
Spironolactone	12.5 mg once	50–100 mg once
Sodium-glucose cotransporter-2 inhibitors[b]		
Canagliflozin	100 mg once	300 mg once
Dapagliflozin[c]	5 mg once	10 mg once
Empagliflozin	10 mg once	25 mg once
Additional therapy		
Ivabradine	5 mg twice daily	7.5 mg twice
Fixed H-ISDN[d]	37.5 mg/20 mg 3 times	75 mg/40 mg 3 times
Digoxin	0.125 mg once	Higher doses (0.375–0.5 mg) are rarely recommended

[a]A maximum dose of 50 mg twice daily can be administered to patients weighing over 85 kg.
[b]No current guideline recommendation.
[c]Dapagliflozin is the only FDA-approved SGLT-2 inhibitor for patients with HFrEF with and without T2DM.
[d]Fixed combination of hydralazine plus isosorbide dinitrate (BiDil).
Modified from Ponikowski P, Voors AA, Anker SD, et al. 2016 ESC guidelines for the diagnosis and treatment of acute and chronic heart failure: The task force for the diagnosis and treatment of acute and chronic heart failure of the European Society of Cardiology (ESC). Developed with the special contribution of the Heart Failure Association (HFA) of the ESC. *Eur Heart J* 2016;18(8):891–975.

Other commonly mentioned noncardiac side effects of β-blockers include exacerbation of reactive airway disease, increased peripheral vascular resistance, depression, fatigue, insomnia, and sexual dysfunction. Hence, despite extensive evidence of clinical efficacy, several HF registries have shown that the use and dose of β-blockers is often suboptimal, possibly due to side effects or intolerance.[136,153] Reasons for β-blocker discontinuation have differed across registries, but generally include worsening of HF symptoms, bradycardia, hypotension, dizziness, and fatigue.

β-Blocker selection may affect tolerability, as patients with reactive airway disease may benefit from β_1-selective blockers, while those with peripheral vascular disease may benefit from carvedilol, given its vasodilatory effects. The CIBIS-ELD trial was designed to compare the tolerability of bisoprolol and carvedilol during attempted titration to guideline-recommended target doses after 12 weeks of treatment in elderly subjects with chronic HF.[154] It showed that adverse bradycardia was more common with bisoprolol, whereas pulmonary events were more common with carvedilol. Lipophilic β-blockers, such as metoprolol, can cause sleep disturbances, insomnia, vivid dreams, and nightmares, due to the high penetration across the blood–brain barrier. Furthermore, intolerance may not be a class effect, as 80% of subjects considered intolerant to one β-blocker might be successfully changed to another. Actually, contrary to early reports, β-blocker therapy is well tolerated by 90% of HF patients, including those with diabetes mellitus, chronic obstructive lung disease, and peripheral vascular disease.[136,155]

Severe bradycardia and asthma with active bronchospasm remain the most important contraindications to β-blockade. The dose of β-blocker should be adjusted if HR decreases to <50 beats/min or in the setting of second- or third-degree heart block. Symptomatic hypotension can be managed by decreasing the diuretic dose. Finally, continuation, but not introduction, of β-blocker treatment during an episode of ADHF is safe, although dose reduction may be necessary.[156]

Angiotensin-Converting Enzyme Inhibitors

The RAAS plays a critical role in the pathophysiology of HF, with effects on cardiac remodeling, vascular tone, endothelial function, sodium retention, oxidative stress, fibrosis, sympathetic tone, and inflammation. The likely mechanisms for RAAS activation include renal hypoperfusion, reduced filtered sodium, and increased SNS stimulation of the kidney, leading to increased renin release from juxtaglomerular apparatus.[128,132]

ACE inhibitors have many short- and long-term biological effects that are beneficial in patients with chronic HFrEF, and the evidence supporting their efficacy has been consistently demonstrated in large randomized clinical trials. These agents prevent the conversion of angiotensin I to angiotensin II, which is formed by the proteolytic action of renin on circulating angiotensinogen. Angiotensin II is a peptide hormone that causes vasoconstriction, modulates SNS activation, and mediates aldosterone and vasopressin secretion, both associated with abnormal fluid retention and volume regulation in HF.[127,157] It also promotes a prothrombotic state and abnormal cellular growth. Through RAAS modulation, ACE inhibitors have a consistent effect in increasing plasma renin while decreasing angiotensin II, aldosterone, NE, epinephrine, and vasopressin. Therefore, they reduce SNS activity and improve arterial tone, endothelial function and ventricular compliance, contributing to a decrease in ventricular afterload and cardiac remodeling. In addition, because ACE is identical to kininase II, ACE inhibitors may also lead to the upregulation of bradykinin, an inflammatory mediator with vasodilator properties. These actions may potentially enhance the effects of angiotensin II suppression and further contribute to the vasodilatory effects of ACE inhibitors.

In the era before ACE inhibitors, the V-HeFT trial demonstrated that a combined vasodilator therapy with hydralazine and isosorbide dinitrate (H-ISDN) conferred a nonsignificant survival benefit in subjects with HFrEF.[158] Subsequently, several prospective, randomized pivotal trials have demonstrated a significant survival benefit with ACE inhibitors in that population. The CONSENSUS trial randomized subjects with NYHA class IV HFrEF to enalapril or placebo in addition to standard medical therapy, which until the late 1980s focused primarily on symptom control through use of digitalis, diuretics, and nitrates. The intervention group had a significant 40% relative risk reduction in 6-month mortality.[130] Enalapril was also associated with significant reductions in NYHA class and is the requirement for further HF therapies.

The SOLVD trial randomized subjects with NYHA class II–IV HFrEF to enalapril or placebo and showed a 16% relative risk reduction in the 4-year mortality in the enalapril group, predominantly due to a reduction in the risk of HF mortality.[159] There was also a reduction in the risk of CV hospitalizations and in the end-diastolic LV volume index, which began a recurring observation that some disease-modifying therapies in HFrEF also cause reverse remodeling.[137,160] Published at the same time as the SOLVD trial, the V-HeFT II showed that enalapril was superior to H-ISDN in patients with NYHA class II–III HFrEF, providing evidence that

ACE inhibition improves HF outcomes through additional mechanisms than just vasodilation.[161]

Enalapril is the only ACE inhibitor that has been used in placebo-controlled mortality trials in HFrEF. However, similar favorable effects were found when captopril, ramipril, and trandolapril were started at least 3 days following MI in the SAVE, AIRE, and TRACE trials, respectively.[125,162,163] Additionally, the GISSI-3 trial also showed a mortality benefit with lisinopril after MI regardless of subsequent LV function.[164] Taken together, these observations suggest a class effect of ACE inhibitors in the treatment of HFrEF. Thus, ACE inhibitors are strongly recommended to all patients with HFrEF, unless contraindicated or not tolerated. Evidence-based doses for ACE inhibitor are listed in Table 3.5.

Most side effects of ACE inhibitors are primarily related to interfering with the conversion of angiotensin I to angiotensin II and degradation of bradykinin. Clinical evaluation prior to ACE inhibitor initiation includes assessment of BP, renal function, and electrolytes.[165] It should be emphasized that patients with hypotension or impaired renal function were excluded from most of the clinical trials, and the efficacy of ACE inhibitors for such patients is less well established. Hypotension, early decrease in renal function, and hyperkalemia are dose-dependent side effects that may be avoided by slow dose titration. Symptomatic hypotension and modest reduction in GFR may be initially managed by reducing the dose of diuretics in the absence of significant fluid retention. However, GFR at reduced renal perfusion pressure ultimately depends upon the postglomerular efferent arteriolar vasoconstrictor effects of angiotensin II. Hence, in subjects with renal-artery stenosis or reduced intravascular volume, RAAS blockade might be capable of reducing filtration pressure at critical levels of kidney perfusion, worsening renal function. Progressive loss of GFR can sometimes recover by withholding ACE inhibitors. An ACE inhibitor therapy should be avoided in nondialysis patients with serum creatinine >3.5 mg/dL or estimated GFR <20 mL/min/1.73 m^2, while dialysis patients can be treated with ACE inhibitors. Hyperkalemia can be prevented by prescription of a low-potassium diet, loop diuretics, and prior discontinuation or dose reduction of other medications that raise serum potassium, such as potassium supplements or a potassium-sparing diuretics.[165] A serum potassium level of up to 5.5 mmol/L is acceptable as long as it is stable. In patients with uncontrollable hyperkalemia and an increase of more than 20% to 30% in creatinine level within a week, the ACE inhibitor should be discontinued or down-titrated. Frequent monitoring is advised, although ACE inhibitors may rarely cause severe hyperkalemia that requires emergency management.

Other side effects, as dry cough and angioneurotic edema, are related to the accumulation of bradykinin. Bradykinin is not only a vasodilator, but it also increases prostaglandin concentrations and vascular permeability with fluid extravasation. This clinical distinction is important as side effects related to reduced angiotensin II, but not those related to increased kinins, are also seen with the ARBs. Persistent dry cough, a recognized side effect that occurs in 5% to 20% of subjects on ACE inhibitors, may be dose-related and is not a true allergic effect. When the ACE inhibitor is discontinued, improvement often begins within 4–7 days. Angioneurotic edema is rare (<1%) and resolves without complications in most cases. However, because endotracheal intubation or emergent tracheostomy may be necessary and fatalities have been reported, an ACE inhibitor should not be prescribed for patients with idiopathic or prior angioneurotic edema. The incidence of ACE inhibitor–induced angioneurotic edema is up to five times greater in individuals of African descent. Actually, there is conflicting evidence on the efficacy of ACE inhibitors in people of African descent, which may be genetically explained by a low-renin system.[166] However, given the available evidence, ACE inhibitor therapy recommendations are the same for all HFrEF patients, regardless of race. Allergic reactions include skin rash, neutropenia, dysgeusia, or anaphylactoid reactions. Both ACE inhibitors and ARBs can cause fetal abnormalities and are absolutely contraindicated in pregnancy in the second and third trimesters.

Angiotensin-converting Enzyme Inhibitors or β-Blockers First

Although the combination of an ACE inhibitor and a β-blocker is more effective in HFrEF than monotherapy with either, the order of initiation is important in clinical practice because patients often cannot tolerate optimum doses of both agents. There are theoretical considerations suggesting it may be more beneficial to initiate the treatment with a β-blocker, as the SNS is systemically activated at an earlier stage than is the RAAS. The CIBIS-III trial addressed this important question and showed that initiating treatment with the selective β_1-receptor blocker bisoprolol is as effective and well tolerated as beginning treatment with the ACE inhibitor enalapril.[167]

In clinical practice, drug initiation and up-titration could be tailored to individual patients and their unique clinical circumstances. The initial treatment strategy with β-blockers first may be better for subjects with ischemic cardiomyopathies and tachycardia, while the strategy of using an ACE inhibitor first should be indicated for patients with hypertension and fluid overload. Current clinical practice guidelines recommend starting with an ACE inhibitor, followed by the addition of a β-blocker. In most cases, β-blockers are then up-titrated to their maximum recommended dose before further increase in the dose of ACE inhibitors.

Angiotensin Receptor Blockers

Long-term treatment with ACE inhibitors leads to a gradual return of circulating angiotensin II concentrations through non-ACE-dependent pathways.[168,169] Any angiotensin II that is produced through such alternative pathways remains available for binding with two types of angiotensin receptors, AT-1 and AT-2. The AT-1 receptors are abundant in the vessels, brain, heart, kidney, adrenal, and nerves, while AT-2 are only available in small amounts in the adult kidney, adrenal, heart, brain, uterus, and ovary. Rather than preventing the conversion of angiotensin I to angiotensin II, the ARBs selectively block the binding of angiotensin II to the AT-1 receptors. Activation of AT-1 leads to increased vasoconstriction, aldosterone and catecholamine release, sodium resorption in the proximal tubules of the kidney, and cell growth in the arteries and heart. Thus, antagonizing AT-1 causes a reduction in both cardiac afterload and preload. Also, ARBs may be better tolerated, since they do not interfere with the degradation of bradykinin and do not appear to induce cough and possibly other side effects that force some patients to discontinue treatment with ACE inhibitors.

Given their different mechanisms, earlier rationale postulated that ARB therapy would provide an advantage over ACE inhibitor therapy. However, despite the theoretical benefits, clinical evidence of ARB effectiveness in HFrEF patients is less robust than that of ACE inhibitors.[168] In the Val-HeFT trial, the addition of valsartan to standard HFrEF therapy that included ACE inhibitors did not improve survival but reduced the incidence of the composite outcome of morbidity and mortality, largely through a decrease in HF hospitalizations.[170] Moreover, a retrospective subanalysis of the Val-HeFT suggested that valsartan might also reduce all-cause mortality in the small subgroup of subjects not receiving an ACE inhibitor. The CHARM program consisted of three independent, parallel, placebo-controlled trials evaluating candesartan in different symptomatic HF populations with the same primary composite outcome of CV death or HF hospitalization.[171] HFrEF subjects who received candesartan had significant better outcomes than those who received placebo in both the CHARM-Alternative and CHARM-Added component trials. Specifically, the CHARM-Alternative trial showed that candesartan was well tolerated in symptomatic HFrEF patients who had previously failed an ACE inhibitor, resulting in a 20% relative risk reduction in CV mortality and fewer HF hospitalization.[172] While similar findings were shown in the CHARM-Added trial, the combination of candesartan with an ACE inhibitor and a β-blocker resulted in higher rates of adverse outcomes including increased creatinine and hyperkalemia.[173] Additionally, a later Cochrane meta-analysis showed that the combination of ARBs and ACE inhibitors increased the risk of withdrawals due to side effects, especially renal dysfunction and hyperkalemia, and did not reduce total mortality or hospitalizations when compared to ACE inhibitors alone.[168] It is noteworthy that only 17% of subjects in the CHARM-Added trial were on an MRA, which might be the preferred next agent to add on to the combination of an ACE inhibitor and a β-blocker in patients with HFrEF. Combined use of MRA, ACE inhibitor, and ARB should be avoided because of concerns about hyperkalemia and lack of evidence of efficacy.

Regarding dosing of ARBs, the HEAAL trial showed that high-dose losartan was associated with a significant reduction in HF admissions when compared to low-dose losartan.[174] Thus, they should be started at low doses and up-titrated to the maximum recommended and tolerated dose. Evidence-based doses for ARBs are listed in Table 3.5. Long-term therapy with ARBs in patients with HFrEF produces hemodynamic, neurohormonal, and clinical effects consistent with those expected after interference with the RAAS. However, controversial results from different meta-analysis cannot confirm their superiority over placebo, particularly when compared to ACE inhibitors.[168,175,176] A direct comparison of ACE inhibitors and ARBs was assessed in the ELITE-II trial, which did not observe any mortality benefit of losartan over captopril in elderly subjects with HFrEF.[177] Furthermore, the VALIANT trial showed that valsartan was noninferior to captopril on all-cause mortality in subjects with post-MI LV dysfunction.[178] Although both classes might have similar effects, the general consensus is that an ARB should only be recommended as an alternative for patients with prior or current symptoms of chronic HFrEF who are intolerant to ACE inhibitors due to cough, skin rash, or angioneurotic edema. It should be stated, however, that other side effects such as hypotension, renal dysfunction, and hyperkalemia appear to be similar for ACE inhibitors and ARBs. Additionally, angioedema has also been reported in some patients taking ARBs, although much less frequently than with ACE inhibitors.

ARBs are also reasonable choices as first-line drugs for HFrEF patients who are already on ARB therapy for other indications, like hypertension, and those who are unable to tolerate an MRA for other reasons than renal dysfunction and hyperkalemia. Both ACE inhibitors and ARBs can cause fetal abnormalities and are absolutely contraindicated in pregnancy in the second and third trimesters.

Angiotensin Receptor Neprilysin Inhibitors

In the context of normal cardiac physiology, both the RAAS and SNS are balanced by the NP system to maintain BP and fluid homeostasis. The NP system consists of structurally similar peptides, such as the atrial, B-type, and C-type NPs, that act through receptor-based generation of cGMP, enhancing diuresis, natriuresis, and vasodilation while countering SNS and RAAS overstimulation.[131] As HFrEF progresses, the effects of the NP system become attenuated by several mechanisms, including reduced availability of active forms of NPs, diminished organ responsiveness, and over-activation of counter-regulatory neurohormones. Therefore, pharmacological approaches to enhance the functional effectiveness of the NP system in chronic HFrEF have been proposed.[179]

Initial efforts focused on the IV administration of synthetic forms of NPs, such as nesiritide and ularitide, in the setting of ADHF, but did not improve clinical outcomes.[62,67] Similar disappointing findings were seen with the lone inhibition of neprilysin (NEP), a neutral endopeptidase responsible for the breakdown of several vasodilator peptides, such as NPs, bradykinin, and adrenomedullin, as well as vasoconstrictors peptides, as angiotensin and endothelin-1.[179,180] By blocking regulators of opposite actions of vasodilation and vasoconstriction, lone NEP inhibition essentially neutralize each effect and further increase RAAS activation stimulated by upregulation of angiotensin II. Later studies tested omapatrilat, a compound that inhibited both ACE and NEP, to further inhibit angiotensin II in addition to NEP. The OVERTURE trial found that the use of omapatrilat in HFrEF patients was not superior to enalapril alone in reducing mortality and hospitalization but was associated with a higher incidence of angioedema (2.17% versus 0.68%).[181] The increased incidence of this life-threatening complication was attributed to the synergism between the ACE and NEP inhibition on the breakdown of bradykinin. In addition, omapatrilat also inhibits a third enzyme involved in the degradation of bradykinin, the aminopeptidase P. Further clinical research on the entire class of ACE-NEP inhibitors were halted.

The strategy that ultimately proved successful in improving HFrEF outcomes was the molecular combination of sacubitril, a NEP inhibitor, with valsartan, an ARB, resulting in the first-in-class ARNI sacubitril–valsartan. The PARADIGM-HF trial showed a highly significant 20% relative risk reduction in the primary composite outcome of CV death or HF hospitalization of sacubitril–valsartan over enalapril in subjects with NYHA class II–IV HFrEF.[182] Sacubitril–valsartan also reduced secondary outcomes of CV death by 20%, first hospitalization for worsening HF by 21%, all-cause mortality by 16%, and prevented deterioration of symptoms and quality of life.

Since all participants of the PARADIGM-HF were required to first tolerate a run-in phase of enalapril, most HFrEF guideline-issuing societies suggested that sacubitril–valsartan should be initiated only in subjects tolerating full-dose ACE inhibitor or ARB. However, given the positive results of the subsequent PIONEER-HF trial, it is now considered a reasonable strategy to initiate sacubitril–valsartan as a first-line component of the long-term RAAS blockade in hemodynamically stable patients with ADHF.[71] To facilitate initiation and titration, the approved ARNI is available in three doses, including a lower one that was not tested in the PARADIGM-HF trial (Table 3.5).

In the PARADIGM-HF trial, symptomatic hypotension was more common in patients receiving sacubitril–valsartan, although there was no increase in the rate of discontinuation. Measures to avoid hypotension include adjusting the dose of diuretics or other concomitant antihypertensive drugs, correcting volume depletion prior to starting sacubitril–valsartan, and starting at a lower dose. Hyperkalemia and renal dysfunction were reported as adverse events in both treatment groups in PARADIGM-HF, although clinically important increases in serum creatinine were less frequent in the sacubitril–valsartan than in the enalapril group. In addition, among MRA-treated patients, severe hyperkalemia was also more likely with enalapril.[183] Nonetheless, the same precautions for renal impairment and hyperkalemia should be applied to all subjects receiving RAAS inhibitors, including careful screening of baseline renal function and serum potassium concentration, followed by close periodic monitoring. Recruiting only subjects who tolerated both enalapril and sacubitril–valsartan during the active run-in phase reduced the risk of angioneurotic edema in the PARADIGM-HF. However, because of the previous experience with Omapatrilat, a 36-hour washout period when switching from an ACE inhibitor to sacubitril–valsartan is advised. Combined treatment with sacubitril–valsartan and an ACE inhibitor, or a lone ARB, is contraindicated. If none of these three agents is tolerated, the combination of H-ISDN is a potential alternative therapy for patients with HFrEF. Sacubitril–valsartan is also contraindicated during pregnancy due to concerns about risk of teratogenicity with ARBs.

There are also additional concerns about the effects of NEP inhibition on the degradation of β-amyloid peptide in the brain, which could theoretically accelerate amyloid deposition, leading to impaired cognitive function. A subanalysis found no increase in dementia-related adverse events in PARADIGM-HF, but long-term follow-up may be necessary to detect such a signal.[184]

Mineralocorticoid-Receptor Antagonists

Aldosterone is a mineralocorticoid hormone produced primarily by the adrenal cortex but also by endothelial and vascular smooth muscle cells in the blood vessels and myocardium in response to angiotensin II, hyperkalemia, and corticotropin.[185] In addition to its classic mineralocorticoid properties, which can lead to hypokalemia and hypomagnesemia, aldosterone has other adverse effects that can contribute to the pathophysiology of HF, such as inflammation, vascular stiffening, collagen formation, and myocardial necrosis.[186] Therefore, chronically elevated aldosterone is associated with coronary and renovascular remodeling, endothelial and baroreceptor dysfunction, myocardial hypertrophy, and reduced HR variability.

Since angiotensin II prevents renin release by negative feedback, a large increase in plasma renin activity occurs with the administration of ACE inhibitors and ARBs. Moreover, plasma aldosterone returns to pretreatment levels after several weeks of therapy in up to 30% to 40% of patients, either through non-ACE-dependent pathways, or high serum potassium concentrations.[157,169] MRAs, often referred to as aldosterone antagonists, block receptors that bind aldosterone and, with different degrees of affinity, other steroid hormone receptors such as corticosteroids and androgens. It has been shown that MRAs provide a more complete inhibition of the RAAS when added to standard HFrEF therapy, preventing many of the maladaptive effects of aldosterone.[185-187] Most of their benefits are mediated by antifibrotic mechanisms, which slows or reverse cardiac remodeling and reduce arrhythmogenesis. In addition, MRAs also preserve serum potassium levels, countering the risk of hypokalemia and further associated arrhythmic risk induced by other diuretics, such as loop diuretics.

The combination of an MRA with standard HFrEF regimen improves survival and reduces morbidity in patients with symptomatic chronic HFrEF, as well as those with LV systolic dysfunction after MI. Such major clinical benefits have been demonstrated in a few well-conducted randomized clinical trials. The first evidence was demonstrated by the RALES trial, which tested spironolactone versus placebo in subjects with NYHA class III–IV HFrEF receiving a background of loop diuretics, ACE inhibitors, and, in most cases, digoxin.[188] RALES demonstrated a 30% relative risk reduction in all-cause mortality with spironolactone, without a significant increase in the risk of serious hyperkalemia or renal failure as hypothesized. HF hospitalization was also 35% lower in the MRA group.

However, although generally well tolerated in RALES, spironolactone was associated with dose-dependent reports of gynecomastia or breast tenderness in 10% of men, compared with 1% in the placebo group. Gynecomastia is clinically defined as benign enlargement of the glandular tissue of male breast due to periductal fibrosis, stromal hyalinization, and increased subareolar fat, while breast pain is caused by inflammatory infiltration of the periductal tissue.[189] Its pathophysiological process usually involves an imbalance between free estrogen and free androgen actions in the breast tissue. Spironolactone induces gynecomastia by decreasing testosterone production in the testicles, increasing its peripheral conversion to estradiol and displacing more estrogen from sex hormone-binding globulin, increasing the bioavailability of estrogen to a greater extent than androgen.[187,189] Other distressing endocrine side effects of spironolactone include menstrual irregularities in premenopausal females and impotence and decreased libido in men.

Shortly after publication of the RALES trial, the MRA eplerenone became available for clinical evaluation. It was postulated that due to its greater specificity for the mineralocorticoid receptor, eplerenone would have fewer antiandrogenic effects than spironolactone, as a greater fraction of free testosterone could tightly bind to sex hormone-binding globulin. This prompted the subsequent EPHESUS trial, which investigated eplerenone in the treatment of LV systolic dysfunction and clinical evidence of HF or diabetes after an MI, as well as the EMPHASIS-HF trial, investigating eplerenone in the treatment of NYHA class II HFrEF.[190,191] Both were positive trials, reinforcing the benefits of MRAs in improving survival and hospitalizations in patients with HFrEF, but with fewer endocrine side effects in comparison to spironolactone. Importantly, both trials were performed in the era of widespread β-blocker use, in contrast to RALES in which only 10% subjects were on β-blocker therapy. In EPHESUS, particularly, eplerenone was beneficial on top of all of the existing therapies for MI at that time, including aspirin, reperfusion, and statin. Prior to EMPHASIS-HF, no clinical trial had evaluated the benefits of aldosterone blockade in HFrEF subjects with mild symptoms, as RALES and EPHESUS randomized a population with higher NYHA classes. Therefore, an MRA is recommended for all patients with HFrEF who remain symptomatic despite treatment with an ACE inhibitor (or ARB or ARNI) and a β-blocker, to reduce the risk of HF hospitalization and death, unless contraindicated. Evidence-based doses for spironolactone and eplerenone are listed in Table 3.5.

The major side effect of MRAs is the development of life-threatening hyperkalemia. Caution should be taken in patients with serum potassium concentrations >5.0 mmol/L or serum creatinine >2.5 mg/dL. In RALES, EPHESUS, and EMPHASIS-HF, hyperkalemia was more common in the active treatment groups, although serum potassium concentration ≥6 mmol/L was rare. The risks of severe hyperkalemia can be mitigated through appropriate patient selection and education, dose adjustments, careful monitoring of serum potassium levels and renal function, and closer follow-up. The development of worsening renal function should prompt therapy discontinuation.

Although eplerenone is associated with fewer endocrine adverse effects, spironolactone is the most widely prescribed MRA, presumably because of its lower cost. Generally, discontinuation of spironolactone results in resolution of such effects. Thus, it may be reasonable to start MRA therapy with spironolactone, and eventually switch to eplerenone case endocrine side effects occurs. Novel, nonsteroidal MRAs, such as the finerenone, combine the potency of spironolactone with the selectivity of eplerenone, resulting in less hyperkalemia and greater decrease in BNP and NT-proBNP levels.[187] Exploratory analysis of the phase 2 ARTS-HF trial suggested a more favorable effect of finerenone on CV mortality and HF hospitalizations when compared to eplerenone.[192] The relative effectiveness of finerenone over eplerenone remains to be determined in a large outcomes trial.

Sodium-Glucose Cotransporter-2 Inhibitors

The SGLT-2 inhibitors, also called "gliflozins," are a class of medications that reduce glucose reabsorption by inhibiting the high-capacity sodium-glucose cotransporter-2 in the proximal tubule of the nephron. This leads to an increased concentration of chloride in the distal tubule and a resetting of the tubulo-glomerular feedback mechanism, which results in a contraction of the plasma volume without activation of the SNS. Empagliflozin, canagliflozin, and dapagliflozin have been shown to reduce the risk of HF hospitalization in three large clinical trials in T2DM patients at high cardiovascular risk: the EMPA-REG Outcomes, the CANVAS Program, and the DECLARE-TIMI 58 trial.[118-120] The DAPA-HF trial was the first outcomes trial with an SGLT-2 inhibitor investigating the treatment of

HFREF irrespective of T2DM status.[193] The DAPA-HF trial randomized subjects with NYHA class II–IV HFrEF to dapagliflozin 10 mg or placebo, in addition to standard care, and showed a statistically significant 26% reduction in the risk of the primary composite outcome of worsening HF or CV death. When analyzed separately, worsening HF was reduced by 30% and the risk of CV death was reduced by 18%. Notably, the treatment effect was consistent across all prespecified subgroups, including patients without baseline T2DM and regardless of hemoglobulin A1c levels. In addition, dapagliflozin reduced the risk for all-cause death by 17% and showed a significant improvement in patient-reported HF symptoms. Adverse events related to volume depletion, renal adverse events, major hypoglycemia, lower limb amputation, and fracture were comparable to placebo, with low rates of discontinuation in both groups (<5%). The potential mechanisms of benefit from gliflozins in HFrEF are likely multifactorial, involving not only glycosuria or osmotic diuresis but also cardio-renal protection through metabolic and hemodynamic effects.

Additional Therapy

Diuretics

Diuretics are the cornerstone of therapy for the treatment of volume overload in patients with HF, relieving clinical symptoms and signs more rapidly than any other drug.[194] They can reduce CVP, pulmonary congestion, peripheral edema, and body weight within hours or days of initiation of therapy, whereas the clinical effects of digoxin, ACE inhibitors, or β-blockers may require weeks or months to become apparent. Additionally, in the intermediate term, diuretics have also been shown to improve cardiac function and exercise tolerance in HF patients.[33] However, the effects of diuretic therapy with long-term follow-up in chronic HFrEF have not been studied in large prospective randomized controlled trials. A Cochrane meta-analysis suggested that in patients with chronic HF, conventional diuretic therapy might reduce the risk of death and worsening of HF compared to placebo and appear to improve exercise capacity compared to active control.[194] However, this meta-analysis included only small-size studies with limited follow-up and cannot be used as formal evidence to recommend the use of diuretics to reduce HF mortality.

Patients at higher risk for fluid overload would benefit from long-term therapy with oral loop diuretics. However, the use of loop diuretics might associate with electrolyte disturbances, arrhythmias, neurohormonal activation, accelerated renal function decline, and hypotension.[33] The latter might be particularly relevant, as it could limit optimal target doses of neurohormonal antagonists. Therefore, it is advised to use the lowest possible dose of loop diuretic, which should be adjusted individually. As previously stated, diuretics do not have a smooth dose-response curve, and natriuresis will only occur when the threshold rate of drug excretion, which is often higher in HF patients, is attained.[30] Hence, if there is little or no response to the initial dose, it is recommended to double it rather than giving the same dose twice a day. Additionally, for patients presenting with an ADHF episode while previously taking a loop diuretic, a higher dose at discharge should be considered.

Thiazide diuretics are widely used for the management of hypertension. Despite structural variation among the heterogeneous group of agents with similar physiological properties, including the thiazide-like diuretics, the term "thiazide diuretic" comprises all diuretics believed to have a primary action in the distal convoluted tubule. Metolazone, a quinazoline sulfonamide, is a thiazide-like diuretic that can be used in combination with furosemide in patients with diuretic resistance. The chronic use of sequential nephron blockade with thiazide diuretics should be avoided in stable patients, as it often induces electrolyte disorders that could go unseen in the ambulatory setting.[30,32]

Since sodium retention occurs in more proximal tubular sites, potassium-sparing diuretics are ineffective in achieving a net negative sodium balance when given alone in HF patients. Besides, the benefit of MRAs in patients with HF is thought to be relatively independent of their diuretic properties and may be due to their ability to antagonize the RAAS.

Vasopressin receptor antagonists modulate the renal actions of AVP by directly blocking its receptors V1A, V1B, and V2.[195] The inappropriate elevation of AVP in HF plays a key role in mediating vasoconstriction, water retention, and electrolyte imbalance. Combined V1A and V2 antagonism causes a decrease in SVR and prevents dilutional hyponatremia. The AVP antagonists, or "vaptans," can either selectively block the V2-receptor or nonselectively block both the V1A- and the V2-receptors. The EVEREST-Outcomes trial randomized subjects admitted with ADHF to the selective V2-receptor antagonist tolvaptan or placebo and showed no difference in long-term mortality or HF-related morbidity at a median follow-up of 9.9 months.[195] Currently, conivaptan and tolvaptan are FDA-approved for the treatment of clinically significant hypervolemic and euvolemic hyponatremia, but they are not officially approved for HF. Although it is reasonable to use these agents after traditional measures to hyponatremia have failed, including fluid restriction and optimal target doses of angiotensin inhibitors, their widespread use might be limited by high costs.

Patients receiving diuretics should be monitored regularly for complications, including electrolyte and metabolic disturbances, volume depletion, and worsening renal function. Even when successful in controlling symptoms and fluid retention, diuretics alone are unable to maintain the clinical stability of patients with chronic HF for long periods of time. Therefore, they should be combined with standard guideline recommended HFrEF therapies, including neurohormonal antagonists.

Combination of Hydralazine Plus Isosorbide Dinitrate

Until the 1970s, standard medical therapy for HF was limited to digitalis and diuretics. A hemodynamic rationale for the combined use of a venous and arterial vasodilator therapy is to reduce both preload and afterload by improving venous capacitance while decreasing SVR.[196] Early pivotal studies found that the combination of two oral vasodilators, hydralazine and isosorbide dinitrate, in patients with NYHA class III–IV HF results in a better hemodynamic response than either drug individually.[197] Additionally, since nitrates are NO donors and hydralazine has antioxidant properties, it is possible that the NO-mediated effects of H-ISDN might also play a complex role in the maintenance of CV health.

The V-HeFT trial was the first major randomized, placebo-controlled HF study, which compared H-ISDN, prazosin, or placebo in subjects with symptomatic HF and LVEF <45%.[158] At a mean follow-up of 2.3 years, there was no statistically significant difference in mortality between the groups, although H-ISDN was associated with a trend toward improved survival when compared to placebo. H-ISDN also improved LVEF at 8 weeks and 1 year, while prazosin was associated neither with mortality nor LVEF improvement. The subsequent V-HeFT II trial was undertaken to compare H-ISDN with enalapril in a similar population to that of V-HeFT and showed a survival benefit with enalapril at the primary specified time point of 2 years but not during the entire follow-up of the trial.[161] The survival benefit was largely driven by a reduction in sudden cardiac death, but there were no significant differences in rates of hospitalizations between the two groups.

Of interest, post hoc subgroup analysis from both V-HeFT and V-HeFT II trials suggested improved survival benefit with H-ISDN among self-identified black subjects, which was the basis of the A-HeFT trial. Based on the rationale that persons of African descent may have less RAAS activity, rendering ACE inhibitors less effective, the A-HeFT trial randomized self-identified black subjects with NYHA class III–IV HFrEF to either placebo or a fixed combination of H-ISDN.[198] The trial was stopped early at a mean follow-up of 10 months due to a significant 43% relative risk reduction in all-cause mortality associated with the use of H-ISDN added to standard therapy with diuretics, ACE inhibitors, β-blockers, digoxin, and spironolactone. H-ISDN was also associated with a lower rate of first and recurrent HF hospitalizations and a significant improvement in quality-of-life assessments. Importantly, the A-HeFT trial tested a fixed-combination single-pill equivalent to the generic H-ISDN, called BiDil, but it is probable that the same benefits can be achieved with a combination of the separate formulations. BiDil has provoked controversy as the first FDA-approved drug marketed for a single racial-ethnic group—those of African descent—in the treatment of HFrEF.

Guideline-issuing professional societies recommend the combination of H-ISDN for self-identified black patients with NYHA class III–IV HFrEF who remain symptomatic despite concomitant use of ACE inhibitors, β-blockers, and MRAs. The results of the A-HeFT trial are difficult to translate to other racial or ethnic origins, and there is less robust evidence supporting the use of H-ISDN as a contemporary first-line therapy for nonblack HFrEF subjects. Nonetheless, based on the V-HeFT trial, which recruited patients who received only digoxin and diuretics, H-ISDN may be considered in symptomatic HFrEF patients who cannot be given an ACE inhibitor, ARB, or ARNI because of drug intolerance, hypotension, or renal dysfunction. Evidence-based doses for H-ISDN are listed in Table 3.5. Concomitant use of any form of nitrate with PDE-5 inhibitors or sGC stimulators is contraindicated due to the increased risk of refractory hypotension.

If Channel Inhibitor

An elevated HR in patients with HFrEF reflects, in part, an imbalance between sympathetic overstimulation and parasympathetic suppression, which are components of the neurohumoral activation. It has been shown that increased HR not only predicts CV death and HF hospitalization but may also be a therapeutic target in patients with chronic HFrEF.[199] Several classes of pharmacological agents can modulate HR, including β-blockers, ivabradine, digoxin, amiodarone, and nondihydropyridine CCBs, such as diltiazem and verapamil. While some agents are associated with clinical benefits in patients with HFrEF, such as β-blockers and ivabradine, others provide no direct benefit and should generally be avoided, such as most CCBs. Choice will depend on heart rhythm, comorbidities, and disease phenotype.[200]

Although the conventional definition of tachycardia is a resting HR over 100 beats/min, the risk of adverse CV outcomes in HFrEF patients appears to increase progressively with HR $\geq$ 70 beats/min.[201-203] β-Blockers reduce HR by antagonizing the adverse effects of the SNS and have become a cornerstone for HFrEF therapy. In some cases, however, recommended target doses cannot be tolerated or are contraindicated, and other drugs should be considered for adequate HR control. Ivabradine is a selective blocker of the cardiac pacemaker If ("funny") channel current that controls the spontaneous diastolic depolarization of the sinoatrial node, approved for the treatment of HFrEF in the United States. Specific blockade of the If channels prolongates the slow depolarization phase, causing a dose-dependent reduction in HR. As a consequence, ivabradine does not affect contractility or SVR.

Initially developed and approved as an antianginal agent in Europe, ivabradine was also shown to improve outcomes in subjects with HFrEF. The BEAUTIFUL trial randomized subjects with IHD to ivabradine or placebo and did not meet its primary outcome of reducing CV death, MI, or HF hospitalization.[201] However, in a post hoc analysis, ivabradine was shown to reduce rates of MI and coronary revascularization in the subgroup with a HR $\geq$70 beats/min, yielding insights into the potential benefits of additional HR reduction in patients with HFrEF.[202] The SHIFT trial randomized symptomatic HFrEF patients with LVEF $\leq$35%, sinus rhythm, and resting HR $\geq$70 beats/min despite maximally tolerated β-blocker therapy to either ivabradine or matching placebo.[204] The primary composite outcome of HF hospitalization or mortality was reduced by 18% in the ivabradine group, driven primarily by 26% fewer HF hospitalizations, since there was no decrease in CV or all-cause deaths. Remarkably, only 26% of subjects in SHIFT were taking optimal target doses of β-blockers and only 56% were on at least half-target doses at inclusion. Given that ivabradine lowered HR by approximately 10 beats/min, and that its benefits were somewhat attenuated in the subgroup of subjects on at least half-target doses of β-blocker therapy, it is possible that titrating β-blockers to recommended doses may have reduced HF hospitalizations to a similar degree.

Overall, ivabradine was well tolerated in the SHIFT trial, with only a modest increase in bradycardia. Transient visual disturbances secondary to effects on the hyperpolarization-activated current within the retina, referred to as phosphenes, were the most common non-CV side effect, but they frequently improved over time. Current HF guidelines recommend considering ivabradine in HFrEF patients with LVEF $\leq$35%, sinus rhythm, and resting HR

≥70 beats/min who remain symptomatic despite β-blocker therapy at maximum tolerated dose. It should be noted that the off-label use of ivabradine for inappropriate sinus tachycardia or other electrophysiological disorders lacks evidence support and remains unapproved.[200] Evidence-based doses for ivabradine are listed in Table 3.5.

Ivabradine is contraindicated in patients with ADHF, hypotension, sinus node dysfunction, sinus bradycardia with a HR <60 beats/min, and sinoatrial (SA) or third-degree atrioventricular (AV) block, unless a functioning demand pacemaker is present. Other contraindications for ivabradine are severe hepatic dysfunction, pacemaker dependence, and known atrial or ventricular arrhythmias. In the SIGNIFY trial, subjects with CAD treated with ivabradine had an increase in relative risk for AF, which is consistent with the findings of a later meta-analysis.[205,206] Ivabradine also has the potential to cause fetal toxicity, and women of reproductive age should therefore be advised.

Digoxin

Digoxin is a purified cardiac glycoside derived from the foxglove plant that has been used for more than 200 years to treat HF. It acts by inhibiting the sodium–potassium (Na-K) ATPase pump in cell membranes, reducing the transport of sodium from the intracellular to the extracellular space in both cardiac and noncardiac cells and contributing to hemodynamic, neurohumoral, and electrophysiologic effects (Fig. 3.7).[207]

In myocytes, inhibition of the Na-K-ATPase pump is associated with a rise in intracellular calcium concentration, which is the pivotal link in excitation-contraction coupling, causing positive inotropy. This results in improved LVEF, CO, and PCWP without causing detrimental effects on HR or BP.[208] In noncardiac cells, digoxin sensitizes Na-K-ATPase activity in vagal afferent nerves, leading to an increase in parasympathetic tone that offsets the deleterious activation of the SNS. In addition to its direct autonomic effects, digoxin indirectly reduces sympathetic outflow by improving carotid baroreflex responsiveness. Thus, at low doses, digoxin acts as a neurohormonal modulator in patients with severe HFrEF. Further dose increases, however, have no additional benefit and may augment sympathetic tone.[209] Also, by increasing vagal tone and decreasing sympathetic outflow, digoxin slows firing at the SA node and prolongs conduction at the AV node, with limited electrophysiological effects on the rest of the conduction system.[207]

Despite its beneficial properties and widespread use in the past, the role of digoxin therapy in patients with chronic HFrEF

INOTROPIC, VAGAL AND SYMPATHETIC EFFECTS OF DIGOXIN

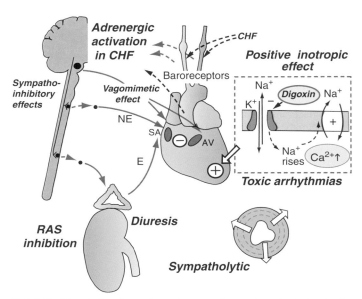

Fig. 3.7 Digoxin has hemodynamic, neurohumoral, and electrophysiologic effects. The inotropic effect of digoxin is due to inhibition of the sodium pump in myocardial cells. Slowing of the heart rate and inhibition of the atrioventricular *(AV)* node by vagal stimulation and the decreased sympathetic nerve discharge are important therapeutic benefits. Toxic arrhythmias are less well understood but may be caused by calcium-dependent afterpotentials. *CHF,* Congestive heart failure; *E,* epinephrine; *NE,* norepinephrine; *RAS,* renin-angiotensin system; *SA,* sinoatrial. (Figure © L.H. Opie, 2012.)

remains controversial. Before the pivotal DIG trial, two digoxin-withdrawal trials from the early 1990s, the PROVED and the RADIANCE, examined the effects of stopping digoxin therapy in subjects with NYHA class II–III HFrEF and normal sinus rhythm.[210-212] Both trials showed that withdrawing digoxin in these subjects significantly worsened HF symptoms and lowered exercise tolerance, with no effects on mortality. In the DIG trial, the largest randomized clinical trial of digoxin efficacy in HF, digoxin therapy reduced hospitalizations by 28% but had no statistically significant effect

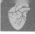

on all-cause mortality.[210] Also, a trend toward survival benefit found in patients with severe HFrEF was offset by an increased risk of sudden and other nonpump-failure cardiac deaths. Of note, most subjects in the DIG were receiving standard therapy with ACE inhibitors and diuretics, while β-blocker therapy was not yet approved for use in HF. Reanalysis of the DIG trial have brought into question the safety of digoxin, including the optimal serum digoxin concentration (SDC) and the role of gender in digoxin therapy. A post hoc analysis of the DIG suggested that the SDC was directly related to mortality, with increased all-cause mortality among subjects with SDC ≥1.2 ng/mL. By contrast, concentrations between 0.5 and 0.8 ng/mL were safe.[213] In another retrospective analysis of the DIG trial, digoxin was associated with a significantly higher risk of death from any cause among women, suggesting a significant treatment-gender interaction.[214] However, further post hoc analyses focusing on subjects with available SDC showed that women with SDC in the lower range of 0.5–0.9 ng/ml had mortality rates similar to those obtained with placebo and a significant 30% relative risk reduction in HF hospitalizations.[215] Conversely, an increased mortality was observed among women with SDC ≥1.2 ng/mL, which is a similar trend to that observed in the general population. Those findings are consistent with a recent post hoc analysis of the ARISTOTLE trial, which examined the association between mortality and digoxin use in subjects with nonvalvular AFib.[216] The retrospective study found that subjects with baseline SDC at 1.2 ng/mL or above had over 50% increased risk of death when compared to those not on digoxin, while subjects with SDC below 0.9 ng/mL showed no increased risk. In addition, patients starting digoxin in the follow-up also had significantly higher mortality risks.

Taken together, the DIG, the PROVED, and the RADIANCE trials prompted the FDA to approve digoxin for use in HFrEF in 1997. However, due to its side effects and a narrow toxic-to-therapeutic window, major clinical practice guidelines currently offer only a secondary recommendation for HFrEF patients with normal sinus rhythm who remain symptomatic despite optimal medical therapy. Evidence-based doses for digoxin are listed in Table 3.5. Importantly, digoxin therapy for patients with chronic kidney dysfunction or those with low lean body mass should be introduced at lower doses or every other day.

Digoxin toxicity typically presents with the combination of cardiac effects and dose-dependent central nervous system or gastrointestinal effects, such as visual changes, anxiety, anorexia, nausea, vomiting, and abdominal pain. While elevated intracellular calcium concentration and increased vagal tone facilitate the development of arrhythmias, digoxin should have minimal proarrhythmic effects when dosed to recommended SDC. However, intoxication through supratherapeutic or therapeutic SDC with concomitant hypokalemia, hypomagnesemia, hypercalcemia, hypothyroidism, or myocardial ischemia can cause sinus bradycardia, SA nodal block, AV block, and escape rhythms. SDC could also be increased by associated use of quinidine, verapamil, flecainide, propafenone, amiodarone, and spironolactone. Consequently, SDC should be closely monitored to minimize side effects.

Iron Supplementation and Anemia

Anemia is a frequent finding in HF patients, with a prevalence ranging from 4% to 55% depending on the population studied.[217] Potential mechanisms of interaction between anemia and HF include inflammation, hemodilution, malnutrition, and renal dysfunction. Acute isovolemic drop of hemoglobin concentration in healthy individuals leads to compensatory changes, including increases in HR, SV, and CI along with tissue oxygen extraction, which are often impaired in patients with reduced CO. Therefore, anemia is associated with worse symptoms and NYHA functional status, greater risk of HF hospitalization, and reduced survival in patients with HFrEF. However, it remains unclear whether anemia is an independent predictor of mortality or simply a marker of more advanced disease and extensive comorbidities.

A standard diagnostic workup should include complete blood count, renal function, occult blood loss, iron and vitamin B12/folate deficiencies, and C-reactive protein. Correctable causes of anemia should be treated according to clinical practice guidelines, but in many cases no specific cause is found. Iron deficiency is very common in HFrEF patients, with an estimated prevalence of over 50% in the ambulatory setting.[218] It is an independent predictor of worse functional status and survival, regardless of anemia. Some studies have evaluated the efficacy and safety of iron supplementation in subjects with HFrEF and iron deficiency, defined as ferritin <100 ng/dl or ferritin of 100–299 ng/dl with transferrin saturation <20%, with mild or no anemia. Early small-size clinical trials and a number of observational studies have provided promising evidence of symptomatic benefit from treating HF with iron, yielding placebo-controlled multicenter trials of IV iron in subjects with chronic HFrEF. The FAIR-HF trial randomized subjects with NYHA class II–III HF and LVEF ≤40%–45% to IV ferric carboxymaltose (FCM) or placebo at regular intervals during correction and maintenance phases. After 24 weeks of follow-up, FCM supplementation resulted in significant improvements in NYHA class, 6-minute walk distance, and several quality-of-life assessments when compared to placebo.[219] Of note, these benefits were similar in patients with hemoglobin concentration ≤ 12 or >12 g/dL, suggesting that an alternate mechanism, rather than anemia, could be associated with the observed outcomes. The second large-scale trial of IV FCM in HFrEF, the CONFIRM-HF trial, showed very similar results to those of the FAIR-HF, with sustained benefits over a 1-year period.[220] The following EFFECT-HF trial further suggested that FCM could improve peak oxygen consumption (VO_2) by ergospirometry at 24 weeks.[221] None of the trials, however, were powered to test for the impact of IV iron on mortality and HF hospitalizations or to evaluate separately its consequences in anemic and nonanemic individuals. In two separate meta-analyses, IV iron supplementation in HFrEF subjects with iron deficiency suggested a reduced composite risk of all-cause mortality and CV hospitalization.[218] The FAIR-HF 2 trial is currently ongoing and aims at examining efficacy of IV iron in reducing CV mortality and recurrent hospitalizations in HF patients.

Oral iron preparations are poorly absorbed due to bowel edema. The IRONOUT-HF trial randomized subjects with NYHA II–IV class HF and LVEF $\leq 40\%$ to oral iron polysaccharide or placebo and showed no significant differences between the treatment groups in VO_2 at 16 weeks.[222] Likewise, there was no significant change for the secondary outcomes of 6-minute walk distance and NT-proBNP levels. Furthermore, oral iron preparations are associated with a higher incidence of gastrointestinal side effects, mostly as a result of direct iron effects on the gut wall. Thus, clinical practice guidelines recommend that iron supplementation with IV, but not oral, preparations might be reasonable in subjects with NYHA class II–III HF and iron deficiency, defined as ferritin <100 ng/dl or ferritin of 100–299 ng/dl with transferrin saturation $<20\%$, to improve functional status and quality of life.

Data on use of blood transfusions in patients with HF are limited. Based upon low-quality evidence and expert opinion, a transfusion threshold for maintaining the hemoglobin above 7 g/dL has been generally accepted, although some symptomatic patients may require transfusion at higher levels.[223] Given the risks of volume overload and the costs of red blood cell transfusion, careful selection of patients is recommended, with adjustment of diuretics doses and transfusion rates as needed. Importantly, the sensitizing effects of transfusion may also affect end-stage HF patients, further limiting their access to heart transplantation. Thus, the routine use of blood transfusion cannot be recommended for treating the anemia that occurs in stable HF patients.

Finally, the best evidence of erythropoiesis-stimulating agents in subjects with HF comes from the RED-HF trial, which randomized HFrEF patients with mild to moderate anemia to receive either darbepoetin alfa or placebo. Darbepoetin alfa did not improve clinical outcomes when compared to placebo but led to an excess of thromboembolic events and is therefore not recommended.[224]

Fish Oil and Marine Omega-3 Polyunsaturated Fatty Acids

Several epidemiological and experimental studies have suggested controversial benefits of dietary omega-3 polyunsaturated fatty acids (PUFAs) on CV health. The three most important omega-3 PUFAs for humans are the α-linolenic acid (ALA), the eicosapentaenoic acid (EPA), and the docosahexaenoic acid (DHA). α-Linolenic acid is an essential fatty acid, mainly obtained from nuts, vegetable oils, flax seeds, and leafy vegetables ingestion, while EPA and DHA can be either synthesized from ALA or obtained from seafood or fish oil supplements.[225] Omega-3 fats are critical in cellular function, influencing cellular structure, signaling, and gene expression. PUFA consumption lowers serum triglyceride concentrations and modestly raises HDL cholesterol. Moreover, various pleotropic effects have been described to be associated with PUFA consumption, including reduction of HR and BP as well as antiinflammatory, antithrombotic, antiarrhythmic, and vasodilatory properties.[225,226]

Supplementation with PUFAs has been of potential interest as a therapy for HF. The GISSI-HF trial randomized subjects with NYHA class II–IV chronic HFrEF to receive 1 g/day of PUFA or matching placebo. At a mean follow-up of 3.9 years, 1 g/day of PUFA was associated with a significant 9% relative risk reduction in mortality from any cause in all of the predefined subgroups, including patients with nonischemic cardiomyopathy.[227] The primary composite outcome of mortality or CV admissions was also reduced. Although the improvements in clinical outcomes were modest, they were additive to those of other therapies that are standard of care in HF, such as ACE inhibitors, β-blockers, MRAs, and diuretics.

While regular dietary seafood consumption can be considered the optimal source of PUFA for many patients, the dose-response for potential HFrEF benefits is not well established. In the GISSI-HF, for example, only preparations containing 850–882 mg of EPA and DHA as ethyl esters at the average ratio of 1:1.2 have shown an effect on the cumulative outcome of death and hospitalization. EPA and DHA have differing effects on lipid oxidation, signal transduction, fluidity, and cholesterol domain formation, potentially due in part to distinct membrane interactions.[228] Therefore, it is unclear if different preparations would have yielded the same results. The CV benefit of lowering triglyceride levels with pure EPA-only preparations is supported by two large clinical trials, the JELIS and the

REDUCE-IT.[229,230] By contrast, many supplements actually contain only the omega-3 ALA, which may also have CV benefits but cannot yet be considered a replacement for marine omega-3 PUFAs.

PUFA therapy is generally safe and well tolerated, with the most common side effects being gastrointestinal abnormalities, such as nausea. In the GISSI-HF trial, there was a similar 30% drop-out rate from both PUFA and placebo groups. The REDUCE-IT found a significant increase in the rates of AFib and peripheral edema in the EPA group, but with no difference in the rates of new HF or HF hospitalization. Thus, current HF guidelines recommend omega-3 PUFA supplementation as a reasonable adjunctive therapy in patients with NYHA class II–IV HFrEF, preferably in preparations containing >850 mg/g of EPA and DHA.

Micronutrient Supplementation

Dietary micronutrient deficiency is common in patients with HFrEF. Deficiencies of L-carnitine, thiamine, and taurine alone are well-known causes of cardiomyopathy.[231,232] Micronutrient supplementation offers the opportunity to correct deficiencies in critical myocyte pathways, including those associated with the provision of ATP, intracellular calcium balance, and reduction of oxidative stress. Although some clinical trials of single micronutrient supplementation, including coenzyme Q10, L-carnitine, thiamine, and taurine, have yielded promising results, their value has been limited by design and inconsistency.[232,233] Because of the inconclusive data, current HF guidelines do not recommend the routine use of nutritional supplements in patients with current or prior HF symptoms. Larger trials of multiple-micronutrient supplementation are needed.

Oral Anticoagulants and Antiplatelet Therapy

HF is considered a major risk factor for thromboembolic events, which is best explained by the elements of the Virchow's triad, hypercoagulability, blood stasis, and endothelial dysfunction. In large clinical HFrEF trials, the rate of thromboembolic events ranged from 1.5% to 2.7% per year. The major thrombotic sources in HF are related to venous thromboembolism (VTE) and AFib. The VTE risk is associated with RV dysfunction, which may reflect previous, often undiagnosed episodes of pulmonary embolism.[234] Likewise, HF is an important risk factor for stroke embolization among patients with AF, as accessed by a variety of risk scores used to guide therapy, including the CHA2DS2-VASc score.[235]

Therapeutic anticoagulation is the mainstay of risk reduction strategies in patients with HFrEF and AFib or a history of systemic or pulmonary emboli, including stroke or transient ischemic attack. However, anticoagulation therapy should be based on an assessment of the risk of thromboembolic events versus the risk of bleeding as recommended by clinical practice guidelines. While warfarin and other vitamin K antagonists (VKA) were the only available class of oral anticoagulants for many decades, their use is limited by a narrow therapeutic index that necessitates frequent monitoring and dose adjustments.[236] Therefore, the direct oral anticoagulants (DOACs) represent a particularly attractive therapeutic option in patients with nonvalvular AFib and concomitant HF, due to a more predictable therapeutic effect. Two meta-analyses of the clinical trials RE-LY, ROCKET AF, ARISTOTLE, and ENGAGE AF-TIMI 48 in patients with nonvalvular AFib suggested that DOACs might have a more favorable risk-benefit profile, with significant reductions in stroke, major bleeding, and intracranial hemorrhage when compared to warfarin.[236,237] DOACs are not approved for use in patients with mechanical heart valves or at least moderate mitral stenosis, because of increased evidence of thromboembolic and bleeding complications as compared with warfarin.[238] In such cases, only VKAs should be used for the prevention of thromboembolic stroke.[1] For patients at high risk of bleeding, a left atrial occlusion device could be considered as an alternative to avoid the risk of anticoagulation-related hemorrhage.

Although anticoagulation in patients with HFrEF and documented AFib is well established, the role of oral anticoagulation in subjects with HFrEF and sinus rhythm is controversial and not recommended for routine use. This recommendation is based on the findings of previous randomized trials, including the WASH, HELAS, WATCH, and WARCEF.[239-242] These trials failed consistently to show the benefit of warfarin for primary outcomes that included death and nonfatal stroke.[243] In both WARCEF and a subsequent meta-analyses including all four trials, warfarin was associated with a significant reduction in the rate of ischemic stroke, which was offset by an increased rate of major bleeding. Interestingly, intracerebral hemorrhage remained very low and was not significantly different from aspirin.[243] Similarly, the COMMANDER-HF trial randomized patients with HFrEF, CAD, and sinus rhythm to the DOAC rivaroxaban or placebo and showed no significant differences in the composite outcome of all-cause mortality, MI, or stroke during a mean follow-up of 21 months.[244] In addition, patients assigned to rivaroxaban had more bleeding events requiring hospitalization than those assigned to placebo.

Evidence supporting anticoagulation in patients with a recent MI and documented LV thrombus is very limited, partially because most data were generated before the contemporary era of thrombolysis, percutaneous coronary intervention, dual antiplatelet therapy, and imaging techniques. Likewise, based on low-quality evidence, there is a weak recommendation for oral anticoagulation in the initial 3 months following a large anterior MI with symptomatic or asymptomatic IHD. Currently, there is no evidence on the benefits of antiplatelet drugs in patients with HFrEF without concomitant CAD, while there is a substantial risk of gastrointestinal bleeding and a potential inhibitory effect of aspirin on ACE inhibitors. Conversely, antiplatelet therapy for patients with CAD and LV systolic dysfunction should be guided by the applicable guidelines.

Statins

Statins, also known as 3-hydroxy-3-methyl-glutaryl-coenzyme A (HMG-CoA) reductase inhibitors, are widely used for both the primary and secondary prevention of atherosclerotic CV disease. In addition to their lipid-lowering action, statins also have a variety of pleiotropic effects including antiinflammatory, antihypertrophic, antifibrotic, and antioxidant properties. Most of these effects can target important components of the complex physiopathology of HFrEF, such as endothelial dysfunction, neurohormonal activation and cardiac arrhythmias.[245] Conversely, statins are associated with a decrease in coenzyme Q10 levels and selenoprotein activity, which could lead to skeletal and cardiac myopathy.[246] Also, low concentrations of LDL cholesterol are associated with a worse prognosis in patients with HFrEF.

The best data on the role of statin therapy in HFrEF comes from two large randomized clinical trials, GISSI-HF and CORONA.[245,246] The CORONA randomized subjects with IHD, NYHA class II–IV, and LVEF ≤35%–40% to either rosuvastatin or placebo and showed no significant difference in the primary composite outcome of CV death, nonfatal MI, or nonfatal stroke at a mean follow-up of 33 months. Following a similar protocol, the GISSI-HF studied this hypothesis among ischemic and nonischemic HF patients, rather than IHD patients only. At a mean follow-up of 47 months, the GISSI-HF investigators found no significant difference in all-cause mortality or in the combined outcome of death or CV hospitalization in both ischemic and nonischemic HF subjects.

Taken together, CORONA and GISSI-HF trials provide reasonably strong evidence against the routine use of statins for NYHA class II–IV HFrEF. Of note, the secondary outcome of all-cause hospitalizations in the CORONA trial was significantly reduced in the rosuvastatin group. Thus, in patients who are already receiving a statin for CAD, a continuation of this therapy may be considered.

Antiarrhythmic Agents

AFib is the most frequent arrhythmia in HF, with a prevalence ranging from <10% of patients with mild disease up to nearly half of those with advanced HF. It can impair myocardial function by several mechanisms, including loss of atrial systole and rapid ventricular HR, both of which can reduce CO and diastolic filling time.[247] Also, persistent tachycardia and irregular heart rhythm can lead to tachycardia-induced cardiomyopathy, a relatively rare though well-recognized condition.

The general management of AFib is rather similar in patients with or without HF and involves three principles: thromboembolic risk assessment, ventricular rate control, and rhythm control in selected cases.[235] Most clinical trials in the general AFib population, such as the AFFIRM, have shown that rhythm control is not superior to rate control in terms of morbidity and mortality.[248] Patients with HF, however, present specific challenges, including a higher risk for side effects from certain antiarrhythmic drug. In a sub-analysis of the CHF-STAT trial, patients with HFrEF and AFib converted to sinus rhythm with amiodarone had significantly lower mortality than those who remained in AFib.[249] The same findings were seen in a substudy of the DIAMOND, with dofetilide.[250] Addressing this controversy, the large prospective randomized trial comparing current strategies for rhythm control among HFrEF with AFib, the AF-CHF trial, showed that higher rates of sinus rhythm did not translate into any clinical benefit.[251] Thus most clinical practice guidelines recommend that rhythm-control strategy should be reserved for patients with HFrEF and AFib-related symptoms or worsening HF despite adequate rate control.

The optimal HR for patients with concomitant AFib and HF is unclear. The RACE II trial found no difference in a composite of clinical outcomes when a strategy of strict rate control, defined as HR <80 beats/min at rest and <110 beats/min during moderate exercise, was compared with lenient rate control, defined as resting HR <110 beats/min.[252] However, a sustained HR >100 beats/min, and particularly >120 beats/min, can lead to tachycardia-induced cardiomyopathy and must be avoided. Available therapies for rate control of AFib include β-blockers, digoxin, nondihydropyridine CCBs, and amiodarone. In the context of HFrEF, β-blockers are recommended as first-line therapy, as individual patient data subgroup meta-analysis of clinical trials suggests no safety concerns.[251] In the event that a second drug is needed to achieve rate control, the combination of digoxin and a β-blocker is more effective than a β-blocker alone. Nevertheless, as previously noted, a direct association between SDC and mortality was consistently reported in observational studies and post hoc analysis of clinical trials.

Routine use of nondihydropyridine CCBs, such as verapamil or diltiazem, should be avoided in patients with HFrEF due to their negative inotropic effects. However, in selected cases, the short-term IV administration of diltiazem can be considered for the acute management of AFib with rapid ventricular response. If rate control has not been achieved with either a β-blocker or a combination of a β-blocker and digoxin, amiodarone may be useful. Of note, there is a small chance that amiodarone may pharmacologically cardiovert patients to sinus rhythm.

Rhythm control can be achieved with pharmacological or electrical cardioversion, catheter ablation, or surgical ablation. Antiarrhythmic drugs for the maintenance of sinus rhythm in patients with AFib and HFrEF are limited to dofetilide or amiodarone. Dofetilide is a class III antiarrhythmic drug that selectively inhibits the rapid component of the late potassium current through cell membranes, increasing the refractory period. In the DIAMOND trial, patients with symptomatic HFrEF and AFib treated with dofetilide were significantly more likely to convert to sinus rhythm when compared to placebo.[250] However, dofetilide requires inpatient stay for loading, and there is a significant risk of torsades de pointes observed in 3.3% of all cases. Because of such risk, dofetilide is not approved in Europe and is only available by mail order or through specially trained local pharmacies in the United States.

Amiodarone is another class III antiarrhythmic with little or no negative inotropic or proarrhythmic effects, particularly when lower doses of 100–200 mg/day are used for maintenance therapy. Despite potentially significant side effects, amiodarone is the ideal antiarrhythmic agent for the rhythm control strategy and may improve the success of electrical cardioversion. Advantages of amiodarone compared to dofetilide include the ability to start therapy as an outpatient, once-a-day dosing and a lower risk of torsades de pointes. Side effects, such as hyperthyroidism, hypothyroidism, pulmonary fibrosis, and hepatitis, are less likely with maintenance therapy at lower doses, but still occur. Amiodarone also increases the serum concentrations of phenytoin and digoxin and prolongs the INR in patients taking VKAs, thus monitoring is advised.

Dronedarone, a derivative of amiodarone with shorter half-life and devoid of iodine moiety, should not be used in patients with advanced HFrEF and long-standing persistent AFib. Strong evidence against its use comes from the ANDROMEDA trial, which had to be discontinued early because of a two fold increase in mortality in the dronedarone-treated HFrEF subjects, mainly due to worsening HF.[253] Other antiarrhythmic drugs, especially class I sodium-channel blockers, are associated with an increased proarrhythmic risk and sudden cardiac death in patients with HF and are contraindicated.

Direct Renin Inhibitors

Based on the observation that long-term therapies with ACE inhibitors or ARBs provoke a compensatory increase in renin and its downstream intermediaries, direct renin inhibitors (DRIs) offer another pharmacologically distinct route of RAAS inhibition. Aliskiren is a first-in-class orally active DRI that provides significant BP-lowering efficacy in patients with hypertension, with no rebound effects after withdrawal. In early preclinical and proof-of-concept studies, aliskiren appeared to produce similar, if not greater, beneficial impact on RAAS inhibition, cardiac hypertrophy, LV wall thickness, and diastolic function when compared to ACE inhibitors and ARBs.[254,255]

Promising results from the ALOFT trial, in which aliskiren was shown to decrease plasma NT-proBNP and urinary aldosterone excretion in HFrEF subjects, yielded several large trials to determine whether adding aliskiren to standard HFrEF therapy would improve clinical outcomes.[256] However, both the ASTRONAUT and the ATMOSPHERE trials failed to improve outcomes in HFrEF subjects.[68,257] In fact, the ASTRONAUT found a tendency toward harm in diabetic patients, and the ATMOSPHERE showed that the addition of aliskiren to enalapril led to more adverse events, as hyperkalemia, renal dysfunction, and symptomatic hypotension. Therefore, DRIs are not recommended as an alternative to an ACE inhibitor or ARB in patients with HFrEF. Fig. 3.8 summarize the 2017 American College of Cardiology (ACC)/AHA/Heart Failure Society of America (HFSA) recommended approach to the treatment of stages C and D HFrEF.

Heart Failure Patients With Preserved Ejection Fraction

Introduction

For many decades, the definition of HF was most commonly associated with LV systolic dysfunction and HFrEF. However, epidemiologic data indicate that at least 50% of all patients with HF have preserved LVEF, a prevalence that has increased over time.[17,258]

The diagnosis of HFpEF requires the presence of symptoms and/or signs of HF, a LVEF $\geq$50%, elevated concentrations of NP, and evidence of diastolic dysfunction or relevant structural heart disease.[1] It should be noted that diastolic dysfunction and HFpEF are not synonymous, as diastolic dysfunction might also be present in HFrEF. Recently, the H2FPEF score was elaborated to estimate the probability of HFpEF versus noncardiac causes of dyspnea.[259]

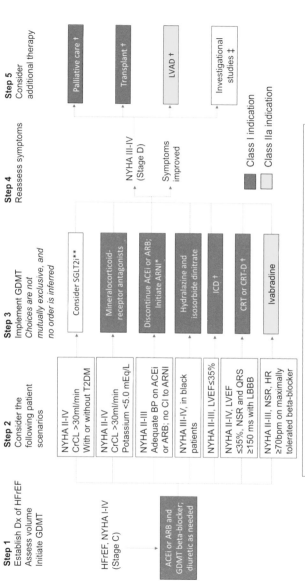

Step 1
Establish Dx of HFrEF
Assess volume
Initiate GDMT

HFrEF, NYHA I-IV
(Stage C)

→ ACEi or ARB and GDMT beta-blocker; diuretic as needed

Step 2
Consider the following patient scenarios

- NYHA II-IV
  CrCL >30ml/min
  With or without T2DM

- NYHA II-IV
  CrCL >30ml/min
  Potassium <5.0 mEq/L

- NYHA II-III
  Adequate BP on ACEi or ARB; no CI to ARNI

- NYHA III-IV, in black patients

- NYHA II-III, LVEF≤35%

- NYHA II-IV, LVEF ≤35%, NSR and QRS ≥150 ms with LBBB

- NYHA II-III, NSR, HR ≥70bpm on maximally tolerated beta-blocker

Step 3
Implement GDMT
Choices are not mutually exclusive, and no order is inferred

- Consider SGLT2i**

- Mineralocorticoid-receptor antagonists

- Discontinue ACEi or ARB; Initiate ARNI*

- Hydralazine and isosorbide dinitrate

- ICD †

- CRT or CRT-D †

- Ivabradine

Step 4
Reassess symptoms

NYHA III-IV
(Stage D)

Symptoms improved

Step 5
Consider additional therapy

- Palliative care †
- Transplant †
- LVAD †
- Investigational studies ‡

■ Class I indication
▢ Class IIa indication

Continue GDMT with serial reassessment and optimized dosing/adherence

Fig. 3.8 See legend on next page

Large outcome trials and registries have demonstrated that the demographics, comorbidities, prognoses, and, most importantly, responses to pharmacotherapy differ between HFpEF and HFrEF. Patients with HFpEF are older, more often females, and have higher rates of hypertension, AFib, obesity, and anemia when compared to those with HFREF. They are also less likely to have IHD, although the prevalence of CAD is not trivial.[4,17,171,260]

All-cause mortality is generally lower in HFpEF than in HFrEF. Nevertheless, the incidence of non-CV deaths is significantly higher for HFpEF patients, reflecting their higher age and increased comorbidity. Also, while survival rates in HFrEF have significantly improved over the past decades, HFpEF prognosis remains the same.[261] No treatment has yet been shown, convincingly, to reduce morbidity or mortality in patients with HFpEF. Therapeutic targets in HFpEF are directed toward associated conditions and include control of congestion, stabilization of HR and BP, and efforts at improving exercise tolerance.[40] Experience has demonstrated that BP control, in accordance with published clinical practice guidelines, is more effective to alleviate symptoms and improve well-being than targeted therapy with specific agents.

Fig. 3.8, Cont'd   Therapeutic approach to heart failure with a reduced ejection fraction stages C and D. For all medical therapies, dosing should be optimized, and serial assessment exercised. *See text for important treatment directions. **No current guideline recommendation. †Palliative care, device-based therapies and surgical management of heart failure are discussed elsewhere. ‡Participation in investigational studies is also appropriate for stage C, NYHA Class II–III heart failure. *ACEi,* Angiotensin-converting enzyme inhibitor; *ARB,* angiotensin receptor-blocker; *ARNI,* angiotensin receptor neprilysin inhibitor; *BP,* blood pressure; *bpm,* beats per minute; *CI,* contraindication; *CrCl,* creatinine clearance; *CRT-D,* cardiac resynchronization therapy-device; *Dx,* diagnosis; *GDMT,* guideline-directed management and therapy; *HFrEF,* heart failure with reduced ejection fraction; *ICD,* implantable cardioverter-defibrillator; *LBBB,* left bundle-branch block; *LVAD,* left ventricular assist device; *LVEF,* left ventricular ejection fraction; *NSR,* normal sinus rhythm; *NYHA,* New York Heart Association; *SGLT-2i,* sodium-glucose cotransporter 2 inhibitor; *T2DM,* type-2 diabetes mellitus. (Modified from Yancy CW, Jessup M, Bozkurt B, et al. 2017 ACC/AHA/HFSA Focused Update of the 2013 ACCF/AHA guideline for the management of heart failure: A report of the American College of Cardiology/American Heart Association task force on clinical practice guidelines and the Heart Failure Society of America. *J Am Coll Cardiol* 2017;23(8):628–651.)

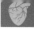

Heart Failure Patients With Mid-Range Ejection Fraction

Despite the widespread adoption of ejection fraction-based classification of HF, the optimal cut-off for group characterization have varied across studies.[5] Medical societies acknowledged that patients with an LVEF in the range of 40% to 49% represent a "grey area," and thus an intermediate group was added to the 2016 ESC HF Guidelines, entitled HF with mid-range ejection fraction (HFmrEF).[1] Because HFmrEF patients have generally been included in trials of HFpEF, the following guidance applies to both phenotypes of HFmrEF and HFpEF. Identifying HFmrEF as a separate group will stimulate research into their unique characteristics. As new evidence demonstrating a prognostic difference between these categories becomes available, it might be possible to make separate recommendations for each one.

Pharmacotherapy

Diuretics

Diuretics are widely used to attenuate symptoms and signs of congestion in both HFrEF and HFpEF, although their effects on long-term survival have never been demonstrated. The goal of decongestive diuretic therapy is similar in all phenotypes of HF, with caution to avoid excessive preload reduction and hypotension.[33] In the small-size Hong Kong Diastolic Heart Failure Study, patients with HFpEF, defined as LVEF >45%, were randomized to diuretics alone or combined with ramipril or irbesartan.[262] Diuretic therapy alone significantly improved quality-of-life assessments, while the addition of ramipril or irbesartan provided only slight additional beneficial effects. Further benefit of diuretics was suggested by an ancillary analysis of the CHAMPION trial, a single-blind clinical trial of a wireless implantable PAP monitor, the CARDIOMEMs, to guide ambulatory management of HF.[263,264] In the ancillary study, treatment decisions driven by the CARDIOMEMs, notably changes in mean loop diuretic dose, were associated with a significant reduction in HF hospitalizations.

Recent preclinical data suggest that empagliflozin reduces myofilament passive stiffness and improves diastolic tension of human end-stage HF ventricular trabeculae, independently of glucose or calcium metabolism modulation.[265] Beneficial diuretic and cardiometabolic effects make SGLT-2 inhibitors particularly attractive for obese HFpEF patients with volume overload and adipose inflammation.[266] Trials such as the EMPEROR-Preserved, DELIVER, and DETERMINE are currently investigating the safety and efficacy of SGLT-2 inhibitors in patients with HFpEF. Current guidelines for the treatment of HFpEF recommend management of volume overload with appropriate diuretic dosing, but do not provide any guidance on therapy choice.

Renin-Angiotensin Blockade: Angiotensin Converting Enzyme Inhibitors and Angiotensin Receptor Blockers

Both angiotensin II and aldosterone are known contributors to LV hypertrophy and myocardial fibrosis, which are important determinants of diastolic dysfunction. The rationale in the use of a RAAS antagonist in HFpEF is to prevent the prohypertrophic and profibrotic effects of angiotensin II. In addition, many underlying risk factors and comorbidities for HFpEF, such as hypertension, T2DM, CAD, and chronic kidney disease, benefit from treatment with ACE inhibitors and ARBs.

The PEP-CHF trial evaluated the effectiveness of perindopril versus placebo on the primary composite outcome of all-cause mortality or HF hospitalization in subjects older than 70 years with HFpEF, defined as LVEF >45%.[267] Despite being the largest trial of ACE inhibitors in HFpEF, PEP-CHF failed to meet sufficient power for its primary composite outcome due to lower than expected enrollment and a high rate of crossover to open-label ACE inhibitor. A post hoc analysis using only the first year of follow-up, when crossover rates were lower, suggested a favorable trend with perindopril, primarily driven by reduction in HF hospitalizations. Other mechanistic studies in the elderly showed conflicting results or no benefits of ACE inhibitors on exercise tolerance, quality-of-life assessments, aortic distensibility, peripheral neurohormone expression, or LV mass.

Two large randomized clinical trials, CHARM-Preserved and I-PRESERVE, addressed the benefit of ARB use in patients with HFpEF. The CHARM-Preserved trial was part of the CHARM program and randomized subjects with NYHA class II–IV HFpEF, defined as LVEF >40%, to either candesartan or placebo.[171,268] After adjustments for nonsignificant covariates in baseline characteristics, the trial showed a reduction in HF hospitalizations with candesartan, but no difference in all-cause mortality. It is unknown whether that benefit was driven by neurohormonal blockade or simply by hypertension management, as the candesartan group achieved better BP control when compared to the placebo control group. The I-PRESERVE trial evaluated irbesartan versus placebo in subjects with NYHA class II–IV HFpEF, defined as LVEF >45%, and found no significant differences for a variety of CV outcomes, including death from any cause and CV hospitalization.[269] However, a doubling of creatinine and serious hyperkalemia occurred more often in the irbesartan group.

According to current ACC/AHA HF guidelines, it is reasonable to use ACE inhibitors or ARBs for BP control in patients with hypertension and HFpEF. Also, based on the CHARM-Preserved, ARBs might be considered to decrease HFpEF admissions.

Mineralocorticoid Receptor Antagonists

Aldosterone has been associated with oxidative stress, endothelial dysfunction, ventricular hypertrophy, and myocardial fibrosis, mechanisms known to influence the progression of HFpEF.[186,270] MRAs antagonize the detrimental effects of aldosterone and can improve diastolic function.

In the ALDO-DHF trial, spironolactone improved echocardiographic indices of diastolic dysfunction in patients with HFpEF, even after adjustment for the effect in systolic BP.[271] However, it had no effect on exercise capacity, symptoms, or other quality-of-life assessments when compared to placebo. The large-scale TOP-CAT trial randomized patients with symptomatic HFpEF, defined as LVEF ≥45%, to receive either spironolactone or placebo.[272] At a mean follow-up of 3.3 years, there was no difference in the primary composite outcome of CV mortality, aborted cardiac arrest, or HF hospitalization. However, spironolactone was associated with a secondary signal of benefit on HF hospitalizations. Further subgroup analysis of the TOPCAT found a controversial heterogeneity of results across regions of enrollment. Eastern European, including Russian and Georgian participants, had roughly equivalent rates of HF hospitalization and CV mortality to age- and gender-matched controls, suggesting that they might not have suffered from HFpEF. They also had no significant changes in BP, creatinine, or potassium levels, and the metabolic product of spironolactone was low or undetected implying nonconsumption of the study medication. By contrast, a post hoc sub-analysis of the Americas, including Canada, United States, Brazil, and Argentina participants, showed that the rates of CV mortality and HF hospitalization were significantly reduced by spironolactone.[273]

Adverse events in the TOPCAT included a higher rate of hyperkalemia and acute kidney injury not requiring dialysis in the spironolactone group. According to current ACC/AHA HF guidelines, MRAs might be considered to decrease hospitalizations in selected patients with HFpEF, defined as LVEF $\geq$45%, with elevated BNP levels or HF admission within 1 year, GFR >30 mL/min/1.73 m^2, creatinine <2.5 mg/dL, and potassium <5.0 mEq/L.

Angiotensin Receptor Neprilysin Inhibitors

Patients with preclinical diastolic dysfunction have an impaired natriuretic and renal endocrine response to acute volume expansion early in the development of HFpEF.[274] The disappointing results of the CHARM-Preserved, PEP-CHF, and I-PRESERVE trials prompted studies with the dual-action agent sacubitril–valsartan, which splits into an ARB and a NEP inhibitor after absorption. NEP inhibition increases NPs and intracellular cGMP, which in turn improves myocardial relaxation and hypertrophy. NPs also stimulate diuresis, natriuresis, and vasodilation, and might have additional antifibrotic and antisympathetic effects.

The proof-of-concept PARAMOUNT-HF trial randomized patients with NYHA class II–III HFpEF, defined as LVEF $\geq$45% and elevated levels of NP, to receive therapy with sacubitril–valsartan or valsartan alone.[275] Sacubitril–valsartan was safe and led to a greater reduction in NT-proBNP at 12 weeks, but not at 36 weeks, along with left atrial reverse remodeling and improvement in NYHA functional class. The PARAMOUNT-HF was followed by the largest clinical trial in HFpEF to date, the PARAGON-HF, which followed a similar protocol to assess the efficacy of sacubitril–valsartan or valsartan alone on the primary composite outcome of CV death and HF hospitalizations. After a median follow-up of 35 months, the sacubitril–valsartan failed to significantly reduce the primary composite outcome. However, exploratory secondary endpoints suggested an improvement in NYHA class and renal function with sacubitril-valsartan. Importantly, there was evidence of a heterogeneous response to treatment, with potential benefit in certain subgroups, such as women and patients in the lower end of the LVEF range included in the study (45% to 57%). Sacubitril–valsartan was associated with a higher rate of hypotension and lower rates of elevated potassium and creatinine compared with valsartan, findings similar to those seen in the PARADIGM-HF trial. Angioedema was also more frequent with sacubitril–valsartan (0.6% vs 0.2%), although none of the cases was associated with airway compromise. Sacubitril–valsartan is currently FDA-approved for use in patients with HF and LVEF ≤40% but has no indication for HFpEF at this time.

β-Blockers

The potential benefits of β-blockers in HFpEF include improvements in BP, HR, diastolic filling time, myocardial oxygen demand, and, with vasodilating agents, arterial stiffness. Conversely, patients with HFpEF have a high prevalence of chronotropic incompetence associated with exercise intolerance, which could be further impaired by β-blockers.

In the SWEDIC study, carvedilol showed echocardiographic improvement in diastolic function from baseline to 6 months when compared to placebo.[276] The SENIORS trial was a placebo-controlled study that tested the effect of nebivolol, a vasodilating β_1-blocker, in both HFpEF and HFrEF patients with a LVEF cut-off of 35% for group characterization.[152] A 14% relative risk reduction was observed in the primary composite outcome of all-cause mortality or CV hospitalization, driven primarily by the effect on hospitalizations, that was not different between patients with LVEF above versus below 35%. However, as very few patients with LVEF ≥50% were included in the trial, no definite conclusion can be drawn about the benefit of nebivolol in HFpEF. The small-size J-DHF trial randomized patients with HFpEF, defined as LVEF >40%, to carvedilol or placebo and found no significant difference in the composite of CV death and unplanned HF hospitalization.[277]

The OPTIMIZE-HF registry found no significant association between β-blocker use and mortality or rehospitalization rates in patients with HFpEF at 60–90 days.[17] However, in a subanalysis including only patients with HR ≥70 beats/min, high-dose β-blocker use was associated with a significantly lower risk of death.[278] Accordingly, the COHERE registry also showed that β-blocker use was associated with a significant reduction in mortality in a cohort of HFpEF patients followed up for 25 months.[279]

There is no definitive evidence for the benefit of β-blockers in patients with HFpEF. According to current ACC/AHA HF guidelines, it is reasonable to use β-blockers for BP control in patients with hypertension and HFpEF.

Digoxin, Calcium Channel Blockers, and Ivabradine

A subgroup analysis of the I-PRESERVE study showed that higher HR was an independent predictor of adverse clinical outcomes among HFpEF patients in normal sinus rhythm.[280] The theory that a reduced diastolic filling time may have detrimental effects in HFpEF led to the investigation of HR-lowering drugs, such as digoxin, nondihydropyridine CCBs, and ivabradine, in that population.

Potential benefits of digoxin in HFpEF include improvements in the active energy-dependent early diastolic function and on neurohormonal profile, as previously described. The DIG ancillary trial was a parallel study to the original DIG trial that included a separate cohort of patients with ambulatory HFpEF, defined as LVEF >45%, and normal sinus rhythm, receiving ACE inhibitors and diuretics.[281] After a mean follow-up of 37 months, digoxin use was not associated with any effect on total, CV, or HF mortality, or total or CV hospitalizations, although a trend toward a reduction of HF hospitalization was observed. To date, the indications for digoxin use in HF are limited to patients with HFrEF. However, it may be considered in patients with HFPEF to slow a rapid ventricular response during AFib.

CCBs may act as third- or fourth-line antihypertensive drugs in patients with HFpEF and hypertension. Data regarding the use of HR-lowering nondihydropyridine CCBs in HFpEF are rare. A small-size placebo-controlled, crossover trial assigned subjects with HFpEF, defined as LVEF >45%, to verapamil or placebo and suggested some improvement of symptoms and exercise tolerance with the CCB.[282] The impact of HR reduction with ivabradine in HFpEF patients is controversial. Small-size randomized trials suggested that short- and long-term treatment with ivabradine is beneficial in terms of diastolic function and exercise capacity improvement in HFpEF patients.[283,284] However, the results of those studies are in contrast with another randomized placebo-controlled trial showing that ivabradine did not improve exercise capacity, but instead worsened VO_2 in the HFpEF cohort.[285] Large randomized trials are required to confirm these observations.

Patients with HFpEF are at greater risk for AFib than the general age-matched population. A rhythm-control strategy is preferred because LV filling in HFpEF occurs largely in late diastole and, consequently, is more dependent on the atrial contraction. When sinus rhythm cannot be achieved, rate control strategy becomes important. The ideal HR in patients with HFpEF and AFib is uncertain, but aggressive HR control might be deleterious and should be avoided. Whether digoxin, β-blockers, or nondihydropyridine CCBs, or a combination of these, should be preferred is unknown. Non-dihydropyridine CCBs should not be combined with a β-blocker.

Nitric Oxide and cGMP Signaling: Phosphodiesterase-5 Inhibitors, Nitrates, and Soluble Guanylate Cyclase Stimulators

PDE-5 inhibitors, nitrates, and sGC stimulators are expected to provide beneficial effects in HFpEF through activation of the NO and cGMP (NO-cGMP) pathway. The NO-cGMP pathway has been shown to play an important role in CV physiology, especially in vasodilation, pulmonary vascular tone, and cardiac remodeling.[286]

The expression of PDE-5 has been proposed to increase in patients with HF. Blockade of cGMP breakdown through PDE-5 inhibition may provide benefits for both vascular and myocardial remodeling, including attenuating hypertrophy, fibrosis, and impaired cardiac relaxation. A small clinical trial demonstrated that after 6 and 12 months, sildenafil significantly improved filling pressures and RV function in patients with HFpEF, defined as LVEF ≥50%, and pulmonary hypertension.[287] Those promising results led to the RELAX trial, which failed to show any difference in exercise capacity or clinical status between sildenafil and placebo in patients with NYHA class II–IV HFpEF, defined as LVEF ≥50%, after 24 weeks of treatment.[288]

Following the neutral results of the RELAX trial, attention had turn to increasing NO availability through use of long-acting nitrates. Nitrates reduce intracardiac filling pressures by lowering both cardiac preload and afterload. Furthermore, high-dose nitrates are effective in improving symptoms and clinical status in patients with ADHF, irrespective of LV systolic function. The NEAT-HFpEF trial was performed on the premise that long-acting isosorbide mononitrate could improve daily activity level in patients with NYHA class II–III HFpEF, defined as LVEF ≥50%.[289] However, at a mean follow-up of 6 weeks, isosorbide mononitrate did not improve quality-of-life, submaximal exercise capacity, or NT-proBNP levels, but instead decreased overall activity levels when compared to placebo.

Although both RELAX and NEAT-HFpEF trials yielded disappointing results, they only observed the short-term effects of each drug in HFpEF patients and did not assess the effects on clinical outcomes. Current ACC/AHA HF guidelines do no recommend the routine use of PDE-5 inhibitors or nitrates to increase activity or quality of life in patients with HFpEF. These recommendations, however, do not apply to patients with angina, for whom nitrates may provide symptomatic relief, or pulmonary arterial hypertension, for whom sildenafil is currently approved.

The oral sGC stimulator riociguat independently activates sGC, the central protein in the NO-cGMP pathway, and also sensitizes it to endogenous NO. The small-size DILATE-1 study tested the hemodynamic effects, safety, and pharmacokinetics of riociguat in patients with HFpEF, defined as LVEF >50%, and pulmonary hypertension.[290] While there was no change in the primary outcome of decrease in mean PAP 6 hours after administration, riociguat significantly improved SV and systolic BP without changing PVR or HR. Large randomized trials are required to confirm these observations.

Other Medications

Contributing factors and comorbidities have an important impact on the clinical course of HFpEF patients. Treatment of hyperlipidemia is recommended for the primary and secondary prevention of CV disease. Besides their lipid-lowering properties, statins also have beneficial effects on LV fibrosis and hypertrophy, endothelial dysfunction, arterial stiffness, and inflammation, all of which contribute to the pathophysiology of HFpEF. While observational data suggest that statins might be of benefit in patients with HFpEF, there are no randomized trials to support its routinely use in clinical practice. In the GISSI-HF trial, no benefit was observed with rosuvastatin in the 10% of patients enrolled with relatively preserved LVEF.[245] Current HF guidelines support the use of statin therapy for patients with known CAD, but do not recommended it for the treatment of HFpEF alone in the absence of other indications.

Ranolazine is a first-in-class anti-anginal drug that selectively inhibits the late sodium current and reduces sodium and calcium overload during ischemia. Data from an HF dog model suggested that ranolazine improves LV end-diastolic pressure. The RALI-DHF trial was a small proof-of-concept study evaluating the effect of ranolazine in patients with HFpEF, defined as LVEF ≥45%, administered intravenously for 24 hours.[291] Ranolazine showed modest improvement in some hemodynamic parameters but had no effect on relaxation. Also, after 14 days of oral administration, there were no significant changes in echocardiographic parameters, NT-proBNP, or exercise performance. Large randomized trials are required to confirm these observations.

Reverse Cardiac Remodeling: Remission Versus Recovery

Advances in medical and device therapies have demonstrated the capacity of the heart to reverse harmful remodeling. Patients who present with improved or recovered LVEF appear to be clinically different from those with persistently reduced or preserved LVEF and have a much better prognosis.[5] Cardiac magnetic resonance findings, specifically the late gadolinium enhancement and the myocardial edema ratio, together with a serial BNP testing may provide a better prediction of LV reverse remodeling than endomyocardial biopsy results or conventional methods of follow-up.[292] Prediction of LV reverse remodeling has important clinical implications, including cost effectiveness of implantable cardioverter-defibrillators and optimal timing for cardiac transplantation referral.

Evidence on whether patients with LV reverse remodeling benefit from indefinite maintenance of therapy is rare, and there are no clear recommendations in guidelines. The TRED-HF trial was an open-label, randomized study of evidence-based medical treatment withdrawal following LV reverse remodeling in patients with a prior diagnosis of DCM taking at least one medication. The primary outcome of HF relapse was met in 44% of subjects in the therapy-withdrawal group compared with none in the control group over a follow-up period of 6 months.[293] During a crossover phase, in which subjects originally assigned to continued treatment underwent therapy withdrawal under the same protocol, the primary outcome was seen in 36% of subjects. Importantly, HF relapse was asymptomatic in all patients over the duration of follow-up. The TRED-HF suggests that, for many patients with LV reverse remodeling, improvement in cardiac function following treatment does not reflect complete recovery but rather reflects remission, which requires indefinite continuation of therapy. Thus, withdrawal of treatment should not be attempted routinely in patients with LV reverse remodeling.

Drugs That Should Be Avoided or Used Cautiously in Heart Failure

Polypharmacy is a significant concern in patients with HF because of the burden of both CV and non-CV conditions. Below is a brief summary of drugs that should be avoided or used with caution in HF. A detailed description of all drug classes that may cause or exacerbate HF is beyond the scope of this document. A 2016

AHA Scientific Statement provides a comprehensive list of such drugs and can be found elsewhere.[294]

Traditional nonsteroidal antiinflammatory drugs (NSAIDs) or cyclooxygenase (COX)-2 inhibitors are not recommended in patients with HF, as they increase the risk of HF precipitation and exacerbation. NSAIDs have the potential to trigger HF through sodium and water retention, increased SVR, and impaired responses to ACE inhibitors and diuretics. They are also associated with increased risk of renal dysfunction and hyperkalemia.

Most anesthetics interfere with cardiac performance either by direct myocardial depression or by impairing hemodynamic responses, such as HR, contractility, preload, afterload, and SVR. Although propofol has both vasodilatory and negative inotropic properties, myocardial depression at clinical doses is minimal. It can decrease BP, SVR, myocardial blood flow, oxygen consumption, and LV preload possibly through direct vasodilation. Such changes may be beneficial in the setting of elevated LV preload, but should be cautiously monitored. Ketamine has both negative inotropic and central sympathetic stimulation effects. In patients with advanced LV dysfunction, the sympathetic stimulation may not be sufficient to overcome its negative inotropic effects, resulting in CV instability.

The oral antidiabetic drugs metformin and thiazolidinediones pose particular risks in patients with HF. Although metformin should be considered the treatment of choice in patients with T2DM and HF, there is an increased risk of potentially lethal lactic acidosis. In 2016, the FDA published a safety warning recommending that metformin should be contraindicated in patients with renal function below 30 mL/min/1.73 m^2. Thiazolidinediones cause sodium and water retention, which may precipitate HF. The 2016 American Diabetes Association standards of medical care recommend avoiding thiazolidinediones in patients with symptomatic HF. There is also limited evidence suggesting that dipeptidyl peptidase-4 inhibitors, including sitagliptin, saxagliptin, alogliptin, and linagliptin, may increase the risk of HF hospitalization. The true mechanism of this potential risk remains unknown, but given their current popularity and growing use, randomized clinical trials in patients with established HF are needed.

Most antiarrhythmics have a negative inotropic activity that can precipitate HF. Some exert an additional proarrhythmic effect, particularly class I sodium-channel blockers and class III ibutilide, sotalol, and dofetilide, and should be contraindicated in patients with HF. Also, as previously discussed, the ANDROMEDA trial was terminated prematurely for increased mortality in the class III dronedarone-treated HF subjects. The latter PALLAS study was also terminated early due to an increase in CV death, stroke, and

HF hospitalization associated with dronedarone. Thus, dronedarone is contraindicated in patients with symptomatic HF with recent decompensation requiring hospitalization, or NYHA class IV HF.

CCBs should generally be avoided in patients with chronic HFrEF. Some dihydropyridine CCBs, such as nifedipine, have both negative inotropic and vasodilating effects and have been associated with higher incidence of HF hospitalization and premature discontinuation of therapy due to clinical deterioration. By contrast, amlodipine, a dihydropyridine CCB without negative inotropic effect, appears to be safe in patients with HF and can be used to treat associated angina or hypertension. Of note, both PRAISE and PRAISE 2 trials assessing the effects of amlodipine in HF reported a higher incidence of peripheral edema and pulmonary congestion that should be considered when prescribing the drug. Nondihydropyridine CCBs, such as diltiazem and verapamil, cause less vasodilation but more contractility depression than dihydropyridine CCBs.

Some antifungal agents, such as itraconazole or amphotericin B, have been associated with reports of cardiotoxicity, premature ventricular contractions, ventricular fibrillation, hypertension, and new-onset cardiomyopathy or worsening HF. Other antimicrobial agents, such as trimethoprim-sulfamethoxazole, should be avoided or used with caution in patients taking ACE inhibitors, ARBs, or MRAs, due to an elevated risk of hyperkalemia.

Limited data are available on the safety and efficacy of neurological and psychiatric medications in patients with HF. Considering the well-recognized risk of sympathetic stimulation in patients with serious cardiac disease, amphetamines should not be used in patients with HF. Among antiepileptic drugs, carbamazepine has been associated with hypotension, AV block, and HF symptoms in patients without CV disease, while pregabalin is possibly related to peripheral edema and HF exacerbation. Several antipsychotic medications have been associated with torsades de pointes secondary to QT prolongation. Tricyclic antidepressants (TCAs) have numerous known adverse CV effects, including sinus tachycardia, postural hypotension, second- and third-degree block, QT prolongation, and direct myocardial depression. While selective serotonin reuptake inhibitors (SSRI) have a lower rate of adverse CV effects than TCAs, some SSRI, like citalopram, may present a dose-dependent risk of QT prolongation, which could lead to torsades de pointes. The largest randomized study of depression in HFrEF, the SADHART-CHF trial, showed that although the use of the SSRI sertraline was safe, it did not provide greater improvement in depression or CV status when compared with nurse-facilitated support.[295]

Concerns have been raised about the safety of PDE inhibitors in patients with HF. Earlier experience with long-term oral milrinone was associated with increased risk of fatal arrhythmias compared with placebo, and thus, none of the currently available oral PDE-3 inhibitors are approved for use in patients with HF.[296] While it is not established if cilostazol, an oral PDE-3 inhibitor used in the treatment of intermittent claudication, impacts mortality in patients with HF, the FDA recommends against its use in HF of any severity. The PDE-5 inhibitors, including sildenafil, vardenafil, and tadalafil, are used in the treatment of erectile dysfunction in men by increasing the amount of cGMP that relaxes the corpus cavernosum smooth muscle. They are potent vasodilators that can also lower pulmonary and systemic arterial pressure. The combined use of PDE-5 inhibitors with any form of nitrate therapy is contraindicated due to the risk of severe hypotension. Combination with other PDE inhibitors, such as milrinone, should be avoided as well.

Several antineoplastic chemotherapy agents are cardiotoxic and can lead to short- and long-term cardiac morbidity. Anthracycline-induced cardiotoxicity has been studied extensively and is associated in large part to the cumulative generation of free radicals leading to LV dysfunction and HF. Antimetabolites, such as 5-fluorouracil, and targeted therapies, including ErbB antagonists, tyrosine kinase inhibitors, and monoclonal antibodies, also have shown to induce cardiomyopathy and myocardial ischemia. In contrast to anthracycline-induced cardiotoxicity, trastuzumab-related cardiac dysfunction is most often reversible and does not appear to increase with cumulative dose, nor is it associated with ultrastructural changes in the myocardium. Cardiac arrhythmias and hypertension have been described with the use of tyrosine kinase inhibitors and antimicrotubule agents, while pericarditis can happen with the use of bleomycin, cyclophosphamide, or cytarabine. Mediastinal radiation can also cause constrictive pericarditis, myocardial fibrosis, valvular lesions, and CAD. Iron-chelating agents that prevent generation of oxygen free radicals, such as dexrazoxane, may confer some cardioprotection in patients receiving anthracyclines. According to current ESC HF guidelines, chemotherapy should be discontinued and HFrEF therapy initiated in patients developing moderate to severe LV systolic dysfunction. If LV function improves, the risks and benefits of further chemotherapy need to be individualized.

Pharmacological Treatment of Selected Cardiomyopathies

Cardiomyopathies are diseases of the heart muscle that may arise from a variety of underlying conditions including genetic abnormalities, myocyte injury, or infiltrative processes of the myocardial and interstitial tissues.[297,298] The term is intended to exclude cardiac dysfunction that results from other structural heart disease, such as CAD, primary valve disease, severe hypertension, and congenital heart disease. The most common classification is based on structural and functional changes, including dilated, hypertrophic, and restrictive cardiomyopathies. The general goals of cardiomyopathy treatment are to manage signs and symptoms, prevent HF worsening, and reduce the risk of complications. In most cases, chronic HF should be treated according to current HF guidelines. However, specific treatment may differ according to underlying disease. Below is a brief summary of the current understanding and specific pharmacological treatment of selected cardiomyopathies. A 2016 AHA Scientific Statement on current diagnostic and treatment strategies for specific cardiomyopathies provides a comprehensive review on the management of most cardiomyopathies.[299]

Cardiac amyloidosis usually starts as restrictive cardiomyopathy with mild LV systolic dysfunction and significant diastolic dysfunction but can progress to severe HF in advanced stages. The most common types of cardiac amyloidosis encountered in clinical practice, defined by their precursor proteins, are primary light-chain (AL) and familial or senile transthyretin (ATTR). Treatment is for the most part supportive. AL amyloidosis may have a very poor prognosis, especially when other organs are affected by progressive amyloid deposition. Patients with important clinical cardiac involvement in AL amyloidosis have been largely excluded from studies with melphalan and hematopoietic cell transplantation. ATTR cardiac amyloidosis is the most common form of cardiac amyloidosis and typically results from deposition of transthyretin, a transport protein that carries thyroxine and retinol-binding protein-retinol complex, in the myocardium. The randomized, placebo-controlled ATTR-ACT trial tested tafamidis, a transthyretin stabilizer, in patients with ATTR cardiomyopathy and showed a significant reduction in overall mortality and CV hospitalization at 30 months when compared to placebo.[300] Tafamidis was also associated with improvements in quality-of-life assessments and functional status. On the strength of those findings, the FDA granted tafamidis a "breakthrough therapy designation" in 2018.

In patients with cardiomyopathy related to substance abuse, total abstinence from cardiotoxic agents and drugs is recommended. There are no studies of specific pharmacotherapies in patients with alcoholic cardiomyopathy other than the standard therapy for HF. However, recovery of ventricular function has been observed in some patients following cessation of alcohol intake, largely in the early course of the disease.

Peripartum cardiomyopathy (PPCM) is an uncommon form of HF that happens during the last month of pregnancy or up to 5 months postpartum. Guideline-recommended HF therapies should be considered, with special attention to specific classes of drugs that are contraindicated during pregnancy and/or breastfeeding. Preliminary data have suggested a potential benefit from prolactin blockade with bromocriptine on the basis of its proposed mechanistic role in PPCM. However, further studies are needed before recommendations on bromocriptine use can be issued.

Corticosteroids are considered the mainstay of therapy for autoimmune cardiomyopathic syndromes, such as cardiac sarcoidosis and eosinophilic endocarditis.[301] However, the optimal dose and duration of treatment have not been well recognized. Chagas cardiomyopathy is a major public health disease in Latin America and, due to migration, is becoming a worldwide health and economic burden. Antiparasitic therapy with benznidazole is recommended for acute and congenital disease, reactivated infections, and chronic disease in patients younger than 18 years, but its role in the chronic phase of Chagas cardiomyopathy remains controversial.[302]

Tachycardia-induced cardiomyopathy (TIC) is a rare but potentially reversible cause of HF, resulting from long-standing tachyarrhythmia or frequent ectopic beats. Although available data suggest that a HR > 100 beats/min can lead to HF, the exact HR at which TIC occurs is not defined. Maintenance of sinus rhythm or control of ventricular rate is indicated in treating patients with TIC, as previously described.

The evidence supporting HF treatment in the pediatric population comes largely from adult studies and includes diuretics, β-blockers, RAAS inhibitors, and other medications as previously described. Lysosomal storage diseases (LSDs) are a group of about 50 rare inherited metabolic disorders that result from deficiencies in catabolic enzymes leading to pathogenic lysosomal accumulation. Each LSD is characterized by the accumulation of specific substrates. Some LSDs, such as Pompe and Fabry diseases, are known to cause cardiomyopathy. Other, like the Gaucher disease, rarely cause cardiac involvement, although allelic variants have been reported, with valvular disease and recurrent pericarditis resulting in constriction. Genetic testing occasionally enables the detection of LSDs for which replacement of defective enzymes is indicated and has been shown to produce substantial clinical benefit.

Iron-overload cardiomyopathy results from the accumulation of iron in the myocardium, and it is the leading cause of death in patients receiving chronic blood transfusion therapy.[303] Definitive treatment is centered on iron removal, usually through phlebotomy in patients with hereditary hemochromatosis or chelation therapy in those with secondary iron overload. The optimal chelation regime must be individualized and will vary according to the current clinical situation.

Future Perspectives

Despite an overwhelming progress in the treatment of HFrEF, HF as a syndrome is still frequently associated with unacceptably high rates of rehospitalization and mortality. In addition, evidence-based medicine with respect to optimal treatment of ADHF and HFpEF remains scarce, with very limited direct data to support any specific drug regimen. The complexity of HF requires a widespread application of best-care practice standards aligned with new medical treatment options.

Research of molecules that modulate contractility accompanied by a growing appreciation of the role of pharmacogenomics may lead to further advances in the field of HFrEF.[34] Ongoing efforts to elucidate the pathobiology of individuals with HF will be better defined by specific expressed microRNAs, which may lead to a tailored therapy with RNA analogues, gene or cell therapy.[304]

To address the knowledge gap in ADHF, the AHA advocates for coordinated international efforts to identify research priorities, conduct clinical trials, and create large population-based registries.[97] Potential therapeutic targets for HFpEF are cardiometabolic abnormalities, microvascular inflammation, and cellular/extracellular structural changes. Ongoing studies are evaluating novel therapies including antiinflammatory drugs, mitochondrial activators, antifibrotic agents, and strategies to enhance the compliance of titin, the elastic sarcomeric protein that regulates cardiomyocyte-derived stiffness.[266]

Summary

1. Drug therapies for HF differ depending on the distinct phenotype and its presentation. Distinctive phenotypes of presentation have different management targets, ranging from acute HF to chronic HF with reduced or preserved ejection fraction.

2. Management of acute HF is largely based on clinical evidence of hypoperfusion or congestion and their combination: Diuretics and vasodilators are often chosen to relieve congestive symptoms. Inotropic agents, such as dobutamine and dopamine, should be considered in patients with low CO syndrome resulting in hypoperfusion, hypotension, and end-organ damage.

3. Cardiogenic shock: vasopressors, such as NE, high-dose dopamine, and high-dose epinephrine, should be reserved for patients with persistent hypotension, especially in the management of cardiogenic shock when persistent hypoperfusion is evident despite optimization of filling pressures.

4. Drugs for chronic HF with reduced ejection fraction: neurohormonal modulation targeting adrenergic, renin–angiotensin–aldosterone and NP systems has become the cornerstone of medical therapy in patients with chronic HF with reduced ejection fraction. β-Blockers, ACE inhibitors, ARBs, MRAs, and angiotensin receptor-neprilysin inhibitors have been shown to improve outcomes and are recommended, unless contraindicated or not tolerated. The combination of nitrates and hydralazine is also a useful adjunct in self-identified blacks, while ivabradine and digoxin should be considered in select patients who remain symptomatic despite standard therapy. The SGLT-2 inhibitors, such as dapagliflozin, have demonstrated improved outcomes irrespective of underlying diabetes mellitus.

5. Associated conditions in chronic HF with reduced ejection fraction: therapeutic anticoagulation is the mainstay of risk reduction strategies in patients with HF and atrial fibrillation or a history of systemic or pulmonary emboli. Amiodarone is the ideal antiarrhythmic drug for rhythm control strategy and may improve the success of electrical cardioversion. Intravenous iron supplementation might be reasonable in subjects with iron deficiency, while erythropoiesis-stimulating agents are associated with an excess of thromboembolic events and should be avoided. Omega-3 polyunsaturated fatty acids are generally safe and well tolerated, with modest improvements in clinical outcomes.

6. Drugs for chronic HF with preserved ejection fraction: at least half of all patients with HF have preserved ejection fraction. No treatment has yet been shown to reduce morbidity in this population. Large randomized clinical trials had conflicting or neutral results. Since these patients are often elderly with a poor quality of life, an important aim of therapy may be to alleviate symptoms and improve well-being.

7. Reverse cardiac remodeling: advances in medical and device therapies have demonstrated the capacity of the heart to reverse

harmful remodeling. For many patients with reverse remodeling, improvement in cardiac function following treatment does not reflect complete recovery, but rather reflects remission, which requires indefinite continuation of therapy. Thus, withdrawal of treatment should not be attempted routinely in this population.

8. Drugs for selected cardiomyopathies: specific therapies for certain cardiomyopathies may differ according to underlying disease. Tafamidis, a transthyretin stabilizer, was associated with reductions in mortality and hospitalizations in patients with transthyretin amyloid cardiomyopathy. Preliminary data have suggested a potential benefit from prolactin blockade with bromocriptine in patients with peripartum cardiomyopathy. Corticosteroids are considered the mainstay of therapy for autoimmune cardiomyopathic syndromes, such as cardiac sarcoidosis and eosinophilic endocarditis. Antiparasitic therapy with benznidazole is recommended for acute, congenital, and reactivated Chagas disease, but its role in the chronic phase of Chagas cardiomyopathy remains controversial. For pediatric patients with lysosomal storage diseases, enzyme replacement is indicated and has been shown to produce substantial clinical benefit.

References

Complete reference list available at www.expertconsult.com.

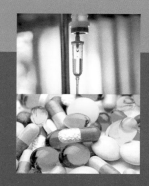

中文导读

第4章
糖尿病的药物治疗

据估计，在美国有1/3的人口会患上2型糖尿病，而2型糖尿病患者更容易出现心血管异常，其发病和死亡的主要原因是动脉粥样硬化性心血管疾病。

本章虽然名为糖尿病的药物治疗，但其实更侧重于阐述治疗糖尿病所用药物的心血管获益。

首先要评估糖尿病患者罹患心血管疾病的风险。目前主流的两个糖尿病指南都建议使用特定种族和性别的合并队列方程来评估首次患动脉粥样硬化性心血管疾病的10年风险。这一风险模型与患者是否患有糖尿病无关，即患者有无糖尿病均适用这一模型。同时，这两个指南还建议评估糖尿病特有的心血管危险因素。在临床实践中，最好评估所有共存的心脏代谢危险因素（包括代谢综合征）、糖尿病病程和发病年龄。

其次是治疗，本章尤其强调以下两点：①客观看待强化血糖控制的价值；②关注体现心血管疾病结局的大型临床试验。

多项随机对照研究证实，强化血糖控制可以减少2型糖尿病患者的微血管并发症。但大型临床试验（ACCORD，ADVANCE，VADT）的结果并未显示更严格的血糖控制可显著减少心血管疾病的不良结局。对于有长期2型糖尿病病史、低血糖病史的患者及老年患者，他们不太可能从严格的血糖控制中受益，且风险可能大于获益。在这种情况下，医师应慎用强化血糖控制。为了制定个体化的血糖控制目标，建议评估以下七项指标：低血糖或药物不良反应的风险、病程、预期寿命、并发症、已存在的血管并发症、患者偏好、医疗资源和支持系统。

本章根据目前临床试验证实的心血管疾病的获益情况，将糖尿病的治疗药物分为以下两大类：①降低心血管疾病风险的药物，包括二甲双胍、钠–葡萄糖协同转运蛋白2抑制剂和胰高血糖素样肽-1受体激动剂；②未降低心血管疾病风险的药物，包括二肽基肽酶4抑制剂、噻唑烷二酮类、磺脲类和胰岛素。本章节从这些药物的作用机制、同类但不同种药物的区别、临床试验数据、心血管结局、不良反应、药物相互作用等多个方面进行了详细介绍。

另外，需要注意的是，糖尿病患者的低血糖发作也会影响心血管健康，多项研究已经观察到低血糖发作和不良心血管结局之间的相关性。

舟　君

Drugs for Diabetes

CARA REITER-BRENNAN · OMAR DZAYE ·
MICHAEL J. BLAHA · ROBERT H. ECKEL

Metabolic Syndrome and Prediabetes

Obesity has become a common problem in Western society, and it is a strong predictor of type 2 diabetes mellitus (T2DM).[1,2] In the United States it is estimated that almost one-third of the population will develop T2DM in their lifetimes. T2DM, in turn, predisposes to cardiovascular abnormalities.[2]

An increased waistline is one of the five criteria of the metabolic syndrome (MetSyn)—a prediabetic state—in addition to fasting hyperglycemia and blood pressure (BP) elevation, increased circulating triglycerides (TGs), and decreased circulating high-density lipoprotein (HDL) cholesterol (HDL-C) (Fig. 4.1).[3] Three of these are required for the diagnosis of the MetSyn (Table 4.1).[4] Abdominal girth, insulin resistance (IR), and insulin response are the three main factors that, each independently, increase the metabolic risk of cardiovascular disease (CVD).[5] However, waist circumference is a better predictor of the risk of myocardial infarction (MI) than body mass index (BMI) is.[6]

Abdominal adipose tissue is now recognized as a metabolically active organ and regarded as the basic abnormality in the MetSyn by the International Diabetes Federation.[7] There are strong links between excessive abdominal fat leading to excessive circulating free fatty acids (FFAs) and cytokines, which contribute to the other four features of the MetSyn and help explain worsening IR (Fig. 4.2).[6] The MetSyn is of clinical importance in that it increases the risk of CVD and especially T2DM, driven almost entirely by the fasting glucose component.[8] Currently an increasing number of patients with the MetSyn obesity or T2DM are being treated by cardiologists, often in close collaboration with primary care physicians and diabetologists.

HDL & TG IN METABOLIC SYNDROME & DIABETES

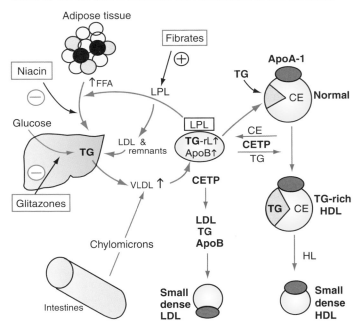

Fig. 4.1   HDL and TG in metabolic syndrome and diabetes. Consistent features (see *right side* of the figure) are the increased circulating levels of triglycerides *(TGs)* and decreased high-density lipoprotein *(HDL)* cholesterol. The basic problem lies in increased levels of the atherogenic particles: very-low density lipoproteins *(VLDLs)*, triglyceride-rich lipoprotein *(TG-rL)*, and apolipoprotein *(Apo)* B. (Apos have detergent-like properties that solubilize the hydrophobic lipoproteins.) Levels of TG-rL and Apo B are increased by (1) excess hepatic synthesis of VLDL, (2) high postprandial TG concentrations after a fatty meal, and (3) low levels of lipoprotein lipase *(LPL)* activity. Adipose tissue releases excess free fatty acids *(FFAs)*, which with hyperglycemia leads to increased hepatic production of VLDL. Cholesterol-ester transfer protein *(CETP)* increases the transfer of TG to HDL particles to form TG-rich HDL, with a simultaneous transfer of cholesteryl esters *(CE)* from the HDL particles to TG-rL. TG-rich HDL is broken down by hepatic lipase *(HL)* to form small, dense HDL particles. A similar process leads to increased formation of small dense low-density lipoprotein *(LDL)* particles.

Table 4.1

Common Definitions for Metabolic Syndrome	
Criterion	NCEP ATP III (3 or more criteria)
Abdominal obesity	Waist circumference
Men	>40 inches (>102 cm)
Women	>35 inches (>88 cm)
Hypertriglyceridemia	>150 mg/dl (≥1.7 mmol/L)
Low HDL	
Men	<40 mg/dl (<1.03 mmol/L)
Women	<50 mg/dl (<1.30 mmol/L)
Hypertension	≥130/85 mm Hg or on antihypertensive medication
Impaired fasting glucose or diabetes	>100 mg/dl (5.6 mmol/L) or taking insulin or hypoglycemic medication

From Floege J, et al.: Comprehensive clinical nephrology, ed 4, Philadelphia, 2010, Saunders.

Risks of Metabolic Syndrome

MetSyn comprises a group of cardiometabolic risk factors, each of which individually may be of only borderline significance, but when taken together indicate enhanced risk of development of overt T2DM or CVD. While a useful tool to communicate underlying pathophysiology and shared risk factors, influential authorities have questioned the independent predictive value of the MetSyn for the future development of T2DM and stress the role of one of the five components alone; glucose.[9] For cardiologists, becoming alert to risk-factor clustering, including abdominal obesity, high TGs, low HDL-C, prehypertension, and hyperglycemia, is an important widening of vision.[10] The risk of developing future CVD is proportional to the number of MetSyn features.[11] With four or five features, the risk of T2DM was 25-fold greater than with no features and still much more than with only one feature.[12] In an analysis of 172,573 persons in 37 studies, MetSyn had a relative risk of 1.78 for future cardiovascular events, and the association remained after adjusting for traditional cardiovascular risk factors (relative risk [RR], 1.54; confidence interval [CI], 1.32–1.79).[13] The International Day for Evaluation of Abdominal Obesity study measured waistlines in 168,000 primary care patients spread worldwide to confirm an association between waist and CVD (RR 1.36) and more so with T2DM (RR 1.59 in men and 1.83 in women).[8]

METABOLIC SYNDROME

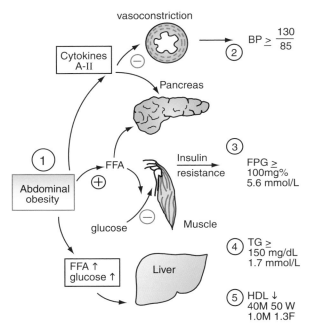

Fig. 4.2 Metabolic syndrome. The adipose tissue releases increased free fatty acids *(FFAs)* into the circulation, thereby inhibiting the uptake of glucose by muscle. Plasma glucose rises and elicits an insulin response. However, the pancreas is damaged by the high FFA levels and increased cytokines. The net effect is increased fasting plasma glucose *(FPG)* despite the increased circulating insulin (insulin resistance). Increased plasma FFA and glucose predispose to increased hepatic synthesis of triglycerides *(TGs)* and increased blood levels of TG, which in turn decrease levels of high-density lipoprotein *(HDL)* cholesterol. Increased release of angiotensin II *(A-II)* from the abdominal fat causes vasoconstriction and increases the blood pressure *(BP).* F, Female; M, male. For details, see Opie LH. Metabolic syndrome. *Circulation* 2007;115:e32.

Insulin Resistance

IR leads to the MetSyn[5] via increased circulating FFA (Fig. 4.2) and elevated glucose production in the liver, which are the precursors of T2DM.[14] There is a dose-response effect of elevated plasma FFA on insulin signaling.[15] Importantly, early life dietary patterns strongly predispose to IR.

How is obesity related to IR? Already modestly elevated FFA often observed in obese persons, and in some increased FFA flux, inhibit insulin signaling[15] and stimulate nuclear factor kappa B (NFκB) to promote IR (Figure 1 in Kim, 2012).[16] NFκB in turn stimulates macrophages to provoke the chronic low-grade inflammatory response (Figure 2 in Kim, 2012)[16] with increased plasma levels of C-reactive protein, and inflammatory cytokines such as tumor necrosis factor–alpha, interleukin (IL) 6, monocyte chemotactic protein 1, and IL-8, and the multifunctional proteins leptin and osteopontin.[14] The "Western" high-fat diet experimentally enhances such cytokine production, whereas exercise diminishes it.[17] The overall sequence is:

$$\text{Obesity} \rightarrow \text{FFA flux} \rightarrow \text{NFκB} \rightarrow \text{macrophages}$$
$$\rightarrow \text{inflammatory cytokines} \rightarrow \text{insulin resistance}$$

Diabetes Prevention

Lifestyle Changes to Slow the Onset of Diabetes

The transition from MetSyn to full-blown T2DM can be significantly lessened by lifestyle intervention. Walking only approximately 19 km per week can be beneficial in treating MetSyn.[18] However, more intense intervention is needed for more substantial change. Tuomilehto et al.[19] studied a group of overweight subjects with impaired glucose tolerance who, on average, also had the features of the MetSyn. Dietary advice and exercise programs were individually tailored. The five aims were weight reduction, decreased fat intake, decreased saturated fat intake, increased fiber intake, and increased endurance exercise (at least 30 minutes daily). Of these, increased exercise was achieved in 86% of participants, and the other components less frequently. After a mean duration of 3.2 years, the relative risk for new T2DM in the lifestyle intervention group was 0.4 ($P < 0.001$).

In the Diabetes Prevention Group,[20] similar subjects were given lifestyle modification or metformin for a mean of 2.8 years. Lifestyle intervention was very intense with a 16-lesson curriculum covering diet, exercise, and behavior modification taught by case managers on a one-to-one basis during the first 24 weeks after enrollment. Lifestyle intervention was more effective than metformin in delaying the onset of T2DM, and both were more effective than placebo in preventing new T2DM.

However, while lifestyle intervention may significantly reduce the severity of DM, lifestyle changes seem to have little effect on the cardiovascular risk seen in T2DM. In the Look-AHEAD study, the National Institute of Health sponsored a randomized controlled trial, assessing if Intensive Lifestyle Intervention (ILI) or Diabetes Support and Education (DSE) would lead to cardiovascular benefits in overweight or obese T2DM patients.[21] Look-AHEAD was stopped prematurely because of futility, as there was no difference in reduction of cardiovascular events between the two groups. For the ILI group, the cardiovascular event rate was 1.83 per 100 patient-years while the DSE group had a similar rate of 1.92 events for 100 patient-years (HR 0.95, 95% CI 0.83–1.09, $P = 0.51$). However, other aspects of DM morbidity were improved in the ILI group, such as glucose and lipid control biomarkers, sleep apnea, liver fat, depression, quality of life, knee pain, inflammation, sexual function, and kidney disease. Overall, these outcomes reduced health care costs of the ILI group.[21,22]

Is the protection from DM found in the Diabetes Prevention Group study sustained? The postintervention 10-year follow-up says no, with an equal incidence of new T2DM in placebo, former lifestyle, and metformin groups. Yet the cumulative incidence of T2DM remained lowest in the lifestyle group. Thus, prevention or delay of T2DM with lifestyle intervention or metformin may persist for at least 10 years.

Blood Pressure and Lifestyle

Modest BP elevation, a component of the MetSyn, is often associated with overweight and obesity. Weight loss and exercise in the setting of intensive behavioral intervention in the MetSyn can reduce systolic blood pressure (SBP) in the range of 8 mmHg with small additional reductions if the Dietary Approaches to Stop Hypertension (DASH) diet is added.[23] When added drugs are required, β-blockers and diuretics should be considered second-line agents and avoided except when there are compelling indications. There is now growing but controversial evidence that new T2DM may develop during the therapy of hypertension, more so with β-blockers and diuretics than with angiotensin-converting enzyme (ACE) inhibitors and angiotensin receptor blockers (ARBs) (Fig. 4.3).[24] There is a "weight of evidence against

DRUG-RELATED NEW DIABETES

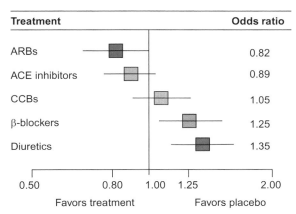

Treatment	Odds ratio
ARBs	0.82
ACE inhibitors	0.89
CCBs	1.05
β-blockers	1.25
Diuretics	1.35

0.50   0.80   1.00   1.25   2.00

Favors treatment   Favors placebo

Fig. 4.3 Drug-related new diabetes. Network meta-analysis of 22 trials with 143,153 patients, using placebo as referent agent, and including earlier higher-dose diuretic trials. *ACE,* Angiotensin conversion enzyme; *ARBs,* angiotensin receptor blockers; *CCB,* calcium channel blocker. (Data from Lam SKH, Owen A. Incident diabetes in clinical trials of antihypertensive drugs. *Lancet* 2007;369:1513–1514.)

β-blockers" as first choice for obese patients with hypertension.[25] A network meta-analysis linked diuretic and β-blocker therapy separately to new T2DM in hypertension (Fig. 4.3).[26] Thus, current European Hypertension Guidelines list MetSyn as a possible contradiction to the use of β-blockers and diuretics (thiazides/thiazide-like).[27] In view of the potential increased risk of new T2DM, it seems prudent to give preference to antihypertensive therapy initially based on ACE inhibitors or ARBs, with low-dose diuretics (hydrochlorothiazide 12.5 to 25 mg) as needed (unless there are compelling indications for β-blocker–diuretic therapy).

Which Drugs Halt the Slide to Diabetes?

Metformin 850 mg twice daily when given in the Diabetes Prevention Study[28] reduced future T2DM, albeit less than vigorous lifestyle changes.

Thiazolidinediones (TZDs) increase hepatic and peripheral insulin sensitivity by activation of peroxisome proliferator-activated receptor-γ (PPAR-γ) receptors. In the ACT NOW trial (Actos Now for Prevention of Diabetes), pioglitazone, as compared to placebo, reduced the risk of conversion of impaired glucose tolerance to T2DM by 72%, but was associated with significant weight gain and edema.[29]

Acarbose inhibits the intestinal absorption of glucose but is often poorly tolerated because of gastrointestinal symptoms. Findings from the Acarbose Cardiovascular Evaluation (ACE) trial, a randomized, double-blind, placebo-controlled phase IV ACE trial of 6522 Chinese adults, demonstrated a reduction of T2DM incidence by 18%.[30] However, there was no significant reduction in the incidence of the composite, five-point major adverse cardiovascular events (MACE).[30]

Because there have been no comparative studies between metformin, acarbose, and TZDs, it is difficult to say with certainty which would be most effective in preventing progression to new T2DM should lifestyle modifications prove inadequate. However, metformin and pioglitazone have convincing data. In light of this, the 2019 Standards of Medical Care of the American Diabetes Association (ADA) recommend metformin for high-risk individuals (patients with gestational diabetes mellitus history or BMI $\geq 35\,kg/m^2$) due to strong evidence, low cost, and safety profile.[31]

What Can Be Achieved?

For lifestyle by itself to be effective in preventing transition to T2DM as well as reducing BP, major behavioral changes have to be affected, requiring intense input from professional personnel such as nutritionists and exercise physiologists. Although this intensive counseling may not be a cost-effective approach when applied to the general population, it is undeniable that the ideal strategy for the whole population is a broad behavior modification that avoids obesity. Drug therapy to prevent the transition to T2DM is both feasible and effective in selected patients, yet not widely applied.

Cardiovascular Disease Risk Assessment

The primary cause of morbidity and mortality of individuals with T2DM is atherosclerotic cardiovascular disease (ASCVD).[32] While T2DM is clearly associated with risk, not all patients with T2DM are at the same risk.[33] A meta-analysis of 45,108 patients in 13 trials showed that patients without T2DM but with a prior MI had a 43% higher coronary heart disease (CHD) risk than individuals with

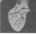

T2DM without previous CVD.[34] This risk heterogeneity argues for the routine use of risk assessment in clinical practice.

Risk Calculators

Both major current DM guidelines, the 2019 guidelines by the American College of Cardiology and the American Heart Association (ACC/AHA) and the 2019 ADA/EASD Standards of Medical Care, recommend evaluating the 10-year risk of first atherosclerotic CVD (10-year ASCVD) using the race-and sex-specific pooled cohort equation (PCE). This risk model is used for patients with as well as without DM. The use of DM-specific risk calculators is questionable, as most studies have shown that risk factors modify CVD risk similarly, irrespective of whether or not the patient suffers from DM.[35] However, when intermediate risk (7.5%–20%) is present, noninvasive imaging such as a coronary calcium score may be useful in decision making to follow, i.e., intensity of statin and aspirin therapy.

Risk Enhancing Factors

In addition to using risk calculators, both guidelines also recommend evaluating CVD risk by assessing each patient's diabetes-specific cardiovascular risk factors (Tables 4.2 and 4.3). The ADA Standards of Medical Care recommend the assessment of these risk factors at least annually. In clinical practice, it is best to assess any comorbid cardiometabolic risk factors (including presence of Met-Syn), the duration of DM, and the age of onset.

Duration of Diabetes

Duration of DM is independently associated with cardiovascular events. Evidence shows that patients with >10-year history of

Table 4.2

Risk-enhancing factors according to the 2019 ACC/AHA Guidelines on the primary prevention of cardiovascular disease
Long duration (>10 years for type 2 diabetes mellitus (S4.3-61) or >20 years for type 1 diabetes mellitus Albuminuria >30 µg albumin/mg creatinine eGFR <60 mL/min/1.73 m^2 Retinopathy Neuropathy ABI <0.9

ABI, ankle brachial index; *eGFR*, estimated glomerular filtration flow.

Table 4.3

Risk-enhancing factors according to 2019 ADA guideline "Standard of Medical Care"
Obesity
Hypertension
Chronic kidney disease
Smoking
Family history of premature coronary disease
Dyslipidemia
Presence of albuminuria

T2DM without history of CHD have similar risk of CHD as patients without DM but with prior CHD.[36] By extension, individuals with less than 10 years of T2DM history are not considered CHD risk equivalents. The 2019 ACC/AHA guidelines of preventive CVD state that a T2DM duration of over 10 years is an independent cardiovascular risk enhancer. [37]

Age of Onset

Age of T2DM diagnosis is an important prognostic factor for cardiovascular risk.

A study using data from the Swedish National Diabetes Registry showed that patients diagnosed with T2DM before the age of 40 had the highest excess relative risk for CVD-related mortality (HR 1.95 [1.68–2.25]), heart failure (HF) (HR 4.77 [3.86–5.89]), and CHD (HR 4.33 [3.82-4.91]) compared to controls. Controls were randomly selected individuals from the general population matched for age, sex, and county. The authors observed that all CVD risks diminished with each additional decade of diagnostic age. Survival of patients with T2DM diagnosed in adolescence was almost a decade less than controls, while patients diagnosed >80 years had the same survival as controls.[38]

Data from a cross-sectional survey of 222,773 T2DM patients showed that early-onset T2DM (mean diagnostic age 35 years) was associated with a higher risk of nonfatal CVD events compared to late-onset T2DM (mean diagnostic age 55 years) (OR, 1.91; 95% CI, 1.81–2.02).[39] While the risk was diminished when adjusted for DM duration, it still remained significant (OR, 1.13; 95% CI 1.06–1.20). This study showed that while duration of T2DM and diagnostic age are associated, age of onset is an independent and significant risk factor for CVD.[39,40]

The ADA 2019 Standards of Medical Care specifically point out that patients with youth-onset T2DM have a particularly high risk of suffering from DM complications.[31] A cross-sectional study of 2733 patients showed that youth-onset T2DM is associated with microvascular as well as macrovascular risk burden.[41] Further, β-cell function in patients with youth onset T2DM seems to deteriorate faster than that of βT2 cells of patients with adult-onset DM.[42]

Coronary Artery Calcium Testing

The CHD and CVD risk variability of patients with T2DM is perhaps best measured by coronary artery calcium (CAC). The CAC score—resulting from a noncontrast cardiac-gated computed tomography scan of the heart—is a marker for atherosclerosis burden, in effect measuring the cumulative effect of a lifetime exposure of measured and unmeasured cardiovascular risk factors.[43] Evidence suggests that CAC can improve risk discrimination of CHD and CVD events more effectively than traditional risk factors.[44] Studies have also shown that the CAC score mirrors the variance in CVD risk of patients with T2DM. For instance, a study by Silverman et al. showed that most individuals with DM <60 years have an extremely low risk at <5 deaths per 1000 person years when CAC = 0.[45] In contrast, CAC was detected in almost all patients with DM with prior CHD (92.5%) and CVD (82.5%) events.[46]

The Diabetes Heart Study suggested that CAC scoring can reclassify risk of patients with T2DM with a heightened risk for CVD mortality.[47] The study showed that CVD mortality risk increased proportionally to CAC score after adjusting for cardiovascular factors. The area under the curve (AUC) without CAC was 0.70 (0.67–0.73) while with CAC was 0.75 (0.72–0.78). After addition of the CAC, the model that classified participants into different risk categories reclassified 28% individuals with a net reclassification index (NRI) = 0.13 (0.07–0.19).[47]

The Multi-Ethnic Study of Atherosclerosis (MESA) evaluated the use of CAC in long-term prognostication of incident CHD and ASVD among patients with T2DM. The addition of CAC to global risk assessment significantly improved risk stratification in individuals with T2DM. CAC was independently associated with CAC (HR 1.3 [1.19–1.43]), and the net reclassification improvement with CAC addition to traditional risk assessment was 0.23 (95% CI, 0.10–0.37).[48] In light of this evidence, current DM guidelines endorse CAC testing for cardiovascular risk assessment for intermediate-risk (7.5%–20%) patients where risk and treatment decisions are uncertain.[31]

Value of Improved Glycemic Control

Guideline Recommendations on Glycemic Control

The major adverse events of T2DM are microvascular and macrovascular complications. Both are affected by the intensity of glycemic control, typically assessed by levels of glycosylated hemoglobin A1c (HbA1c).

While it is established that effective management of all levels of gylcemia reduces microvascular complications,[49–51] results from the large outcome trials (ACCORD, ADVANCE, VADT—Table 4.4) have not shown that more intensive glycemic control significantly reduces CVD outcomes. In response to this evidence, the 2019 ADA/EASD Standards of Medical Care acknowledge the complexity of adequate glycemic control and strongly endorse the importance of shared decision making to incorporate the individual characteristics and preferences of each patient to find optimal glycemic targets.[31] A general target of <7% HbA1c for nonpregnant adults is still recommended. However, in individuals just diagnosed with T2DM, without CVD, patients with long life expectancy or individuals treated with lifestyle therapy and metformin only, more aggressive glycemic management(<6.5%) is reasonable and can prevent microvascular complications.[31] For patients with short life expectancy who may not profit from the long-term benefits of more aggressive glycemic management, or suffer from serious comorbidities and poor self-management, an HbA1c up to 8% is more suitable.[31] Where tight HbA1c levels cannot be achieved safely, higher HbA1c levels are acceptable. In order to personalize

Table 4.4

Rates of hypoglycemia in the ACCORD, ADVANCE, and VADT clinical trials				
	HbA1c target, %	Standard glucose control arm%	Intensive glucose control arm %	*P* value
ACCORD	<6	5.1	16.2	<0.001
ADVANCE	< 6.5	1.5	2.7	<0.001
VADT	If >6, insulin added	9.9	21.2	<0.001

Modified from Connelly KA, Yan AT, Leiter LA, Bhatt DL, Verma S. Cardiovascular implications of hypoglycemia in diabetes mellitus. *Circulation* 2015; 132(24):2345–2350.

glycemic targets for each patient, the Standards of Medical Care recommend assessing seven categories to decide on the stringency of the glycemic target; risks of hypoglycemia/drug adverse effects, disease duration, life expectancy, comorbidities, established vascular complications, patient preference, and resources and support system.[31]

Microvascular Complications

Multiple randomized controlled studies have repeatedly established that intensive glycemic control can reduce microvascular complications in T2DM.[49–51] The Diabetes Control and Complications Trial (DCCT) reported that a 60% reduction of development of diabetic retinopathy, nephropathy, and neuropathy was achieved in the intensive treatment group (mean HbA1c of 7%) than in the standard group (HbA1c of 9%)[52] in early-onset youths and younger adults with T1DM. The landmark trial, UK Prospective Diabetes Study (UKPDS), which included over 7600 subjects with T2DM and a median follow-up of 10 years, assessed the effects of intensive glycemic control on incidence of complications. One of the major conclusions drawn from the study showed that the microvascular complication rate was reduced by 25% more in the intensive treatment arm (median HbA1c of 7.0%) compared to the control treatment arm (median HbA1c of 7.9%). [49]

Macrovascular Complications

However, the microvascular benefits of more aggressive glycemic management may be offset by the effects on cardiovascular outcomes. The current discussion of glycemic control on cardiovascular risk is shaped by recent major outcome studies including the ACCORD,[53] ADVANCE,[7] and VADT[54] (Table 4.4).

ACCORD. In patients with T2DM at high cardiovascular risk, perhaps similar to those that a cardiologist might see, the NID-supported Action to Control Cardiovascular Risk in Diabetes (ACCORD) study compared intense versus standard glycemic control. Mean HbA1c levels were 6.4% in the intense and 7.5% in the standard arms. ACCORD ended the glycemic control study early after results showing an increased mortality in individuals belonging to the very intense glycemic control arm, with an HbA1c target of <6%, compared to the standard arm (1.41 versus 1.14% per year; 257 versus 203 deaths over a mean 3.5 years of follow-up; hazard ratio [HR] 1.22 [95% CI 1.01–1.46]). As a result, the ACCORD study researchers wrote, "Such a strategy cannot be recommended for high-risk patients with advanced T2D."[53] As a result of the ACCORD study, the subsequently published ADA Standards of Care in Diabetes 2013 guidelines only recommended intensive glycemic control in low 10-year ASCVD risk patients.[55]

ADVANCE. The ADVANCE trial (Action in Diabetes and Vascular Disease: Preterax and Diamicron MR Controlled Evaluation) was launched with a similar motivation to ACCORD: to evaluate more aggressive glycemic management on the risk of CVD in patients with T2DM. The primary outcome of ADVANCE combined macrovascular (MI, stroke, and cardiovascular death) and microvascular (nephropathy and retinopathy) events.[56] While intensive glycemic control resulted in a significant reduction of this combined primary endpoint (18.1% intensive versus 20.0% conventional therapy—HR 0.90; 95% CI 0.82–0.98; $P = 0.01$), this decrease was mainly driven by the reduction of microvascular events (mainly albuminuria). There was no significant reduction in major macrovascular events (10.0% intensive versus 10.6% conventional therapy; HR 0.94; 95% CI 0.84–1.06; $P = 0.32$). Unlike ACCORD, ADVANCE did not observe an elevated risk in mortality for patients with intensive glucose control.[57]

VADT. The Veterans Affairs Diabetes Trial (VADT), a prospective-randomized trial in patients with advanced T2DM, also failed to demonstrate a significant benefit in terms of overall or cardiovascular mortality, herein from lowering HbA1c to 6.9% in the intensive-therapy group versus 8.4% in the standard-therapy group.[54] The VADT trial's population included predominantly (98%) older men with poorly controlled T2DM (median entry HbA1c 9.4%). CVD risk factors such as BP, smoking cessation, aspirin therapy, and statin therapy were treated intensively. While the tight glycemic control group reduced HbA1C levels to 6.9% within the first year of the study, the primary outcome, time to first cardiovascular event, was not significantly reduced in the intensive group (HR 0.88 [95% CI 0.74–1.05], $P = 0.12$). The study also reported more CVD deaths in the intensive glycemic control group than in the standard control group (38 versus 29); however, this difference was not statistically significant. More recent analysis has demonstrated that VADT participants randomly assigned to intensive glycemic control over 5.6 years had fewer CVD events only during the prolonged period in which the glycated hemoglobin curves were separated.[58]

Summary. Results from these outcome studies suggest that patients with a long history of T2DM, history of hypoglycemia, advanced atherosclerosis, and old age are less likely to benefit from tight glycemic control.[59,60] In all three trials, significantly more hypoglycemic episodes occurred in tight glycemic control groups than in others. In response to ACCORD, VADT, and ADVANCE, the 2019 ADA/EASD Standards of Medical Care state that physicians should be cautious of intensive glucose control for patients with long history of T2DM and cardiovascular risk factors.[31] The risks associated with intensive glycemic control might outweigh its benefits.

Importance of Large Cardiovascular Disease Outcome Trials

Until 2008, antidiabetic drugs were exclusively approved on the basis of lowering of HbA1c, as trials with intensive glycemic control demonstrated lower rates of microvascular complications. Most participants in trials evaluating effects of certain glycemic targets had no established ASCVD or very low cardiovascular risk and were generally drug naïve. This study design limited the ability to adequately assess cardiovascular effects of these drugs. Over time, a range of evidence demonstrated that some diabetic drugs might pose risks to cardiovascular safety (Table 4.5).[61]

Perhaps the most famous trial that initiated the debate on cardiovascular safety of antidiabetic drugs was the study showing that rosiglitazone was associated with an elevated risk of MI and risk of death from cardiovascular causes.[62] Ironically, later studies did not confirm the adverse cardiovascular effects of rosiglitazone,[63] and the FDA since lifted safety regulations against this agent.[64]

In response to the overall rosiglitazone trial data[62] and other trials questioning cardiovascular safety of antidiabetic agents, in 2008 the US Food and Drug Administration (FDA) published guidance for industry recommending the inclusion of enough patients with high CVD risk in order for trials to adequately assess the cardiovascular risks of diabetic drugs.[65] In order for novel drugs to demonstrate sufficient cardiovascular safety and win FDA approval, the agency mandated that a premarketing outcomes trial show that the upper bound of the two-sided 95% confidence interval of the estimated hazard ratio is less than 1.8 for composite three-point MACE (cardiovascular death, nonfatal MI, and nonfatal stroke) or four-point MACE (cardiovascular death, nonfatal MI, nonfatal stroke, and hospitalization for unstable angina).[65] For approved drugs, the FDA also required a postmarketing safety trial that must demonstrate that the estimated risk ratio of the upper bound of the two-sided 95% confidence interval is less than 1.3 for the composite MACE outcome.[65] To achieve this, most enrolled patients must have established CVD or high ASCVD risk.

Table 4.5

Cardiovascular data for selected type 2 diabetes mellitus drugs before guidance

Class	Medication	Trial phase	Outcomes	Events	Subjects	Other outcomes
GLP-1 RA	Exenatide	Phase 2 and 3	Cardiac disorders SAEs	27	2371	⋮
DPP-4i	Liraglutide	Phase 3	Custom MACE SMQ	38	6638	⋮
	Saxagliptin	Phase 3	Custom MACE SMQ	40	4607	⋮
	Alogliptin	Phase 3	Custom MACE SMQ	18	4702	⋮
	Sitagliptin	Pooled phase 3	Cardiac disorders SAEs	12	2342	⋮

DPP-4, Dipeptidyl peptidase 4;
Modified from Cecilia C, Low Wang M, Brendan M, et al. Cardiovascular safety trials for all new diabetes mellitus drugs? Ten years of FDA guidance requirements to evaluate cardiovascular risk. *Circulation* 2019;139:1741–1743.

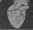

Drug manufacturers quickly adapted to this new regulatory climate. While most trials were designed to only demonstrate the antidiabetic agent's noninferiority to placebo, some drugs were powered to show superiority compared to standard treatment.[66]

As a result, a multitude of large CVOTs for antidiabetic agents were published after 2008 (Table 4.6). Categorically, the drugs tested demonstrated cardiovascular safety (noninferior cardiovascular outcomes compared to placebo). These post-2008 FDA mandated CVOTs led to a paradigm shift in T2DM treatment; therapies now are not primarily aimed at HbA1c reduction but are focused on other aspects of T2DM comorbidities as well, such as the effects on cardiovascular health. In addition, the information of these CVOTs led to great insights, such as the demanding issue of HF in older patients with T2DM[67] and the effects of these agents on kidney function.[66] In response to the outcome of these trials, the FDA for the first time approved label changes to drugs used to treat patients with diabetes for lower risk of MACE (liraglutide,[68] canagliflozin[69]) and cardiovascular death (empagliflozin[70]).[71]

After a decade under the 2008 guidance, in October 2018, the FDA Endocrinologic and Metabolic Drugs Advisory Committee discussed whether to provide updated guidance. Perhaps the most important critique about the past CVOTs is the lack of generality of the trial's results.[66] Most participants had high baseline CVD risk, and this limits how much the results can be extrapolated onto the entire population.[66] Further, some point out that focusing new T2DM drugs on atherosclerotic cardiovascular safety is too limited.[71] For instance, members of the committee emphasized the importance of drug development for outcomes such as HF, peripheral artery disease, and fatty liver disease, and these comorbidities are all important to individuals with T2DM.[61] In addition, the high cost and rigor of these large outcome trials might deter the development of novel drugs by pharmaceutical companies.[71]

The committee voted 10 to 9 to continue the 2008 guidance; the close decision demonstrates the complexity of the subject.[72] While the new guidelines have not been finalized, a possible outcome of the committee's discussion is that trials assessing new drugs should be more strict than before the implementation of the FDA 2008 guidance for industry, but more lenient than 2008 recommendations.[61] For instance, there were discussions on modifying the approval procedure to a one-step process and altering the preapproval hazard ratios from 1.8 to <1.5, while removing the 1.3 postapproval limit.[61] If implemented by the FDA, this simplified approach to diabetes related CVOT trial design would allow more resources to be directed to development of drugs that show efficacy against outcomes like peripheral artery disease, HF, glycemic variability, quality of life, or kidney disease.[61]

Table 4.6

Cardiovascular data for selected type 2 diabetes mellitus drugs after guidance

Class	Medication	Trial	Cardiovascular safety signals or MACE-three-Point CVD Risk, Hazard Ratio (95% CI)	Events	Subject	Other outcomes
GLP-1 RA	Lixisenatide	ELIXA[a] (2015)	1.02 (0.89–1.17)[b]	805	6068	...
	Liraglutide[c]	LEADER (2016)	0.87 (0.78–0.97)[D]	1302	9340	...
	Semaglutide	SUSTAIN-6 (2016)	0.74 (0.58–0.95)[D]	254	3297	Retinopathy 1.76 (1.11–2.78)[D]
	Exenatide	EXSCEL (2017)	0.91 (0.83–1.00)	1744	14752	...
	Albiglutide	HARMONY OUTCOMES (2018)	0.78 (0.68–0.90)[D]	766	9463	...
	Dulaglutide	REWIND (2019)	0.88 (0.79–0.99)[D]	1257	9901	...
	Oral semaglutide	PIONEER-6 (2019)	0.79 (0.57–1.11)[D]	137	3183	...
SGLT-2i	Empagliflozin[d]	EMPA-REG (2015)	0.86 (0.74–0.99)[D]	772	7020	...
	Canagliflozin[d]	CANVAS program (2017)	0.86 (0.75–0.97)[D]	1011	10142	Amputation 1.97 (1.41–2.75)[D]
	Dapagliflozin	DECLARE-TIMI 58 (2018)	0.93 (0.84–1.03)	1559	17160	Diabetic ketoacidosis 2.18 (1.10–4.30)[D]
	Canagliflozin	CREDENCE (2019)	0.80 (0.67–0.95)[D]	486	4401	...
DPP-4i	Saxagliptin	SAVOR-TIMI 53 (2013)	1.00 (0.89–1.12)	1222	16492	HF hospitalization 1.27 (1.07–1.51)[D]
	Alogliptin	EXAMINE[a] (2013)	0.96 (0.80–1.16)	621	5380	HF hospitalization 1.19 (0.90–1.58)

| Sitagliptin | TECOS (2015) | 0.98 (0.89–1.08)[B] | 1690 | 14671 | HF hospitalization 1.00 (0.83–1.20) |
| Linagliptin | CARMELINA (2018) | 1.02 (0.89–1.17) | 854 | 6979 | HF hospitalization 0.90 (0.74–1.08) |

CANVAS, Canagliflozin cardiovascular assessment study; CARMELINA, Cardiovascular and renal microvascular outcome study with linagliptin in patients with type 2 diabetes mellitus; CVD, cardiovascular disease; DECLARE-TIMI 58, Dapagliflozin effect on cardiovascular events–thrombolysis in myocardial infarction 58; DPP-4, Dipeptidyl peptidase 4; ELIXA, Evaluation of lixisenatide in acute coronary syndrome; EMPA-REG, Empagliflozin, cardiovascular outcomes, and mortality in type 2 diabetes trial; EXAMINE, Cardiovascular outcomes study of alogliptin in patients with type 2 diabetes and acute coronary syndrome; EXSCEL, Exenatide study of cardiovascular event lowering trial; HARMONY OUTCOMES, Effect of albiglutide, when added to standard blood glucose lowering therapies on major cardiovascular events in subjects with type 2 diabetes mellitus; GLP-1, glucagon-like peptide-1; HF, heart failure; LEADER, Liraglutide effect and action in diabetes: evaluation of cardiovascular outcome results; MACE-3-point, major adverse cardiovascular event: myocardial infarction, stroke, or cardiovascular death; REWIND, Researching cardiovascular events with a weekly incretin in diabetes; SAVOR-TIMI 53, Saxagliptin assessment of vascular outcomes recorded in patients with diabetes mellitus–thrombolysis in myocardial infarction 53; SGLT, sodium glucose transporter; SMQ, Standardized medical query (of adverse event terms); SUSTAIN-6, Trial to evaluate cardiovascular and other long-term outcomes with semaglutide in subjects with type 2 diabetes; TECOS, Trial evaluating cardiovascular outcomes with sitagliptin.

Modified from Cecilia C, Low Wang M, Brendan M, et al. Cardiovascular Safety Trials for All New Diabetes Mellitus Drugs? Ten Years of FDA guidance requirements to evaluate cardiovascular risk. Circulation 2019;139:1741–1743.

Drugs That Lower Cardiovascular Disease Risk

Metformin

Drug Class Overview

Singly or in combination, metformin is the standard of care to promote glycemic control and is the first-choice agent in international T2DM guidelines.[31,73] Importantly, it also suppresses appetite, is associated with modest (2%–3%) weight reduction, appears to be devoid of cardiovascular harm, and may benefit when given to patients with T2DM and HF.[74] In the prolonged UKPDS study, metformin was the only drug to reduce T2DM-related and all-cause mortality, although the number of events was low.[75] Since then, it has been the first-line treatment in overweight patients with T2DM.

Mechanisms of Action

Most of the metabolic effect of metformin occurs in the liver wherein it reduces glucose production.[76] Although the *in vivo* effects in patients with T2DM or at risk for T2DM remain unproven, in skeletal muscle, metformin phosphorylates, and activates 5' AMP-activated protein kinase (AMPK), which facilitates many of the observed cellular effects of metformin, such as inhibition of glucose and lipid synthesis. AMPK activation also leads to the glucose transporter-4 mediated glucose uptake (Fig. 4.4). Overall, metformin leads to a higher systemic insulin sensitivity.[77] Another putative mechanism of metformin relates to the impact on the intestinal microbiome.[78]

Differences Among Drugs in Class

Metformin can be administered twice daily in the short-release form or once daily in the long-release form.[31] Both forms are equally effective. However, the long release is associated with fewer gastrointestinal effects than the short-release form.[79]

Data for Use

Overall, the initial treatment with metformin shows many benefits on clinical outcomes, such as less hypoglycemia and weight gain compared to insulin or sulfonylureas.[50]

Glycemic control. Metformin is the first-choice agent for T2DM primarily because of its glycemic efficacy in the absence of side effects seen with other glucose-lowering agents. The United States Multicenter Metformin Study group showed that after 29 weeks,

CELLULAR GLUCOSE METABOLISM

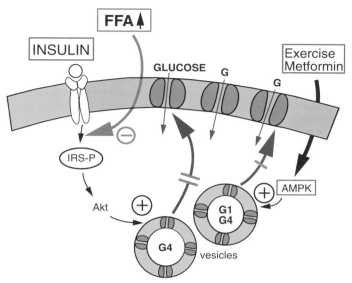

Fig. 4.4 Cellular glucose metabolism. Excess free fatty acid *(FFA)* entering the muscle cell is activated to long-chain acyl coenzyme A, which inhibits the insulin signaling pathway so that there is less translocation of glucose transporter vesicles (GLUT-4 and GLUT-1 glucose) to the cell surface. Glucose uptake is decreased, and hyperglycemia is promoted. The increased uptake of FFA promotes lipid metabolites accumulation in various organs, including the heart and pancreas. Metformin and exercise, by stimulating adenosine monophosphate protein kinase *(AMPK)*, promote the translocation of transport vesicles to the cell surface to promote glucose entry and to oppose insulin resistance. Protein kinase B, also called *Akt*, plays a key role. *AMPK*, 5' AMP-activated protein kinase; *G*, glucose; *IRS-P*, insulin receptor substrate–phosphatidyl. (Modified from Opie LH. *Heart Physiology, from Cell to Circulation.* 4th ed. Philadelphia: Lippincott, Williams and Wilkins; 2004: 313.)

patients randomly assigned to metformin had a mean HbA1c concentration of 7.1% compared to 8.6% in the placebo group.[80]

Weight loss. An additional advantage over other antidiabetics is the weight loss associated with metformin. In the Diabetes Prevention Program, study participants reduced their body weight by $2.06 \pm 5.65\%$ when taking metformin, compared to the $0.02 \pm 5.52\%$ weight loss of the placebo group ($P < 0.001$).[81] In a meta-analysis, when combined with insulin, metformin reduced HbA1c by 0.5% and weight gain by 1 kg, whereas the insulin dose fell by 5 U/day.[82]

Cardiovascular outcomes. Trials on cardiovascular outcomes of metformin preceded the FDA guidance, and as a result there are no definitive CVOTs similar to those with SGLT-2 (sodium-glucose cotransporter-2) inhibitors, GLP-1 receptor agonists, and DPP-4 (dipeptidyl peptidase 4) inhibitors. Evidence on cardiovascular effect of metformin relies on a number of smaller studies that, even though controversial, overall point toward cardiovascular benefits. Evidence from a meta-analysis of 179 trials and 25 observational studies concluded that cardiovascular mortality was lower for metformin compared to sulfonylureas.[83] For example, compared to sulfonylureas, metformin was associated with a lower all-cause mortality (HR 0.5–0.8), lower CVD mortality (HR 0.6–0.9), and lower CVD morbidity (HR 0.3–0.9),[83] In a Danish retrospective national cohort study, Andersson et al. demonstrated that patients with T2DM with HF treated with metformin had a lower risk of mortality compared with sulfonylureas and/or insulin.[84]

REMOVAL (Reducing with Metformin Vascular Adverse Lesions), the largest and longest double-blinded randomized control study assessing metformin, observed the progression of atherosclerosis in patients with T1DM. Atherosclerosis progression was measured by average maximal carotid intima-media thickness (CIMT). In the group treated with metformin, CIMT was significantly reduced (-0.013 mm/year, -0.024 to -0.003; $P = 0.0093$), suggesting cardiovascular benefits. There is also evidence that metformin may protect against coronary atherosclerosis in prediabetes and early T2DM in men. This hypothesis is currently being examined in the study VA-IMPACT (Investigation of Metformin in Pre-Diabetes on Atherosclerotic Cardiovascular Outcomes), testing if metformin reduces mortality and cardiovascular morbidity in patients with prediabetes and established ASCVD compared to placebo.

Cancer incidence. In addition, observational studies have observed that metformin may lower cancer incidence.[85,86]

Side Effects

The major side effects of metformin are gastrointestinal intolerances such as bloating or diarrhea. A very rare observed occurrence is lactic acidosis at very high circulating metformin levels if patients suffer from overdose, or acute renal failure. Consequently, metformin should be avoided in patients with a predisposition to lactic acidosis. Such factors include an estimated glomerular filtration rate (eGFR) <30 mL/min/1.73 m^2 or severe illness with vomiting and dehydration.[87,73] Additionally, metformin is potentially associated with Vitamin B12 deficiency.[88] The 2019 ADA Standards of Medical Care state that Vitamin B levels should be routinely measured in patients treated with metformin, especially in patients with anemia or peripheral neuropathy (Level B recommendation).[31]

Drug Interactions or Major Restriction

Metformin demonstrates synergistic effects when coadministered with SGLT-2 inhibitors. In comparison to the application of metformin alone, the combination of metformin and SGLT-2 inhibitors improved arterial stiffness in T1DM patients.[89] Endothelial dysfunction is improved through the combination of metformin and saxagliptin in T2DM.[90]

Metformin and kidney disease. Metformin is renally excreted. Bearing in mind that moderate to severe renal disease with eGFR <60 mL/min occurs in 20%–30% of patients with T2DM, metformin dose reduction should be considered at an eGFR <45 mL/min and at an eGFR <30 mL/min, metformin should not be used.[31,73] If eGFR is 30–60 mL/min, the 2019 ADA Standards of Medical Care additionally advise to pause metformin treatment before iodinated contrast imaging procedures.[31]

SGLT-2 Inhibitors

Drug Class Overview

The 2019 ADA Standards of Medical Care state that if the HbA1c target is not achieved after 3 months of metformin and lifestyle intervention alone, metformin can be combined with additional drugs. For patients with ASCVD, HF, or CKD, the guidelines recommend the addition of SGLT-2 inhibitors or glucagon-like peptide 1 (GLP-1) receptor agonists.[31]

Mechanisms of Action

SGLT-2 inhibitors work by decreasing glucose levels through urinary excretion (Fig. 4.5). Their glucosuric effect, coupled with a diuretic-mediated antihypertensive effect and hemoconcentration, may explain their cardiovascular benefits.[91] The inhibition of SGLT-2 receptors in the kidneys result in increased urinary excretion of glucose, which reduces postprandial glycemic excursions and leads to more effective glycaemic control and weight loss. The weight loss associated with SGLT-2 inhibitors, which was confirmed in a meta-analysis that compared SGLT-2 inhibitors with placebo showing that SGLT-2 inhibitors, were associated with a mean of 2.99 kg reduction in weight over 2 years (95% CI −3.64 to −2.34[92]), may also contribute CVD risk reductions. These effects

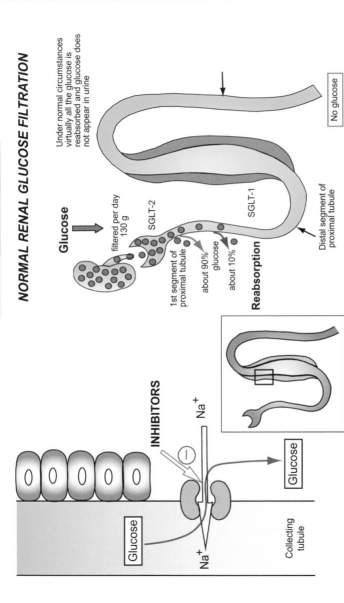

Fig. 4.5 SGLT-2 inhibitors effect on renal glucose filtration. *SGLT*, Sodium glucose transporter.

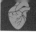

improve insulin sensitivity. The negative energy balance associated with glycosuria leads to ketone body metabolization by cardiac myocytes, which are a more efficient energy fuel.[93] The osmotic diuresis contributes to the BP reduction associated with SGLT-2 inhibitors. For example, the CANTATA-M (Canagliflozin Treatment and Trial Analysis – Monotherapy) trial showed that SBP and diastolic blood pressure (DBP) values were reduced with 300 mg canagliflozin by −5.4 mmHg and −2 mmHg, respectively.[94]

Differences Among Drugs in Class

While canagliflozin and empagliflozin have demonstrated cardiovascular and renal benefits, canagliflozin was associated with a higher risk of lower limb amputations and fractures.[69] The ADA 2019 Standards of Medical Care state that for patients with established ASCVD, evidence for empagliflozin is the strongest.[73] Dapagliflozin showed significant benefits for individuals with HF.[95]

Data for Use

Multiple large FDA mandated CVOTs have since reported on the cardiovascular effects of SGLT-2 inhibitors (Table 4.6). The two FDA-approved SGLT-2 inhibitors, empagliflozin and canagliflozin, showed significant reductions in cardiovascular events.

EMPA-REG. EMPA-REG, a randomized double-blinded trial, evaluated the effect of empagliflozin on a composite of cardiovascular death, nonfatal MI, or nonfatal stroke.[70] Even though designed for noninferiority, the study concluded that empagliflozin was superior to placebo. Empagliflozin reduced risk of the primary outcome, with a relative risk reduction of 14% (10.5% empagliflozin vs 12.1% placebo - HR 0.86 [95% CI 0.74–0.99. $P = 0.04$]. In individuals using empagliflozin, cardiovascular death was reduced by 38% (absolute rate 3.7% versus 5.9%, HR 0.62 [95% CI 0.49–0.77], $P < 0.001$). Due to the significant decrease in cardiovascular death associated with empagliflozin, the FDA approved empagliflozin in 2016 "to reduce the risk of cardiovascular death in adult patients with T2DM and cardiovascular disease," even though cardiovascular death reduction was only a secondary outcome.

In addition, empagliflozin reduced risk of HF both in patients with and without HF at baseline. The ACC/AHA 2019 Standards of Care recognized empagliflozin's potential for primary prevention of HF.[38] Within the first few months, reduction in cardiovascular mortality was observed in EMPA-REG.[70] This posits that the increased diuresis and improved hemodynamics associated with empagliflozin may result in the cardiovascular benefits, which are independent of glycemic control.[96] The hypothesis that glycemic control is not the only cause of empagliflozin's beneficial cardiovascular effect is further established by the observation that patients with HF benefited from empagliflozin, within a large range of HbA1c values.[96] In order to assess if SGLT-2 inhibitors prevent HF independent of glycemic control, the effect of SGLT-2 inhibitors on HF will be measured in EMPEROR HF for empagliflozin (ClinicalTrials.gov trial number NCT03057977) and DAPA HF for dapagliflozin (ClinicalTrials.gov trial number: NCT03036124) in patients without T2DM.

CANVAS. The CANVAS trial evaluated the cardiovascular effects of canagliflozin. Here, canagliflozin reduced the rate of three-point MACE from 31.5 to 26.9 participants per 1000 patient-years (HR 0.86; 95% CI 0.75 to 0.97; $P < 0.001$ for noninferiority; $P = 0.02$ for superiority). However, there were no significant findings for cardiovascular death or death by any cause. Of note, the rate of lower limb amputations almost doubled in the canagliflozin group compared to the control group 6.3 versus 3.4 per 1000 patient years (HR 1.97 [1.41–2.75]).

CREDENCE. The CREDENCE trial also studied canagliflozin, but the authors evaluated the renal effects of this drug. The primary outcome was a composite of end-stage kidney disease, doubling of serum creatinine and death from renal/cardiovascular disease. Compared to the placebo group, the rates of the primary outcome were lower in the canagliflozin group (43.2 and 61.2 per 1000 patient-years HR: 0.70; 95% CI 0.59–0.82; $P = 0.00001$). CREDENCE also showed that canagliflozin positively impact patients with chronic kidney disease (CKD).[97] According the most current guidelines, SGLT-2 inhibitors are not recommended for patients with GFR < 45 mL/min but results from CREDENCE suggest that for precisely these patients, SGLT-2 inhibitors are most beneficial. Even though the CREDENCE population consisted of a population which had slightly higher risk profiles than CANVAS, there was no increase in amputation or fracture as observed as adverse events in the CANVAS participants. [97]

DECLARE-TIMI-58. The impact of dapagliflozin on cardiovascular outcomes was studied in the DECLARE-TIMI-58 trial.[96] This was the first CVOT SGLT-2 inhibitor trial to enroll a majority (59%) primary prevention patients. Only 41% had established ASCVD. While dapagliflozin achieved noninferiority, it was not superior to placebo in the primary outcome, three-point MACE (HR = 0.93, 95% CI 0.84–1.03, $P = 0.17$). However, dapagliflozin did result in lower rates of hospitalization of HF (4.9% versus. 5.8%; HR 0.83; 95% CI 0.73–0.95; $P = 0.005$).

Summary. The conclusion from a meta-analysis studying all-cause mortality and cardiovascular mortality was that SGLT-2 inhibitors are the most beneficial to cardiovascular outcomes compared to the other drug classes that underwent the FDA-mandated trials (GLP-1 receptor agonists and DPP-4 inhibitors). SGLT-2 inhibitors were also associated with lower rates of HF and MI outcome, compared to GLP-1 receptor agonists and DPP-4 inhibitors.[96]

Side Effects

The FDA-mandated outcome studies showed that SGLT-2 inhibitors were associated with an increased risk of genital infections due to the glucosuria. In a recent report, the FDA identified 55 cases of Fournier Gangrene receiving SGLT-2 inhibitors.[98] Other adverse events, such as an increase in LDL-C (1.09 ± 2.3 mg/dL) and an increase in total cholesterol (2.14 ± 3.7 mg/dL), have also been noted.[99] Ten cases of bladder cancer have been noted among patients prescribed dapagliflozin. As the result, the FDA initiated postmarketing surveillance studies for this rare outcome. SGLT-2 inhibitors may cause symptomatic hypotension in older adults when taken simultaneously with ACE inhibitors, ARBs, or diuretics.[100] Postmarketing reports also observed cases of acute kidney injury in patients taking canagliflozin and dapagliflozin.[101] SGLT-2 inhibitors should not be prescribed when eGFR <30 mL/min/1.73 m². Although some studies reported a higher incidence in bone fractures, this could not be confirmed in a meta-analysis of dapagliflozin or empagliflozin.[102] In the CVOTs, the fracture risk was only increased in the CANVAS trial but not in the other SGLT-2 inhibitor trials.[103] Cases of euglycemic ketoacidosis have also been reported with patients taking SGLT-2 inhibitors, and patients with T2DM treated with insulin may be at higher risk. In the post-2008 CVOTs, only canagliflozin showed an elevated risk of lower limb amputation.[69] As a result, the FDA issued a warning that canagliflozin should not be issued to patients at risk of foot amputations. Patients prescribed canagliflozin should be observed for any signs of foot ulceration.[104]

Drug Interactions or Major Restrictions

Overall, SGLT-2 inhibitors show little drug interactions with other drugs used to treat patients with diabetes or other usual concomitant drugs. Only canagliflozin should be given in a higher dose when patients simultaneously are taking UDP-glucuronosyltransferase inducer like rifampicin, phenytoin, or ritonavir.[105]

Experimental Drugs

Sotagliflozin is a dual SGLT-1 receptor (expressed in the gastrointestinal tract) and SGLT-2 (expressed in the kidneys) inhibitor.[107]

Thus, the agent reduces absorption of glucose in the kidneys as well as in the gastrointestinal tract.[106] Sotagliflozin currently completed phase III trial testing for T1DM patients, while phase III trial testing for T2DM patients is ongoing.[106] In April 2019, the European Union approved the use of sotagliflozin in addition to insulin in T1DM patients with a BMI >27 when insulin therapy is insufficient.[107] In the US, during the January 2019 FDA Endocrinologic and Metabolic Drug Advisory Committee meeting, the committee raised concerns regarding incidence of diabetic ketoacidosis with sotagliflozin. As a result, the FDA deferred approval and issued a complete response letter for sotagliflozin.[108]

GLP-1 Receptor Agonists

Drug Class Overview

GLP-1 receptor agonists stimulate insulin secretion and suppress glucagon release while also reducing appetite and promoting weight loss. For patients with ASCVD, HF, or CKD, the ADA/EASD Standard of Care recommend the addition of SGLT-2 inhibitors or GLP-1 receptor agonists if HbA1c targets are not achieved through metformin or lifestyle intervention alone.[31]

Mechanism of Action

GLP-1 receptor agonists and DPP-4 inhibitors are drugs developed on the basis of the incretin system. Incretins are gastrointestinal peptide hormones released during absorption of nutrients to augment insulin secretion. GLP-1 is a hormone secreted into the circulation by the intestinal L-cells in response to ingested food (Fig. 4.6).[109] The incretin response system is disturbed in T2DM. The incretin axis also includes the enzyme DPP-4, a serine protease that rapidly degrades GLP-1 and other proteins. Ultimately, this "arc of discovery" has led to new approved diabetes therapies: GLP-1 analogs (exenatide, liraglutide) and DPP-4 inhibitors (saxagliptin, sitagliptin, and others).[109] Incretin mimetics are GLP-1 receptor agonists. GLP-1 regulates glucose levels by stimulating glucose-dependent insulin secretion and biosynthesis, and by suppressing glucagon secretion, delayed gastric emptying, and promoting satiety (Fig. 4.6). They regulate glucose metabolism through multiple mechanisms and have beneficial cardiovascular effects, possibly independent of the glucose-lowering activity, which include changes in BP, endothelial function, body weight, cardiac metabolism, lipid metabolism, left ventricular function, atherosclerosis, and the response to ischemia-reperfusion injury.[102]

METHOD OF ACTION: GLP-1 RECEPTORS AGONISTS AND DPP-4 INHIBITORS

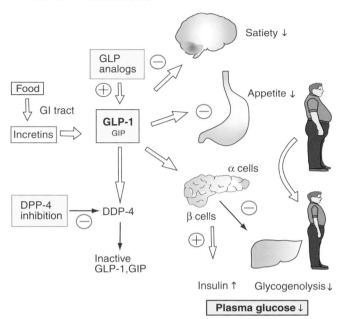

Fig. 4.6   Method of action: GLP-1 receptor agonists and DPP-4 inhibitors. *DPP-4*, Dipeptidyl peptidase 4; *GIP*, gastric inhibitor polypeptide; *GLP-1*, glucose like peptide-1.

Differences Among Drugs in Class

GLP-1 receptor agonists are divided into short-and long-acting drugs. Exenatide and lixisenatide are shorter acting and have a more marked effect on postprandial glucose and gastric emptying but less on fasting glucose.[110] Lixisenatide is administered once daily, while exenatide is given twice daily. After the initial short-acting GLP-1 receptor agonists were produced, longer-acting versions were developed. Dulaglutide, exenatide extended release (ER), liraglutide, and semaglutide are all long-acting GLP-1 receptor agonists. In contrast to short acting, long-acting agents have a greater effect on fasting glucose and less on gastric emptying.[111] A review of 17 trials assessing the effects of multiple GLP-1 receptor agonists showed that compared to active comparators, liraglutide and exenatide led to greater weight loss.[112] Unlike other GLP-1 receptor agonists, semaglutide may be associated with retinopathy through its potent glucose-lowering effects.[113]

Data for Use

Glycemic control. GLP-1 receptor agonists improve glycemic control. A meta-analysis of 17 trials showed that GLP-1 receptor agonists reduce HbA1c by approximately 1% compared to placebo.[112] In patients who require greater glycemic efficacy of injectable therapies, GLP-1 may be a reasonable option versus insulin because the glycemic efficacy is similar with a lower risk of hypoglycemia and more weight loss.[114] In comparison to other glucose-lowering agents, GLP-1 receptor agonists have a higher glycemic efficacy compared to TZDs and sulfonylureas.[114]

Weight loss. Weight loss is a beneficial therapeutic effect of GLP-1 receptor agonists. A systematic review of 17 randomized trials showed that individuals had a weight reduction of approximately 1.5–2.5 kg over 30 weeks on a GLP-1 receptor agonist compared to a placebo or active comparator (insulin glargine, DPP-4 inhibitor, TZD, sulfonylurea).[112]

Cardiovascular outcomes. The cardiovascular safety of GLP-1 receptor agonists was reviewed in a total of eight large CVOTs (Table 4.6).

   ELIXA. ELIXA assessed the effect of lixisenatide on cardiovascular outcomes in T2DM patients with recent acute coronary events.[116] Notably, lixisenatide was the only short-acting GLP-1 receptor agonist drug tested in the immediate post 2008 FDA mandated trials. However, while noninferior, lixisenatide did not prove to be superior to the placebo regarding the primary composite outcome of the study. The composite of MI, stroke, cardiovascular death, or hospitalization for unstable angina occurred in 13.4% of the lixisenatide group compared to 13.2% of the placebo group (HR 1.02; 95% CI 0.89 to 1.17; $P < 0.001$ for inferiority; $P = 0.81$ for superiority).

   LEADER. LEADER, evaluating the effects of liraglutide, showed a dramatic reduction of cardiovascular mortality. In participants taking liraglutide, MI, stroke, and cardiovascular death occurred in 13% compared to 14.9% in the placebo group (HR 0.87; 95% CI 0.78–0.97; $P = 0.01$).[68] This reduction in primary composite outcome was mainly due to the significant reduction of cardiovascular death (4.7% liraglutide versus 6.0% placebo, HR 0.78; 95% CI 0.66–0.93). While liraglutide was already approved for the reduction of blood glucose in patients with T2DM, in response to the LEADER study, the FDA additionally approved liraglutide "to reduce the risk of MACE in adults with T2DM and established cardiovascular disease" in 2017.

SUSTAIN-6. SUSTAIN-6 examined the weekly GLP-1 receptor agonist semaglutide for cardiovascular safety.[113] Despite a fewer number of events in a smaller sample, results were similar to LEADER; semaglutide was noninferior to cardiovascular safety compared to placebo. 6.6% of the semaglutide group suffered from the primary outcome (first occurrence of cardiovascular death, nonfatal MI or nonfatal stroke), compared to 8.9% in the placebo group (HR 0.74; 95% CI 0.58–0.95; $P < 0.001$ for noninferiority).

EXSCEL. Exenatide ER, observed in the EXSCEL study, demonstrated a borderline statistical benefit in the primary outcome but did not significantly lower cardiovascular events compared to the placebo.[116] The primary outcome (cardiovascular death, MI or stroke) occurred in 11.4% of the Exenatide group compared to the 12.2% of the placebo group (HR 0.91; 95% CI 0.83–1.00; $P = 0.06$ for superiority; $P < 0.001$ for noninferiority).

HARMONY OUTCOMES. HARMONY OUTCOMES showed that albiglutide significantly reduced major cardiovascular events when added to standard care of T2DM patients.[117] The incidence rate of three-point MACE was 7% in the albiglutide group compared to 9% in the placebo group (HR 0.78; 95% CI 0.68–0.90; $P < 0.0001$ noninferiority; $P = 0.0006$ for superiority). However, 2017 sales of albiglutide were discontinued due to limited prescriptions of the drug.

REWIND. The REWIND study was the CVOT trial with the longest follow-up time of 5.5 years.[118] Noteworthy is also REWIND's inclusion of a high proportion of women (47%), lower baseline HbA1c (7.2%), and higher proportion of primary prevention patients (70%). REWIND showed that dulaglutide is superior to placebo regarding cardiovascular events. Twelve percent of participants of the dulaglutide group suffered three-point MACE events compared to 13.4% in the placebo group (HR 0.88; 95% CI 0.79–0.99; $P = 0.026$). Further, REWIND suggests that dulaglutide may be beneficial for primary prevention.

In summary, the results of the CVOTs for GLP-1 receptor agonists showed somewhat heterogenous results. Only four of the trials (LEADER, SUSTAIN-6, REWIND, HARMONY OUTCOMES) significantly reduced the risk of the primary outcome, major cardiovascular events. In addition, only REWIND suggested that GLP-1 receptor agonists may be applicable to primary prevention. ELIXA, HARMONY, LEADER, SUSTAIN-6, and EXSCEL included a majority of patients with a history of CVD, suggesting that these drugs primarily reduce cardiovascular events in individuals with established ASCVD. After reflection on the CVOT trials for GLP-1 receptor agonists, the 2019 ADA/EASD Standards of Care state that liraglutide has strongest evidence for cardiovascular benefit.[31] The 2018 ADA/EASD Standards of Care also noted that evidence is also favorable for semaglutide.[73]

Side Effects

The most common side effects of GLP-1 receptor agonists are gastrointestinal. A meta-analysis showed that diarrhea, vomiting, and nausea occur in 10%–50% of patients.[112] Events of acute pancreatitis have also been associated with GLP-1 receptor agonist treatment. However, the incidence is extremely low; a meta-analysis of 14,562 individuals enrolled in trials reported only 16 cases of acute pancreatitis.[119] Injection site reactions may also occur. A study concluded that local site reactions were more common (10%) in albiglutide and exenatide compared to insulin (1%–5%).[120,121] GLP-1 receptor agonists are also associated with risk of gallbladder events, an adverse effect that may relate to the weight reduction.[122] Patients administered semaglutide in the SUSTAIN-6 trial showed complications of diabetic retinopathy more frequently than the placebo group (HR 1.76; 95% CI 1.11–2.78).[113] However, currently it is unclear if this is a direct effect of the drug or only consequence of the glycemic control through semaglutide. The FDA advises that exenatide should not be used with severe renal impairment, after receiving reports from 78 individuals with acute renal failure or renal insufficiency.[123] Rodent studies also showed that liraglutide and dulaglutide were associated with benign and malignant thyroid C tell tumors.[124] Further, GLP-1 receptor agonists may modestly increase risk of hypoglycemia when added to insulin and sulfonylureas.[125]

Experimental Drugs

Tirzepatide, a GLP-1 receptor agonist developed for T2DM patients with increased cardiovascular risk, is currently undergoing phase III testing. The phase II trial showed that tirzepatide was associated with greater weight loss and HbA1c reduction compared to Trulicity (standard GLP-1 agonist).[126] SURPASS-4, a phase III trial initiated in 2018, demonstrated the safety and efficacy of tirzepatide in participants with elevated cardiovascular risk.[127]

Drugs That Do Not Lower Cardiovascular Disease Risk

DPP-4 Inhibitors

Drug Class Overview

DPP-4 inhibitors are chemically derived, selective, competitive inhibitors of DPP-4 and can be administered orally.

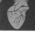

Mechanisms of Action

DPP-4 inhibitors counteract the degradation of plasma GLP-1 and GIP after eating (Fig. 4.6). Like GLP-1 agonists, these agents have antidiabetic activity by stimulating the release of insulin from the pancreas and by inhibiting that of glucagon. However, DPP-4 inhibitors only elevate GLP-1 by a modest amount, compared to when administering GLP-1 receptor agonists directly. This could account for the greater beneficial effects on weight, fasting glucose levels, and reduction of HbA1c of GLP-1 compared to DPP-4 inhibitors.[96,128]

Differences Among Drugs in Class

All DPP-4 inhibitors are excreted renally and need to be adjusted according to renal function. Linagliptin is an exception, as it is excreted via the enterohepatic system. Thus, linagliptin dosage does not need to be adjusted for patients with CKD.[73]

Data for Use

Glycemic control. All DPP-4 inhibitors moderately lower HbA1c to a similar extent.[129] As a second-line treatment, DPP-4 inhibitors are inferior to GLP-1 receptor agonists, but had no advantage over sulfonylureas in a meta-analysis.[130] DPP-4 inhibitors and pioglitazone were associated with the same change in HbA1c from baseline, but pioglitazone was associated with a higher chance of reaching <7% (goal HbaA1c value of the study).[130]

Cardiovascular effect. In CVOTs examining the cardiovascular outcomes of DPP-4 inhibitors (Table 4.6), no agents were associated with cardiovascular benefit. However, saxagliptin[131] and alogliptin[132] demonstrated an elevated risk for hospitalization from HF, with saxagliptin showing the greater risk. As a consequence of these results, the American Heart Association and Heart Failure Society of America (HFSA) concluded that for patients with HF or at high risk of HF, the use of DPP-4 inhibitors is not justified.[133] In 2017, the FDA issued package insert warnings regarding the increased risk of HF for saxagliptin and alogliptin.

    EXAMINE. The EXAMINE trial evaluated the cardiovascular safety of alogliptin on T2DM with recent acute coronary syndrome. Alogliptin was noninferior to placebo in regard to the primary endpoint, three-point MACE (HR 0.98; 95% CI 0.86–1.12).[134] However, a post hoc analysis showed that alogliptin increased the risk of hospitalization from HF contrast to placebo (HR 1.07; 95% CI 0.79–1.46).[132]

    TECOS. The authors of the trial TECOS concluded that sitagliptin did not increase the risk of cardiovascular events compared to placebo (HR 0.98; 95% CI 0.88–1.09).[135]

SAVOR TIMI-53. Saxagliptin did not increase or decrease the rate of ischemic events in the SAVOR-TIMI-53 trial (HR 1.00; 95% CI 0.89–1.12; $P = 0.99$ for superiority and $P < 0.001$ for noninferiority).[131] However, the authors noted an increase in the rates of hospitalization for HF (3.5% saxagliptin versus 2.8% placebo) in the saxagliptin group compared to the control arm.

CARMELINA. The CARMELINA study examined the cardiovascular safety of linagliptin. Linagliptin was noninferior with regard to risk of major cardiovascular events.[136] Notably, the CARMELINA study included a patient population who were at high vascular risk. This is significant, as it provides important information on the use of linagliptin with high-risk patients.

Side Effects

As a group, DPP-4 inhibitors are well tolerated, and rates of weight gain, gastrointestinal adverse effects, and hypoglycemia are minimal.[137] In contrast to GLP-1 receptor agonists, they are weight neutral rather than promoting weight loss.[130] Importantly, in monotherapy, the incidence of hypoglycemia in DPP-4 inhibitor–treated patients in clinical trials was similar to placebo.[139] Moreover, in older patients on stable insulin doses, linagliptin improved glycemic management without an excess of hypoglycemia.[139] While nasopharyngitis was more prevalent with the DPP-4 inhibitors than with placebo, rates of pancreatitis were lower than with other oral antihyperglycemic agents.[99] Incidences of musculoskeletal side effects have also been noted.[140]

Drug Interactions or Major Restrictions

The addition of DPP-4 inhibitors to sulfonylureas increases the risk of hypoglycemia by 50% compared to monotherapy.[141]

Thiazolidinedione

Drug Class Overview

Pioglitazone and rosiglitazone belong to the class of TZDs, also called *glitazones.* TZDs are oral agents that improve insulin sensitivity and lower glucose levels very effectively. While they are inexpensive, show atherosclerotic benefits, and have a high glucose efficacy, these benefits have to be balanced with safety concerns like weight gain,[142] fracture risk,[143] HF,[144,145] and possible increased risk for bladder cancer.[146]

Mechanisms of Action

TZDs activate the PPAR-γ (gamma) transcriptional system, thereby promoting the metabolism of glucose (Fig. 4.7). Evidence also

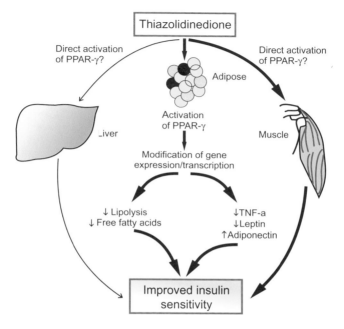

Fig. 4.7 Thiazolidinediones. *PPAR-γ*, Peroxisome proliferator activated receptor γ; *TNF-a*, tumor necrosis factor alpha. (Modified from Cheng AYY, Fantus IG. Oral antihyperglycemic therapy for type 2 diabetes mellitus. *CMAJ* 2005;172(2):231–226.)

suggests that TZDs slow the rate of β-cell function loss more than oral antidiabetics do.[147]

Differences Among Drugs in Class

The main drugs are rosiglitazone—the first, but now suspended in Europe—and the safer pioglitazone.[148] The FDA restricted access to rosiglitazone in September 2010.

Data for Use

Glycemic control. In the ACT NOW trial, pioglitazone reduced the risk of conversion of impaired glucose tolerance to T2DM by 72% but was associated with significant weight gain and edema.[29] However, TZDs may achieve glycemic control without excessive risk of hypoglycemia.[149]

Cardiovascular benefits. Pioglitazone (Actos) although found to increase CHF, was associated with decreased mortality, MI, and stroke.[145,150] In the IRIS (Insulin Resistance Intervention after Stroke) trial, patients with a recent history of ischemic stroke or transient ischemic attack receiving pioglitazone had lower risk of stroke or MI (HR 0.76; 95% CI 0.62–0.93; $P = 0.007$). While the PROACTIVE (Prospective Pioglitazone Clinical Trial In Macrovascular Events) trial also demonstrated a potential beneficial cardiovascular effect by reducing the risk of the composite primary endpoint (death from any cause, nonfatal MI, coronary revascularization, or revascularization of the leg) compared to placebo (HR 0.90; 95% CI 0.80–1.02; $P = 0.095$), this result was nonsignificant.[145] However, the secondary endpoint, three-point MACE, was significantly reduced by 16% (HR 0.84, $P = 0.027$).[145] In a large UK general practice research database on 91,521 people with a mean follow-up of 7.1 years, pioglitazone was associated with reduced all-cause mortality compared with metformin and with rosiglitazone.[150]

Side Effects

Cardiovascular. While cardiovascular benefits of pioglitazone have been observed, multiple publications suggest possibly harmful cardiovascular effects of the now infrequently used drug rosiglitazone.

Fluid retention seems to be an important side effect of TZDs, which is associated with HF.[152] This explains the results of the two large outcome trials, DREAM (Diabetes Reduction Assessment with Ramipril and Rosiglitazone Medication)[144] and ProACTIVE,[145] which reported relative risk increase of HF. The ADA/EASD 2019 Standards of Care suggest avoiding TZDs in patients with symptomatic HF.[31] This advice was also issued in a scientific statement from the HFSA.[133] Here the authors stated that even in patients with T2DMs without HF, TZDs may increase the risk of HF events.[133]

Weight gain. In addition, TZDs are associated with weight gain.[142]

Bladder cancer. There is conflicting evidence on whether pioglitazone is linked to bladder cancer. Nevertheless, the FDA has issued a warning that physicians should not subscribe pioglitazone to patients with active bladder cancer.[146]

Bone fractures. TZDs may increase the risk of fractures due to reduction in bone mineral density, especially in women.[143] The 2019 ADA/EASD Standards of Care also state that TZDs should be used with care in patients at risk of falls or fractures.[31]

Lipid profiles. Glitazones favorably increase HDL-C by 19%, potentially offsetting an LDL-C increase of 8%, while reducing

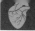

TGs and glycemia (Fig. 4.1).[153] Total LDL-C rose more with rosiglitazone, whereas pioglitazone increased HDL-C levels much more than rosiglitazone.[154] Pioglitazone decreased fasting TGs, which was increased by rosiglitazone.[154] These changes may help to explain why rosiglitazone but not pioglitazone monotherapy was associated with increased MI[62,155] and mortality.[149]

Drugs Interactions or Major Restriction

Rosiglitazone and pioglitazone are metabolized via cytochrome P450. Consequently, simultaneous subscription with rifampicin decreases the AUC, while the addition to gemfibrozil increases the AUC by almost three fold.[156,157]

Experimental Drugs

In the last decade, dual PPAR α/γ agonists have gained international attention due to their combination of insulin-sensitizing and lipid-lowering capabilities. While many dual PPAR α/γ agonists failed during preclinical stages due to safety issues or efficacy, saroglitazar is approved in India for the treatment of diabetic dyslipidemia. The phase III trial PRESS V (Prospective Randomized Efficacy and Safety of Saroglitazar V) demonstrated the reduction of plasma TG levels with 2 mg saroglitazar by 26.4% and with 4 mg by 45%. In this trial HbA1c levels were also decreased by $-0.3\% \pm 0.6\%$ with saroglitazar 4 mg.[159] Another phase III trial, PRESS VI, also showed that 2 mg and 4 mg saroglitazar reduced HbA1c TG levels by $-45.5\% \pm 3.03\%$ and $-46.7\% \pm 3.02\%$, respectively.[159] However the reduction of HbA1c levels in this trial was not significant.[159]

Sulfonylureas

Drug Class Overview

Sulfonylureas are oral antidiabetic drugs known for their high glucose-lowering efficacy while being relatively inexpensive. However, they are also associated with significant weight gain and risk of hypoglycemia. If cost is a determining factor in a patient without known CVD, sulfonylureas may be a reasonable choice.[73]

Mechanisms of Action

These are insulin secretagogues that stimulate insulin secretion by inhibiting adenosine triphosphate (ATP)–sensitive potassium channels of β-cells.[160]

Differences Among Drugs in Class

Sulfonylureas can be distinguished between the older first-generation (tolbutamide) and newer agents belonging to the second generation (glipizide, glibenclamide, [glyburide], gliclazide, and glimepiride). Overall, hypoglycemia is less common with short-acting agents (gliclazide) compared to long-acting sulfonylureas (glibenclamide)[161]; however, in contrast with other sulfonylureas, glibenclamide is associated with the highest risk of hypoglycemia.[162] As a result, the ADA/EASD 2019 Standards of Care state that short-acting agents like glipizide are preferred. Glibenclamide is contraindicated in older adults, as these individuals have a higher risk of hypoglycemia.[31] For patients with renal impairment, it is important to keep in mind that glibenclamide and gliquidone are predominantly excreted biliary, while other agents are excreted through urine.[163]

Data for Use

Glycemic control. Sulfonylureas have a high glucose-lowering efficacy. In a systematic review of 31 double-blind randomized controlled trials, sulfonylureas lowered HbA1c levels by 1.51% compared to placebo. In comparison to other oral glucose-lowering agents, sulfonylureas lowered HbA1c by 1.62%, and compared to insulin by 0.46% (mean baseline HbA1c varied from 4.6% to 13.6% between the individual trials).[164] However, it is also known that sulfonylureas do not have a lasting effect on lowering glucose levels.[165]

Side Effects

Cardiovascular effects. Because the sulfonylurea receptor SUR2a is also expressed on cardiomyocytes, it has long been held that these drugs might also interfere with cardiac function. Indeed, several smaller-scale clinical trials and experimental studies have suggested an impairment of ischemic preconditioning with sulfonylurea drugs.[166] Besides these potential direct effects of sulfonylureas on cardiac and vascular functions, hypoglycemia, as commonly seen during sulfonylurea therapy, is associated with cardiac arrhythmias, thereby providing an additional potential mechanism linking these drugs to increased cardiovascular events.[167] There are few prospective studies on the long-term major clinical effect of these agents on outcomes in T2DM. The University Group Diabetes Program (UGDP) study from the 1960s initially suggested a high incidence of cardiovascular mortality in patients treated with the sulfonylurea agent tolbutamide.[168] In contrast, the UKPD study revealed no significant effect of glibenclamide on either mortality or the incidence of cardiovascular events.[49] There are few

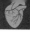

prospective studies on the long-term major clinical effect of these agents on outcomes in T2DM. Monotherapy with the most-used agents, including glimepiride, glibenclamide, glipizide, and tolbutamide, was associated with increased mortality and cardiovascular risk compared with metformin in a large prospective registry trial.[169] Findings from a more recent meta-analysis observed no increase in all-cause mortality in comparison to other treatment plans.[170] In addition, the recently published CAROLINA study affirmed the cardiovascular safety of sulfonylureas; CAROLINA observed no major differences in cardiovascular risk between glimepiride (sulfonylurea) and linagliptin (DPP-4 inhibitor) (three-point MACE occurred in 11.8% of participants subscribed linagliptin and 12.0% of individuals taking glimepiride (HR 0.98; $P = 0.7625$).[171]

Weight gain. In addition, sulfonylureas are also associated with weight gain. Patients prescribed glibenclamide in the UPKDS study gained 4 kg of weight in the first 3 years.[49] In the ADOPT study (A Diabetes Outcome Progression Trial), glyburide resulted in a 1.6 kg weight gain after 12 months (95% CI 1.0–2.2).[172]

Hypoglycemia. A systematic review of a population-based study concluded sulfonylureas had a prevalence of mild/moderate (defined as no third-party assistance needed during the episode) hypoglycemic events of 30% and a severe prevalence (third-party assistance was needed) of 5%. Nevertheless, sulfonylureas still had less hypoglycemic incidences than insulin.[174] Evidence suggests that especial care should be taken prescribing sulfonylureas to elderly patients with low HbA1c or impaired renal function, as in these patients hypoglycemic episodes occur more frequently.[174–176]

Drug Interactions or Major Restriction

Evidence suggests that sulfonylureas interact with drugs that utilize CYP2C9 substrates, such as nonsteroidal antiinflammatory drugs and increase risk of hypoglycemia.[177]

Insulin

Drug Class Overview

After failed oral or GLP-1 receptor agonists (GLP-1 RA) therapy, insulin is the remaining requirement, as in the current Standards of Care.

The current 2019 ADA Standards of Care suggest administering insulin if patients show signs of catabolism like weight loss, hyperglycemia, HbA1c levels >10% (86 mmol/mol), or blood glucose levels over 300 mg/dL (16.7 mmol/L).[31]

Mechanisms of Action

Long-acting insulin preparations (degludec, insulin glargine) inhibit endogenous glucose production (mostly liver) after meals.[31,178] Rapid-acting insulins, on the other hand, are used if/when basal insulin therapy is not sufficient to achieve or maintain level of glycemia.[73] Bolus insulins (lispro, aspart, glulisine) help to limit postprandial increases in plasma glucose after meals. Inhaled insulin is more rapid in onset and, along with bolus insulins, can be used to correct hyperglycemia; however, larger studies are needed to confirm any benefits compared to injectable insulins. These insulins are the preferred agents for T2DM according to the 2018 EASD-ADA Standards of Care.[73] Decludec's insulin mechanism is particularly interesting. The long-acting flat profile of degludec forms a deposit of soluble subcutaneous multihexamers from which insulin is slowly and continuously absorbed into the circulation, thus being "not a revolution but an evolution" of insulin therapy for T1DM and T2DM.[180]

Differences Among Drugs in Class

As the most basic difference, insulins differ in their action profile between rapid-, short-, intermediate-, and long-acting agents. Combination insulins include basal and prandial insulin types, which cover a patient's basal and bolus insulin needs simultaneously by one injection. Evidence suggests that long-acting insulins offer a modest advantage compared to neutral protamine Hagedorn (NPH) insulin regarding risk of hypoglycemia but are more costly.[180] Increases in the cost of insulins have been a major issue for patients and treating health care professionals.[181] However, in real-world hospital settings there was no hypoglycemia risk differences in NPH and long-acting insulins.[182] Clinicians should also keep in mind that in patients with high CVD risk, decludec is associated with lower risk of sever hypoglycemia compared to glargine U100.[183]

Data for Use

Glycemic control. When added to metformin, insulins can reduce HbA1c levels up to 4.9% in patients with T2DM.[184] Well established in clinical practice is the addition of insulin to oral agents for therapy intensification. In a study in which participants were prescribed metformin and insulin, HbA1c was significantly reduced compared to insulin monotherapy. In addition, patients in the insulin-metformin group gained less weight and had fewer incidences of hypoglycemia.[185] A meta-analysis confirmed that not only the combination of metformin and insulin but also the addition of TZDs and sulfonylureas to insulin improve glycemic control.[186] In all studies, the average insulin-sparing effect of the addition of oral agents was 62%.[186]

Side Effects

Cardiovascular. The often presumed increased risk of HF caused by fluid retention with insulin treatment has not been translated into a consistent increase in the rate of mortality or hospitalization for HF.[74] In addition, the Outcome Reduction with Initial Glargine Intervention trial (ORIGIN) showed that the addition of the basal insulin glargine and an oral agent in patients with prediabetes or new-onset T2DM does not increase the risk of cardiovascular events. The incident rates of cardiovascular outcomes were similar in the glargine group versus the standard care (2.94 glargine and 2.85 standard care per 100 person-years).[187] A meta-analysis of four trials (ACCORD, ADVANCE, VADT, and UKPDS) evaluating outcomes of tight glycemic control showed an overall 9% reduction in major cardiovascular events (HR 0.91; 95% CI 0.84–0.99) in the intensive glucose-lowering arm compared to the standard arm, mainly due to 15% reduction of MI.[188]

Hypoglycemia. The major problem with insulin is that hyperglycemia control may be bought at the cost of hypoglycemia. A meta-analysis of glucose-lowering drugs showed that basal insulins and sulfonylureas had the highest risk of hypoglycemia (OR, 17.9 [95% CI 1.97–162]; RD, 10% [95% CI 0.08%–20%]).[189]

Weight gain. A particularly pressing issue is the weight gain associated with insulin therapy. The UKPDS study demonstrated that after 10 years after insulin therapy initiation, patients gained on average 7kg of weight.[49] Of note, combination injection therapy of GLP-1 receptor agonists and insulin is associated with less weight gain and hypoglycemia, compared to intensified insulin plans, while maintaining the same glucose lowering efficacy.[190]

Drug Interactions or Major Restriction

Numerous agents have adverse reactions with insulin. Several substrates have glucose-lowering effects and should not be administered with insulin to avoid the risk of hypoglycemia. Glucose-lowering effects have been observed when insulin is combined with some antibiotics,[191] β-blockers, salicylates, and alcohol. Diuretics,[192] steroids, and oral contraceptives promote peripheral IR and reduce insulin release and thereby may reduce the amount of exogenous insulin needed.

Inhaled insulins should not be prescribed to patients who are smokers or suffer from asthma, chronic obstructive pulmonary disease, or other chronic lung diseases.[31]

Hypoglycemia

Not only do microvascular and macrovascular complications of DM pose risks to DM patients, but hypoglycemic episodes equally enhance risks of diabetic morbidity.

Hypoglycemia and Cardiovascular Risk

Hypoglycemia seems to especially affect cardiovascular health. Episodes of hypoglycemia promote platelet aggregation,[193] inflammation,[193] endothelial dysfunction,[194,195] and proarrhythmogenic processes[196] that increase the risk of adverse cardiovascular events (Table 4.7).

Table 4.7

Rates of change in HbA1c and hypoglycemia with antihyperglycemic agents		
	Change in HbA1c, %	Hypoglycemia, odds ratio
Sulfonylureas	−0.82[a]	8.86 [a]
Meglitinides	−0.71 [a]	10.518 [a]
DPP-4 Inhibitors	−0.69 [a]	1.13
GLP-1 receptor agonists	−1.02 [a]	0.92
Basal insulin	−0.88 [a]	4.77 [a]
Premixed insulin	−1.07 [a]	17.78 [a]
SGLT-2 inhibitors	−0.66 [a]	1.28 [a]

[a]Significant versus placebo.

DPP-4, Dipeptidyl peptidase 4; *GLP-1*, glucagon-like peptide-1; *HbA1c*, hemoglobin A1c; *SGLT*, sodium glucose transporter.

Modified from Liu SC, Tu YK, Chien MN, Chien KL. Effect of antidiabetic agents added to metformin on glycaemic control, hypoglycaemia and weight change in patients with type 2 diabetes: a network meta-analysis. *Diabetes, Obes Metab* 2012;14(9)810–820.

Connelly KA, Yan AT, Leiter LA, Bhatt DL, Verma S. Cardiovascular implications of hypoglycemia in diabetes mellitus. *Circulation* 2015;132(24):2345–2350.

Vasilakou D, Karagiannis T, Athanasiadou E, et al. Sodium-glucose cotransporter 2 inhibitors for type 2 diabetes: a systematic review and meta-analysis. *Ann Intern Med* 2013;159(4):262–274.

Trial Data

Multiple studies have observed the relationship between cardiovascular outcomes and hypoglycemic episodes. In a study including 11,140 patients examining the association between severe hypoglycemia and adverse clinical outcome, patients with severe hypoglycemia had a significantly higher incidents of macrovascular events (HR 2.88; 95% CI 2.01–4.12) compared to patients without episodes of hypoglycemia.[197] This was confirmed in the EXAMINE trial, in which patients with severe hypoglycemia had a HR of 2.42 (95% CI 1.27–4.60; $P = 0.007$) for risk of major adverse cardiovascular events.[198] Hypoglycemia has also been shown to affect development of atherosclerosis, as a study reported association between hypoglycemia and higher CAC scores (CAC > 100 Agatston units).[199] Data from the Atherosclerosis Risk in Communities (ARIC), a prospective cohort analysis including 1209 individuals, concluded that participants with severe hypoglycemic events had higher rates of cardiovascular disease, CHD, HF, atrial fibrillation, peripheral artery disease, and all-cause mortality. The risk of all-cause mortality (HR 1.73; 95% CI 1.38–2.17), cardiovascular mortality (HR 1.64; 95% CI 1.15–2.34), and CHD (HR 2.02; 95% CI 1.27–3.2) reached statistical significance.[200]

However, some suggest that this relationship may be explained due to confounding factors. Individuals who experience hypoglycemic episode are older, more likely to suffer from comorbid illnesses, and are also more vulnerable cardiovascular disease.[198] On the other hand, a bias analysis including data from over 900,000 patients in observational studies showed that there is a strong direct relationship between hypoglycemia and cardiovascular disease.[199] Even though this meta-analysis concluded that a moderate heterogeneity across the included studies exists, in the stratified analysis most subgroups showed similar results.[199]

Diabetes Drugs and Hypoglycemia

A marked difference exists between glucose-lowering drugs and their individual risk of hypoglycemia. In a meta-analysis of second-line T2DM agents, only insulins, sulfonylureas, and glinides increased risk of hypoglycemia compared to placebo (OR of 8.86 [95% CI 4.63–17.83], 10.51 [95% CI 3.59–38.32], 4.77 [95% CI 1.35–18.3] and 17.78 [95% CI 4.84–69.98], respectively).[202] Newer antidiabetic drugs like SGLT-2 inhibitors, GLP-1 receptor agonists, and DPP-4 inhibitors have a very low risk or even reduce risk of hypoglycemia.

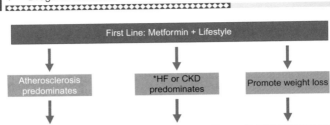

Fig. 4.8 2019 Guidelines "Standard of Medical Care in Diabetes". Avoid TZDs in patients with heart failure *(HF)*. *CKD*, Chronic kidney disease; *GLP-1*, glucagon-like peptide-1; *SGLT*, sodium glucose transporter. (Data from American Diabetes Association. Standards of medical care in diabetes-2019. *Diabetes Care*. 2019;42(suppl 1):S13–S28. https://doi.org/10.2337/dc19-Sint01).

Guidelines

Overall, the 2019 ADA/EASD Standards of Care endorse an individualized approach to pharmacological DM therapy (Fig. 4.8). Key comorbidities (ASCVD, HF, and CKD), effect on weight gain, risk of hypoglycemia, cost, and patient preference should all be taken into consideration when deciding on the antidiabetic agent.

Metformin is still recommended as the primary agent for T2DM. If HbA1c target is not achieved after 3 months, the choice of add-on therapy to metformin can be guided by comorbidities. Due to the cardiovascular benefit demonstrated for GLP-1 receptor agonists and SGLT-2 inhibitors, these agents should be used for patients with established ASCVD. If HF or CKD predominates, SGLT-2 inhibitors should be initiated, which demonstrated inhibition of HF and CKD progression in CVOTs, if the eGFR is acceptable. Empagliflozin, dapagliflozin, and canagliflozin have proven to reduce HF incidence and CKD development in CVOTs. If patients do not tolerate SGLT-2 inhibitors or the eGFR is not adequate, GLP-1 receptor agonists should be used with evidence of reducing CVD events. For GLP-1 receptor agonists, liraglutide was shown to have the strongest evidence.

TZDs should be avoided in patients with HF. If weight loss is a therapeutic goal, then physicians can prescribe GLP-1 receptor agonists. Semaglutide had the greatest evidence for weight loss. Due to the moderate glucose-lowering efficacy of DPP-4 inhibitors and the possible elevated risk of HF associated with some DPP-4 inhibitor agents, it is only second-line therapy in the guidelines.

Future Directions

Cardiometabolic Specialist

The strong relationship between DM and CVD has long been established. T2DM medication now also can affect cardiovascular health, as recent large outcome trials of GLP-1 receptor agonists and SGLT-2 inhibitors have demonstrated. In light of this, some argue that T2DM cannot be allotted to one specialty but be described as a cardiometabolic disease requiring expert clinical knowledge of both endocrinologists and cardiologists. Initiation of "cardiometabolic" specialist training programs combining fields of expertise of endocrinologist, cardiologists, and primary care doctors is currently under discussion. The cardiometabolic specialist integrating these disciplines offers the most benefit to the increasingly aging and obese patients with T2DM and cardiovascular disease.[203] The cardiometabolic specialist integrates disciplines that offer the most benefit to the increasingly aging and obese patients with T2DM and cardiovascular disease.[203]

Vitamin D

Current research has posited low 25-hydroxyvitamin D levels as a risk factor for T2DM, and observational studies have supported this association.[2–4] However, a trial randomizing 2423 participants to 4000 IU of vitamin D per day did not find a significantly lower risk of T2DM than placebo.[205]

Oral Semaglutide

A novel development in GLP-1 research is the development of an oral formulation of semaglutide that proved successful in multiple trials. The series of PIONEER (Peptide Innovation for Early Diabetes Treatment) trials compared oral semaglutide to placebo,[206] sitagliptin,[207] and liraglutide,[208] and concluded that oral semaglutide was superior to all of these agents in terms of weight loss and HbA1c reduction. In addition, oral semaglutide proved safe for patients with T2DM with renal impairment.[209] Current studies have demonstrated promising results regarding cardiovascular outcomes. Oral semaglutide was shown to be noninferior to placebo by reducing the risk of the primary outcome by 21% ($P < 0.001$) in PIONEER 6, but due to the small scale of the trial (PIONEER 6 enrolled 3183 patients), it was too underpowered to demonstrate superiority. The study also showed oral semaglutide's cardiovascular benefit by extensively lowering the risk of multiple secondary endpoints; oral semaglutide significantly reduced death from cardiovascular cause (HR 0.49; 95% CI 0.27–0.92) and all-cause mortality (HR 0.51; 95% CI 0.31–0.84) compared to placebo. The oral form of GLP-1 receptor agonists will hopefully improve therapy adherence compared to injectable medication.

References

Complete reference list available at www.expertconsult.com.

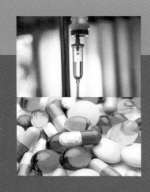

第5章
肥胖症的药物治疗

肥胖症是一个全球性的社会和医学问题。根据2017年的统计，全球有超过19亿人超重（BMI为25～29 kg/m²），超过6.5亿人肥胖（BMI≥30 kg/m²）。自1975年以来，全球人口肥胖率增加了两倍。从BMI>25 kg/m²开始，人群总死亡风险将随BMI的增加而持续增加。据估计，全球每年有超过280万人死于肥胖。减重对人体健康很重要，特别是对于预防糖尿病、患有与肥胖相关疾病的人群，即使是相对较小的减重（5%～10%）也能给人体带来良好的代谢改善。

纵观各减重治疗手段，主要有三大类：①饮食及生活方式调节，该方法操作简单，但效果有限且难以长期坚持；②减重手术，该方法疗效最为显著，但属于有创操作，仅适用于一小部分年轻、并发症少且显著肥胖的人群，不具有普适性；③居于两者之间的为药物治疗，该方法理论上似乎能平衡前两者的优缺点，从而兼顾疗效和普适性，但在过去的数十年中，多种减重药物的尝试均以失败告终，如非选择性5-羟色胺受体激动剂（芬氟拉明-芬特明组合药丸）、大麻素受体拮抗剂（利莫那班）、拟交感神经药（西布曲明）等，这些药物实际减重效果有限，且均因其严重的心血管或神经系统不良反应而下架。这些药物治疗失败的经验，也导致美国食品药品监督管理局对减重药物的审批政策更严格，即必须有明确的减重效果和心血管安全证明。

但既往药物试验的失败，并不代表药物治疗这一策略的错误，强烈的临床需求仍然推动着减重药物的持续研发，并更加注重安全性及心血管获益，至今已有多种减重药物获批用于肥胖症的治疗。

本章全面介绍了肥胖症治疗的各类方法及已有的临床证据，着重介绍了近年来减重药物的治疗进展，并详细列举了这些药物的作用机制、减重效果和不良反应，包括脂肪酶抑制剂（奥利司他）、拟交感神经药（苯丙氨酸、二乙基丙酮、苯非他明和苯二甲肼）、选择性5-羟色胺2C受体激动剂（氯卡色林）、胰高血糖素样肽-1受体激动剂（利拉鲁肽、度拉糖肽、司美格鲁肽）、芬特明、托吡酯、纳曲酮、安非他酮等多种已获批用于肥胖症的药物。

本章重点介绍了胰高血糖素样肽-1受体激动剂及其相关临床证据。虽然目前还没有任何药物显示出对非糖尿病肥胖症患者的心血管获益，但越来越多的证据表明，胰高血糖素样肽-1受体激动剂对糖尿病患者（其中大部分也是肥胖症患者）有心血管获益，这使得胰高血糖素样肽-1受体激动剂成为目前最具临床吸引力的减重药物选择，特别是对糖尿病或心血管风险较高的患者。未来需要更多的研究以确定这类药物的获益机制，以及开发出其他安全有效的治疗方式，为解决肥胖症这一全球性问题提供支持。

舟　君

Drugs for Obesity

BENJAMIN M. SCIRICA

Drug Class Overview and Guidelines

Obesity is a worldwide societal and medical problem. The most recent estimates (2017) suggest that more than 1.9 billion people in the world are overweight (body mass index [BMI] 25–29 kg/m^2) and over 650 million are obese (BMI $\geq$ 30 kg/m^2).[1] In the United States, over 39% of the adult population are obese and 33% are overweight, and obesity rates have doubled over the last 20 years.[2] Globally, rates of obesity have tripled since 1975 with most of the global population living in countries where overweight and obesity kills more people than poor nutrition. There is a well-accepted relationship between BMI and overall mortality with a steady increase in risk starting at a BMI greater than 25. It is estimated that there are between 115,000 and 300,000 obesity-related deaths in the United States each year and over 2.8 million deaths attributable to obesity worldwide. The costs associated with obesity are estimated to be almost $150 billion a year in the United States alone.

There is a consensus that losing weight is important to improve health, in particular for prevention of diabetes and other obesity-related diseases such as sleep apnea, fatty liver, and polycystic ovary disease.[3] Even relatively small weight loss (5%–10%) will result in favorable metabolic improvements. However, it has been challenging to identify either weight loss strategies or specific medical therapies that achieve meaningful and sustained weight loss. Moreover, the history of pharmacotherapy for weight loss includes many instances of drugs that caused serious side effects and therefore limited the interest in the clinical use of pharmacotherapy for the treatment of obesity. More challenging is the fact that no study of the weight loss strategy or therapy has definitively demonstrated cardiovascular benefit. While multiple weight loss studies have improved glycemic indices or reduced cardiac risk factors, none resulted in reductions in cardiovascular events such as myocardial infarction, stroke, revascularization, heart failure, or cardiovascular death. The absence to date of any study demonstrating cardiovascular benefit of weight loss has raised the question whether there is truly a causal relationship between obesity and cardiovascular outcomes, or whether obesity simply exacerbates other known cardiovascular risk factors, or is just a marker of worse metabolic health.

Weight Loss Intervention

The clinical challenge in choosing weight loss therapies is that the most effective weight loss strategy is bariatric surgery, which is invasive and only available to a relatively small proportion of patients. Bariatric surgery tends to be used in younger patients with fewer comorbidities but significant burden of obesity-related risks. At the other end of the therapeutic spectrum for obesity therapy are the diet and lifestyle interventions, for which there are many different programs (some with better evidence than others) but that in general attain modest weight loss that is difficult to maintain over time. Pharmacologic therapy falls in between the ends of the therapeutic spectrum but historically provided only modest weight loss at relatively high cost and with treatment-limiting side effects. There is therefore great clinical need to bridge this spectrum by discovering more effective weight loss pharmacotherapy that can achieve greater and sustained weight loss without safety concerns and therefore expand the potential patients population that could achieve significant and sustained weight loss (Fig. 5.1).

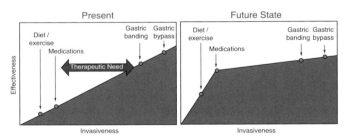

Fig. 5.1 Obesity treatment options. Currently, there is a large gap between diet/lifestyle/pharmacologic therapy on the left and bariatric surgery on the right in terms of effectiveness. Ideally, on the right, pharmacologic therapy will safely achieve greater weight loss and expand treatment options.

Historical and Regulatory Perspective

The past several decades unfortunately witnessed several notable failures among pharmacologic weight loss therapy. In 1997, the combination pill fenfluramine–phentermine, a nonselective serotonin agonist, was found to increase the risk of valvulopathy and pulmonary hypertension after a relatively short treatment duration, leading to its removal from the market. Rimonabant, a cannabinoid antagonist, received approval for use in Europe. A large randomized study subsequently demonstrated an unacceptable increase in neuropsychiatric side effects that led to its withdrawal. Another drug, Sibutramine, a sympathomimetic, facilitates weight loss; however, in a randomized trial, it increased myocardial infarction and stroke. A full list of drugs withdrawn or not approved in the United States is presented in Table 5.1.[4]

Based on this history, the US Food and Drug Administration (FDA) provided new guidance for the industry developing products for weight management, which required that to achieve approval, a drug must first demonstrate efficacy for weight loss, defined as both (1) greater than or equal to 5% weight loss compared to placebo, and (2) that the proprotion of patients who achieve at least 5% weight loss must be overall greater than 35% and twice the rate of placebo. In addition, the FDA required that any new agent must demonstrate cardiovascular safety through a post-marketing cardiovascular outcome trial, where the trial must exclude an excess risk defined by a noninferiority boundary of the upper amount of the 95% confidence interval (CI) <1.4 for a composite major adverse cardiovascular endpoint.[5] As in the diabetes area, this guidance has dramatically changed the development programs for obesity-related medications.

Guidelines

Weight loss treatment must be multimodal and address underlying medical, behavioral, and lifestyle conditions that can often prevent adequate and sustained weight loss. Guidelines recommend that all obese and overweight patients receive lifestyle therapy (reduced-calorie healthy meal plan/physical activity/behavioral interventions). For all obese patients (BMI ≥ 30 kg/m^2) and those overweight patients (BMI ≥ 25 kg/m^2) with adiposity-related complications, weight loss medications are recommended if lifestyle therapy does not achieve adequate weight loss. Bariatric surgery is recommended for those overweight and obese patients with at least one severe complication.[6-9]

Table 5.1

Drug	Year introduced or withdrawn	Comments
Thyroid	1892	Mimics endogenous thyroxine/triiodothyronine. Associated with tachycardia and increase in metabolic rate
Dinitrophenol	1932	Uncouples oxidative phosphorylation. Associated with cataracts, neuropathy, and death
Amphetamine	1937	Noradrenergic-dopaminergic drug. Associated with recreational abuse and pulmonary hypertension
Aminorex	1965	Noradrenergic drug. Associated with pulmonary hypertension
Fenfluramine, dexfenfluramine	1997	Serotonergic drugs. Both associated with cardiac valvulopathy and primary pulmonary hypertension
Phenylpropanolamine	1998	Noradrenergic agonist. Associated with strokes and cardiovascular deaths
Ephedra alkaloids	2003	Noradrenergic drugs. Associated with heart attacks, strokes, and death
Rimonabant	2008	Cannabinoid receptor antagonist. Associated with depression and suicidality
Sibutramine	2010	Norepinephrine-serotonin reuptake inhibitor. Associated with elevated blood pressure and death
Locaserin	2020	Selective serotonin (5HT) C2 receptor agonist. Concern for increased cancer risk

Adapted from Bray GA Heisel WE, Afshin A, et al. The science of obesity management: an Endocrine Society scientific statement. *Endocr Rev.* 2018; 39(2):79–132.

Obesity Pathophysiology

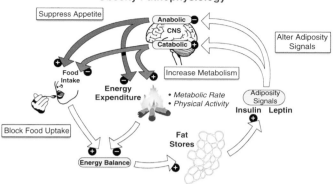

Fig. 5.2 Pathophysiology of obesity. (Modified from Cummings DE, Schwartz MW. Genetics and pathophysiology of human obesity. *Annu Rev Med* 2003;54: 453–471.)

Pathophysiology and Mechanism of Action

The pathophysiology of obesity is a complex lifelong interplay between genetic, societal, cultural, behavioral, psychological, and medical factors, to name just a few, that result in the final heterogeneous manifestation of excess weight gain. The simplest calculation for obesity is the relationship between energy (caloric) intake and energy expenditure. However, each side of this balance becomes much more complicated based on nutritional content, central signaling, metabolic set points, and hormonal variations. Fig. 5.2 provides a broad overview of energy balance together with potential areas for prevention. In general, one can tilt this scale by (1) blocking food uptake, (2) suppressing appetite, (3) increasing metabolism, or (4) altering adiposity signaling.

Centrally Acting Drugs

Centrally acting drugs affect a variety of pathways within the hypothalamus. Fig. 5.3 reviews the complex interplay between anorexigenic (loss of appetite) and orexigenic (appetite stimulant) signaling in the key areas such as the nucleus accumbens neuron, the dorsal vagal complex, paraventricular nucleus, lateral hypothalamic area, and the arcuate nucleus.[4] Different therapeutic

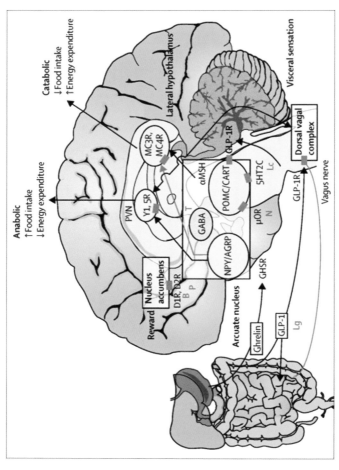

Fig. 5.3 See legend on facing page.

agents will inhibit orexigenic or augment anorexigenic pathways, but the redundancy in the different pathways highlights why single agents are often ineffective in achieving significant weight loss.

Lifestyle and Diet Interventions

ifestyle and diet can typically achieve a clinically relevant 5% to 10% weight loss, though it requires dedicated interventions to activate and sustain patients over time. Current guidelines recommend that a program have at least 14 direct patient–provider interventions to activate and sustain a patient in a program of calorie-reduced diet, increased exercise, and physical activity as well as the behavioral support. Most patients will achieve the greatest weight loss over the first 6 months; however, sustaining long-term weight loss is challenging and generally requires increased physical activity[4,7,8]

Fig. 5.3, Cont'd   **Sites of action of anti-obesity drugs.** Schematic depiction of the regions of the brain involved in regulation of appetite and energy expenditure, showing the sites of action of US Food and Drug Administration-approved anti-obesity drugs. Red text indicates anti-obesity drugs. The primary brain region involved in the regulation of energy balance is the arcuate nucleus of the hypothalamus. The dorsal vagal complex in the brainstem receives input from the vagus nerve. Several drugs modulate the activity of pro-opiomelanocortin neurons in the arcuate nucleus and in areas of the hypothalamus and other regions of the brain with the overall effect of reducing food intake and increasing energy expenditure. GLP-1 is made in the intestine and seems to act on vagal afferents, the brainstem, and also the hypothalamus. The nucleus accumbens is involved in rewarding aspects of food intake and responds to neural signals, including those regulating homoeostatic feeding to alter the perception of reward associated with food stimuli. Black arrows indicate stimulatory signals and red arrows indicate inhibitory signals. *αMSH*, melanocyte-stimulating hormone. *AGRP*, agouti-related peptide; *B*, bupropion; *CART*, cocaine and amphetamine related transcript; *D1R*, dopamine 1 receptor; *D2R*, dopamine 2 receptor; *GABA*, γ-aminobutyric acid; *GHSR*, growth hormone secretagogue (ghrelin) receptor; *GLP-1*, glucagon-like peptide-1; *GLP-1R*, glucagon-like peptide-1 receptor; *Lc*, lorcaserin; *Lg*, liraglutide; *MC3R*, melanocortin-3 receptors; *MC4R*, melanocortin-4 receptors; *N*, naltrexone; *NPY*, neuropeptide Y; *P*, phentermine; *POMC*, pro-opiomelanocortin; *PVN*, paraventricular nucleus; *T*, topiramate; *μOR*, μ-opioid receptor. (From Bessesen DH, Van Gaal LF. Progress and challenges in anti-obesity pharmacotherapy. *Lancet Diabetes Endocrinol.* 6(3):237–248.)

Several studies have evaluated the intermediate to long-term effect of diet and lifestyle on cardiovascular outcomes. The Diabetes Prevention Program (DPP) randomized 3234 patients with impaired glucose tolerance and a mean baseline BMI of 34 kg/m^2 to placebo, metformin, or a lifestyle-modification program that included a goal of at least 7% weight loss and 150 minutes of physical activity per week. Over an average of 2.8 years of follow-up, the incidence of diabetes was 11.0, 7.8, and 4.8 cases per 100 person-years in the placebo, metformin, and the lifestyle groups, respectively. The lifestyle intervention was significantly more effective than metformin for preventing diabetes, though both strategies were superior to placebo.[10] After 15 years of follow-up, the incidences of diabetes were 55%, 56%, and 62%, respectively, though there was no difference in the aggregate rates of microvascular disease.[11]

One of the most rigorous lifestyle intervention study, the Look AHEAD (Action for Health in Diabetes) Study, randomized 5145 obese or overweight patients with type 2 diabetes to either an intensive lifestyle intervention or a control group report that received education only.[12] Over a median follow-up of almost 10 years, the intervention group achieved greater weight loss (8.6% versus 0.7% at 1 year; 6% versus 3.5% at study end), and had greater reductions in glycemic indices; however, much of this early benefit deteriorated over the subsequent years such that the early improvement was attenuated by year 3. There was no corresponding effect on the primary outcome of cardiovascular death, myocardial infarction, stroke or hospitalization for angina (hazard ratio [HR] 0.95; 95% CI 0.83–1.09; $P=0.51$). Unfortunately, much of the early benefit in terms of weight loss, reductions in waist circumference, and improved physical fitness deteriorated after the first year such that one cannot tell if the absence of cardiovascular benefit was because weight loss does not affect cardiovascular events or if weight loss was not sustained sufficiently to assess benefit.

The longest follow-up of a randomized lifestyle and diet intervention is from the Da Qing Study, which started in 1986 in China. Five hundred seventy-seven adults with impaired glucose tolerance were randomized to either control or one of three interventions (diet, exercise, or diet plus exercise). The latest update is now 30 years from the start of the study, with 94% follow-up. The combined intervention group had a median delay of diabetes by 3.96 years, and fewer cardiovascular events (HR 0.74, 95% CI 0.59–0.92, $P=0.006$), cardiovascular deaths (HR 0.67, 95% CI 0.48–0.94; $P=0.022$), and all-cause deaths (0.74, 95% CI 0.61–0.89; $P=0.0015$), and an average increase in life expectancy of 1.44 years (95% CI 0.20–2.68; $P=0.023$) (Fig. 5.4).[13]

Lifestyle and diet will always be the cornerstone of the management of weight loss and a key component to an overall healthy

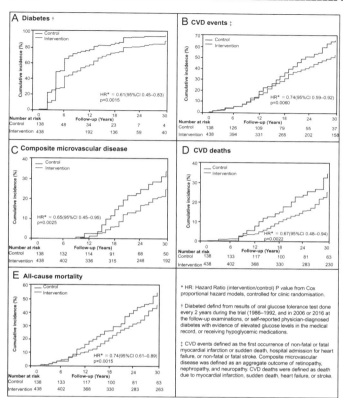

Fig. 5.4 Prevention of diabetes over 30 years from intense lifestyle intervention – The Da Qing Study. Kaplan-Meier plot of cumulative incidence of diabetes (A), cardiovascular disease (CVD) events (B), composite microvascular disease (C), CVD deaths (D), and all-cause mortality (E) in the control and intervention groups during the 30-year follow-up (From Gong, Q, Zhang P, Wang J, et al. Morbidity and mortality after lifestyle intervention for people with impaired glucose tolerance: 30-year results of the Da Qing Diabetes Prevention Outcome Study. *Lancet Diabetes Endocrinol* 2019;7(6): 452–461.)

life, but multiple studies demonstrate that this alone is unlikely to meaningfully alter the major complications associated with obesity. Economic, societal, and regulatory interventions that encourage and support large populations to eat more healthily and increase overall physical activity are likely the only methods by which population-level weight loss management can be achieved and sustained, in particular among the younger population.

Bariatric Surgery and Medical Devices

The two most common surgical interventions for weight loss are sleeve gastrectomy and Roux-en-Y gastric bypass. Roux-en-Y gastric bypass is the most effective weight loss therapy available, with up to 40% of weight loss at 1 year and sustained weight loss of over 25% by 5 years. The weight loss with sleeve gastrectomy is slightly less than Roux-en-Y, but still achieves up to 30% weight loss at 1 year and 20% over 5 years. Sleeve gastrectomy is a less complex surgery than the Roux-en-Y, with fewer complications, and therefore is performed more commonly.

There has been one randomized trial of bariatric surgery versus medical therapy together with several large observational studies. The Surgical Treatment and Medications Potentially Eradicate Diabetes Efficiently (STAMPEDE) study randomized 150 patients with diabetes to receive either intensive medical therapy alone or medical therapy plus Roux-en-Y gastric bypass or sleeve gastrectomy. The primary outcome of the study was an achieved glycated hemoglobin (hemoglobin A1c) of less than 6% with or without the use of diabetes medications. After 5 years of follow-up only 2% of the medical therapy group achieved the primary endpoint compared to 29% of patients who had gastric bypass and 23% with sleeve gastrectomy. The absolute reduction in hemoglobin A1c was 2.1% with surgery versus 0.3% with medical therapy ($P = 0.003$). Gastric bypass surgery resulted in the greatest weight loss (23.3 kg), followed by sleeve gastrectomy (18.6 kg), which was much more than medical therapy alone (5.3 kg, $P < 0.05$ for all comparisons).[14] This study was not powered for clinical outcomes and the cardiovascular event rates were low; however, the favorable metabolic effects of sustained weight loss are clinically impressive.

Two large observational studies have reported an association between bariatric surgery and lower risk of cardiovascular events. The Swedish Obese Subjects (SOS) study was a prospective nonrandomized study of 4047 subjects who underwent either bariatric surgery or conventional standard of care. Over 15 years of follow-up, patients in the surgical group had 16% more weight loss, 78% lower risk of developing incident diabetes, a 33% lower risk of cardiovascular death, myocardial infarction, or stroke, and a 24% lower risk of all-cause mortality.[15,16] Another observational study, a cohort study of 2287 patients who underwent surgery and 11,435 controls matched for diabetes and BMI, found that metabolic surgery was associated with almost 15% weight loss and more than 1% absolute reduction in hemoglobin A1c, 41% reduction in all-cause mortality, and a 62% reduction in the risk of heart failure.[17] Despite the large numbers and extended follow-up, the studies were observational and cannot prove a causal association between surgery and outcomes. Bariatric surgery should be considered in obese patients with diabetes and is recommended in most guidelines for appropriate patients because of the improvement in glycemic indices, hypertension, dyslipidemia, and overall quality of life metrics.

There are several medical devices approved for the treatment of obesity that achieve weight loss through different mechanisms, including intragastric balloons, neural stimulation systems to increase satiety, and external drainage systems. These tend to lead to weight loss of less than 10% compared to placebo and have a variety of complications depending on the actual device.[18]

Pharmacologic Therapy

Pharmacotherapy should be considered for either obese patients (BMI $\geq$ 30 kg/m^2) or overweight patients (BMI $\geq$ 25 kg/m^2) with a weight-related comorbidity such as diabetes, fatty liver, or sleep apnea. Unfortunately, there are very few head-to-head studies of weight loss drugs so that determining which agent is the most "effective" remains a clinical challenge. Moreover, most weight loss studies are performed in relatively young and healthy populations, are often not more than a year in duration, and are plagued by high rates of drug discontinuation (either due to lack of weight loss or side effects). In practice, if a patient does not achieve at least a 5% weight loss by 12 weeks, then they are unlikely to benefit from longer-term treatment. Pharmacotherapy has only been studied in addition to diet and lifestyle modification. Because obesity is a heterogeneous disease with multiple underlying pathophysiologic axes, individual patients may respond differently based on the drugs' mechanism of action. Thus it is common for patients to cycle through several different classes of agents to identify the most effective.

Orlistat

Orlistat inhibits gastric and pancreatic lipases, thus preventing fat hydrolysis and absorption and increasing fecal fat excretion. With a normal diet, orlistat inhibits the absorption of 25% to 30% of the calories from fat. The 1-year placebo-subtracted weight loss with orlistat is only about 3%, but in one randomized trial of 3304 obese or overweight patients, orlistat reduced the incidence of diabetes after 4 years (6.2% with orlistat versus 9% in the placebo).[19] In another study of 892 subjects, orlistat 120 mg three times daily led to an 8 mg/dL reduction in fasting low-density lipoprotein (LDL) cholesterol levels compared to placebo.[20] Patients must take multivitamins to compensate for the malabsorption of fat-soluble vitamins. While there are no systemic side effects of orlistat because it is not absorbed, its mechanism of action will lead to fecal urgency, incontinence, and flatus, which often limits adherence. Oxalate-induced acute kidney injury has also been reported with orlistat and may be due to the binding of intraintestinal calcium leading to higher oxalate absorption.

Sympathomimetic Drugs

Sympathomimetic drugs induce weight loss by promoting early satiety through increased norepinephrine release or inhibiting its reuptake in the central nerve terminals that signal satiety in the hypothalamus. Because these drugs are all related to amphetamines, they also increase blood pressure and heart rate. There are four sympathomimetic drugs approved by the FDA for the short-term treatment (12 weeks) of obesity: phentermine, diethylpropion, benzphetamine, and phendimetrazine. Sibutramine, another sympathomimetic drug that also blocks serotonin reuptake, was withdrawn from the market because of the higher risk of myocardial infarction and stroke, despite promoting weight loss.[21] Long-term use of sympathomimetic drugs is discouraged because of side effects and potential for abuse. Phentermine is by far the most commonly prescribed drug in this class, and overall is the most commonly used weight loss drug in the United States. In short-term randomized control trials, phentermine 30 mg/day led to about 4% to 6% weight loss relative to placebo. In addition to increase in heart rate and blood pressure, this class of drugs can cause insomnia, nervousness, and dry mouth.

Phentermine/Topiramate

In 2012, the FDA approved a combination capsule of phentermine and the extended-release antileptic drug topiramate for obese patients with a BMI ≥ 30 kg/m^2 or with a BMI ≥ 27 kg/m^2 with at least one weight-related comorbidity. Topiramate, an inhibitor of sodium and calcium channels that also inhibits the effect of gamma-aminobutyric acid (GABA), was noted to facilitate weight loss in other disease areas. In several dedicated weight loss studies, this combination appeared to be the most potent oral obesity therapy on the market, with placebo-subtracted 1-year weight loss from 8.6% to 9.3%. The CONQUER study randomized 2487 patients to placebo or the combination phentermine/topiramate for 56 weeks.[22] A total of 70% of patients in the higher-dose group achieved a 5% weight loss compared to 62% in the lower-dose group and 21% in the placebo group. The corresponding rates for 10% weight loss at 56 weeks were 48%, 37%, and 7%, respectively (Fig. 5.5). The most common side effects were dry mouth, constipation, insomnia,

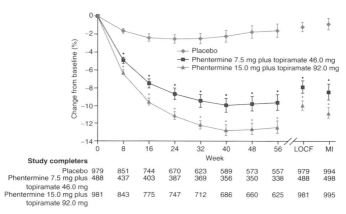

Study completers

	0	8	16	24	32	40	48	56	LOCF	MI
Placebo	979	851	744	670	623	589	573	557	979	994
Phentermine 7.5 mg plus topiramate 46.0 mg	488	437	403	387	369	356	350	338	488	498
Phentermine 15.0 mg plus topiramate 92.0 mg	981	843	775	747	712	686	660	625	981	995

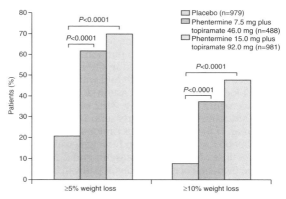

Fig. 5.5 Effects of phentermine plus topiramate on body weight. (A) Least squares mean change (95% CI) derived from three different statistical analyses. Weight change curves are plotted for completers by visit; shown to the right of the graph are data derived from the analyses of the intention-to-treat LOCF and MI. (B) Patients with at least 5% and at least 10% weight loss. *LOCF,* Last observation carried forward; *MI,* multiple imputation (From Gadde KM, Allison DB, Ryan DH, et al. Effects of low-dose, controlled-release, phentermine plus topiramate combination on weight and associated comorbidities in overweight and obese adults (CONQUER): a randomised, placebo-controlled, phase 3 trial. *Lancet* 2011;377 (9774):1341–1352.)

and dizziness. Because of the sympathomimetic actions of phentermine, this combination increases heart rate and should be used cautiously in patients with established cardiovascular disease or hypertension. This combination is contraindicated in pregnancy because of an increased risk of cleft palate for infants exposed during the first trimester. Women of childbearing age are required to have a pregnancy test before starting and monthly thereafter. The drug should be prescribed within a Risk Evaluation and Medication Strategy (REMS), which requires formal training and certification for physicians and pharmacies.

Lorcaserin

Lorcaserin is a selective serotonin (5HT) C2 receptor agonist. It was approved in 2012 for the treatment of obesity in addition to a reduced calorie diet and exercise. In contrast to nonselective serotonergic agonists such as fenfluramine and dexfenfluramine, lorcaserin is highly selective for the 2C receptor, which is centrally located in the hypothalamus, as compared with the 2A and 2B receptors, which are present on cardiac valves which is thought to be the mechanism by which fenfluramine and dexfenfluramine precipitate valve disease and pulmonary hypertension.

Lorcaserin was evaluated in three dedicated weight loss randomized trials in patients with and without diabetes. In the Behavioral Modification and Lorcaserin for Overweight and Obesity Management (BLOOM) Study, 3182 obese or overweight subjects were randomized either to lorcaserin 10 mg twice daily or placebo. At 1 year 47.5% of the patients on lorcaserin and 23.3% of patients on placebo lost 5% or more body weight, which corresponded to an average loss of 5.8 kg for lorcaserin and 2.2 kg for placebo. There was no evidence of cardiac valvulopathy in 2472 patients with serial echocardiograms at 1 year and in 1127 patients at 2 years.[23] The BLOSSOM study randomized 4008 obese or overweight patients to lorcaserin twice daily, lorcaserin once daily, or placebo. More patients treated with lorcaserin achieved at least 5% weight loss compared to placebo (47.2%, 40.2%, and 25%, $P < 0.001$). The corresponding rates for at least 10% weight loss were 22.6%, 17.4%, and 9.7% ($P < 0.001$). There was no evidence of an excess in FDA-defined valvulopathy with lorcaserin compared to placebo.[24] In a dedicated study of 604 patients with diabetes (BLOOM-DM) there was a 4.5% weight loss with lorcaserin 10 mg twice daily, 5.0% weight loss with lorcaserin once daily, and 1.5% with placebo ($P < 0.001$ for each). Corresponding reductions in hemoglobin A1c were 0.9%, 1.0%, and 0.4% ($P < 0.001$ for each).[25]

Lorcaserin is to date the only obesity drug to fulfill the FDA guidance for excluding excess of cardiovascular risk. The

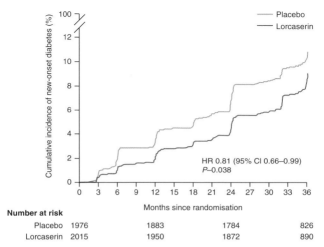

Fig. 5.6 Prevention of incident diabetes with lorcaserin versus placebo. Cumulative incidence of incident diabetes. Incidence is assessed in patients with prediabetes at baseline according to the intention-to-treat method. *HR,* Hazard ratio (From Bohula EA, Scirica BM, Inzucchi SE, et al. Effect of lorcaserin on prevention and remission of type 2 diabetes in overweight and obese patients (CAMELLIA-TIMI 61): a randomised, placebo-controlled trial. *Lancet* 2018;392(10161): 2269–2279.)

CAMELLIA–TIMI 61 study randomized 12,000 obese or overweight patients with established cardiovascular disease, or diabetes with other cardiovascular risk factors, to lorcaserin 10 mg twice daily or placebo.[26] The primary safety endpoint was the composite of cardiovascular death, myocardial infarction, or stroke. The co-primary efficacy endpoints were (1) an expanded clinical endpoint that included cardiovascular death, myocardial infarction, stroke, hospitalization for heart failure, unstable angina, or coronary revascularization; and (2) the incidence of type 2 diabetes in patients with prediabetes. At 12 months, there was a net weight difference of 2.8 kg between arms of the study. This led to a significant reduction in the incidence of diabetes in patients with prediabetes (8.5% versus 10.3%, HR 0.81, 95% CI 0.66–0.99, $P=0.038$) (Fig. 5.6).[26] Lorcaserin fulfilled the primary safety endpoint of cardiovascular death, myocardial infarction, or stroke (HR 0.99, 95% CI 0.85–1.14, P for noninferiority <0.001), but did not demonstrate superiority for the expanded cardiovascular endpoint (12.8% in lorcaserin versus 13.3% in placebo, HR 0.97, 95% CI 0.87–1.07, $P=0.55$).[26] Lorcaserin also reduced the primary composite renal end point, which included a combination of new or worsening albuminuria and evidence of other renal dysfunction (HR 0.87, 95% CI 0.79–0.96, $P=0.006$).[27] In February 2020, the FDA requested that the manufacturer of lorcaserin voluntarily withdraw the weight loss drug from the U.S. market because a safety clinical trial shows an increased occurrence of cancer (462 patients [7.7%] with diagnosis of cancer in the lorcaserin group vs. 423 patients [7.1%] in placebo). (https://www.fda.gov/drugs/drug-safety-and-availability/fda-requests-withdrawal-weight-loss-drug-belviq-belviq-xr-lorcaserin-market)

Naltrexone/Bupropion

The combination of naltrexone, an opioid antagonist, and bupropion, a norepinephrine–dopamine reuptake inhibitor and nicotinic receptor antagonist, was approved by the FDA in 2014 for the management of obesity. The Contrave Obesity Research I (COR-I) study randomized 1742 patients to two doses of naltrexone/bupropion versus placebo.[28] Only 50% of patients actually completed the 56 weeks of treatment. The main change in body weight was −1.3% for placebo, −6.1% for the high-dose combination group, and −5.0% for the low-dose combination group. A total of 16% of patients in the placebo group had a body weight decrease of 5% or more compared to 48% in the high-dose and 39% in the low-dose treatment arms (Fig. 5.7). The most common side effects were nausea, headaches, constipation, dizziness, vomiting, and dry mouth. There was also transient increase in systolic blood pressure by 1.5 mmHg.

Naltrexone/bupropion was evaluated in the LIGHT Study, a cardiovascular outcome trial that randomized 8910 patients to placebo or naltrexone/bupropion. Almost one-third of the patients had established cardiovascular disease and the majority had type 2 diabetes. The trial was adequately powered to exclude the FDA-mandated upper bound of the 95% CI of 1.4 for a composite endpoint of cardiovascular death, myocardial infarction, or stroke. Unfortunately, during the trial, unblinded interim data was released publicly and thus compromised the scientific integrity of the study requiring its early termination. In the final analysis, the early benefit of active therapy noted after only 25% of the events attenuated to no treatment difference by the time the trial was completed. The rate of discontinuation of study drug exceeded 60% of the patients by 26 weeks, further compromising the scientific integrity of the study.[29] Because of these fundamental breaches of trial integrity, the FDA mandated that a new trial be performed, though it is unclear whether this will ever happen.

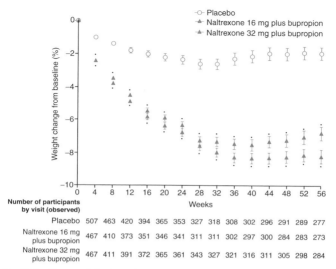

Fig. 5.7 Change in body weight with naltrexone plus bupropion versus placebo. Observed least squares mean percentage change from baseline in body weight and number of participants at each visit over 56 weeks. *$P < 0.0001$ compared with placebo (From Greenway FL, Fujioka K, Plodkowski RA, et al. Effect of naltrexone plus bupropion on weight loss in overweight and obese adults (COR-I): a multicentre, randomised, double-blind, placebo-controlled, phase 3 trial. *Lancet* 2010;376(9741):595–605.)

Glucagon-Like Peptide (GLP)-1 Receptor Agonist

GLP-1 is an incretin hormone secreted by the intestinal neuroendocrine L cells in response to food, and stimulates glucose-dependent insulin secretion. GLP-1 has a variety of actions in addition to increasing insulin release, including inhibition of glucagon release, slowing gastric emptying, decreasing central appetite satiety, and increasing heart rate. Several different GLP-1 receptor agonists are approved for the treatment of diabetes as daily or once-weekly injectable formulations, and most recently as a daily pill. Among the GLP-1 receptor agonists approved for diabetes, several (liraglutide, dulaglutide, semaglutide, and albiglutide) have been shown to reduce cardiovascular events, specifically cardiovascular death, myocardial infarction, and stroke, in cardiovascular outcome trials of patients with diabetes.[30] Among GLP-1 receptor agonists, the degree of weight loss appears to be both drug and dose dependent, with some agents appearing to be more potent than others in terms of weight loss and hemoglobin A1c reduction in patients with diabetes.

One GLP-1 receptor agonist, liraglutide, has been approved for the treatment of obesity in patients with and without diabetes using a higher dose than used in the treatment of diabetes. The SCALE trial randomized 3731 overweight or obese patients without diabetes for 56 weeks to either liraglutide 3.0 mg daily or placebo. Liraglutide reduced weight by a placebo-subtracted reduction 5.6 kg and lowered blood pressure by 2.8 mmHg. More than 63% of patients in the liraglutide group lost at least 5% of body weight compared to 27.1% in placebo, with rates of 33.1% versus 10.6%, respectively, for >10% weight loss.[31]

The SCALE Diabetes trial randomized three regimens in addition to low-calorie diet—the 3.0 mg daily obesity dose, the 1.8 mg daily obesity dose, or placebo—in 846 patients with diabetes. Achieved weight loss was 6.0% with 3.0 mg, 4.7% with 1.8 mg, and 2.0% with placebo, resulting in estimated placebo-subtracted values of 4% and 2.7% for the two dosing regimens. Weight loss of greater than 5% occurred in 54.3% with 3.0 mg, 40.4% with 1.8 mg, and 21% with placebo. The corresponding numbers for 10% weight loss were 25.2%, 15.9%, and 6.7%. In general across several weight loss agents, patient with diabetes tend to achieve less weight loss than those patients without diabetes.[32]

In the SCALE Obesity and Prediabetes study, 2254 patients were randomized to the obesity dose of 3 mg daily versus placebo and followed for 160 weeks. After 3 years of follow-up, liraglutide reduced the incidence of diabetes by almost 80% (HR 0.21, 95% CI 0.13–0.34). Almost 50% of patients treated with liraglutide had a 5% weight loss compared to 24% with placebo, 25% had a 10% weight loss compared to 10% placebo, and 11% had greater than 15% weight loss compared to just 3% in placebo (Fig. 5.8).[33] The most common side effects of liraglutide (and all GLP-1 receptor agonists) are nausea, diarrhea, constipation, and vomiting.

Several other GLP-1 receptor agonists are being evaluated for the treatment of obesity. In a dose-ranging study in 957 patients with or without diabetes, increasing doses of subcutaneous semaglutide resulted in more significant weight loss than placebo or liraglutide 3.0 mg. The highest dose of semaglutide resulted in a 16.3% change in body weight compared to 7.8% with liraglutide 3.0 mg and 2.3% in placebo. There was a corresponding increase in heart rate by approximately 4 to 6 bpm and a decrease in systolic blood pressure by 4 mmHg compared to placebo (Fig. 5.9).[34] The potential for cardiovascular benefit of once-weekly semaglutide in patients *without* diabetes is being tested in the 17,500 patient Semaglutide Effects on Cardiovascular Outcomes in People With Overweight or Obesity (SELECT) trial (ClinicalTrials.gov Identifier: NCT03574597).

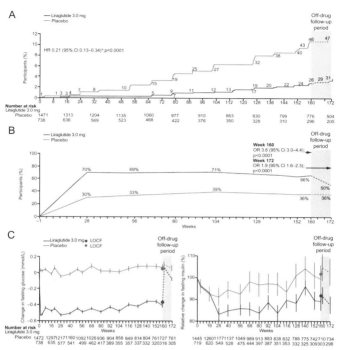

Fig. 5.8   Liraglutide 3.0 mg and glycemic status. (A) Kaplan-Meier estimates of the proportion of participants who received a diagnosis of type 2 diabetes during the course of the trial. Glycemic status was defined according to American Diabetes Association 2010 criteria. All individuals for whom diabetes was diagnosed had prediabetes at screening, except for one in the placebo group, who had normoglycemia. The numbers along the graph lines show the cumulative number of individuals who received a diagnosis of diabetes over the course of 172 weeks. (B) Proportion of participants with prediabetes at screening who regressed to having normoglycemia during the 172 weeks. (C) Changes in fasting plasma glucose and fasting serum insulin during the 172 weeks. Changes in fasting glucose translated into a similar corresponding pattern for glycated hemoglobin changes. Data shown are the observed means with least squares mean (fasting glucose) or with 95% CI (fasting insulin). *LOCF,* Last-observation-carried-forward; *OR,* odds ratio. *Derived from the primary Weibull analysis (From le Roux CW, Astrup A, Fujioka K, et al. 3 years of liraglutide versus placebo for type 2 diabetes risk reduction and weight management in individuals with prediabetes: a randomised, double-blind trial. *Lancet* 2017;389(10077): 1399–1409.)

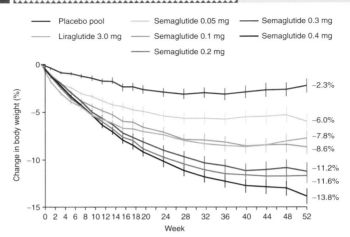

Fig. 5.9 Weight loss with semaglutide. Estimated mean changes (A) and observed mean changes (B) in body weight from baseline to week 52. Error bars are SEMs. Estimated changes (primary endpoint) are ANCOVA-modeled with jump-to-reference multiple imputation of missing data. Observed changes are without imputation and use either all available data at week 52 (in-trial) or only data from those still on treatment. *FE,* Fast (2-weekly) dose escalation (From O'Neil PM, Birkenfeld AL, McGowan B, et al. Efficacy and safety of semaglutide compared with liraglutide and placebo for weight loss in patients with obesity: a randomised, double-blind, placebo and active controlled, dose-ranging, phase 2 trial. *Lancet* 2018;392(10148):637–649.)

The compound LY3298176, a dual GLP-1/glucose-dependent insulinotropic polypeptide (GIP) agonist, was tested in a phase 2 dose-ranging study in 555 patients with diabetes and a BMI between 23 and 50 kg/m^2. At 26 weeks the highest dose of LY3298176 led to a weight loss of 11.3% compared to 0.4% in placebo. In comparison, the active comparator of the GLP-1 receptor agonist dulaglutide had a 2.7% weight loss. The highest dose of LY3298176 reduced hemoglobin A1c by 2.4% compared to no change in placebo (Fig. 5.10).[35]

Conclusion

There are multiple weight loss agents available, all with differing mechanisms of action, degrees of efficacy for weight loss, and side effects (Table 5.2). While no agent has yet demonstrated cardiovascular benefit in obese patients without diabetes, the extensive evidence of cardiovascular benefit of GLP-1 receptor agonist in

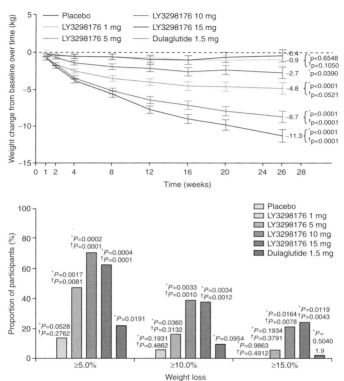

Fig. 5.10 Weight and HbA1c effects with the dual GLP-1/GIP agonist LY3298176. Body weight outcomes of treatment with LY3298176 at week 26. (A) Mixed-effect model for repeated measures analysis of the modified intention-to-treat (mITT) on treatment dataset. Data are least squares mean, with SE error bars. (B) Last observation carried forward endpoint data of the mITT on treatment dataset. *HbA1c*, Glycated hemoglobin. *P values versus placebo. †P values versus dulaglutide 1.5 mg (From Frias JP, Nauck MA, Van J, et al. Efficacy and safety of LY3298176, a novel dual GIP and GLP-1 receptor agonist, in patients with type 2 diabetes: a randomised, placebo-controlled and active comparator-controlled phase 2 trial. *Lancet* 2018;392(10160):2180–2193.)

patients with diabetes (most of whom are also obese) positions GLP-1 receptor agonists as the most clinically appealing pharmacologic weight loss option at this time, especially for patients with diabetes or at higher cardiovascular risk. Future research to identify potential mechanisms of benefit of this class of drug and the

Table 5.2

Cardiovascular considerations: effect of obesity therapies on heart rate and blood pressure

	Heart rate	Blood pressure	Cardiovascular effect	Prevention of diabetes
Phentermine/ topiramate	↑	↓	Unknown	Unknown
Sibutramine	↑	↑	Increased risk of myocardial infarction and stroke	Unknown
Buboprion/ naltrexone	↑	↑	Unknown	Unknown
Liraglutide	↑	↓	Cardioprotective at diabetes dosing	Yes
Lorcaserin	↓	↓	Neither increases nor reduces cardiovascular risk	Yes

development of additional safe and effective therapies are needed as part of a more societal approach to obesity and its related comorbidities.

References

Complete reference list available at www.expertconsult.com.

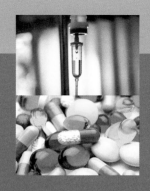

中文导读

第6章
调脂药物

　　血脂水平与动脉粥样硬化性心血管疾病密切相关。血脂主要包括总胆固醇、低密度脂蛋白胆固醇、高密度脂蛋白胆固醇、甘油三酯、其他脂蛋白及脂蛋白载体。低密度脂蛋白是导致动脉粥样硬化的重要因素。炎症与动脉粥样硬化的关系错综复杂，降脂治疗的作用靶点、脂蛋白在动脉粥样硬化形成中的作用与动脉粥样硬化的发病机制密不可分。当然，血脂异常的危险因素有很多，因此在特定人群中进行一级和二级预防十分必要。

　　人群的血脂代谢具有异质性，特殊人群的血脂代谢尤其值得关注，通过学习本章节可以了解代谢综合征、继发性血脂异常（特别是降血压药物对血脂的影响）、糖尿病患者及其他成年人（如妊娠女性等）的血脂代谢特点。

　　本章还涵盖了血脂异常的治疗方案，如一般的饮食治疗及非药物治疗，通过改变生活方式和减少危险因素而达到治疗效果。当然，药物治疗仍然占据重要地位，当下药物研发快速迭代，调脂药物也迎来了新的发展机遇。除应用较广泛的他汀类及贝特类药物外，读者还将了解胆固醇吸收抑制剂（依折麦布）、前蛋白转化酶枯草溶菌素9、贝培多酸、ω-3脂肪酸、胆汁酸螯合剂（树脂）、烟酸等多种药物的临床用法及注意事项。另外，本章还介绍了目前仍处于发展中的针对非低密度脂蛋白的治疗进展。

陈安天

6

Lipid-Modifying Drugs

ALIZA HUSSAIN · CHRISTIE M. BALLANTYNE

Serum cholesterol level is known to be related to incident atherosclerotic cardiovascular disease (ASCVD), with low-density lipoprotein cholesterol (LDL-C) found to be a dominant contributor to atherosclerosis. Multiple large landmark randomized controlled trials of lipid-lowering therapy have consistently shown that LDL-C lowering reduces risk of incident ASCVD.[1-3] The widespread availability, convincing clinical evidence, and relative safety of the statins have established pharmacologic control of blood lipids as an increasingly acceptable strategy. Furthermore, aggressive reduction in LDL-C, via intensified statin therapy, has been shown to yield greater reduction in cardiovascular morbidity and mortality. Therefore, measurement of cholesterol level, especially LDL-C, is an important step both for assessing cardiovascular risk and as an indicator of effectiveness of lipid-lowering therapy.

Cardiovascular risk assessment involves a thorough knowledge of both the serum lipid profile and other "traditional" risk factors that have been shown to play a pivotal role in atherosclerosis. The Pooled Cohort Equation, incorporated first in the 2013 American College of Cardiology (ACC)/American Heart Association (AHA) cholesterol guidelines,[4] is a risk prediction tool that integrates the major "traditional" risk factors, which include cigarette smoking, hypertension, dysglycemia, and advancing age along with blood lipid profile, to calculate 10-year risk for ASCVD (Table 6.1). This equation has been derived from five community-based cohorts that provide a broad and diverse representative sample of the U.S. population. The European guidelines recommend the use of the Systematic Coronary Risk Evaluation (SCORE) system for 10-year ASCVD risk prediction, as it was derived from a large representative European cohort data set.[5] The patient's absolute risk for developing cardiovascular disease (CVD) in the next 10 years determines the aggressiveness of lipid intervention. Since the 2013 ACC/AHA guidelines were published, immense research in individualized risk assessment has resulted in the emergence of several additional risk factors that are strongly associated with atherosclerosis and confer a higher-risk state. These "risk-enhancing factors" (see Table 6.1), as defined in the

Table 6.1

Traditional risk factors and risk-enhancing factors for ASCVD[6]

Traditional risk factors (used in the Pooled-cohort Equation)

Age
Cigarette smoking
Blood pressure
Presence or absence of diabetes mellitus
Serum TC
Serum HDL-C

Risk-enhancing factors

Family history of premature ASCVD (males, age <55 years; females, age <65 years)
Primary hypercholesterolemia (LDL-C, 160–189 mg/dL [4.1–4.8 mmol/L]; non–HDL-C 190–219 mg/dL [4.9–5.6 mmol/L])
Metabolic syndrome
CKD
Chronic inflammatory conditions such as such as psoriasis, RA, or HIV/AIDS
ABI <0.9
History of premature menopause (before age 40) and history of pregnancy-associated conditions that increase later ASCVD risk such as preeclampsia
High-risk race/ethnicities (e.g., South Asian ancestry)
Lipid/biomarkers: Associated with increased ASCVD
  – Persistently elevated, primary hypertriglyceridemia (≥175 mg/dL);
  – If measured:
    ○ Elevated high-sensitivity C-reactive protein (≥2.0 mg/L)
    ○ Elevated Lp(a) (≥50 mg/dL or ≥125 nmol/L)
    ○ Elevated apoB (≥130 mg/dL)

ABI, Ankle-brachial index; *AIDS;* Acquired immunodeficiency syndrome; *apoB,* apolipoprotein B; *ASCVD,* atherosclerotic cardiovascular disease; *CKD,* chronic kidney disease; *eGFR,* estimated glomerular filtration rate; *HDL-C,* high-density lipoprotein cholesterol; *HIV:* human immunodeficiency virus; *LDL-C,* low-density lipoprotein cholesterol; *Lp(a),* lipoprotein (a).
Adapted from AHA/ACC/AACVPR/AAPA/ABC/ACPM/ADA/AGS/APhA/ASPC/NLA/ PCNA Guideline on the management of blood cholesterol,[6] page 34.

2018 AHA/ACC guidelines for the management of blood cholesterol,[6] allow for more individualized risk assessment and care for patients. Conditions associated with systemic inflammation, e.g., metabolic syndrome, chronic renal disease, and elevated high-sensitivity C-reactive protein (hs-CRP), contribute to the pathogenesis of atherosclerosis and predispose to atherosclerotic events. Additionally, certain individual characteristics, such as premature menopause, certain ethnicities, and family history of premature ASCVD, confer higher risk. In addition to the standard lipid profile, two additional lipid-related measures, apolipoprotein B (apoB)[7] and lipoprotein(a) [Lp (a)],[8] can also be useful in risk assessment, especially in circumstances such as hypertriglyceridemia and/or LDL-C >160 mg/dL. Additional characteristics that can increase risk mentioned in the 2019 European Society of Cardiology (ESC)/European Atherosclerosis Society (EAS) Guidelines for the Management of Dyslipidaemias[9] include social deprivation, obesity and central obesity, physical inactivity, psychosocial stress including vital exhaustion, major psychiatric disorders, atrial fibrillation, left ventricular hypertrophy, obstructive sleep apnea syndrome, and nonalcoholic fatty liver disease.

Physicians may help guide younger patients toward long-term cardiovascular health by addressing early risk factors, whereas middle-aged and older patients may need a more-intensive approach because of their near-term risk for coronary heart disease (CHD). Effective strategy for lipid-lowering therapy therefore involves the following important considerations: (1) detailed evaluation of individualized risk for CVD based on lipid parameters as well as genetic and acquired risk factors; (2) review of lifestyle habits (e.g., diet, exercise, tobacco use) and development of individualized recommendations regarding healthy diet and body mass index and regular physical activity; (3) potential benefit of high-intensity therapy to achieve very low LDL-C levels, i.e., *"lower is better"*; and (4) growing recognition of newer lipid-lowering therapies and their role in CVD risk reduction. These developments and their translation into clinical practice hold the potential to improve patient outcomes.

Lipid-modifying therapy encompasses several classes of drugs: statins, cholesterol absorption inhibitors, proprotein convertase subtilisin/kexin type 9 (PCSK9) inhibitors, bile acid sequestrants, fibrates, and nicotinic acid (Fig. 6.1). These all have been shown to reduce LDL-C.

Inflammation and Atherogenesis

Atherosclerosis is characterized by a chronic inflammatory process of the arterial wall that results from unbalanced lipid accumulation and the ensuing maladaptive immune responses.[10] Atherosclerosis is triggered when circulating LDL enters the arterial wall and is retained in the subendothelium through interaction with proteoglycans in the extracellular matrix (Fig. 6.2). LDL modification within the arterial wall occurs through a series of oxidative steps, as reactive oxygen species or enzymes such as myeloperoxidase and

SITES AND TARGETS OF LIPID-LOWERING THERAPIES

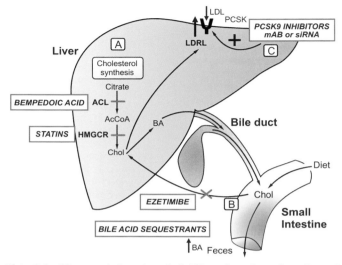

Fig. 6.1 Sites and targets of lipid-lowering therapies. Several cholesterol-lowering medications act through their respective mechanisms of actions to increase the number of low-density lipoprotein receptors (LDLR). Sites of action of individual therapies in boxes. (A) Liver. Citrate is converted to acetyl-CoA (AcCoA) by ACL (ATP citrate lyase) for fatty acid (FA) and cholesterol (Chol) biosynthesis; bempedoic acid blocks its activity. Statins inhibit 3-hydroxy-3-methylglutaryl coenzyme A reductase (HMGCR). (B) Small intestine. Absorption of dietary cholesterol into enterocytes is blocked by ezetimibe. Bile acid sequestrants bind luminal bile acids (BA) and block their enterohepatic circulation in the terminal ileum, thereby reducing cholesterol delivery to the liver. Reduced levels of intracellular cholesterol in A and B lead to upregulation of LDLR synthesis. (C) Recycling of LDLRs is increased by inhibiting proprotein convertase subtilisin kexin type 9 (PCSK9) either through monoclonal antibodies (mAB) or small interfering RNA (siRNA). *ASCVD,* atherosclerotic cardiovascular disease; *apo B,* apolipoprotein B; *CAC,* coronary artery calcium; *CHD,* coronary heart disease *hsCRP,* high-sensitivity C-reactive protein; *LDL-C,* low-density lipoprotein cholesterol; *Lp(a),* lipoprotein(a).

lipoxygenases are released from inflammatory cells. Oxidized LDL in turn damages the endothelium, which stimulates an immune and inflammatory response, with increased production of chemoattractant molecules, cytokines, and adhesion molecules, driving intimal immune cell infiltration.[11] Subsequently, the dysfunctional

ROLE OF LIPOPROTEINS IN ATHEROSCLEROSIS

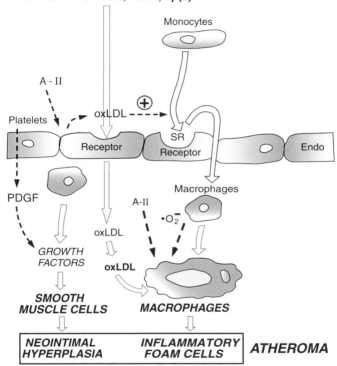

ATHEROGENIC, APOB-CONTAINING LIPOPROTEINS: LDL, TGRL, Lp(a)

Monocytes

A - II

Platelets

oxLDL ⊕

SR

Receptor

Receptor

Endo

PDGF

Macrophages

A-II

•O₂⁻

GROWTH FACTORS

oxLDL

oxLDL

SMOOTH MUSCLE CELLS

MACROPHAGES

| **NEOINTIMAL HYPERPLASIA** | **INFLAMMATORY FOAM CELLS** | **ATHEROMA** |

Fig. 6.2 Role of lipoproteins in atherosclerosis. Atherosclerosis is an inflammatory process that involves atherogenic, apolipoprotein B *(apoB)*–containing lipoproteins (low-density lipoprotein *[LDL]*, triglyceride-rich lipoprotein [*TGRL*; chylomicrons, very-low-density lipoprotein, and their remnants), and lipoprotein(a) [*Lp(a)*]) and proinflammatory agents such as oxidized LDL *(oxLDL)* and angiotensin-II *(A-II)*. OxLDL is taken up by scavenger receptors (SR), and circulating monocytes infiltrate into vascular endothelium and differentiate to macrophages, which take up oxLDL and become lipid-laden foam cells. Platelet-derived growth factor *(PDGF)* induces smooth muscle cell proliferation, which leads to neointimal hyperplasia.

endothelium is more permeable to circulating monocytes and T cells; both are transported into the intima, where the monocytes are converted into macrophages. Activated macrophages and T cells release a variety of mediators that collectively exacerbate inflammation and oxidation within the vessel wall.[12] Foam cells are formed when macrophages ingest oxidized LDL through receptors, including CD36. Elevated levels of circulating LDL therefore promote atherosclerosis and ASCVD.[13] Patients with severe hyperlipidemia and postprandial lipemia have been shown to have lipid uptake in circulating monocytes known as "foamy monocytes," which are activated and accelerate atherosclerosis.[14] Growth of the atherosclerotic lesion is characterized by smooth muscle cell proliferation and increased production of matrix metalloproteinases, which can cause deterioration of elastin and collagen within the extracellular matrix. Mature plaques typically consist of a lipid-rich necrotic core encased by a weakened fibrous cap. Inflammatory cells, such as macrophages, T cells, and mast cells, produce enzymes and proinflammatory mediators, promote the deterioration of fibrous caps, and may make mature plaques more prone to rupture.[15]

C-Reactive Protein

Much interest has centered on CRP, a general measure of inflammation that is produced in the liver in response to interleukin-6. This inflammatory marker is one of the "risk-enhancing factors" and is useful in assessment of patients at borderline or intermediate risk (5%–20% 10-year risk) according to traditional risk factors.[6] hs-CRP level <1 mg/L is considered low risk, and >3 mg/L is high risk, with an approximate doubling of the relative risk compared with the low-risk category. Elevated CRP is associated with obesity and the metabolic syndrome, and levels can be reduced through weight loss, increased physical activity, and smoking cessation. The Justification for the Use of Statins in Prevention: an Intervention Trial Evaluating Rosuvastatin (JUPITER) trial[16] (see later), which studied apparently healthy persons at increased ASCVD risk because of age, elevated hs-CRP (>2 mg/L), and one additional ASCVD risk factor, demonstrated the utility of hs-CRP in identifying individuals at increased risk despite having low to normal levels of LDL-C. Patients in this trial who attained LDL-C levels <50 mg/dL with rosuvastatin 20 mg daily had greater reductions in cardiovascular morbidity and mortality than the rest of the cohort.[17]

Prevention and Risk Factors

Primary Prevention

Assessment of global CVD risk is a fundamental step in primary prevention. In general, patients without known CHD have a much lower baseline risk of CVD events than patients with known CVD, and their potential absolute risk reduction with treatment for hypercholesterolemia will usually be smaller than for patients with established CVD. Hence, the decision of whether to initiate LDL-C treatment relies heavily on determination of global CVD risk. Based on the 2018 AHA/ACC cholesterol guidelines[6] and 10-year ASCVD risk as estimated by the Pooled Cohort Equation, adults 40–75 years of age in primary prevention can be classified as low risk (10-year risk of ASCVD <5%), borderline risk (5% to <7.5%), intermediate risk (7.5% to <20%), and high risk (≥20%). The 2019 ESC/EAS dyslipidemia guidelines,[9] on the other hand, divide patients into low risk (calculated SCORE <1%), moderate risk (calculated SCORE ≥1% but <5%), high risk (calculated SCORE ≥5% but <10%), or very high risk (calculated SCORE ≥10%). Individuals with markedly elevated single risk factors such as familial dyslipidemias (LDL-C >190 mg/dL or total cholesterol >310 mg/dL), severe hypertension (blood pressure ≥180/110 mmHg), or moderate chronic kidney disease (CKD) with estimated glomerular filtration rate <60 mL/min/1.73 m^2 are classified as high risk irrespective of SCORE in the ESC/EAS guidelines. Individuals with very high risk are treated similar to secondary prevention. Lifestyle interventions (dietary modification, smoking cessation, and physical activity) are first-line treatment and may achieve meaningful cholesterol reduction in many patients. Clinical trials of statins in the past decade have demonstrated safety and clinical event reduction across a spectrum of cardiovascular risk, even in populations with low baseline risk such as the Japanese.[18] The current 2018 AHA/ACC guidelines[6] recommend statin therapy along with lifestyle intervention for intermediate- to high-risk individuals; the absolute risk for developing CVD in the next 10 years determines the aggressiveness of lipid-lowering therapy. For individuals with intermediate risk, moderate-intensity statin to reduce LDL-C by 30%–49% is recommended, whereas for high risk, high-intensity statin to reduce LDL-C by ≥50% is recommended. The 2019 ESC/EAS dyslipidemia guidelines[9] recommend consideration of lipid-lowering therapy in addition to lifestyle interventions in individuals at moderate risk if LDL-C remains >100 mg/dL and in those at low risk if LDL-C remains >116 mg/dL. In patients at high risk, statin therapy along with lifestyle intervention is recommended to achieve LDL-C reduction of ≥50% from baseline and goal LDL-C goal of <70 mg/dL (Class IIa). The Heart Outcomes Prevention Evaluation–3 (HOPE-3) trial showed that ASCVD risk reduction in a large diverse population with intermediate risk outweighs the observable risk of treatment.[19] Furthermore, individuals in the high-risk category or with risk-enhancing factors as seen in the JUPITER trial[16,20] benefit from maximal statin therapy to achieve greater reductions in LDL-C level and ASCVD events. Still debated, however, are the fiscal and ethical issues related to the cost effectiveness of lipid drug therapy in lower-risk primary prevention.[21]

Secondary Prevention

The 2018 AHA/ACC guidelines[6] support aggressive lipid-lowering therapies for patients with established CHD or other ASCVD (including peripheral vascular disease, stroke, and aortic aneurysm) and recommend an LDL-C threshold of 70 mg/dL (1.8 mmol/L) to consider further LDL-C–lowering therapy, with the addition of ezetimibe or, in very-high-risk ASCVD patients, a PCSK9 inhibitor. Very high risk ASCVD was defined as either a history of multiple major ASCVD events or one major ASCVD event and multiple high-risk conditions (age >= 65 years, history of familial hypercholesterolemia, history of CABG or primary cutaneous intervention outside of the major ASCVD event, DM, HTN, CKD (eGFR 15–59 mL/min/1.73 m^2), current tobacco smoking, persistently elevated LDL-C >=100 mg/dL despite maximally tolerated statin and ezetimibe or history of congestive HF.

In contrast, the 2019 ESC/EAS dyslipidemia guidelines[9] adopted a broader definition of individuals at very high risk to include anyone with documented ASCVD, either clinically or on imaging. This group includes all of those identified in the 2018 AHA/ACC guideline as secondary prevention but additionally patients with diabetes mellitus and end organ damage, moderate to severe CKD (estimated glomerular filtration rate <30 mL/min/1.73 m^2) even in the absence of ASCVD, familial hypercholesterolemia with ASCVD or with another major risk factor, or a calculated SCORE of ≥10% (roughly equivalent to a 30% risk of 10-year ASCVD events according to the Pooled Cohort Equation). Furthermore, unlike the "threshold" of 70 mg/dL set by the AHA/ACC guidelines for considering the addition of a nonstatin lipid-modifying agent in very-high-risk patients, the ESC/EAS guidelines recommend a more aggressive approach: ≥50% reduction in LDL-C with an absolute "goal" of <55 mg/dL (Class IIa), with first ezetimibe and then PCSK9 inhibitors in all patients with ASCVD, even without a recent ASCVD event. This goal is based on LDL-C levels achieved in large-scale trials of PCSK9 inhibitors.[22,23] For patients with ASCVD who have a second vascular event within 2 years, a more aggressive LDL-C goal of <40 mg/dL may be considered.

While maximally tolerated high-intensity statin remains the cornerstone of lipid lowering, more recent trials such as the Improved Reduction of Outcomes: Vytorin Efficacy International Trial (IMPROVE-IT),[24] Further Cardiovascular Outcomes Research with PCSK9 Inhibition in Subjects with Elevated Risk (FOURIER),[22] and Evaluation of Cardiovascular Outcomes after an Acute Coronary Syndrome During Treatment with Alirocumab (ODYSSEY Outcomes)[23] now provide convincing evidence of clinical benefit with the addition of ezetimibe or PCSK9 inhibitors to statin to reduce LDL-C levels further. Although drug-induced LDL-C reduction remains an essential component of cardiovascular risk factor management, total risk can also be reduced through blood pressure control, dietary changes, increased exercise, weight loss, smoking cessation, and treatment of diabetes.

Blood Lipid Profile

Total Cholesterol and Low-Density Lipoprotein Cholesterol

Optimal total blood cholesterol levels are <150 mg/dL (3.9 mmol/L),[6] but it bears reemphasizing that cholesterol level is only part of the patient's absolute global risk. Furthermore, LDL-C, not total cholesterol, is the real target of therapy. Both the 2018 AHA/ACC guidelines[6] and 2019 ESC/EAS guidelines[9] emphasize lowering LDL-C as the primary target of therapy.

Every reduction in LDL-C of 40 mg/dL (1 mmol/L) is accompanied by a 22% reduction in vascular events.[25] There is now an overall consensus that "lower LDL is better." In a large meta-analysis, the Cholesterol Treatment Trialists' (CTT) Collaboration[25] suggested that lower LDL-C levels with more-intensive statin therapy resulted in greater reductions in cardiovascular events and proposed that aggressive reduction of LDL-C by 2–3 mmol/L (about 80–120 mg/dL) would reduce risk by about 40%–50%. Similarly, the Pravastatin or Atorvastatin Evaluation or Infection Therapy (PROVE IT) trial[26] showed that in patients with recent acute coronary syndrome (ACS), LDL-C levels of 62 mg/dL (1.60 mmol/L) led to convincingly better clinical outcomes than levels of 95 mg/dL (2.46 mmol/L). In primary prevention, the JUPITER study also supported this theory: a subgroup of patients achieving LDL-C levels <50 mg/dL had a 65% reduction in cardiovascular events compared with placebo, whereas risk reduction was 44% in the study overall.[16] In a study involving patients with stable coronary disease and much lower values of hs-CRP, high-dose atorvastatin reduced atheroma volume at an LDL-C of 79 mg/dL.[27] In another study, an LDL-C value of approximately 75 mg/dL (2 mmol/L) marked the point at which progression and regression of the atheroma volume were in balance.[28]

There had been debate in the past about whether there is a lower limit of LDL-C beyond which no further benefit occurs; this argument is now largely settled with the recent trials. In IMPROVE-IT,[24] mean LDL-C level of 54 mg/dL led to convincingly better clinical outcomes than mean LDL-C level of 70 mg/dL. Furthermore, LDL-C reduction even to very low levels (<30 mg/dL) appeared to be safe; these patients, in fact, had the lowest event rates. Similarly, in the FOURIER trial[22] (discussed later), the absolute event rate of cardiovascular death, myocardial infarction (MI), or stroke was lowest in patients achieving LDL-C level <20 mg/dL compared with the group with LDL-C >100 mg/dL (5.7% versus 7.8%; hazard ratio [HR] 0.69; 95% confidence interval [CI] 0.56–0.85; $P < 0.0001$). From a safety perspective, there were no differences in drug discontinuation rates or serious adverse events regardless of the achieved LDL-C at 4 weeks. Of the 1839 subjects who achieved ultralow LDL-C levels (<15 mg/dL), cardiovascular events further declined without any major safety concerns. However, it is important to note these data are limited to only 2.2 years of follow-up. An open-label extension study (FOURIER-OLE; NCT02867813)[29] is currently ongoing in the United States and Europe to determine safety over a 5-year follow-up period.

Based on these substantial data, the 2018 AHA/ACC Guideline on the Management of Blood Cholesterol[6] reintroduced thresholds for LDL-C in secondary prevention. An LDL-C threshold of ≥70 mg/dL is recommended for consideration of combination therapy to lower LDL-C further in patients with ASCVD.

High-Density Lipoprotein Cholesterol

High-density lipoprotein (HDL) is postulated to aid in clearing cholesterol from the foam cells that develop in diseased arteries, either by returning cholesteryl esters directly to the liver through scavenger receptor class B type I (SR-BI) or through transfer to the apoB-containing lipoproteins in exchange for triglycerides (reverse cholesterol transport mediated by cholesteryl ester transfer protein). HDL is also hypothesized to exert antiinflammatory and antioxidant effects.[30]

Low HDL-C level is an independent risk factor that is strongly associated with risk for CHD.[31] Many observational studies have shown an inverse relationship between HDL-C levels and incident cardiovascular events.[32] In the Cholesterol and Recurrent Events (CARE) study, every 10 mg/dL decrease in HDL-C led to a 10%

increase in risk.[33] HDL-C ≥60 mg/dL (1.6 mmol/L) is a negative (protective) risk factor, although it remains to be proven that raising HDL-C is cardioprotective. Low HDL-C is often associated with other lipid abnormalities such as high triglycerides, but there is insufficient evidence to support treating these lipid components separately. The Atherothrombosis Intervention in Metabolic Syndrome with Low HDL/High Triglycerides: Impact on Global Health Outcomes (AIM-HIGH) study, which investigated the effect of raising HDL-C with niacin, did not show cardiovascular benefit in CHD patients who were already treated with a statin to a baseline mean LDL-C of 71 mg/dL.[34] Furthermore, genetic studies do not show that genetic variants that can raise HDL-C lower cardiovascular events.[35] Although American and European guidelines do not propose a target value for HDL-C, they do recommend raising low HDL-C when possible by lifestyle modification (exercise, modest alcohol intake, weight loss, smoking cessation).

A low HDL-C level is often part of *atherogenic dyslipidemia*, with the other two components being elevated triglycerides and small, dense LDL particles. Atherogenic dyslipidemia is a risk factor in its own right[36] and is commonly found in patients with the metabolic syndrome, type 2 diabetes, and premature CHD. Lifestyle modification, combined with omega-3 fatty acids or fibrates, are the recommended treatments for patients with atherogenic dyslipidemia.

Triglycerides

Although triglyceride levels are commonly high in patients with CHD, the specific role of hypertriglyceridemia in atherogenesis remains controversial because it often occurs in conjunction with obesity, hypertension, and diabetes mellitus. Epidemiologically, an elevated triglyceride level can be an independent risk factor, even with adjustment for HDL-C,[37] and in PROVE IT, triglyceride <150 mg/dL (1.6 mmol/L) was associated with reduced cardiovascular risk even after major reduction of LDL-C.[38] AHA defines normal triglycerides as fasting level <150 mg/dL and optimal as <100 mg/dL.[39] The 2018 AHA/ACC guidelines[6] define two categories of elevated triglycerides: moderate hypertriglyceridemia (fasting or nonfasting triglycerides 150–499 mg/dL [1.6–5.6 mmol/L]) and severe hypertriglyceridemia (fasting triglycerides ≥500 mg/dL [≥5.6 mmol/L]) (Fig. 6.3). The guidelines recommend treatment with intensive dietary and lifestyle therapy for patients with moderate hypertriglyceridemia prior to initiating medications to lower triglyceride levels. A severely elevated triglyceride level (>500 mg/dL [2.3 mmol/L]) may be viewed with special concern for risk of pancreatitis and should be treated with therapy shown to lower triglycerides most reliably, i.e., fibrates or omega-3 fatty acids.[39]

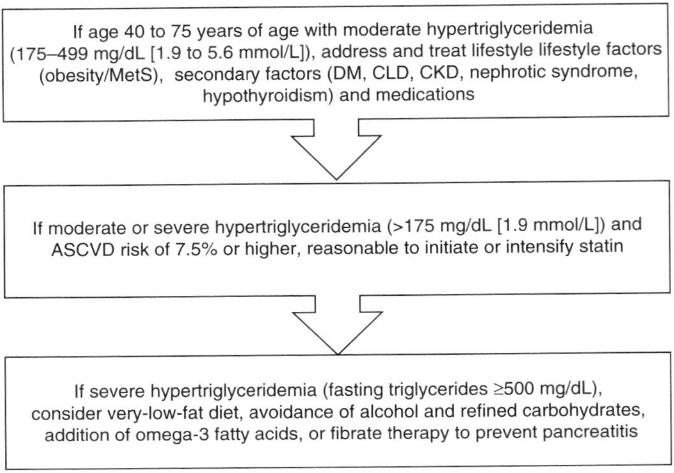

If age 40 to 75 years of age with moderate hypertriglyceridemia (175–499 mg/dL [1.9 to 5.6 mmol/L]), address and treat lifestyle lifestyle factors (obesity/MetS), secondary factors (DM, CLD, CKD, nephrotic syndrome, hypothyroidism) and medications

If moderate or severe hypertriglyceridemia (>175 mg/dL [1.9 mmol/L]) and ASCVD risk of 7.5% or higher, reasonable to initiate or intensify statin

If severe hypertriglyceridemia (fasting triglycerides ≥500 mg/dL), consider very-low-fat diet, avoidance of alcohol and refined carbohydrates, addition of omega-3 fatty acids, or fibrate therapy to prevent pancreatitis

Fig. 6.3 Management of hypertriglyceridemia: 2018 AHA/ACC cholesterol guidelines. For ASCVD prevention, treatment of elevated triglycerides includes lifestyle modification, controlling secondary dyslipidemias, and, if needed, drug therapy. Patients with severe hypertriglyceridemia are also at risk for pancreatitis and should be treated accordingly. *ASCVD,* Atherosclerotic cardiovascular disease; *CLD,* chronic liver disease; *CKD,* chronic kidney disease; *DM,* diabetes mellitus; *MetS,* metabolic syndrome; *TG,* triglycerides. (Data from Grundy SM, Stone NJ, Bailey AL, et al. 2018 AHA/ACC/AACVPR/AAPA/ABC/ACPM/ADA/AGS/APhA/ASPC/NLA/PCNA Guideline on the management of blood cholesterol: A report of the American College of Cardiology/American Heart Association task force on clinical practice guidelines. *J Am Coll Cardiol* 2019;73:e285–e350.)

The Reduction of Cardiovascular Events with Icosapent Ethyl–Intervention Trial (REDUCE-IT; discussed later), which was published after the AHA/ACC guidelines and hence was not included in the guidelines, showed favorable reduction in cardiovascular events, including cardiovascular mortality, in patients with established ASCVD or diabetes and moderately elevated triglyceride levels treated with icosapent ethyl.[40] The 2019 ESC/EAS guidelines, which came out afterwards, however, did recommend the addition of omega-3 fatty acids (icosapent ethyl 4 g/day) to statins in high-risk patients with triglyceride of 135–499 mg/dL) despite statin treatment (Class IIa).[9] Similar recommendations are endorsed by both the National Lipid Association (NLA)[41] and American Diabetes Association (ADA)[42] (see below).

Other Lipoproteins and Lipoprotein Carriers

The combination of cholesterol in LDL and very-low-density lipoprotein (VLDL) is known as non-HDL-C and is a strong predictor of cardiovascular risk,[43] especially in patients with elevated triglycerides or diabetes. Elevated triglycerides result from accumulation of VLDL and other triglyceride-rich lipoproteins, which are highly atherogenic.[43] In such cases, non-HDL-C provides a more accurate measure of the cholesterol content of all atherogenic lipoproteins than LDL-C alone. The 2018 AHA/ACC guidelines[6] support a non-HDL-C threshold of 100 mg/dL (2.6 mmol/L), along with LDL-C, to guide therapy and enhance identification of those at increased ASCVD risk, especially in very-high-risk patients with ASCVD.

Similarly, measurement of apoB may be valuable in patients with moderately elevated triglycerides, as it may be a more accurate indicator of atherogenic potential in these individuals.[6] ApoB level ≥130 mg/dL, especially in patients with elevated triglycerides, denotes a high lifetime risk and is a risk-enhancing factor (see Table 6.1) in the 2018 AHA/ACC guidelines.[6]

Lp(a), which is structurally similar to LDL with the addition of apo(a) covalently linked to apoB, may also be useful in risk assessment. The 2018 AHA/ACC guidelines define Lp(a) ≥50 mg/dL as a risk-enhancing factor and consider family history of premature ASCVD a relative indication for measurement of Lp(a) level.[6] The 2019 ESC/EAS dyslipidemia guidelines recommend Lp(a) measurement in all adults at least once to identify individuals with very high inherited Lp(a) levels >180 mg/dL, whose lifetime ASCVD risk may be equivalent to individuals with heterozygous familial hypercholesterolemia.[9]

Lipids in Special Population Groups

Metabolic Syndrome

Metabolic syndrome is a cluster of risk factors (Fig. 6.4) that greatly enhances the risk for coronary morbidity and mortality at any level of LDL-C.[44-46] The underlying pathology of the metabolic syndrome appears to be linked to obesity and insulin resistance, and its prevalence increases with age and with presence of type 2 diabetes mellitus. The 2018 AHA/ACC cholesterol guidelines incorporate metabolic syndrome in the risk-enhancing factors (see Table 6.1), which influence initiation or up-titration of lipid-lowering therapy in primary prevention. First-line therapy for metabolic syndrome is weight control and increased physical activity. LDL-C and non-HDL-C should be controlled; achieving a significant increase in HDL-C, although desirable, has not proven to be clinically useful.

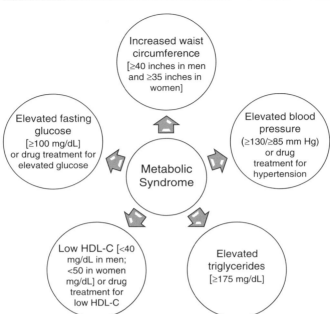

Fig. 6.4   Metabolic syndrome. Metabolic syndrome is a constellation of risk factors, including central obesity, insulin resistance, hypertriglyceridemia, low HDL-C, and hypertension, that increases risk for ASCVD and diabetes. In the 2018 AHA/ACC cholesterol guidelines, metabolic syndrome is diagnosed by ≥three of the risk factors shown. *ASCVD*, Atherosclerotic cardiovascular disease; *HDL-C*, high-density lipoprotein cholesterol. (Data from Grundy SM, Stone NJ, Bailey AL, et al. 2018 AHA/ACC/AACVPR/AAPA/ABC/ACPM/ADA/AGS/APhA/ASPC/NLA/PCNA Guideline on the management of blood cholesterol: A report of the American College of Cardiology/American Heart Association task force on clinical practice guidelines. *J Am Coll Cardiol* 2019;73:e285–e350.)

Secondary Dyslipidemias

Diabetes mellitus, hypothyroidism, nephrotic syndrome, and alcoholism should be remedied if possible. Among drugs causing adverse lipid changes are β-blockers and diuretics (Table 6.2),[47-52] progestogens, and oral retinoids. Nonetheless, cardiac drugs known to be protective should not be withheld on the basis of their lipid effects alone, especially in postinfarct patients when there is clear indication for the expected overall benefit.

Table 6.2

Effects of antihypertensive agents on blood lipid profiles

Agent	TC	LDL-C	HDL-C	TG
	Change, %			
Diuretics				
TZ[47]	14	10	2	14
Low-dose TZ[48] a	0	0	0	0
Indapamide[49]	0 (+9)	0	0	0
Spironolactone[50]	5	?	?	31
β-Blockers				
Grouped (>1 year)[51]	0	0	−8	22
Propranolol[47]	0	−3	−11	16
Atenolol[47]	0	−2	−7	15
Metoprolol[47]	0	−1	−9	14
Acebutolol[48] a	−3	−4[b]	−3	6
Pindolol[47]	−1	−3	−2	7
α-Blockers				
Grouped	−4	−13	5	−8
Doxazosin[48] a	−4[b]	−5[b]	2	−8
αβ-Blocker				
Labetalol[47]	2	2	1	8
Carvedilol[52]	−4	?	7	−20
CCBs				
Grouped[47]	0	0	0	0
Amlodipine[48] a	−1	−1	1	−3
ACE inhibitors				
Grouped	0	0	0	0
Enalapril[48]	−1	−1	3	−7
Angiotensin receptor blockers				
Losartan[49]	(0)[c]	(0)[c]	(0)[c]	(0)[c]
Central agents				
MD + TZ	0	0	0	0

[a]Chlorthalidone 15 mg/day; acebutolol 400 mg/day; doxazosin 2 mg/day; amlodipine 5 mg/day; enalapril 5 mg/day; data placebo-corrected.
[b]<0.01 versus placebo over 4 years.
[c]no long-term data.
ACE, Angiotensin-converting enzyme; CCBs, calcium channel blockers; HDL-C, high-density lipoprotein cholesterol; LDL-C, low-density lipoprotein cholesterol; MD, methyldopa; TC, total cholesterol; TG, triglyceride; TZ, thiazide.

β-Blockers

β-Blockers tend to reduce HDL-C and to increase triglycerides. β-blockers with high intrinsic sympathomimetic activity or high cardioselectivity may have less or no effect (as in the case of carvedilol with added α-blockade). The fact that β-blockers also impair glucose metabolism is an added cause for concern when giving these agents to young patients. Nonetheless, strong evidence supports the protective effects of β-blockers in postinfarct and heart failure patients. Statins appear to counter some of the effects of β-blockers on blood lipids. In stable effort angina, calcium channel blockers may have a more favorable effect on triglycerides and HDL-C than β-blockers. In hypertensive patients, angiotensin-converting enzyme inhibitors, angiotensin receptor blockers, and calcium channel blockers are all lipid neutral.

Diuretics

Diuretics increase triglycerides and tend to increase total cholesterol unless used in low doses. In the Antihypertensive and Lipid-Lowering Treatment to Prevent Heart Attack Trial (ALLHAT), chlorthalidone 12.5–25 mg daily over 5 years increased total cholesterol by 2–3 mg/dL.[53] In the Antihypertensive Treatment and Lipid Profile in a North of Sweden Efficacy Evaluation (ALPINE) study, hydrochlorothiazide 25 mg, combined with atenolol in most patients, increased blood triglycerides and apoB, while decreasing HDL-C.[54]

Oral Contraceptives

When oral contraceptives are given to patients with ischemic heart disease or with risk factors such as smoking, possible atherogenic effects of high-dose estrogen merit attention. In postmenopausal women, the cardiovascular benefits of hormone replacement therapy have not been supported by clinical trials.

Diabetic Patients

Patients with diabetes constitute a high-risk group and warrant aggressive risk reduction. Risk for MI is increased almost fivefold in diabetic women aged 35–54 years and more than twofold in diabetic men aged 35–54 years, compared with age-matched women and men, respectively, without diabetes.[55] In line with this, type 2 diabetes is regarded as a risk category in its own right in the 2018 AHA/ACC cholesterol guidelines,[6] and in the 2019 ESC/EAS guidelines,[9] type 2 diabetes is considered a high-risk category, irrespective of calculated SCORE. Both guidelines recommend initiation of statin therapy along with lifestyle modification in these patients. In recent years, growing awareness of the overlapping pathophysiologic characteristics of

CHD and type 2 diabetes has led to increased coordination between cardiologists and endocrinologists in addressing the joint risk.[56] Patients with type 2 diabetes may have a preponderance of smaller, denser, more atherogenic LDL particles, even though the LDL-C level may be relatively normal.

Meta-analysis of 14 randomized trials with a follow-up of at least 2 years indicated that lipid-lowering drug treatment significantly reduced cardiovascular risk in both diabetic and nondiabetic patients.[57] The Collaborative Atorvastatin Diabetes Study (CARDS),[58] a multicenter, randomized primary-prevention trial in patients with type 2 diabetes and at least one other risk factor who were treated with atorvastatin, 10 mg/day, or placebo, was stopped early because of a favorable clinical benefit of statin therapy. Taken together with a large subgroup analysis from the Heart Protection Study (HPS)[59] and Anglo-Scandinavian Cardiac Outcomes Trial–Lipid-Lowering Arm (ASCOT-LLA),[60] there are strong arguments for considering statin therapy, in addition to lifestyle modification and blood pressure control, in all patients with type 2 diabetes. A meta-analysis of all four double-blinded primary-prevention randomized controlled trials with large cohorts with diabetes found that use of moderate-intensity statin therapy in a total of 10,187 participants was associated with a risk reduction of 25%, with no apparent difference in benefit between type 1 and type 2 diabetes mellitus.[61]

Recent trials have provided evidence for the role of nonstatin lipid-lowering therapy in combination with statin to reduce cardiovascular risk among patients with diabetes. In IMPROVE-IT, which evaluated the addition of ezetimibe to statin therapy in patients with recent ACS (27% of whom had diabetes), individuals with diabetes had significantly greater relative and absolute benefit on cardiovascular outcomes than those without diabetes.[62] Subanalysis of the diabetic subgroup in the FOURIER trial showed that median LDL-C levels were reduced to a similar degree with evolocumab relative to placebo (57% in those with diabetes mellitus versus 60% in those without diabetes mellitus).[63] In the ODYSSEY OUTCOMES trial, a similar subgroup analysis compared patients with diabetes (n = 5444; 29%), prediabetes (n = 8246; 43%), and normoglycemia (n = 5234; 28%). Over a median follow-up of 2.8 years, treatment with alirocumab resulted in twice the absolute reduction in cardiovascular events among patients with diabetes as in those without diabetes given higher baseline risk.[64] Similarly, in REDUCE-IT, 30% of subjects enrolled had diabetes and at least one other traditional risk factor, along with elevated triglycerides, and had significant reduction in risk of ischemic events, including cardiovascular death, with icosapent ethyl compared to placebo.[40] Based on this study, the American Diabetes Association updated its comprehensive evidence-based recommendations to endorse the use of icosapent ethyl in patient with diabetes already on statin with elevated triglyceride level (134–499 mg/dL).[42] Similar endorsements were made by the NLA[41] and 2019 ESC/EAS guidelines.[9]

Older Adults

Although the relation between cholesterol and CHD weakens with age, physicians should continue to consider lipids as a modifiable risk factor in older adults. The absolute risk for clinical CHD in older adults is much higher because age is a powerful risk factor and because blood pressure, another risk factor, often increases with age. Furthermore, consider the cumulative effect of lifetime exposure to a coronary risk factor on an older adult patient. While the Prospective Study of Pravastatin in the Elderly at Risk (PROSPER) found coronary but not overall mortality benefit with statin treatment in older adults (see section on pravastatin), this trial may have been too short (3 years) to show major decreases in cerebrovascular disease.[65] In a recent meta-analysis of JUPITER and HOPE-3, benefits on ASCVD reduction with rosuvastatin were similar among those ≥70 years of age versus <70 years of age, with relative risk reduction for nonfatal MI, nonfatal stroke, or cardiovascular death of about 26% and no difference in adverse events between the two age groups.[66] Furthermore, those ≥70 years of age had much higher event rates, which along with the comparable relative risk reductions, would mean that larger absolute risk reductions can be achieved with statin treatment and hence a smaller number needed to treat (NNT) to prevent an event in older compared with younger patients. Other meta-analyses[67-69] similarly support primary prevention for adults in their 70s. The Study Assessing Goals in the Elderly (SAGE) confirmed the safety and benefit of intensive treatment with atorvastatin, 80 mg/day, in older adult patients with stable coronary syndromes, but failed to demonstrate the superiority of intensive versus moderate treatment in reducing the primary endpoint of total ischemia duration from baseline to 1 year.[70] However, data on older subsets (≥80 years of age) remain sparse. Furthermore, older adults may be more susceptible to statin-related risk, owing to increasing frailty, multiple comorbidities, cognitive impairment, polypharmacy, and altered pharmacodynamics in older adults. The 2018 AHA/ACC guidelines[6] therefore recommend judicious use of statin therapy in higher-risk older adults and support clinical judgment and thorough risk and benefit discussion between patient and clinician prior to initiating statin. The 2019 ESC/EAS dyslipidemia[9] guidelines recommend initiation of statin in older adults >75 years old with high risk or above, and suggest that statin be started at a low dose and titrated upwards to achieve LDL-C treatment goals. In individuals whose cumulative risk outweighs benefit or with limited lifespan, the guidelines recommend not initiating therapy and, in individuals already taking statin, deprescription.

Women

Women have a lower baseline risk for CHD than men at all ages except perhaps beyond 80 years. Risk lags by about 10–15 years, perhaps because of a slower rate of increase in LDL-C, higher levels of HDL-C, or ill-understood protective genetic factors in the heart itself. It is not simply a question of being pre- or postmenopausal. In large statin trials such as HPS, women had relative risk reduction comparable to that in men.[59] In the Management of Elevated Cholesterol in the Primary Prevention Group of Adult Japanese (MEGA) trial of low-dose pravastatin (10–20 mg daily) in low-risk Japanese patients, 69% of whom were women, women had marginally less CHD risk reduction than men, possibly because of their lower initial risk.[18] The JUPITER trial,[16] which enrolled 6801 women (38% of the study population), showed that women had similar risk reduction as men, primarily because of reductions in risk for revascularization and unstable angina. A meta-analysis conducted by the JUPITER investigators found that statins reduced cardiovascular events in women in primary prevention trials by one-third.[71]

The 2018 AHA/ACC guidelines[6] address certain conditions specific to women that may augment their baseline risk for CVD and may help clinical decision-making regarding lifestyle intervention and lipid-lowering therapy. These conditions include pregnancy-related complications (hypertensive disorders during pregnancy, preeclampsia, gestational diabetes mellitus, delivering a preterm or low-birth weight infant) and premature menopause, all of which have been shown to increase future risk of CVD and portend increased cardiovascular morbidity and mortality.[72-75]

Pregnant Women

As a group, lipid-lowering drugs are either completely or relatively contraindicated during pregnancy because of the essential role of cholesterol in fetal development. Bile acid sequestrants may be safest, whereas statins should not be used (see "Contraindications and Pregnancy Warning" in the later section on statins).

Dietary and Other Nondrug Therapy for Dyslipidemia

Lifestyle and Risk Factor Reduction

Nondrug dietary therapy is fundamental to the management of all primary hyperlipidemias and frequently suffices as basic therapy when coupled with weight reduction, exercise, ideal (low) alcohol intake, and treatment of other risk factors such as smoking, hypertension, or diabetes. Regular exercise may also increase insulin sensitivity and lessen the risk of type 2 diabetes. If lifestyle recommendations, including diet, were rigorously followed, CHD would be dramatically reduced in those younger than age 70.[76] However, high-intensity lifestyle modification is required to prevent progression or even to achieve regression of CHD.

Diet

Changes in diet are an absolute cornerstone of lipid-modifying treatment. The 2018 AHA/ACC Guideline on the Management of Blood Cholesterol provides practitioners with evidence-based dietary recommendations to improve cardiovascular health.[6] They stress including nutrient-dense foods with cardioprotective fats while avoiding intake of excessive calories, saturated and *trans* fats, and refined carbohydrates. The two most commonly employed dietary patterns, also supported by the ACC/AHA, are the Mediterranean dietary pattern and Dietary Approaches to Stop Hypertension (DASH) diet.[77]

The DASH dietary pattern was initially developed for blood pressure management. It puts emphasis on intake of fruits, vegetables, and low-fat dairy products; includes whole grains, poultry, fish, and nuts; and reduces saturated fats, red meat, sweets, and beverages containing added sugars. The Optimal Macronutrient Intake Trial for Heart Health (OmniHeart) study[78] compared three variants of the DASH diet: a diet rich in carbohydrate (like the original DASH diet), a diet higher in protein (about half from plant sources), and a diet higher in unsaturated fat (predominantly monounsaturated fat). Each of the diets was similar to the original DASH diet, and all led to reductions in LDL-C and triglycerides.

In comparison, the typical Mediterranean dietary pattern is lower in dairy products and red and processed meats, higher in olive oil and seafood, and includes moderate wine intake. Total dietary fat is in the range of 32% to $\geq$35% of total energy intake. Similar to the DASH diet, the Mediterranean diet limits saturated fats but includes relatively high amounts of monounsaturated and polyunsaturated fats, with an emphasis on omega-3 fatty acids, instead. Fruits, vegetables, and whole grains provide a high dietary fiber intake. In the Prevención con Dieta Mediterránea (PREDIMED) trial,[79] in nearly 7500 adults with high cardiovascular risk, strict adherence to a Mediterranean diet with added olive oil or nuts reduced the incidence of major cardiovascular events—stroke or heart attack—by nearly one-third. The better the adherence to this diet, the better the survival rate.[80]

Physical Activity

Along with dietary modification, physicians should counsel patients on staying active and incorporating regular physical activity in their weekly routines to help reduce risk of CVD. The 2018 AHA/ACC guidelines[6] recommend at least 120 minutes a week of aerobic physical activity (3–4 sessions per week, ~40 minutes per session) and including moderate- to vigorous-intensity physical activity. The Diabetes Prevention Program (DPP) showed that intensive lifestyle interventions focusing on exercise and weight loss prevented the development of diabetes and future microvascular complications over a 15-year follow-up.[81]

Drug Therapy for Dyslipidemia

Statins: 3-Hydroxy-3-Methylglutaryl Coenzyme A Reductase Inhibitors

Statins are well established as the first drugs of choice in primary and secondary prevention of CHD because of their favorable clinical outcomes, predictable effects on LDL-C, and relatively few side effects across multiple large clinical trials. Available statins include lovastatin, pravastatin, simvastatin, fluvastatin, atorvastatin, rosuvastatin, and pitavastatin. All the statins decrease hepatic cholesterol synthesis by inhibiting 3-hydroxy-3-methylglutaryl coenzyme A (HMG-CoA) reductase. They are highly effective in reducing total cholesterol and LDL-C, they usually increase HDL-C, and long-term safety and efficacy is well established. Many are now available in generic form. The landmark Scandinavian Simvastatin Survival Study (4S) showed that simvastatin used in secondary prevention achieved a reduction in total mortality and in coronary events.[82] This was soon followed by a successful primary-prevention study with pravastatin in high-risk men (CARE).[83] Successful primary prevention of common events has been found in patients with LDL-C values near the U. S. national average.[84] An interesting concept is that lipid-lowering drugs may act in ways beyond regression of the atheromatous plaque, for example, by improving endothelial function, stabilizing platelets, reducing fibrinogen (strongly correlated with triglyceride levels), or inhibiting the inflammatory response associated with atherogenesis.[85]

Class Indications for Statins

ASCVD Prevention. In general, depending on the drug chosen, the large statin trials (Table 6.3) show beyond doubt that cardiovascular endpoints are reduced, total mortality is reduced in primary and secondary prevention, and the NNT to prevent any given major endpoint makes statins cost effective, especially in secondary prevention. In patients with clinical ASCVD, statins may be used to slow the progression of coronary atherosclerosis, again as part of an overall treatment strategy. In patients with primary hypercholesterolemia, homozygous familial hypercholesterolemia, or mixed dyslipidemias, statins reduce levels of total cholesterol, LDL-C, apoB, and triglycerides.

Stroke Prevention and Transient Ischemic Attack. Patients with a history of stroke or CHD equivalent should be considered for statin therapy. In CARDS, stroke risk in diabetic patients was reduced by 48% with only a 10-mg daily dose of atorvastatin.[58] In the Stroke Prevention by Aggressive Reduction in Cholesterol Levels (SPARCL) study, high-dose atorvastatin (80 mg/day) reduced fatal and nonfatal strokes (2.2% absolute risk reduction; HR 0.84) and major cardiovascular events (3.5% absolute risk reduction; HR 0.80) in patients with a history of stroke or transient ischemic attack but no clinical ischemic heart disease.[87] These benefits outweighed the slight increase in nonfatal hemorrhagic stroke (22 in 2365 patients; absolute increase 0.9%).[87] A meta-analysis of more than 120,000 persons found powerful statin-related reductions of ischemic stroke and associated mortality that were not linked to the degree of LDL-C reduction,[88] which suggested that stroke reduction was related to pleiotropic effects of statins. However, PCSK9 inhibitors have also been shown to reduce stroke (discussed later).

How Intensive Should Statin Therapy Be?

A meta-analysis of more than 90,000 subjects with clinical vascular disease on standard statin therapy showed significant reduction in cardiovascular events with statin use.[3] The authors estimated that, for every 1-mmol/L decrease in LDL-C (approximately 40 mg/dL), the 5-year relative risk for major coronary events is reduced by about one-fifth, with the absolute risk reduction dependent on the initial level of risk, and they projected that sustained statin therapy for 5 years might reduce the incidence of major vascular events by

Table 6.3

Key statin trials with major significant outcomes

Trial, statin, 1° or 2° prevention	Initial blood cholesterol (mean)	Duration and numbers	Comparator events per trial (%)	Statin events per trial (%)	Absolute risk reduction per trial	Number needed to treat per trial
4S[82] Simvastatin 40 mg 2° prevention	260 mg/dL (6.75 mmol/L)	5.4 yr, median (Placebo: 2223; statin: 2221)	Total deaths 1° end point: 256 (11.5%) 2° end point: 502 (22.6%)	182 (8.2%) 353 (15.9%)	74 (3.3%) 149 (30%)	30 (162/yr) 15 (80/yr)
WOSCOPS[83] Pravastatin 1° prevention	272 mg/dL (7.03 mmol/L)	4.9 yr (mean) (Placebo: 3293; statin: 3302)	Deaths: 135 (4.1%) 1° end point: 248 (7.5%)	106 (3.2%) 174 (5.3%)	29 (0.9%) 74 (2.2%)	114 (558/yr) 45 (217/yr)
AFCAPS/ TexCAPS[84] Lovastatin 1° prevention	221 mg/dL (5.71 mmol/L)	5.2 yr (mean) (Placebo: 3301; statin: 3304)	CAD deaths: 15 (0.5%) AMI[a] 81 (2.5%) 1° end point: 183 (5.5%)	11 (0.3%) 45 (1.4%) 116 (3.5%)	4(0.12%) 39 (1.3%) 67 (2.0%)	826 (4295/yr) 85 (441/yr) 49 (256/yr)
HPS[58] Simvastatin 40 mg 65% with CHD	228 mg/dL (5.9 mmol/L)	5 yr (mean) (Placebo: 10,267; statin: 10,269)	Mortality: 1507 (14.7%) Vascular deaths: 937 (9.1%) Total MI: 1212 (11.8%)	1328 (12.9%) 781 (7.6%) 898 (8.7%)	179 (1.8%) 156 (1.5%) 314 (3.1%)	56 (280/yr) 66 (330/yr) 32 (160/yr)
PROSPER[65] Pravastatin High-risk older adults	221 mg/dL (5.7 mmol/L)	3.2 yr (mean) (Placebo: 2913; statin: 2891)	Primary end point CHD death, nonfatal MI, + stroke: 473 (16.2%)	408 (14.1%)	65 (2.1%)	48 (152/yr)

Continued on following page

Table 6.3

Key statin trials with major significant outcomes (Continued)

Trial, statin, 1° or 2° prevention	Initial blood cholesterol (mean)	Duration and numbers	Comparator events per trial (%)	Statin events per trial (%)	Absolute risk reduction per trial	Number needed to treat per trial
ASCOT-LLA[86] Atorvastatin 10 mg 1° prevention; hypertensive	212 mg/dL (5.48 mmol/L)	3.3 yr (median) (Placebo: 5137; statin: 5168)	Primary end point nonfatal MI + CHD death: 154 (3.0%)	100 (1.9%)	54 (1.1%)	90 (297/yr)
PROVE IT[26b] Atorvastatin 80 mg; pravastatin 40 mg Recent ACS, 2° prevention	180 mg/dL (4.65 mmol/L)	2 yr (median) (Pravastatin: 2063; atorvastatin 2099)	Primary composite endpoint (death plus cardiovascular events): pravastatin, 543 (26.3%)	Atorvastatin, 470 (22.4%)	73 (3.7%)	29 (58/yr)
JUPITER[16] Rosuvastatin 20 mg 1° prevention	186 mg/dL (4.81 mmol/L)	1.9 yr (median) (Placebo: 8901; rosuvastatin: 8901)	Primary composite endpoint (MI, stroke, revascularization, hospitalization for angina, CV death): 251 (2.8%)	142 (1.6%)	109 (1.2%)	29 (5/yr)[c]

[a]Estimated.

[b]PROVE IT compares atorvastatin versus pravastatin, not versus placebo.

[c]Endpoint of myocardial infarction, stroke, or death.[16]

ACS, Acute coronary syndrome; AMI, (nonfatal) acute myocardial infarction; CAD, coronary artery disease; CHD, coronary heart disease; CV, cardiovascular; MI, myocardial infarction.

approximately one-third. An updated meta-analysis of trials comparing intensive- versus moderate-intensity statin therapy from the same group, including 170,000 subjects, found that intensive statin treatment further reduced the risk of major vascular events, so that the relation between absolute LDL-C reduction and proportional risk reduction remained consistent in the trials of intensive statin therapy.[25] These findings support a strategy to achieve the largest LDL-C reduction possible in high-risk patients without increasing risk for myopathy.

Benefit Versus Possible Harm With Very-High-Dose Statins. A retrospective analysis of possible adverse effects with very-high-dose statin therapy suggested a small increased risk of cancer, equivalent to only 1.5% per 5 years.[89] However, in an analysis of more than 6000 patients with LDL-C levels <60 mg/dL, those with very low levels (<40 mg/dL) had improved survival without any increased risk of cancer or rhabdomyolysis.[90] Myopathy remains a definite risk, especially in the case of high-dose simvastatin, and new diabetes is more common in high- than in medium-dose statin therapy (see "Class Warnings").

Class Warnings

Liver Damage, Myopathy, New Diabetes, and Cognitive Side Effects. The package inserts for statins were revised by the U.S. Food and Drug Administration (FDA) in early 2012.[91,92] Pretreatment *liver function tests* are recommended, but routine periodic monitoring of liver enzymes is not, as it was in the past, because serious liver injury with statins rarely occurs. Warnings regarding myopathy and rhabdomyolysis remain in place. Skeletal muscle effects range from muscle pains to objective myopathy to severe myocyte breakdown that in turn can cause potentially fatal renal failure by way of myoglobinuria. *Myopathy* is diagnosed when creatine kinase blood levels exceed 10 times normal. The patient should be warned that muscle pain, tenderness, or weakness must immediately be reported to the physician and the statin stopped. Abnormal enzyme values usually resolve with cessation of treatment. Thereafter follows a monitored rechallenge at a lower dose or a change to low-dose fluvastatin or alternate-day low-dose rosuvastatin (because these may cause less myopathy) or nonstatin therapy.[93] A trial of added coenzyme Q10 may help. However, in HPS, with more than 10,000 patients in each treatment group, enzyme-diagnosed myopathy over 5 years occurred in only 0.11% of statin-treated patients versus 0.06% in controls, and rhabdomyolysis in only 0.05% versus 0.03% in controls.[59] The absolute rates of myopathy, much less rhabdomyolysis, are low in reported clinical surveys,[94] although in clinical practice, these complaints are more common.[89,93] Fatal cases are extremely rare, occurring in only 0.2 or fewer instances per million prescriptions.[95] Risk for myopathy is greater with high-dose simvastatin (see section on simvastatin) and coadministration with fibrates, niacin, cyclosporine, erythromycin, or azole antifungal agents. Although not contraindicated, the combination of a statin and a fibrate increases the risk for myopathy to an incidence of approximately 0.12%,[96] and physicians are cautioned to be mindful of this risk.

Interactions with protease inhibitors are potentially myopathic. The FDA warns as follows (statins in alphabetical order):[92]

- **Atorvastatin:** caution with telaprevir and ritonavir; use lowest dose with lopinavir + ritonavir; limit dose to 20 mg/day with darunavir + ritonavir, fosamprenavir, fosamprenavir + ritonavir, saquinavir + ritonavir; limit dose to 40 mg/day with nelfinavir

- **Fluvastatin:** no data available

- **Lovastatin:** contraindicated with human immunodeficiency virus (HIV) protease inhibitors, boceprevir, telaprevir

- **Pitavastatin:** no dose limitations

- **Pravastatin:** no dose limitations

- **Rosuvastatin:** limit dose to 10 mg/day with atazanavir ± ritonavir, lopinavir + ritonavir

- **Simvastatin:** contraindicated with HIV protease inhibitors, boceprevir, telaprevir

Thus, pravastatin and pitavastatin are the safest and simvastatin the least safe to use with HIV and hepatitis C protease inhibitors.

New-onset diabetes is a more recently discovered side effect, first reported with rosuvastatin and now recognized as a generalized problem of high-dose statins. In a meta-analysis of 91,140 persons in 13 trials, statin therapy was associated with a slightly increased risk of new diabetes (9%, odds ratio 1.09; 95% CI 1.02–1.17).[97] Based on these data, statin therapy used in 255 patients for 4 years led to one extra case of diabetes and prevented 5.4 coronary events (coronary deaths, nonfatal MI). In another meta-analysis, which compared intensive- with moderate-dose statin therapy in five studies that included 32,752 persons without diabetes at baseline, the NNT annually was 498 for new-onset diabetes versus 155 for reduced cardiovascular events.[98] Thus, the approximate ratio of benefit to harm for high versus medium doses was approximately 3:1. An observational study of 161,808 postmenopausal women found an increase in risk for diabetes (48%, multivariate-adjusted HR 1.48; 95% CI 1.38–1.59).[99] As a result of this cumulative evidence, the FDA has added information concerning an effect of statins on incident diabetes and increases in hemoglobin A1c and fasting plasma glucose to all statin labels.[91]

Additional information about potential nonserious and reversible *cognitive side effects* (memory loss, confusion, etc.) were also added to statin labels, based on postmarketing reports.[91] However in the PROSPER trial,[100] cognitive function was assessed repeatedly in all 5804 participants, and no difference was found in cognitive decline in subjects treated with pravastatin compared with placebo during a 3-year follow-up period. Similarly, a systematic review and meta-analysis found no difference in cognitive performance related to procedural memory, attention, or motor speed.[101]

Contraindications and Pregnancy Warning. Statins are contraindicated in patients with active liver disease or unexplained persistent elevations of serum transaminases. Statins must not be prescribed to women who are pregnant or who are planning to become pregnant because cholesterol is essential to fetal development. Statins are excreted in the mother's milk, so women taking statins should not breast feed. Women desiring to become pregnant should stop statins for approximately 6 months before conception. If a patient becomes pregnant while taking statins, therapy should be discontinued, and the patient apprised of the potential hazard to the fetus.

Lovastatin (Altoprev, Mevacor)

Lovastatin (Altoprev, Mevacor) was the first statin to be approved and marketed in the United States and was the first generically available. In the landmark primary prevention Air Force/Texas Coronary Atherosclerosis Prevention Study (AFCAPS/TexCAPS), lovastatin reduced clinical cardiac events, including MI, by 37% in individuals with baseline LDL-C values considered "normal" within the general American population (221 mg/dL; 5.71 mmol/L), but with low HDL-C levels (36 mg/dL; 1.03 mmol/L).[84]

Dose, Effects, and Side Effects. The usual starting dose for lovastatin is 20 mg once daily with the evening meal, going up to 80 mg in one or two doses. In 2012, the FDA revised the labeling of lovastatin with new contraindications and dose limitations for concomitant medications, because of an increased risk for myopathy with strong inhibitors of the hepatic cytochrome P-450 3A4 (CYP3A4) substrate.[91] Lovastatin is contraindicated with itraconazole, ketoconazole, posaconazole, erythromycin, clarithromycin, telithromycin, HIV protease inhibitors, boceprevir, telaprevir, and nefazodone. Regarding *drug interactions*, concomitant therapy with cyclosporine and gemfibrozil should be avoided; a 20-mg dose of lovastatin should not be exceeded when the patient is taking danazol, diltiazem, or verapamil; and the 40-mg dose should not be exceeded with amiodarone. Large quantities of grapefruit juice should also be avoided. There are no significant interactions between lovastatin and the common antihypertensive drugs, nor with digoxin. The same cautions concerning hepatotoxicity, myopathy, and rhabdomyolysis that affect other statins also apply to lovastatin.

Fluvastatin (Lescol, Lescol XL)

Fluvastatin was the first synthetic statin approved by the FDA. In the Lipoprotein and Coronary Atherosclerosis Study (LCAS), fluvastatin in patients with mildly to moderately elevated LDL-C reduced CHD progression,[102] and the Lescol Intervention Prevention Study (LIPS) showed reduced risk for cardiac events with early initiation of fluvastatin in patients with average cholesterol levels following percutaneous coronary intervention.[103]

Dose, Effects, and Side Effects. The dosing range of fluvastatin is 20–80 mg/day, taken in the evening or at bedtime, and the recommended starting dosage may be determined by the degree of LDL-C reduction needed. Fluvastatin is metabolized mainly by the CYP2C9 isoenzyme, making it less likely to interact with drugs that compete for the CYP3A4 pathway, such as the fibrates. However, phenytoin and warfarin share metabolism by CYP2C9, raising the risk for interactions. The same cautions concerning hepatotoxicity, myopathy, and rhabdomyolysis that affect other statins also apply to fluvastatin.

Pravastatin (Pravachol, Lipostat)

In the primary-prevention West of Scotland Coronary Prevention Study (WOSCOPS), pravastatin reduced the risk for coronary morbidity and mortality in high-risk men.[83] In the secondary-prevention Long-term Intervention with Pravastatin in Ischemic Disease (LIPID) trial, pravastatin therapy reduced the risk for death from any cause by 22% ($P < 0.001$) and also decreased the risks for nonfatal MI or CHD death, stroke, and coronary revascularization.[104] In PROVE IT, pravastatin at 40 mg daily was inferior to atorvastatin at 80 mg daily in the reduction of LDL-C and clinical events.[26] The PROSPER trial, which enrolled older adult patients with a mean cholesterol of 212 mg/dL (5.7 mmol/L) and high coronary risk, found that pravastatin, 40 mg/day, reduced the relative risk for CHD death by 24% ($P = 0.043$), chiefly when given for secondary prevention; results for primary prevention were nonsignificant.[65] There was, however, an increased incidence of cancer in PROSPER. Longer-term follow-up from WOSCOPS found no increase in cancer at 10^{105} or 20^{106} years after the trial.[3]

Indications. Besides its class indications (see previous), pravastatin is approved for primary prevention in patients with hypercholesterolemia to reduce the risk for MI, revascularization, and cardiovascular mortality. In patients with previous MI, it is indicated to reduce total mortality by reducing coronary deaths and to reduce recurrent MI, revascularization, and stroke or transient ischemic attack.

Dose and Effects. The recommended starting dose for pravastatin is 40 mg at any time of the day, increasing to 80 mg if needed. As with the other statins, liver damage and myopathy are rare but serious *side effects. Cautions and contraindications* are similar to other statins. There is no drug interaction with digoxin. Pravastatin is not metabolized by the CYP3A4 pathway, so there may be a lower risk for interactions with agents such as erythromycin and ketoconazole. Importantly, there is no interaction with antiretrovirals.

Simvastatin (Zocor)

Major Trials. The landmark 4S paved the way to widespread acceptance of statins as the cornerstone of lipid-lowering drug therapy. In this study in 4444 patients with severely elevated cholesterol levels, mostly men with past MI, simvastatin reduced LDL-C by 35% over 4 years, total mortality by 30%, cardiac death rate by 42%, and revascularization by 37%.[82] There was no evidence of increased suicide or violent death, previously thought to be a potential hazard of cholesterol reduction. Differences between simvastatin and placebo arms started to emerge after 1–2 years of treatment, and most curves were still diverging at 4 years. Longer-term follow-up (up to 8 years) after the trial suggested that benefits were maintained.[107]

HPS evaluated the role of simvastatin versus placebo in 20,536 high-risk patients for whom guidelines at the time would not have recommended drug intervention.[59] Included patients were 40 to 80 years of age and had total serum cholesterol concentrations of at least 135 mg/dL (3.49 mmol/L). Only 65% of the patients had a history of CHD at baseline, and HPS included many high-risk "primary-prevention" individuals who had never had a coronary event (n = 7150), although a significant number had a CHD risk equivalent: diabetes, peripheral vascular disease, or cerebrovascular disease. Simvastatin reduced the risk for any major vascular event by 24% ($P < 0.0001$) and all-cause mortality by 13% ($P = 0.0003$), with a 17% reduction in deaths attributed to any vascular cause. No safety issues were observed with treatment, and myopathy incidence was only 0.01%. The similar clinical benefit in patients with baseline LDL-C level of less than 116 mg/dL (3 mmol/L) and those with higher levels supports treatment decisions based on clinical risk rather than baseline lipids, and initiation of statin therapy in high-risk patients regardless of initial LDL-C level. In the Study of the Effectiveness of Additional Reductions in Cholesterol and Homocysteine (SEARCH), 12,064 participants were randomized to either 80 mg or 20 mg simvastatin daily.[108] The 6% reduction in major vascular events with a further 13.5 mg/dL (0.35 mmol/L) reduction in LDL-C was consistent with previous trials. However, myopathy was increased with 80 mg simvastatin daily, which led to new FDA recommendations (see later).

Indications. Simvastatin has additional, specific indications in patients with CHD and hypercholesterolemia, for (1) reduction of coronary and total mortality, (2) reduction of nonfatal MI, (3) reduction of myocardial revascularization procedures, and (4) reduction of stroke or transient ischemic attack. Simvastatin is also indicated for increasing HDL-C in patients with hypercholesterolemia or combined dyslipidemias, without claiming an effect independent of LDL-C lowering. Based on the results of HPS, the FDA approved revised labeling for simvastatin in 2003 that emphasized high-risk status rather than LDL-C alone as the primary determinant of treatment. Essentially, the labeling states that simvastatin may be started simultaneously with dietary therapy in patients with CHD or at high risk for CHD.

Dose, Side Effects, and Safety. The usual starting dosage for simvastatin is 20 mg once daily in the evening. In 4S, the initial dose was 20 mg once daily just before the evening meal, increased to 40 mg if cholesterol lowering was inadequate after 6 weeks (37% of subjects).[82] For patients at high risk, the starting dosage is 40 mg/day as in HPS. The previous maximum dosage of 80 mg daily is now linked to a substantial risk of myopathy; therefore, the FDA recommends that patients should not be started on or switched to this dose, and patients already on this dose should be carefully monitored for myopathy. *FDA recommendations to reduce myopathy with simvastatin*, which is broken down by the hepatic enzyme CYP3A4 system, are that simvastatin should not be used with the conazole group of drugs (itraconazole, ketoconazole, posaconazole), some antibiotics (erythromycin, clarithromycin, telithromycin), nefazodone, gemfibrozil, cyclosporine, and danazol.[91,92] Specifically contraindicated by the FDA are the HIV protease inhibitors, boceprevir, and telaprevir.[92] The 10-mg dose should not be exceeded in patients taking amiodarone, verapamil, and diltiazem. The 20-mg dose should not be exceeded with amlodipine and ranolazine (Ranexa). The 80-mg dose should not be started.[91,109]

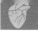

The 11-year follow-up study of HPS found no increase in cancer incidence, cancer mortality, or other nonvascular mortality with simvastatin.[110] The original concerns about the long-term safety of statins have thus been dispelled.[111]

Atorvastatin (Lipitor)

Secondary Prevention. Atorvastatin is one of the best tested and most prescribed of the statins. The Myocardial Ischemia Reduction and Aggressive Cholesterol Lowering (MIRACL) trial[112] and PROVE IT[26] examined the premise that early treatment with high-dose (80 mg daily) atorvastatin therapy following ACS would give clinical benefits. In MIRACL, atorvastatin, compared to placebo, produced modestly significant relative risk reductions for symptomatic ischemia.[112] In the large PROVE IT study in more than 4000 patients, atorvastatin reduced LDL-C to 62 mg/dL (1.60 mmol/L) and decreased the composite primary endpoint when compared with pravastatin 40 mg daily.[26] In patients with stable coronary disease in the Reversal of Atherosclerosis with Aggressive Lipid Lowering (REVERSAL) study, a similar vigorous reduction of LDL-C with atorvastatin versus pravastatin decreased atheroma volume.[27] In the Treating to New Targets (TNT) trial, high-dose atorvastatin (80 mg daily) reduced mean LDL-C from approximately 100 mg/dL (2.6 mmol/L) to 77 mg/dL (2 mmol/L), and major cardiovascular events fell by 22% versus low-dose atorvastatin (10 mg daily).[113] In the Incremental Decrease in Endpoints through Aggressive Lipid lowering (IDEAL) study[114] in 8888 patients with prior MI, atorvastatin 80 mg daily reduced the secondary endpoint of any coronary event, when compared with simvastatin taken at mostly 20 mg daily. However, the primary endpoint of major coronary events was not different between treatment groups nor was mortality reduced. The final lower LDL-C level of 81 mg/dL (2.1 mmol/L) in the atorvastatin group versus 100 mg/dL (2.6 mmol/L) in the simvastatin group modestly supports the "lower is better" hypothesis, at the cost of approximately double the rate of adverse events leading to drug discontinuation (9.6% for atorvastatin versus 4.2% for simvastatin).[114]

Primary Prevention. ASCOT-LLA assessed the clinical effect of atorvastatin, 10 mg/day, versus placebo in 10,305 hypertensive patients with mean total cholesterol of 212 mg/dL (5.5 mmol/L), mean LDL-C of 130 mg/dL (3.4 mmol/L), and a high-risk profile.[86] Originally planned with a follow-up of 5 years, ASCOT ended early because of clear benefit. Atorvastatin reduced the relative risk for cardiovascular events by 36% ($P = 0.0005$) and for stroke by 27% ($P = 0.024$). There was no effect on the low total mortality rate, and the adverse event rates did not differ between the treatment groups. CARDS, in high-risk diabetics, was similarly stopped early because of improved clinical endpoints in those treated with atorvastatin, 10 mg daily, versus placebo.[58] An analysis from TNT suggests that atorvastatin may improve glomerular filtration rate in patients with kidney disease.[115]

Indications. Besides class indications (see previous), atorvastatin is approved by the FDA for primary prevention in patients with multiple risk factors to reduce the risk for MI, stroke, revascularization, or angina. For primary prevention in those with type 2 diabetes and multiple risk factors, atorvastatin is indicated for reduction of MI and stroke. For patients with CHD, atorvastatin is indicated for reduction of nonfatal MI, stroke, revascularization, hospitalization for congestive heart failure, and angina.

Dosage, Effects, and Side Effects. Atorvastatin is available as 10-, 20-, 40-, and 80-mg tablets, which can be given once daily at any time of the day, with or without food. ASCOT[86] and CARDS[58] suggested that a dosage of only 10 mg daily may help prevent clinical events.[4] The PROVE IT study showed that high-dose atorvastatin, 80 mg/day, reduces LDL-C to very low levels and reduces clinical events in patients with recent ACS.[26] A 10-mg starting dose of atorvastatin provides good reductions in total cholesterol, LDL-C, apoB, and triglyceride, and a modest increase in HDL-C. Blood lipid levels should be checked 2–4 weeks after starting therapy and the dosage adjusted accordingly. As with the other statins, liver damage and myopathy are rare but serious *side effects*.

Drug Interactions. Patients on potent inhibitors of hepatic CYP3A4, such as ketoconazole, erythromycin, or HIV protease inhibitors, should in principle not be given any statin that is metabolized through this enzyme (atorvastatin, fluvastatin, lovastatin). Specifically, the FDA warns as follows: avoid atorvastatin with tipranavir and ritonavir, use lowest dose with lopinavir and ritonavir, and use care with other antiretrovirals.[92] *Erythromycin* inhibits hepatic CYP3A4 to increase blood atorvastatin levels by approximately 40%. The interaction with clopidogrel has not been clinically evident.[116] Atorvastatin increases blood levels of some *oral contraceptives*. There is no interaction with warfarin. Other drug interactions are similar to the other statins, including cotherapy with fibrates and niacin.

Rosuvastatin (Crestor)

Rosuvastatin is a hydrophilic compound with high uptake into and selectivity for its site of action in the liver, leading to substantial reductions in total cholesterol and LDL-C. Rosuvastatin's half-life is approximately 19 hours, and it can be taken at any time of the day. It is not metabolized by the CYP3A4 system, thus lessening the risk for certain key drug interactions. However, there are interactions with antiretrovirals.

Major Trials. A Study to Evaluate the Effect of Rosuvastatin on Intravascular Ultrasound-Derived Coronary Atheroma Burden (ASTEROID), conducted in 349 patients with coronary atherosclerosis, found that high-intensity rosuvastatin, 40 mg/day, achieved a mean LDL-C of 61 mg/dL (1.6 mmol/L) and increased HDL-C by 14.7%, with regression of coronary atherosclerosis as measured by intravascular ultrasound.[117] In Measuring Effects on Intima-Media Thickness: an Evaluation of Rosuvastatin (METEOR), in low-risk men with modest carotid intimal–medial thickening and mean LDL-C values of 154 mg/dL, 40-mg/day rosuvastatin for 2 years substantially reduced the rate of progression of carotid atherosclerosis.[118] Results from the JUPITER study have established the efficacy of rosuvastatin in primary prevention, particularly for individuals at increased risk because of elevated levels of hs-CRP but with low levels of LDL-C.[16] JUPITER, which enrolled 17,802 middle-aged adults free of heart disease and diabetes with LDL-C <130 mg/dL and hs-CRP ≥2 mg/L, compared rosuvastatin 20 mg versus placebo and was stopped after 1.9 years because of efficacy. Rosuvastatin reduced LDL-C levels by 50% to a median of 55 mg/dL and decreased hs-CRP levels by 37%, which translated to a 44% relative reduction in major cardiovascular events and a 20% reduction in all-cause mortality compared with placebo.[16]

Indications. In addition to its class indications, rosuvastatin has a favorable effect on triglycerides in patients with elevated serum triglyceride levels and is indicated to slow the progression of atherosclerosis. In primary prevention, based on JUPITER, rosuvastatin is indicated to reduce the risk for stroke, MI, and revascularization in patients at increased risk because of age, hs-CRP of at least 2 mg/L, and one additional cardiovascular risk factor. Rosuvastatin can be safely used in systolic heart failure without any specific antifailure benefit.[119]

Dosage, Effects, and Side Effects. Rosuvastatin is supplied in 5-, 10-, 20-, and 40-mg tablets. The usual starting dosage is 10 mg/day (5 mg for Asian patients) taken any time with or without food. At this dosage, in patients with primary hypercholesterolemia, the expected LDL-C reduction is 52%, with approximately 10% increase in HDL-C and 24% decrease in triglycerides. For patients of advanced age or with renal insufficiency, the recommended starting dose of rosuvastatin is 5 mg/day. In renal patients, rosuvastatin may be titrated up to 10 mg/day; at this dose, rosuvastatin did not increase adverse events and reduced lipid parameters in patients with end-stage renal disease, although it had no effect on cardiovascular outcomes.[120] In patients receiving concomitant cyclosporine, rosuvastatin should be limited to 5 mg/day. In combination with gemfibrozil, rosuvastatin should be limited to 10 mg/day. Its *side effects* and warnings are similar to those of other statins. The maximum 40-mg dose of rosuvastatin is reserved for patients who have an inadequate response to 20 mg/day. Findings of increased risk for new diabetes were first observed with rosuvastatin in the JUPITER trial and subsequently extended to the other statins.[16] Whereas a large meta-analysis of statin trials found a 9% increased risk for incident diabetes with statin treatment over a 4-year period, the risk with rosuvastatin was 18%, based on the results of JUPITER and two other clinical trials.[97] Uncommon instances of proteinuria with microscopic hematuria have been reported, and the frequency may be greater at the 40 mg dose.

Drug Interactions. Like fluvastatin, rosuvastatin is metabolized by way of the CYP2C9 isoenzyme and therefore may be less likely to interact with common drugs that use the CYP3A4 pathway, such as ketoconazole or erythromycin. The FDA warns that the rosuvastatin dose should be limited to 10 mg daily with atazanavir with or without ritonavir, or lopinavir with ritonavir.[92] *Warfarin* interaction is a risk. The standard statin warnings against cotherapy with fibrates or niacin remain, although fenofibrate appears safe. Coadministration of cyclosporine or gemfibrozil with rosuvastatin results in reduced rosuvastatin clearance from the circulation; therefore, the rosuvastatin dose should be reduced. An antacid (aluminum and magnesium hydroxide combination) decreases plasma concentrations of rosuvastatin and should be taken 2 hours after and not before rosuvastatin.

Pitavastatin (Livalo)

Pitavastatin, a low-dose statin, has shown in noninferiority studies of equivalent doses to produce LDL-C reductions comparable to those of atorvastatin and simvastatin and greater than those of pravastatin.[121] It also favorably affects HDL-C and triglycerides. The Japan Assessment of Pitavastatin and Atorvastatin in Acute Coronary Syndrome (JAPAN-ACS) study demonstrated that pitavastatin reduced plaque volume similar to atorvastatin.[122] In the Stabilization and Regression of Coronary Plaque Treated with Pitavastatin Proved by Angioscopy and Intravascular Ultrasound (TOGETHAR) trial,[123] pitavastatin improved plaque composition as assessed by intravascular ultrasound in coronary segments in patients with ACS. High-Dose Versus Low-Dose Pitavastatin in Japanese Patients with Stable Coronary Artery Disease (REAL-CAD), a large prospective, multicenter clinical trial in which 13,054 Japanese patients with stable CHD were randomized to receive pitavastatin 4 mg/day (high dose) or pitavastatin 1 mg/day (low dose), confirmed that high-dose

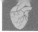

pitavastatin compared to low-dose pitavastatin safely and significantly reduced cardiovascular events in Asian patients.[124]

Indications, Dose, Effects, and Side Effects. Pitavastatin is indicated as an adjunct to diet to reduce elevated total cholesterol, LDL-C, apoB, and triglyceride levels and to increase HDL-C in patients with primary hyperlipidemia or mixed dyslipidemia. It is supplied in 1-, 2-, and 4-mg tablets, with a usual starting dose of 2 mg/day taken at any time of day and a maximum dose of 4 mg/day. For patients with renal disease, the recommended starting dose is 1 mg/day up to a maximum of 2 mg/day. Depending on the dose, pitavastatin can be expected to reduce LDL-C by 31%–45%, reduce triglycerides by 13%–22%, and increase HDL-C by 1%–8%. The *side effects* and warnings for pitavastatin are similar to those of other statins.

Drug Interactions. Pitavastatin is not a substrate for CYP3A4, so it may be less likely to interact with drugs that inhibit the CYP3A4 system. It is minimally metabolized by CYP2C9, which appears to have little clinical effect on drug clearance. Importantly, there is no interaction with antiretrovirals. It is primarily metabolized via glucuronidation, so concomitant treatment with gemfibrozil and other fibrates should only be used with caution, as gemfibrozil has the potential to inhibit the glucuronidation and clearance of statins.[125] Coadministration of cyclosporine is contraindicated because of reduced clearance of pitavastatin, and dosages of pitavastatin should be reduced with coadministration of erythromycin and rifampin for the same reason. Pitavastatin has not been studied with the protease inhibitor combination lopinavir–ritonavir, so should not be used with this combination. As with other statins, combination treatment with niacin and fibrates increases risk for myopathy.

Combination Therapy

Despite the widespread availability of effective statin therapy, observational studies have shown that 16%–53% of patients fail to attain their recommended LDL-C targets in clinical practice,[126,127] and even in patients on ideal statin dosing the risk of major vascular events is reduced by only around one-third.[3] These limitations may be due to suboptimal treatment because of insufficient starting doses or failure to up-titrate therapy, poor LDL-C response to statin, or issues with medication adherence, especially among patients who cannot tolerate the recommended intensity of statin because of adverse effects.[128] The recent large outcome studies combining statin with ezetimibe (IMPROVE-IT[24]), PCSK9 inhibitor (FOURIER[22] and ODYSSEY[23]), and most recently icosapent ethyl (REDUCE-IT[40]) provide strong support for combination strategies in secondary prevention. Both the 2018 AHA/ACC guidelines[6] and 2019 ESC/EAS guidelines[9] recommend the sequential addition of nonstatin lipid-modifying agents, ezetimibe and then PCSK9 inhibitors, to maximally tolerated statin in high-risk statin-intolerant or statin-unresponsive secondary-prevention patients. Furthermore, though increased risk of myopathy was previously a feared complication of combination therapy, myopathy is a rare event with combination therapy.[129,130] Two reservations regarding combination therapy are the lack of data on primary prevention and, for PCSK9 inhibitors, economic feasibility and long-term safety, which is still being established (discussed later).

Cholesterol Absorption Inhibitors: Ezetimibe (Zetia, Vytorin, Nexlizet)

Although statins remain the mainstay for treatment of hypercholesterolemia and secondary prevention of ASCVD, recent data suggest that ezetimibe may serve as a valuable addition to the armamentarium of lipid-lowering drugs. Cholesterol absorption inhibitors selectively interrupt intestinal absorption of cholesterol and phytosterols. Ezetimibe acts at the brush border of the small intestine and inhibits the absorption of cholesterol, leading to decreased delivery of intestinal cholesterol to the liver,[131] which reduces hepatic cholesterol and increases cholesterol clearance from the blood. This mechanism is complementary to that of statins. Ezetimibe has a half-life of 22 hours and is not metabolized by the CYP system.

A meta-analysis of eight randomized, double-blind, placebo-controlled trials found that ezetimibe significantly reduced LDL-C levels by 18.5% when used as monotherapy.[132] The use of ezetimibe in conjunction with a statin has been shown to be an effective strategy for not only reducing LDL-C levels but also preventing cardiovascular events. Early trials demonstrated that statin and ezetimibe combination therapy reduced LDL-C by 12%–19% more than statin monotherapy.[133] The Plaque Regression With Cholesterol Absorption Inhibitor or Synthesis Inhibitor Evaluated by Intravascular Ultrasound (PRECISE-IVUS) trial[134] in patients with CHD demonstrated greater coronary plaque regression, assessed by serial volumetric intravascular ultrasound, in patients treated with ezetimibe in combination with atorvastatin than in patients treated with atorvastatin monotherapy (78% versus 58%; $P = 0.004$). However, the Ezetimibe and Simvastatin in Hypercholesterolemia Enhances Atherosclerosis Regression (ENHANCE) study[135] did not find significant reduction of carotid atherosclerosis in patients with familial hypercholesterolemia with combined ezetimibe and simvastatin compared with simvastatin monotherapy, despite greater LDL-C reduction.

The Study of Heart and Renal Protection (SHARP)[136] was the first major trial that assessed cardiovascular outcomes using combination therapy of statin and ezetimibe. In a wide range of patients with CKD, simvastatin 20 mg daily plus ezetimibe 10 mg daily compared to placebo significantly reduced both the LDL-C levels (33-mg/dL [0.85-mmol/L] difference between treatment groups) and the rate of cardiovascular events (11.3% versus 13.4%; rate ratio 0.83; absolute risk reduction 2.1%; NNT 48) at median 5-year follow-up. However, because the study lacked a statin-only comparison arm, it was unclear whether the benefit of adding ezetimibe was independent of the LDL-lowering effects of the statin. Note that this study could equally well argue for lipid lowering with a statin in dialysis patients.[137] The FDA updated the prescribing information for ezetimibe to include data from SHARP. Although the FDA approved the ezetimibe–simvastatin combination for use in CKD as a new indication, ezetimibe without simvastatin was not approved because the relative contributions of simvastatin and ezetimibe were not assessed in the trial.

IMPROVE-IT was the first trial to provide compelling evidence that a nonstatin medication, ezetimibe, resulted in greater reduction in cardiovascular events when added to statin therapy than statin monotherapy in high-risk patients.[24] Patients with known CHD, within 10 days of a recent MI or ACS and with low LDL-C levels (<125 mg/dL [3.2 mmol/L]), were randomized to ezetimibe therapy in conjunction with simvastatin or to simvastatin monotherapy and followed for a median of 6 years. The combination therapy group had a significantly lower rate of major cardiovascular events (32.7% versus 34.7% in the simvastatin monotherapy group; absolute risk reduction 2.0%; HR 0.936; 95% CI 0.89–0.99; $P = 0.016$) but no difference in mortality. Adverse effects were similar in the two groups, demonstrating the safety profile of ezetimibe. The application of the findings of IMPROVE-IT are twofold. First, it supports the theory of "lower is better" for LDL-C levels to reduce cardiovascular risk. Second, it demonstrated a significant add-on effect of ezetimibe to statin in terms of both LDL-C reduction and reduction of cardiovascular events.

Subanalysis of IMPROVE-IT demonstrated greater reduction in LDL-C among patients with diabetes within the first year of the trial: 43 mg/dL (1.1 mmol/L) reduction in the simvastatin–ezetimibe arm versus 23 mg/dL (0.6 mmol/L) reduction in the simvastatin monotherapy arm.[62] Addition of ezetimibe also conferred a larger protective cardiovascular benefit in high-risk patients with diabetes. Therefore, combination therapy of statin and ezetimibe may be an effective option for patients with diabetes who are unable to tolerate high-intensity statin or those requiring large LDL-C reductions.

The results of the open-label Ezetimibe Lipid Lowering Trial on Prevention of Atherosclerosis in 75 or Older (EWTOPIA75) showed that in 4000 elderly Japanese patients, without prior history of CHD but with LDL-C level $\geq$140 mg/dL and one or more other cardiovascular risk factors (including diabetes, hypertension, prior cerebral infarction, or peripheral artery disease), patients receiving ezetimibe monotherapy had significantly lower cardiovascular events, including strokes, over a 5-year follow-up than patients not receiving ezetimibe.[138]

Indications

Current indications for ezetimibe approved by the FDA include use in primary hypercholesterolemia (heterozygous familial and nonfamilial), as monotherapy or as combination therapy with statins, as adjunctive therapy to diet for the reduction of elevated total cholesterol, LDL-C, and apoB. Combination therapy with atorvastatin or simvastatin is approved for lipid-lowering treatment in homozygous familial hypercholesterolemia, as an adjunct to other lipid-lowering treatments (e.g. LDL apheresis), or used if such treatments are unavailable. Ezetimibe can be combined with fenofibrate for reduction of elevated total cholesterol, LDL-C, apoB, and non-HDL-C in patients with mixed hyperlipidemia. The FDA also approved ezetimibe as adjunctive therapy to diet for the reduction of elevated sitosterol and campesterol levels in patients with homozygous familial sitosterolemia. Both the 2018 AHA/ACC guidelines[6] and 2019 ESC/EAS guidelines[9] recommend the use of ezetimibe as add-on therapy in patients with ASCVD who are unable to achieve recommended LDL-C with maximally tolerated statin therapy, especially very-high-risk patients. The 2019 ESC/EAS guidelines[9] extend the use of ezetimibe as an add-on therapy to statin even in primary-prevention patients unable to achieve the individualized LDL-C goals set for the specific level of risk (Class Ib).

Dosage and Effect

The recommended dosage of ezetimibe is 10 mg once daily, administered with or without food. It may be taken at the same time as a statin. As fixed-dose monotherapy, ezetimibe produces an approximate 18% reduction in LDL-C and modest beneficial effects on triglycerides and HDL-C, with no apparent safety concerns. No dosage adjustment is necessary in patients with mild hepatic insufficiency, but the effects of ezetimibe have not been examined in patients with moderate or severe hepatic insufficiency. No dosage adjustment is necessary in patients with renal insufficiency or in geriatric patients. As *cotherapy*, the lipid effects of ezetimibe and a statin appear to be additive. For example, with pravastatin, 10–40 mg, LDL-C fell by 34%–41% and triglycerides by 21%–23%, and HDL-C rose by 7.8%–8.4%, with a safety profile similar to pravastatin alone.[139] Coadministration of a resin may decrease the bioavailability of ezetimibe; therefore, ezetimibe should be administered either 2 or more hours before or 4 or more hours after administration of the resin.

The FDA recommendations to reduce myopathy with simvastatin are also applicable to combined simvastatin–ezetimibe (Vytorin). In brief, simvastatin–ezetimibe should not be used with the conazole group of drugs, some antibiotics, HIV protease inhibitors, cyclosporine, and gemfibrozil.[93]

Proprotein Convertase Subtilisin/Kexin Type 9 (PCSK9) Inhibitors (Repatha, Praluent)

PCSK9 inhibitors have been shown to be the most potent LDL-lowering class of drug. The FDA has approved two monoclonal antibodies in this class of drugs for LDL-C reduction and secondary prevention: evolocumab (Repatha) and alirocumab (Praluent).

PCSK9 is a hepatic protease that attaches to and internalizes LDL receptors into lysosomes, promoting LDL receptor degradation.[140] PCSK9 inhibitors bind and inactivate extracellular PCSK9 and prevent its interaction with the LDL receptor, thereby preventing trafficking of LDL receptors to lysosomes and therefore increasing the number of LDL receptors on the surface of liver cells available to clear LDL,[141] which in turn lowers LDL-C levels in the blood. Additionally, PCSK9 inhibitors significantly reduce total cholesterol, apoB, triglycerides, and Lp(a).

Despite widespread use of the statins, a large proportion of high-risk patients are not able to achieve targeted LDL-C levels and have residual risk. Previously, options were limited for patients who develop CVD despite being on maximally tolerated statin therapy, were intolerant to statin therapy, or had severe hypercholesterolemia. The PCSK9 inhibitors evolocumab and alirocumab have been shown in multiple phase III and IV clinical trials to provide consistent and substantial LDL-C reductions of 50%–70% across a broad range of CVD risk, pretreatment LDL-C levels, and background therapy and have been studied as monotherapy (MENDEL-2,[142] ODYSSEY COMBO I[143]), as an add-on to statin therapy (LAPLACE-2,[144] ODYSSEY CHOICE I[145]), or in individuals with heterozygous familial hypercholesterolemia (RUTHERFORD-2,[146] ODYSSEY-FH[147]). The Goal Achievement After Utilizing an Anti-PCSK9 Antibody in Statin

Intolerant Subjects 3 (GAUSS-3) randomized clinical trial also demonstrated tolerability of PCSK9 inhibitor therapy in patients with muscle-related statin intolerance.[148] These agents can be used as both adjunctive and alternative therapy for reducing LDL-C and have ushered in a new era of lipid-lowering therapy

Data from two large landmark outcome trials, FOURIER[22] and ODYSSEY OUTCOMES,[23] provided robust proof of the clinical safety and efficacy of evolocumab and alirocumab in reducing ASCVD events when used in combination with a statin compared to statin monotherapy. FOURIER was a large randomized, double-blind, placebo-controlled clinical trial investigating the efficacy and safety of evolocumab when added to high-intensity or moderate-intensity statin therapy in patients with stable clinical ASCVD.[22] Patients were randomized to receive evolocumab or matching placebo as subcutaneous injections for 26 months. The majority of the 27,564 patients (69.3%) were on a high-intensity statin, 30.4% were on moderate-intensity statin, and 5.2% were on ezetimibe. At 48 weeks, evolocumab reduced LDL-C levels by 59% from baseline compared with placebo for a mean absolute reduction of 56 mg/dL. The primary efficacy endpoint (composite of cardiovascular death, MI, stroke, hospitalization for unstable angina, or coronary revascularization) occurred in 9.8% of patients in the evolocumab group and 11.3% of patients in the placebo group, indicating a 15% risk reduction with evolocumab (HR 0.85; 95% CI 0.79–0.92; $P < 0.001$) and NNT of 74. No effect was observed on hospitalization for unstable angina, cardiovascular death, or all-cause death but there were significant reductions in the risk for nonfatal MI (HR 0.73; 95% CI 0.65–0.82; $P < 0.001$), nonfatal stroke (HR 0.79; 95% CI 0.66–0.95; $P = 0.01$), and coronary revascularization (HR 0.78; 95% CI 0.71–0.86; $P < 0.001$).

ODYSSEY OUTCOMES assessed the efficacy of adding alirocumab to maximally tolerated statins on cardiovascular outcomes in 18,924 patients who had an ACS within a year of enrolling in the trial.[22] At 48 weeks, alirocumab reduced LDL-C levels by 54.7% compared to placebo for an absolute reduction of 48.1 mg/dL. Patients who received alirocumab had significant reduction in major cardiovascular events; the primary composite endpoint (composite of cardiovascular death, MI, stroke, or hospitalization for unstable angina) occurred in 9.5% of patients in the alirocumab group and 11.1% of patients in the placebo group, resulting in a 15% risk reduction (HR 0.85; 95% CI 0.78–0.93; $P = 0.0003$) and NNT of 62. There were also significant reductions in nonfatal MI (6.6% versus 7.6%; $P = 0.006$), stroke (1.2% versus 1.6%; $P = 0.01$), and all-cause death (3.5% versus 4.1%; nominal $P = 0.026$) but no difference in cardiovascular death. This was the first trial to show mortality benefit with the addition of a nonstatin medication. Whereas alirocumab significantly reduced total deaths, cardiovascular death or noncardiovascular death analyzed separately was not significantly reduced. Patients with nonfatal cardiovascular events were at increased risk for both cardiovascular and noncardiovascular deaths. Because alirocumab reduced total nonfatal cardiovascular events ($P < 0.001$), the authors postulated that this may have attenuated the number of cardiovascular and noncardiovascular deaths and thus led to a reduction in total mortality.[149]

Patients with peripheral artery disease are a very-high-risk group and often undertreated. A subanalysis[150] from FOURIER demonstrated that evolocumab reduced both major adverse cardiovascular events and major adverse limb events, defined as acute limb ischemia, major amputation, or urgent peripheral revascularization in patients with history of peripheral artery disease. Furthermore, the subgroup of patients with peripheral artery disease were shown to derive the most benefit from alirocumab therapy, as this subgroup achieved the highest absolute risk reduction in both adverse cardiovascular and adverse limb events. Evolocumab also reduced the risk of major adverse limb events in all patients, regardless of peripheral artery disease diagnosis at baseline, with reduction in lower limb events shown to be directly proportional to achieved LDL-C level, down to an LDL-C level of 10 mg/dL. Thus, PCSK9 inhibitor therapy should be strongly considered to reduce risk for cardiovascular and peripheral artery disease events.

Indications

FDA approved use of alirocumab (Praluent) and evolocumab (Repatha) for adult patients with heterozygous familial hypercholesterolemia or in patients with clinically significant ASCVD requiring additional LDL-C lowering after diet and maximally tolerated statin therapy. Evolocumab has also been approved for use in patients with homozygous familial hypercholesterolemia. The FDA has also approved use of both alirocumab and evolocumab to reduce the risk of MI, stroke, and unstable angina requiring hospitalization in adults with established CVD based on FOURIER and ODYSSEY OUTCOMES. The 2018 AHA/ACC Guideline on the Management of Blood Cholesterol reserve PCSK9 inhibitors for the treatment of patients with very high ASCVD risk on maximally tolerated statins and ezetimibe (Class IIa recommendation) and for primary prevention patients with heterozygous familial hypercholesterolemia on maximally tolerated statins and ezetimibe (Class IIb recommendation).[6] These conservative recommendations are based on issues related to cost effectiveness, insurance coverage, affordability, and patient acceptance of subcutaneous administration.

However, after publication of the guideline, the price of both drugs was reduced by >60% by their respective pharmaceutical companies. The subsequently published 2019 ESC/EAS dyslipidemia guidelines,[9] on the other hand, recommend the use of PCSK9 inhibitors in any patients with a documented ASCVD event, even if the event is not recent, if unable to achieve goal LDL-C <55 mg/dL with statin and ezetimibe (Class IIa).

Dosage and Side Effects

Alirocumab is administered subcutaneously 75 mg every 2 weeks and can be titrated to 150 mg every 2 weeks; alternatively, alirocumab can also be administered 300 mg once every 4 weeks (monthly), according to patient preference. Evolocumab is administered subcutaneously 140 mg every 2 weeks or 420 mg every 4 weeks. Pooled data from multiple large clinical trials[151] showed that these agents are well tolerated with no difference in serious adverse effects compared to placebo. For both alirocumab and evolocumab, the most common adverse events reported in clinical trials were injection-site reactions (erythema, itchiness, swelling, pain, or tenderness), nasopharyngitis, and upper respiratory tract infection. The most common adverse events that led to drug discontinuation were allergic reactions with alirocumab and myalgia, nausea, and dizziness with evolocumab. PCSK9 inhibitors seem to provoke fewer muscle-related adverse effects than statins and do not appear to cause muscle toxicity or elevated liver enzymes. The Evaluating PCSK9 Binding Antibody Influence on Cognitive Health in High Cardiovascular Risk Subjects (EBBINGHAUS) study[152] in a subgroup of patients from FOURIER found no significant difference in cognitive function in patients who received evolocumab or placebo in addition to statin over a median of 19 months.

In Development: Inclisiran

In contrast with these monoclonal antibodies against PCSK9, inclisiran is a novel, synthetic, small interfering double-stranded RNA (siRNA) molecule that inhibits intracellular PCSK9 synthesis in hepatocytes. siRNA binds intracellularly to RNA-induced silencing complex, affecting the degradation of mRNA posttranscription, thus preventing translation. Inclisiran is a long-acting, synthetic siRNA directed against mRNA coding for PCSK9. It is conjugated to triantennary N-acetylgalactosamine carbohydrates, which specifically bind to abundant liver-expressed asialoglycoprotein receptors, leading to the uptake of inclisiran specifically into the hepatocytes.[152a] As mentioned for the previous PCSK9 inhibitors, any therapeutic approach to reduce circulating levels of PCSK9 offers an additional route through which plasma LDL-C levels can be controlled. This is especially important in clinical practice because of significant variability in individual responses to statins, with many individuals at risk for or with ASCVD failing to achieve LDL-C goals or exhibiting intolerance to statins. Such individuals may benefit from additional LDL-C lowering by other therapeutic means, as evidenced in the FOURIER and ODYSSEY OUTCOMES trials.[22,23]

In two randomized, single-blind, placebo-controlled, phase I studies of inclisiran in healthy adult volunteers, significant, dose-dependent, long-term mean reductions in circulating PCSK9 and LDL-C levels were demonstrated, with similar safety profile and tolerability to placebo.[152b,152c] ORION-1 was the first phase II, multi-center, double-blind, placebo-controlled, multiple-ascending-dose trial of inclisiran, conducted in 501 patients at high risk for or with history of ASCVD.[152d] The greatest reductions in LDL-C and PCSK9 levels were attained with the two-dose 300-mg regimen of inclisiran: 52.6%, and 69.1%, respectively, at 180 days. Serious adverse events occurred in 11% of the patients who received inclisiran and in 8% of the patients who received placebo. A follow-up study of ORION-1, in which participants were followed up to 1 year after initial injection, showed that treatment with inclisiran resulted in durable reductions in LDL-C over 1 year, with similar incidence of adverse events between inclisiran and placebo.[152e]

Three phase III clinical trials, ORION-9 (NCT03397121), ORION-10 (NCT03399370), and ORION-11 (NCT03400800), designed to evaluate the safety and efficacy of inclisiran in people with ASCVD and elevated LDL-C despite the maximum tolerated dose of LDL-C–lowering therapies, as well as in individuals with familial hypercholesterolemia, have been completed.[152f–152h] All three studies demonstrated that inclisiran produced significant reductions in LDL-C and PCSK9 levels with an acceptable side effect profile, as compared to placebo. In ORION-9, a randomized trial in 482 patients with heterozygous familial hypercholesterolemia who were already taking statins and ezetimibe, inclisiran 300 mg administered as a subcutaneous injection on days 1, 90, 270, and 450 was superior to placebo in reducing LDL-C.[152f] In ORION-10, a randomized, parallel-group, double-blind, clinical trial in 1561 US patients with ASCVD who were taking maximally tolerated statin therapy, twice-yearly inclisiran injections (300 mg) reduced LDL-C by 56% over a follow-up of 18 months; serious and treatment-emergent side effects were similar between the two groups.[152g] ORION-11 showed similar results in 1617 European patients with ASCVD or at high risk for ASCVD who received inclisiran 300 mg on days 1, 90, 270, and 450 and had 50% reduction in LDL-C over 18 months; the overall adverse event profiles of the placebo- and inclisiran-treated groups in ORION-11 were similar.[152h] The ongoing ORION-4 trial (NCT03705234; HPS-4/TIMI 65/ORION-4) is designed to evaluate cardiovascular outcomes in 15,000 people with ASCVD; primary results are expected in 2024 and final completion in 2049.[152i]

Bempedoic Acid (Nexletol, Nexlizet [US]; Nilemdo, Nustendi [EU])

Bempedoic acid is a recently approved nonstatin therapy designed to inhibit cholesterol biosynthesis primarily in the liver. Bempedoic acid is administered as a prodrug that is converted to its active moiety primarily in the liver and inhibits adenosine triphosphate citrate lyase (ACL), an enzyme two steps upstream from HMG-CoA reductase along the cholesterol biosynthesis pathway,[152j] thereby effectively reducing cholesterol synthesis, resulting in LDL receptor upregulation and increased clearance of LDL from the bloodstream. Bempedoic acid can only converted to its active moiety by the enzyme ACSVL1, which is present in hepatocytes but not present in skeletal muscle[152k]; therefore, based on its pharmacological profile, bempedoic acid may have fewer serious muscle adverse effects.

Five randomized, double-blind, placebo-controlled, parallel-group, multicenter phase III clinical trials known as Cholesterol Lowering via Bempedoic Acid, an ACL-inhibiting Regimen (CLEAR) have established safety, tolerability, and LDL-C–lowering efficacy of bempedoic acid in a total 3623 participants.[152l] In the largest of these trials, CLEAR Harmony, which studied bempedoic acid only in 2230 patients with ASCVD and/or heterozygous familial hypercholesterolemia on background statin therapy (85% using moderate- to high-intensity statin), bempedoic acid resulted in a significant 16.5% reduction in LDL-C and did not lead to higher incidence of overall adverse events compared to placebo over 52 weeks' follow-up.[152m] In CLEAR Tranquility, in which 269 statin-intolerant patients on stable background therapy and open-label ezetimibe 10 mg were randomized to receive bempedoic acid 180 mg or placebo for 12 weeks, bempedoic acid + ezetimibe resulted in 28.5% greater LDL-C reduction than placebo + ezetimibe.[152n] In another phase III clinical trial (not part of the CLEAR program), the safety and efficacy of a fixed-dose combination tablet containing bempedoic acid 180 mg and ezetimibe 10 mg was evaluated in 301 patients with hypercholesterolemia and ASCVD and/or heterozygous familial hypercholesterolemia on background maximally tolerated statin therapy (35% on high-intensity statin, 35% on no statin). Fixed-dose combination therapy lowered

LDL-C by 38% compared with placebo at week 12 and had a generally similar safety profile compared with bempedoic acid, ezetimibe, or placebo.[152o]. The ongoing CLEAR Outcomes trial (NCT02993406) is a cardiovascular event–driven, multinational, randomized, double-blind, placebo-controlled study in approximately 12,600 patients, with an estimated study duration of 4.75 years.[152p]

Indications

Bempedoic acid is indicated as an adjunct to diet and maximally tolerated statin therapy for the treatment of adults with heterozygous familial hypercholesterolemia or established ASCVD who require additional lowering of LDL-C. The European Medicines Agency indications also include use in patients who cannot tolerate statins.

Dosage, Effects, and Side Effects

Bempedoic acid is available as a tablet containing 180 mg of bempedoic acid or as a combination tablet containing 180 mg of bempedoic acid and 10 mg of ezetimibe. Either tablet is taken orally once a day with or without food.

The combined tablet is contraindicated in individuals with a known hypersensitivity to ezetimibe. Bempedoic acid may increase blood uric acid levels and may lead to gout, especially in patients with a history of gout. Bempedoic acid therapy may also be associated with an increased risk of tendon rupture, which may occur more frequently in patients over 60 years of age, patients taking corticosteroid or fluoroquinolone drugs, patients with renal failure, and patients with previous tendon disorders. In clinical trials of bempedoic acid, the most commonly reported adverse events were upper respiratory tract infection, muscle spasms, hyperuricemia, back pain, abdominal pain or discomfort, bronchitis, pain in extremity, anemia, and elevated liver enzymes; events reported less frequently, but still more often than with placebo, included benign prostatic hyperplasia and atrial fibrillation. For the combination bempedoic acid/ezetimibe tablet, the most commonly reported adverse events that were not observed in clinical trials of bempedoic acid or ezetimibe and occurred more frequently than with placebo were urinary tract infection, nasopharyngitis, and constipation.

Treatment with bempedoic acid has been associated with persistent changes in laboratory tests within the first four weeks of treatment, including increases in creatinine, blood urea nitrogen, platelet counts, liver enzymes, and creatine kinase and decreases in hemoglobin and leukocytes. Laboratory abnormalities generally return to baseline after discontinuation of treatment.

Bempedoic acid should not be taken during breastfeeding. Pregnant patients should consult their healthcare provider about whether to continue treatment during pregnancy. The safety and efficacy of bempedoic acid has not been established in patients under the age of 18. No adjustments in dosing are required for advanced age, mild or moderate renal impairment, or mild hepatic impairment; in patients with moderate hepatic impairment, no dosing adjustment is required for bempedoic acid, but the combination bempedoic acid/ezetimibe tablet is not recommended for patients with moderate or severe hepatic impairment.

Drug Interactions

Concomitant use of bempedoic acid with simvastatin or pravastatin results in increased statin concentration and increased risk for statin-related myopathy. Use of bempedoic acid with >20 mg of simvastatin or >40 mg of pravastatin should be avoided. Caution should be exercised when using combination bempedoic acid/ezetimibe with cyclosporine because of increased exposure to both ezetimibe and cyclosporine; cyclosporine concentrations should be monitored, and the potential risk/benefit ratio of concomitant use should be carefully considered. Coadministration of combination bempedoic acid/ezetimibe with fibrates other than fenofibrate is not recommended. Fenofibrate and ezetimibe may increase cholesterol excretion into the bile, leading to cholelithiasis; if cholelithiasis is suspected, gallbladder studies are indicated and alternative lipid-lowering therapy should be considered. Concomitant use of combination bempedoic acid/ezetimibe with cholestyramine decreases ezetimibe concentration, which may reduce efficacy; bempedoic acid/ezetimibe should be administered at least 2 hours before or at least 4 hours after bile acid sequestrants.

Omega-3 Fatty Acids (Fish Oils; Lovaza, Vascepa, Epanova)

Omega-3 fatty acids are a major class of polyunsaturated fatty acids. Studies show that omega-3 fatty acids in general decrease blood triglyceride and VLDL levels in hyperlipidemic individuals but may have no effect or may increase LDL-C in patients with very high triglycerides. These effects are most prominently seen with high-dose supplements (>2 to 44 g/day). Eicosapentaenoic acid (EPA) and docosahexaenoic acid (DHA) are two major types of omega-3 fatty acids. EPA and DHA have been shown to reduce inflammation, with production of resolvins[153] and decrease in proinflammatory compounds.[154,155] A number of other beneficial actions for atherosclerosis prevention have been reported, relating to endothelial function, oxidative stress, foam-cell formation, plaque formation/progression, platelet aggregation, thrombus formation, and plaque rupture.[156,157] DHA is the major polyunsaturated fatty acid found in the brain and is important for brain development and function.

In the Multi-center, Placebo-controlled, Randomized, Double-blind, 12-Week Study with an Open-label Extension (MARINE) trial,[158] in adult patients with very high fasting triglyceride levels between 500 mg/dL and 2000 mg/dL, patients treated with EPA ethyl ester (icosapent ethyl) 4 g/day for 12 weeks had a statistically significant placebo-adjusted median triglyceride reduction of 33% ($P < 0.0001$) and a small reduction in LDL-C levels (5%). In addition, treatment with icosapent ethyl 4 g/day led to statistically significant placebo-adjusted median reductions from baseline in non-HDL-C (18%), total cholesterol (16%), VLDL-C (29%), and apoB (8.5%).

The efficacy of icosapent ethyl was also evaluated in ANCHOR,[159] a phase III placebo-controlled randomized clinical trial in high-risk statin-treated patients (n = 702) with triglyceride levels between 200 mg/dL and 500 mg/dL and with LDL-C levels of 40–100 mg/dL. After 12 weeks, treatment with icosapent ethyl 4 g/day resulted in a significant median placebo-adjusted change from baseline in triglyceride levels of 21.5% ($P < 0.0001$).

Historically, clinical trials assessing the role of fish oil supplementation or low-dose prescription omega-3 fatty acids showed variable results without clear benefit in prevention of cardiovascular events. However, both the Japan EPA Lipid Intervention Study (JELIS)[160] and REDUCE-IT[40] provided valuable findings to support clinical benefit of EPA as an add-on to statins in high-risk patients. In JELIS,[160] 18,645 Japanese patients with hypercholesterolemia were randomly assigned to receive either low-intensity statin therapy plus EPA 1.8 g/day or statin therapy alone (there was no placebo group). The risk of major coronary events was significantly reduced by 19% in the group that received EPA plus statin therapy compared with the group that received statin therapy alone. Additional evidence was obtained from REDUCE-IT,[40] which was the first large multinational cardiovascular outcomes study that evaluated the effect of prescription EPA therapy as an add-on to statins. Over 8000 patients with high cardiovascular risk who, despite stable statin therapy, had residual hypertriglyceridemia (fasting triglyceride of at least 135 mg/dL) were randomized to 2 g of icosapent ethyl twice daily (total daily dose, 4 g) or placebo. Patients in the icosapent ethyl group had significantly reduced risk for the primary endpoint of cardiovascular events (cardiovascular death, nonfatal MI, nonfatal stroke, coronary revascularization, or unstable angina), which occurred in 17.2% of the icosapent ethyl group versus 22.0% of

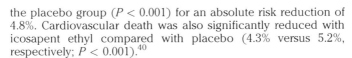

the placebo group ($P < 0.001$) for an absolute risk reduction of 4.8%. Cardiovascular death was also significantly reduced with icosapent ethyl compared with placebo (4.3% versus 5.2%, respectively; $P < 0.001$).[40]

Indications

Two prescription-strength omega-3 fatty acids, omega-3-acid ethyl esters (Lovaza) and icosapent ethyl (Vascepa), are approved by the FDA to treat severe hypertriglyceridemia (triglycerides levels 500 mg/dL or more) at a dose of 4 g/day. A third formulation, omega-3 carboxylic acids (Epanova), was being evaluated in A Long-Term Outcomes Study to Assess Statin Residual Risk Reduction with Epanova in High Cardiovascular Risk Patients with Hypertriglyceridemia (STRENGTH), which was discontinued due to low likelihood of benefit.[161]

Each 1-g capsule of omega-3-acid ethyl esters contains ≥900 mg of ethyl esters of omega-3 fatty acids, predominantly a combination of ethyl esters of EPA (~465 mg) and DHA (~375 mg), whereas icosapent ethyl contains only EPA and no DHA. The suggested daily dosage of both omega-3-acid ethyl esters and icosapent ethyl is 4 g twice a day with food. Each gram of omega-3 carboxylic acids contains 850 mg of polyunsaturated fatty acids, including multiple omega-3 fatty acids (EPA and DHA being most abundant). Both EPA and DHA reduce triglyceride levels; however, DHA also raises LDL-C.[162]

Icosapent ethyl is also approved by the FDA as an adjunctive therapy to statins to reduce the risk of ASCVD events among adults with established ASCVD or with diabetes and ≥ 2 risk factors who also have elevated triglyceride levels ≥150 mg/dL. It is the first and only FDA-approved medication to reduce cardiovascular risk beyond cholesterol-lowering therapy in high-risk patients. The 2019 ESC/EAS guidelines[9] recommend the addition of icosapent ethyl 4 g/day in high-risk patients with triglyceride of 135–499 mg/dL despite high-intensity or maximally tolerated statin treatment (Class IIa). The NLA issued a scientific statement[41] and the ADA amended its Standard of Care[42] to endorse the use of icosapent ethyl in individuals with clinical ASCVD or diabetes mellitus with other cardiovascular risk factors to treat elevated triglycerides, as an add-on to statin therapy.

Side Effects

Because omega-3 fatty acids are obtained from the oil of fish, they should be used cautiously in patients with a fish allergy and/or shellfish allergy. Some data suggest that omega-3 fatty acids may prolong bleeding time; therefore, patients receiving omega-3 fatty acids with other drugs that affect coagulation should be monitored periodically. In clinical trials, treatment-emergent adverse events were similar in those treated with omega-3 fatty acids compared with placebo. In REDUCE-IT,[40] the most common reported adverse reaction was arthralgia (2.3% for icosapent ethyl, 1.0% for placebo); other common adverse events occurring more frequently with icosapent ethyl than placebo were peripheral edema (6.5% versus 5.0%, respectively), constipation (5.4% versus 3.6%), and atrial fibrillation (5.3% versus 3.9% placebo). A larger percentage of patients in the icosapent ethyl group than in the placebo group were hospitalized for atrial fibrillation or flutter (3.1% versus 2.1%, $P = 0.004$). Icosapent ethyl patients had reductions in rates of cardiac arrest, sudden death, and myocardial infarctions. Serious adverse bleeding events occurred in 2.7% of the icosapent ethyl group and 2.1% of the placebo group ($P = 0.06$), but the rate of anemia was significantly lower in the icosapent ethyl group than in the placebo group (4.7% versus 5.8%; $P = 0.03$).

Fibrates: Fibric Acid Derivatives

Fibrates are highly effective in reducing triglycerides, but as a rule, none of the fibrates reduce LDL-C as much as do the statins or PCSK9 inhibitors. Unlike statins, which have demonstrated clinical efficacy across a broad range of LDL-C levels, fibrates have primarily shown reductions in cardiovascular events in a subset of patients with high triglycerides ($\geq$200 mg/dL [2.2 mmol/L]) and low HDL-C (<40 mg/dL [1.0 mmol/L]). The primary role of fibrates is to decrease triglyceride level, atherogenic triglyceride-rich lipoproteins, and concentration of small, dense LDL particles. They are therefore suitable for use in atherogenic dyslipidemia.[163] Fibrates are first-line therapy to reduce the risk for pancreatitis in patients with very high levels of plasma triglycerides[164] and may be useful with more modest triglyceride elevations or when the primary dyslipidemia is low HDL-C.[165]

At a molecular level, fibrates are agonists for the nuclear transcription factor peroxisome proliferator–activated receptor–α (PPAR-α), which stimulates the synthesis of the enzymes of fatty acid oxidation, thereby reducing VLDL triglycerides.[163] Although all fibrates belong to the same class of drugs, structural differences between the compounds seem important because of the very different results between large-scale trials of clofibrate (unfavorable) and gemfibrozil (favorable; see below).

Combined Statin Plus Fibrate

In primary prevention, for patients with severe hypercholesterolemia or familial combined hyperlipidemia with marked triglyceride elevations, combination of a statin with a fibrate is an option.

The statin is effective in the reduction of LDL-C, whereas the fibrate reduces triglycerides and triglyceride-rich lipoproteins. Statins metabolized through CYP3A4 have a greater risk of adverse interaction with fibrates during cotherapy with erythromycin, azole antifungals, and antiretrovirals.[166] A logical combination would be a statin and a fibrate that are metabolized by noncompeting pathways, for example, fluvastatin or rosuvastatin combined with fenofibrate.

Class Warnings

There are five warnings or reservations for this class of drugs. First, the early experience with clofibrate suggested that fibrates may increase mortality. This fear has not been borne out by trials of other fibrates, and gemfibrozil has demonstrated significant coronary benefits. Second, hepatotoxicity may occur, with a pooled analysis of 10 placebo-controlled trials showing elevated transaminases in 5.3% of patients given fenofibrate compared to 1.1% on placebo.[167] Third, cholelithiasis is a risk, because fibrates act in part by increasing biliary secretion of cholesterol; however, this was not found in the Veterans Affairs High-Density Lipoprotein Cholesterol Intervention Trial (VA-HIT).[165] Fourth, fibrates have an important drug interaction with concomitant oral anticoagulants; therefore, warfarin dose needs to be reduced by about 30%. Fifth, combined therapy with statins should be avoided unless the potential beneficial effect on lipids outweighs the increased risk for myopathy via competitively inhibiting CYP3A4, which leads to a reduction in statin metabolism.

Fenofibrate (Tricor, Trilipix, Lipofen, Antara, Lofibra)

Fenofibrate is a prodrug converted to fenofibric acid in the tissues. The FDA-approved indications are as adjunctive therapy to diet to reduce LDL-C and total cholesterol, triglycerides, and apoB and to increase HDL-C in severe hypertriglyceridemia or mixed dyslipidemia. Although indicated for treatment of hypertriglyceridemia, its effect on the risk for pancreatitis in patients with very high triglyceride levels, typically exceeding 1000 mg/dL, has not been well studied. The Trilipix formulation, which contains fenofibric acid rather than the ester, has an indication for mixed dyslipidemia in combination with statin therapy. Tricor is available in 48- and 145-mg tablets and is dosed at 48–145 mg once daily (half-life of 20 hours), taken with food to optimize bioavailability. Other formulations have slightly altered dosing. Predisposing diseases such as obesity, diabetes, CKD, chronic liver disease, nephrotic syndrome, and hypothyroidism need to be excluded and treated prior to initiating treatment.[6] The Diabetes Atherosclerosis Intervention Study (DAIS) suggests that treatment with fenofibrate in patients with type 2 diabetes reduces progression of atherosclerosis, with a nonsignificant trend toward cardiovascular event reduction.[168] The Fenofibrate Intervention and Event Lowering in Diabetes (FIELD) study similarly attempted to assess the effect of fenofibrate on CVD events in patients with type 2 diabetes, but failed to show a benefit on the primary endpoint of coronary events (MI and CHD death), possibly because the study design allowed for initiation of statin therapy in both the placebo and fenofibrate treatment arms.[169] Despite these null findings, FIELD did show a decrease in total cardiovascular events, primarily caused by significant reductions in nonfatal MI and revascularizations, as well as a significant benefit on the primary endpoint in the subgroup with high triglycerides and low HDL-C. The Action to Control Cardiovascular Risk in Diabetes Lipid (ACCORD Lipid) trial was conducted in 5500 patients with type 2 diabetes on statin therapy who were randomized to receive fenofibrate or placebo.[170] Combination therapy with fenofibrate and statin did not significantly reduce major cardiovascular events (HR 0.92; 95% CI 0.79–1.08; $P = 0.32$) as compared to statin alone, and no cardiovascular benefit was found with the drug combination, except in a subgroup of individuals with low HDL-C and high triglycerides at baseline. Post hoc analyses of three other fibrate trials, including the Helsinki Heart Study, the Bezafibrate Infarction Prevention study (BIP), and FIELD, similarly suggested benefit with a fibrate in a subgroup of patients with atherogenic dyslipidemia.[170] Thus the cumulative body of evidence indicates that the prime lipid-lowering therapy for prevention of macrovascular complications in most diabetic patients remains a statin.

Weight reduction, increased exercise, and elimination of excess alcohol are essential steps in the overall control of triglyceride levels. Fenofibrate coadministered with cyclosporine may cause renal damage with decreased excretion of fenofibrate and increased blood levels. Use with caution in patients taking oral coumarin-type anticoagulants; anticoagulant dosage may need to be adjusted. Animal data suggest a deleterious effect in pregnancy. Avoid in nursing mothers (carcinogenic potential in animals). Use with caution in older adults or patients with renal dysfunction (renal excretion).

Gemfibrozil (Lopid)

Major Trials. Gemfibrozil was used in the large primary-prevention Helsinki Heart Study in 4081 apparently healthy men with modest hypercholesterolemia (non-HDL-C $\geq$200 mg/dL) observed for 5 years.[171] Gemfibrozil 600 mg twice daily led to a major increase in HDL-C (10%), decreases in total cholesterol, LDL-C, and non-HDL-C (11%, 10%, and 14%, respectively), and a substantial reduction in triglycerides (43%), with a 34% reduction in coronary events (fatal and nonfatal MI and cardiac death). Although the total death rate was not different between treatment groups, the study was not powered to assess mortality. An open-label follow-up study found mortality reduction after 13 years.[172] Despite the theoretical risk of gallstone formation with fibrate therapy, none was reported during the study.

VA-HIT was a secondary-prevention trial in 2531 men with CHD whose primary abnormality was low HDL-C: <40 mg/dL (1 mmol/L), with a mean of 32 mg/dL.[165] The entry criterion for LDL-C was ≤140 mg/dL (3.6 mmol/L), with a mean of 112 mg/dL. Over 5 years, mean HDL-C was 6% higher, mean triglyceride 31% lower, and total cholesterol 4% lower with gemfibrozil than with placebo, whereas mean LDL-C level was not different between treatment groups. The primary outcome of nonfatal MI or coronary death was reduced by 22% with gemfibrozil (event rates 17.3% in the gemfibrozil group versus 21.7% in the placebo group, $P < 0.001$). The 5-year NNT was 23, which compared well with that of the major statin trials. It must be noted that gemfibrozil was only studied as monotherapy and not as an add-on to statin in this clinical trial. Therefore, with statins currently the first-line option and multiple other drugs showing benefit as an add-on therapy (discussed previously), gemfibrozil probably has limited clinical utility.

Dose, Side Effects, Contraindications. Gemfibrozil is currently approved in the United States for treatment of severe hypertriglyceridemia and mixed dyslipidemia (elevated LDL-C, decreased HDL-C, and increased triglycerides). The dose is 1200 mg given in two divided doses 30 minutes before the morning and evening meals. *Contraindications* are hepatic or severe renal dysfunction, preexisting gallbladder disease (possible risk of increased gallstones, not found in VA-HIT), and coadministration with simvastatin, repaglinide, dasabuvir, or selexipag. There are *drug interactions* to consider. Because it is highly protein bound, gemfibrozil potentiates warfarin. When combined with statins, there is an increased risk for myopathy with myoglobinuria and a further rare risk for acute renal failure

Bezafibrate

Bezafibrate (Bezalip in the United Kingdom; not available in the United States) resembles gemfibrozil in its overall effects, side effects, and alterations in blood lipid profile. Uniquely among fibrates, bezafibrate is also a PPAR-γ agonist, thereby theoretically stimulating the enzymes that regulate glucose metabolism. Hence, plasma glucose tends to fall with bezafibrate, which may be useful in patients with diabetes or abnormal glucose metabolic patterns. In patients with CHD, bezafibrate slows the development of insulin resistance.[173] As with other fibrates, warfarin potentiation is possible, and cotherapy with statins should ideally be avoided. In addition, myositis, renal failure, alopecia, and loss of libido have occurred. Bezafibrate is dosed at 200 mg two to three times daily; however, once daily is nearly as effective, and a slow-release formulation is available (in the United Kingdom: *Bezalip-Mono*, 400 mg once daily). Some increase in plasma creatinine is very common and of unknown consequence. The major limitation with bezafibrate is that, unlike gemfibrozil and the statins, no major long-term outcome trials have provided clear results. In BIP,[174] conducted in 3090 patients with previous MI or angina and low HDL-C combined with modestly elevated LDL-C, HDL-C was increased by 18% and triglyceride decreased by 21% with bezafibrate, but the primary endpoint of fatal or nonfatal MI or sudden death was not significantly different between treatment groups (13.6% with bezafibrate versus 15.0% with placebo; $P = 0.26$), except post hoc in a subgroup of patients with initial triglyceride levels ≥ 200 mg/dL.[174]

Bile Acid Sequestrants: Resins (Questran, Welchol, Colestid)

Bile acid sequestrants—*cholestyramine (Questran), colesevelam (Welchol)*, and *colestipol (Colestid)*—bind to bile acids to promote the secretion of bile acids into the intestine, resulting in increased loss of hepatic cholesterol into bile acids and hepatic cellular cholesterol depletion. The latter leads to a compensatory increase in hepatic LDL receptors, increasing the removal of LDL from the circulation and decreasing total cholesterol and LDL-C. There may be a transitory compensatory rise in plasma triglycerides that is usually mild but may require cotherapy or discontinuation of the agent. Colesevelam has an additional FDA indication for glycemic control in the treatment of type 2 diabetes, as combination therapy with metformin, sulfonylureas, or insulin. The major outcome trial conducted with resins was the Lipid Research Clinics Coronary Primary Prevention Trial, in which cholestyramine modestly reduced CHD (primary endpoint: CHD death or nonfatal MI) in hypercholesterolemic patients and improved blood lipid profiles but had no effect on overall mortality.[175] *Drug interactions* include interference with the absorption of digoxin, warfarin, thyroxine, and thiazides, which need to be taken 1 hour before or 4 hours after the sequestrant. Impaired absorption of vitamin K may lead to bleeding and sensitization to warfarin. Poor palatability is the major problem. *Combination therapy* is often undertaken, and coadministration with a statin may exploit the complementary mechanisms of action of these two drug classes. Resins may increase triglycerides, so a second agent such as nicotinic acid or a fibrate may be required to lower triglycerides. Resins should be used with caution in patients with hypertriglyceridemia.

Nicotinic Acid (Niacin; Niaspan)

Nicotinic acid was the first hypolipidemic drug shown to reduce overall mortality, in 15-year follow-up from the Coronary Drug Project.[176] The basic effect of nicotinic acid may be decreased mobilization of free fatty acids from adipose tissue, so that there is less substrate for hepatic synthesis of lipoprotein lipid. Consequently, there is less secretion of lipoproteins so that LDL particles, including triglyceride-rich VLDL, are reduced. Nicotinic acid also increases HDL-C and reduces Lp(a).

In the angiographic Familial Atherosclerosis Treatment Study (FATS), men with apoB ≥ 125 mg/dL, CHD, and family history of CVD received either lovastatin (20 mg BID) or nicotinic acid (1 g QID), combined with colestipol (10 g TID). Both regimens were equally effective on blood lipids, and angiographically measured coronary stenosis was lessened, although side effects were worse, with nicotinic acid.[177]

The AIM-HIGH study, an outcomes study examining the effect of adding extended-release niacin to simvastatin in patients with cardiovascular disease, was stopped early because of lack of clinically meaningful efficacy.[34] Niacin failed to demonstrate incremental benefit in cardiovascular event reduction for patients already optimally treated with lipid-lowering therapy to a mean LDL-C of 71 mg/dL at baseline; in addition, an unexplained increase in ischemic stroke was observed in the niacin arm. After 36 months, the difference in HDL-C between treatment groups was only 4 mg/dL; the study may have been underpowered to show benefit of niacin on top of statin therapy.

Laropiprant was developed in an attempt to reduce the side effects of niacin that led to poor patient compliance but was discontinued. In the Heart Protection Study 2–Treatment of HDL to Reduce the Incidence of Vascular Events (HPS2-THRIVE),[178] a large multicenter, double-blind, controlled clinical trial, 25,673 patients with prior CVD, all on LDL-lowering therapy with simvastatin 40 mg, were randomized to receive either extended-release niacin–laropiprant combination tablets (a total of 2 g of niacin and 40 mg of laropiprant) daily or matching placebo. Over a median follow-up of 4 years, HDL-C levels increased by 6 mg/dL, triglycerides levels decreased by 33 mg/dL, and LDL-C levels decreased by 10 mg/dL in the niacin–laropiprant group. However, no significant difference in the incidence of major vascular events (nonfatal MI, stroke, coronary or noncoronary revascularization, or death from coronary causes) was demonstrated between patients assigned to niacin–laropiprant and those assigned to placebo (13.2% versus 13.6%, respectively, $P = 0.29$). Lack of efficacy was uniform in all subgroups defined according to different types of vascular disease or diabetes. Patients assigned to niacin–laropiprant were more likely to have disturbances in diabetes control (11.1% versus 7.5%; $P < 0.001$) and a new diagnosis of diabetes (5.7% versus 4.3%; $P < 0.001$) than those assigned to placebo. Study drug was discontinued in 25.4% of the niacin–laropiprant group compared with 16.6% of the placebo group ($P < 0.001$). Furthermore, the niacin–laropiprant group had a significant excess in serious adverse events associated with the gastrointestinal system (mostly bleeding and ulcerations; 4.8% versus 3.8%; $P < 0.001$), myopathy (3.7% versus 3.0%; $P < 0.001$), and skin rash/ulceration (0.7% versus 0.4%; $P = 0.003$), as well as excess bleeding events (mostly gastrointestinal and intracranial; 2.5% versus 1.9%; $P < 0.001$) and infections (8.0% versus 6.6%; $P < 0.001$).

Both AIM-HIGH[34] and HPS2-THRIVE[178] failed to show any incremental clinical benefit from niacin added to standard LDL-lowering therapy and raised doubts about the safety profile of niacin. With widespread acceptance of statin therapy and recent landmark trials supporting the safety and clinical benefit of ezetimibe and PCSK9 inhibitors, the role of niacin as lipid-modifying therapy has become very limited.

Dose, Side Effects, and Contraindications

The dosage required for lipid lowering is up to 4 g of immediate-release (crystalline) niacin daily, achieved gradually with a low starting dose (100 mg twice daily with meals to avoid gastrointestinal discomfort) that is increased until the lipid target is reached, or side effects occur. The extended-release formulation (Niaspan) is available in an initiation package that up-titrates the dose to reduce side effects. The recommended dose of extended-release niacin is 1–2 g once daily at bedtime. Because of the difference in dosing, care must be taken in switching patients between immediate-release and extended-release formulations.

Niacin has numerous *side effects*, which can be lessened by carefully building up the dose. Nicotinic acid causes prostaglandin-mediated symptoms such as flushing, dizziness, and palpitations. Flushing, which is very common, lessens with time and with use of the extended-release formulation; flushing is also reduced by taking niacin with food. *Caution* should be used in patients with peptic ulcer, diabetes, liver disease, or a history of gout. Impaired glucose tolerance and increased blood urate are reminiscent of thiazide side effects, also with an unknown basis. Hepatotoxicity may be linked to some *long-acting preparations* (sustained-release formulations), whereas flushing and pruritus are reduced. Myopathy is rare. Use in pregnant women is questionable.

Non–LDL-C Therapies in Development

Considerable residual cardiovascular persists despite well-controlled LDL-C levels, and epidemiological and genetic studies have established the role of other lipid parameters, most notably triglycerides,[179] triglyceride-rich lipoproteins (VLDL, chylomicrons, and remnants),[180] and Lp(a),[181] in residual cardiovascular risk, especially among patients on maximal statin therapy. Advances in gene-silencing technology through antisense oligonucleotide inhibition or siRNA provide novel approaches to target lipid parameters, by degrading mRNA transcripts of specific genes to reduce protein production and plasma lipoprotein levels. As discussed previously with inclisiran, the most recently developed agents have been modified to target the liver, allowing much lower doses to be used, for improved safety profiles compared with prior delivery approaches. Pharmacological use of monoclonal antibodies is also being examined for non–LDL-C targets.

Targeting Lp(a)

Therapies targeting Lp(a) currently in development include an siRNA to apo(a) called AMG 890 (formerly ARO-LPA; Amgen), which is currently completing phase I testing (NCT03626662[182]) and beginning phase II trials, and an antisense oligonucleotide targeted to apo(a) called TQJ230 (formerly AKCEA-APO(a)-L$_{Rx}$; Novartis). Results of a phase II clinical study of TQJ230 in 286 patients with established CVD and elevated levels of Lp(a) showed significant Lp(a) reductions that were dose dependent and without any serious adverse effects such as thrombocytopenia.[183] Novartis is conducting a phase III cardiovascular outcomes trial called Lp(a) HORIZON (NCT04023552[184]).

Targeting Triglycerides

To reduce triglycerides, gene silencing can be employed to target proteins that are involved in the production or clearance of triglyceride-rich lipoproteins, such as apoC-III (present on triglyceride-rich lipoproteins) and angiopoetin-related protein 3 (ANGPTL3, which inhibits lipoprotein lipase and catabolism of triglyceride-rich lipoproteins), thereby reducing circulating triglyceride levels. Antisense oligonucleotides and siRNAs that target each of these proteins are in development.

Volanesorsen (AKCEA-APOCIII$_{Rx}$) is a second-generation antisense oligonucleotide developed to reduce circulating apoC-III and triglyceride levels. In the phase III, double-blind, randomized, 52-week APPROACH Study trial conducted in 66 patients with familial chylomicronemia syndrome, volanesorsen reduced mean triglyceride level by 77%, compared with an 18% increase in triglyceride level with placebo; thrombocytopenia and injection-site reactions were significant adverse events.[185] Another phase III study of volanesorsen, the COMPASS Study conducted in patients with severe hypertriglyceridemia (triglycerides ≥500 mg/dL),[186] also included patients with familial chylomicronemia syndrome, and based on these studies, volanesorsen was approved for treatment of familial chylomicronemia syndrome in the European Union but not the United States. Volanesorsen is undergoing further phase III testing in the ongoing APPROACH Open-Label Study in patients with familial chylomicronemia syndrome[187] and the BROADEN Study in patients with familial partial lipodystrophy.[188]

AKCEA-APOCIII-L$_{Rx}$, a modified version of volanesorsen, is a second-generation ligand-conjugated antisense oligonucleotide that targets the liver; it is more potent and has a much better safety profile than volanesorsen. In a phase I/IIa study in 67 healthy volunteers, triglyceride levels were significantly reduced by up to 77%, with one injection-site reaction and no platelet count reductions.[189] Phase II results are expected in 2020,[190] and a phase III study is under way.

ARO-APOC3 is a hepatocyte-targeted siRNA to apoC-III. Results of a phase I/IIa trial showed that single doses in 40 healthy volunteers reduced serum apoC-III levels by 70%–91% and reduced serum triglycerides by 41%–55% at week 16.[191] A phase I trial that includes patients with hypertriglyceridemia and patients familial chylomicronemia syndrome is under way.[192]

ANGPTL3 is another promising protein target for triglyceride reduction. Evinacumab (REGN1500; Regeneron) is a human monoclonal antibody against ANGPTL3 that reduced fasting triglyceride levels by up to 70% and LDL-C levels by up to 23% in a phase I trial in healthy adults.[193] In a small phase II study in nine patients with homozygous familial hypercholesterolemia, evinacumab reduced LDL-C by 49% and triglycerides by 47%.[194] Another phase II clinical trial (NCT03175367), in 252 patients with heterozygous familial hypercholesterolemia or with hypercholesterolemia and ASCVD, is currently under way.[195]

AKCEA-ANGPTL3-L$_{Rx}$ (Pfizer), an antisense therapy against hepatic ANGPTL3, similarly reduced triglycerides by up to 63% and LDL-C by 33% without any serious adverse events in a phase I, randomized, double-blind, placebo-controlled trial in 44 healthy adults.[196] It is currently being evaluated in phase II studies in patients with familial chylomicronemia syndrome,[197] familial partial lipodystrophy,[198] or type 2 diabetes, hypertriglyceridemia, and nonalcoholic fatty liver disease.[199]

ARO-ANG3 is a hepatocyte-targeting siRNA against ANGPTL3 under development by Arrowhead. Phase I/IIa safety and efficacy data showed that a single dose in normal healthy volunteers led to dose-dependent reductions in ANGPTL3 levels of 43%–75%

and in triglyceride levels of 47%–53% by week 16, with no serious adverse events reported.[200]

Although the findings for these developing drugs are promising, evidence from large cardiovascular outcome studies and long-term safety trials is needed before these novel, targeted, gene-silencing technologies can be evaluated for use in clinical practice.

Summary

Primary Prevention

In primary prevention of CVD, global risk factor assessment and correction are the recommended approach. The atherogenic components of blood lipids, especially LDL-C, are an important part of an overall risk factor profile that includes factors that cannot be changed, such as age, sex, and family history of premature disease, and those that can, such as blood pressure, diet, smoking, exercise, and weight (see Table 6.1). The Pooled Cohort Equation should be used to guide treatment and identify individuals for whom aggressive lifestyle modification and statin therapy are indicated. For a heart-healthy diet, a Mediterranean or DASH diet is currently recommended. Risk-enhancing factors (see Table 6.1) can help identify individuals at increased risk who may benefit most from initiating or maximizing statin therapy. The ideal blood cholesterol and LDL-C levels appear to be falling lower and lower, based on clinical trial results.

Secondary Prevention

In secondary prevention, strict LDL-C lowering with high-intensity statin therapy, along with lifestyle modification, is an essential part of a comprehensive program of risk-factor modification. The 2018 AHA/ACC guidelines make strong recommendation to use a threshold of LDL-C ≥70 mg/dL in patients with established ASCVD for augmenting statin therapy with add-on ezetimibe or (in very-high-risk patients) PCSK9 inhibitor therapy. In individuals already on statin therapy who have residual hypertriglyceridemia, strong evidence supports add-on icosapent ethyl. Strict dietary modification and exercise (minimum of 150 minutes of moderate- or 75 minutes of high-intensity exercise per week) must be emphasized in all patients.

Diabetes

Diabetes is regarded as a risk category in its own right in the 2018 AHA/ACC cholesterol guidelines, as this high-risk group warrants aggressive risk reduction. Guidelines recommend initiation of moderate-intensity statin irrespective of LDL-C levels in patients with diabetes aged 40–75 years.

Statins as Initial Treatment

Statin trials have shown substantial reductions in total and cardiac mortality as well as major adverse cardiovascular events, and statins are recommended for four patient management groups (according to the 2018 AHA/ACC guidelines): 1) secondary prevention for patients with established ASCVD; 2) patients with severe hypercholesterolemia (LDL-C $\geq$190 mg/dL); 3) patients with diabetes; and 4) primary prevention. Statins have few serious side effects or contraindications. In primary prevention, the Pooled Cohort Equation can be used to stratify risk, with 10-year risk <5% considered low, 5 to <7.5% borderline, 7.5 to <20% intermediate, and $\geq$20% high. In intermediate- and high-risk groups, statin therapy is appropriate, with high-intensity statin preferred for the latter group (Class I recommendation). In the borderline-risk group, risk-enhancing factors (see Table 6.1) may be considered to guide risk discussion.

Combination Therapy

Combination therapy is now increasingly used to achieve reductions in LDL-C and non-HDL-C. The principle is to combine two different classes of agents with different mechanisms of action, such as a statin and ezetimibe or a statin and a PCSK9 inhibitor. Recent trials have shown overwhelming evidence of efficacious LDL lowering as well as reduction of adverse cardiovascular events with these combined agents. The consensus is that judicious use of combination therapy, when required, is likely to confer more benefit than harm.

Other lipid-regulating agents, which are used less frequently because they lack clinical trial evidence of incremental clinical benefit and increase risk for adverse events, include fibrates, bile acid sequestrants, and niacin. The combination of fibrates and statin increases risk of myopathy and hepatotoxity. Niacin is usually not well tolerated because of multiple side effects including flushing, pruritus, skin rashes, and gastrointestinal issues. Bile acid sequestrants require caution in patients with high triglycerides.

Hypertriglyceridemia

Intensive diet and lifestyle modification remains the cornerstone of therapy for elevated triglycerides, especially in patients with moderate hypertriglyceridemia (triglycerides 150–499 mg/dL

[1.7–2.3 mmol/L]). Secondary causes of elevated triglycerides, including obesity, metabolic syndrome, chronic kidney or liver disease, nephrotic syndrome, diabetes, or hypothyroidism, must be evaluated and addressed. Triglyceride levels of more than 1000 mg/dL (11.3 mmol/L) confer increased risk for pancreatitis and require treatment with prescription-strength omega-3 fatty acids or a fibrate (see Fig. 6.4).

References

Complete reference list available at www.expertconsult.com.

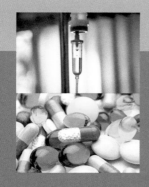

中文导读

第7章
抗炎药物

炎症反应在一定意义上涵盖了机体的一系列防御与修复机制。炎症反应在机体与微生物、病毒的对抗及组织稳态调节中发挥重要作用，因此炎症通路对于个体和种族的生存具有重要意义。鉴于炎症反应在宿主对外防御和维持组织稳态中的关键作用，炎症干预措施需要十分精细，以免产生超过潜在获益的不良后果，导致弊大于利。虽然抗炎策略早已在关节及气道相关疾病中得到应用，但其在心血管系统疾病中的前景才初见端倪。

本章详细阐述了炎症生物学的基本概念、调节慢性炎症性疾病的潜在治疗靶点、缺血性心血管疾病中白细胞连接局部和系统性炎症反应的机制、与移植相关的动脉粥样硬化发病过程的多种机制、心脏移植的免疫抑制治疗等。同时，克隆性造血近期被认为是动脉粥样硬化性血栓及心力衰竭事件的危险因素。读者还可以进一步探索炎症信号转导的中心枢纽，了解各种介质及信号通路在其中的关键作用，如白细胞介素-6在心脏代谢通路中的枢纽作用等。

炎症生物学的基础和丰富的实验数据，使得炎症及免疫反应成为心血管疾病的潜在治疗靶点。凭借坚实的科学研究基础及丰富多样的潜在治疗靶点，也许在不远的将来，随着治疗手段的进一步发展，心血管系统疾病中的抗感染治疗的应用前景会更加光明。

陈安天

Drugs Targeting Inflammation

PETER LIBBY · AHMED A.K. HASAN* · ANJU NOHRIA

Inflammatory responses encompass a series of host defense and repair mechanisms.[1] Inflammatory processes fight off microbial and viral invaders. They aid the repair of injured tissues. Thus, the operation of inflammatory pathways proves essential to survival of the individual and of the species. Yet, these very processes that can protect from infection or injury, when unleashed inappropriately, or if the inflammatory response fails to resolve, can cause disease. The aging of the population favors the development of chronic diseases. The control of communicable diseases by sanitation, vaccination, antibiotic treatment, and other societal measures permits more individuals to survive to the point of developing chronic diseases of many organ systems. Inflammatory pathways contribute to many of the chronic conditions that currently challenge successful aging. Inflammation contributes to the pathogenesis of diseases as diverse as forms of dementia, the arthritides, chronic lung and kidney diseases, and of course cardiovascular conditions. Thus, understanding and combatting inflammation holds a key for the prevention and treatment of many chronic conditions associated with aging. Moreover, recognition has increased that oncogenesis, and the growth, invasion, and metastasis of many cancers hijack inflammatory pathways.[2]

Given the critical role of inflammation in host defenses and tissue homeostasis, interventions that modulate inflammatory processes require careful targeting and modulation, lest adverse consequences outweigh potential benefits. While antiinflammatory strategies have long contributed to the management of forms of arthritis and airways disease, the advent of strategies that modulate inflammation have just begun to show promise in cardiovascular conditions. Given the delicate balance required to intervene

---

*Dr. Hasan works for the NHLBI/NIH, but any opinions, findings, and conclusions expressed in this review are those of the author and do not reflect the views of the NHLBI or the NIH.

successfully to modulate therapeutically inflammation, a background in the basics of inflammation biology provides a framework for this undertaking.

Basic Concepts of Inflammation Biology

Inflammatory pathways encompass two major sets of responses that have evolved in an interdependent manner (Fig. 7.1). The innate immune response arose early in evolution. Marine invertebrates such as the starfish and limulus crab have innate immune responses. The innate pathways mobilize rapidly. Their triggers include products of infectious agents known as pathogen-associated molecular patterns (PAMPs). Damaged or dead cells can release triggers for innate immunity known as damage-associated molecular patterns (DAMPs). These signals interact with a series of pattern recognition receptors, prominently the class known as Toll-like receptors (TLRs). These receptors recognize hundreds or just a few thousand different DAMPs or PAMPs. Thus, although innate immune responses mobilize rapidly, they are relatively blunt, as they recognize a fairly restricted set of patterns.

In contrast, the adaptive immune response arose much later in evolution. Most arms of adaptive immunity require "education." Specific structures can serve as antigens for instigating cellular or humoral immune responses. Defined structural features of proteins, carbohydrates, and some lipids can engender adaptive immune responses. Rather than hundreds or thousands of structures as triggers, adaptive immunity can recognize millions or even billions of structures. The "education" of the adaptive immune response helps to limit recognition of self structures, to minimize autoimmune responses. Also, the affinity of antibodies and specificity of cellular responses to antigens can increase with time. Thus, in contrast to the innate immune response, adaptive immunity shows exquisite specificity and considerable power, given the fine-tuning of adaptive immune responses over time after encountering an initial antigenic stimulus.[3]

While the mononuclear phagocyte exemplifies the main cellular mediator of innate immunity, lymphocytes give rise to the adaptive immune response. T lymphocytes comprise the afferent limb of cellular immunity. Several important subclasses of T lymphocytes subserve specific functions. T helper 1 (Th1) cells, characterized by secretion of a signature cytokine immune interferon or interferon-gamma (IFN-γ), promote adaptive immune responses. Th2 lymphocytes tend to mediate allergic responses. Th2 cells secret interleukin (IL) -4 and -10 as signature cytokines. Regulatory T cells (T_{reg}) secrete transforming growth factor-beta (TGF-β) and

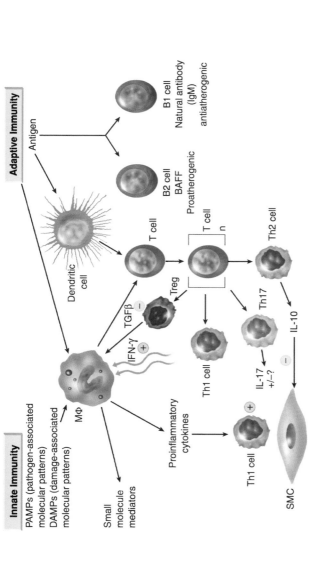

Fig. 7.1 Innate and adaptive immunity in atherosclerosis. A diagram of the pathways of innate (*left*) and adaptive (*right*) immunity operating during atherogenesis. *BAFF*, B cell–activating factor; *IFN*, interferon; *IL*, interleukin; *MΦ*, macrophage; *SMC*, smooth muscle cell; *TGF*, transforming growth factor; *Th*, T helper; *Treg*, regulatory T cell. (From Libby P. The vascular biology of atherosclerosis. In: Zipes DP, Libby P, Bonow RO, Mann DL, Tomaselli GF, eds. *Braunwald's Heart Disease*, 11th ed. Philadelphia: Elsevier; 2018: 859–875; after Hansson G, Libby P, Schoenbeck U, Yan ZQ: Innate and adaptive immunity in the pathogenesis of atherosclerosis. *Circ Res* 2002;91:281.)

can calm immune responses and promote tissue repair through fibrosis. B lymphocytes mediate humoral immunity and give rise to plasma cells that produce large quantities of antibody. In an exception to the rule that adaptive immune responses require "education," B1 lymphocytes secrete "natural" antibodies, some of which can mitigate experimental atherosclerosis. B2 lymphocytes tend to aggravate adaptive immune responses.

Although innate immunity evolved before the adaptive response, adaptive immune factors regulate innate immunity. Innate immune cells such as the dendritic cell (a relative of the mononuclear phagocytes) serve to present antigens to the T cell, initiating the adaptive immune response. IFN-γ elaborated by Th1 cells can activate macrophages strongly. Cytokines derived from Th2 cells such as IL-10 can dampen innate immune responses mediated by macrophages. These examples provide an illustration of the complex crosstalk underway in any moment in complex organisms (Fig. 7.1). The inflammatory status of an individual can vary immensely and depends on an intricate balance of proinflammatory, antiinflammatory, and proresolving pathways.

In acute bacterial infections the rapidly mobilized innate immune system responds rapidly, causing fever and a series of host defense mechanisms that help to fight off the invaders including mobilization of polymorphonuclear leukocytes. The extreme example of an acute inflammatory response, Gram-negative bacterial sepsis, familiar to all clinicians, illustrates the rapidity and devastating nature of an undampened acute inflammatory response. Fulminant myocarditis illustrates another acute inflammatory response that affects the cardiovascular system.

On the other end of the spectrum, the chronic conditions that plague the cardiovascular system often involve much more muted inflammatory responses that play out over months and years rather than hours and days as in the case of acute inflammation. An example of a chronic immune response mediated by macrophages, tuberculosis, illustrates the long-term and indolent nature of the chronic immune response. The intersection of innate and adaptive immune responses that give rise to chronic diseases of many organ systems, including atherosclerosis, exemplifies the ravages of a chronic immune response in the cardiovascular system.

Stimuli for the Inflammatory Response

A number of stimuli can initiate inflammatory responses in the context of cardiovascular disease (Fig. 7.2). Atherosclerosis represents the best-studied chronic inflammatory condition of the

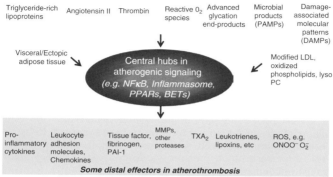

Fig. 7.2 Diagram summarizing some of the potential therapeutic targets for modifying chronic inflammatory diseases. These overlapping categories fall into three major categories: proximal triggers *(top)*, central hubs *(middle)*, and distal effectors *(bottom)*. *BETs,* Bromodomain and extraterminal domain proteins; *LDL, low-density lipoprotein; MMP,* matrix metalloproteinase; *NF-κ B,* nuclear factor κ B; *PAI-1,* plasminogen activator inhibitor-1; *PPARs,* peroxisome proliferation activation receptors; *ROS,* reactive oxygen species; TXA_2, thromboxane A_2. (Adapted from Libby P. How our growing understanding of inflammation has reshaped the way we think of disease and drug development. *Clin Pharm Ther* 2010;87:389–391.)

cardiovascular system. Although low-density lipoprotein (LDL) doubtless plays a pivotal permissive role in atherosclerosis, it does not appear to exert most of its proatherogenic actions primarily by instigating inflammation.[4-6] While macrophages of the innate immune system accumulate lipid and become foam cells when exposed to excessive concentrations of atherogenic lipoproteins, unmodified LDL itself does not lead to lipid overload. The LDL receptor responds exquisitely to intercellular cholesterol concentrations. Hence, loading cells with cholesterol requires uptake of cholesterol-containing lipoproteins via receptors besides the classical LDL receptor. Such scavenger receptors tend to recognize modified LDL particles that have undergone oxidation or glycation. Foam cell formation may thus depend less on native LDL than on cholesterol derived from other atherogenic lipoproteins.

Although initial evidence pointed to oxidized LDL as a possible antigen triggering the adaptive immune response in the context of atherosclerosis, more recent data suggest that the T cells recognize native LDL more readily than modified LDL.[7,8] Finally, an intervention that lowers LDL by augmenting activity of the LDL receptor, inhibitors of proprotein convertase subtilisin/kexin type 9 (PCSK9), can mitigate atherosclerotic events without decreasing biomarkers of inflammation. This observation underscores the contention that LDL itself has modest proinflammatory properties at best.

Hypertension and mediators of high blood pressure can involve both adaptive and innate immunity. High concentrations of angiotensin II, a prototypical vasoconstrictor hormone implicated in the pathogenesis of many forms of hypertension, can elicit the production of the proinflammatory cytokine IL-6 from various cell types involved in atherosclerosis, including smooth muscle cells.[9,10] Considerable experimental evidence supports the involvement of adaptive immunity in hypertension.[11] Yet, antiinflammatory drugs tend not to improve blood pressure in hypertensive individuals. Indeed, nonsteroidal antiinflammatory agents tend to increase blood pressure modestly. These findings argue against inflammation as a major contributor to chronic forms of hypertension.

Many have invoked oxidative stress, and oxidatively modified lipoproteins in particular as instigators of both innate and adaptive immune responses in the context of atherosclerosis. Yet, all antioxidant vitamins tested, and a number of inhibitors of oxidative pathways including the production of oxidized LDL, have failed to reduce cardiovascular events in rigorously conducted clinical trials. Once again, despite considerable preclinical evidence and the results of observational studies, oxidative stress and lipoprotein oxidation have not shown promise as therapeutic targets. These observations demote the clinical relevance of oxidative pathways as instigators of immune and inflammatory responses.

A large body of experimental and observational epidemiologic literature support associations between various infectious agents and atherosclerosis.[12-14] While viral myocarditis indubitably represents an example of an inflammatory trigger for cardiovascular disease, targeting infectious agents has not proven actionable in general in atherosclerosis. While bacteria and viruses can stimulate both innate and adaptive immunity, and microbial products can serve as PAMPs, rigorously conducted and appropriately sized antibiotic intervention studies have failed to show reduced cardiovascular events.[15,16] These studies have used several classes of antibiotic agents that target microorganisms implicated by experimental and seroepidemiologic studies in atherosclerosis, e.g., Chlamydia pneumoniae. The types of agent used in the larger randomized clinical trials include macrolides (e.g., azithromycin) and fluoroquinolones (e.g., gatifloxacin). While various viruses, notably Herpesviridae, can inhabit many human tissues including atheromata, rigorous evidence implicating viral agents as triggers to innate and adaptive immunity in usual forms of human atherosclerosis has not emerged. Experimentally, a herpes virus can cause an atherosclerotic-like disease in avian species (Marek disease),[17] and cytomegalovirus can also enhance arterial disease in rodents.[18]

Considerable recent interest has highlighted the potential of the microbiome as a contributor to cardiovascular disease.[19] The clinical extrapolation of intriguing experimental results showing the ability of intestinal microbiota to produce metabolites that putatively potentiate atherosclerosis, such as trimethylamine N-oxide (TMAO), to humans still requires reinforcement.

Tissue damage can instigate innate immune responses through the production of DAMPs (Fig. 7.1). Experimental evidence substantiates the possibility that DAMPs elaborated from the infarcted myocardium can augment innate immune responses. For example, dying cardiac myocytes can release DNA that can initiate an inflammatory response through a pathway mediated by interferon regulatory factor 3 (IRF3).[20] Myocardial infarction can mobilize systemic inflammatory responses that can augment remote inflammatory responses, including in preexisting atherosclerotic lesions.[21] These pathways involve mobilization of macrophages and their activation in response to tissue injury (Fig. 7.3). These examples show how ischemic damage to myocardium produced by preexisting atherosclerotic plaques can elicit and amplify immune responses. Yet, these pathways likely participate in the potentiation of inflammatory responses to preexisting disease, rather than proving pathogenic in initiation of primary atherosclerotic plaques.

A good deal of recent work has firmly established that adipose tissue can contribute to inflammatory states. In particular, ectopic fat deposition around the viscera, associated with the android fat distribution (male or "apple" pattern), associates with markers of innate immune activation such as C-reactive protein (CRP).[22,23] Such ectopic depots of adipose tissue team with inflammatory cells including macrophages and T lymphocytes. Ectopic adipose tissue elaborates proinflammatory mediators such as tumor necrosis factor that can mediate insulin resistance. Perivascular adipose tissue may participate in local "outside in" inflammatory signaling that can potentiate vascular disease.[23] Thus, weight loss either pharmacologic or through bariatric surgery might mitigate inflammation in cardiovascular diseases. The use of pharmacologic agents in this regard has proved quite challenging due to adverse or off-target effects. For example, certain classes of weight loss drugs can produce pulmonary hypertension or valvular heart disease. The thiazolidinediones that activate peroxisome proliferation activation receptor gamma (PPAR-γ) may cause a redistribution of adipose tissue away from the visceral depot, but also can cause fluid retention and exacerbate heart failure. These limitations have frustrated pharmacologic management of adiposity and as antiinflammatory strategies in cardiovascular disease.

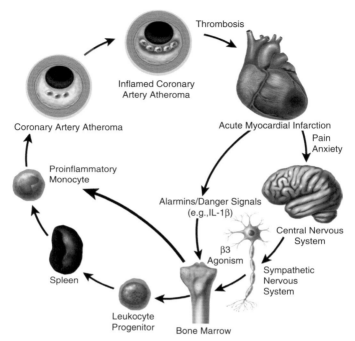

Fig. 7.3 Leukocytes link local and systemic inflammation in ischemic cardiovascular disease. The stress of acute myocardial infarction produces an "echo" in atherosclerotic plaques. Acute myocardial infarction causes pain and anxiety that triggers sympathetic outflow from the central nervous system. β_3 adrenergic stimulation mobilizes leukocyte progenitors from their bone marrow niche. These progenitor cells can migrate to the spleen, where they can multiply in response to hematopoietic growth factors. The proinflammatory monocytes then leave the spleen and enter the atherosclerotic plaque, where they promote inflammation that can render a plaque more likely to provoke thrombosis and hence acute myocardial infarction. *IL*, Interleukin. (From Libby P, Nahrendorf M, Swirski FK. Leukocytes link local and systemic inflammation in ischemic cardiovascular disease. *J Am Coll Cardiol* 2016;67:1091–1103.)

Exposure to foreign tissues, such as transplanted organs, can also lead to activation of the immune response (Fig. 7.4). Such adaptive immune reactions to foreign tissues known as the allogeneic immune response, clearly contribute to rejection of solid organ transplants. This is one arena where therapies that mitigate immune and inflammatory responses have proven of daily applicability in the practice of cardiovascular medicine. Allograft

Cytolytic injury by CD8+ T cells

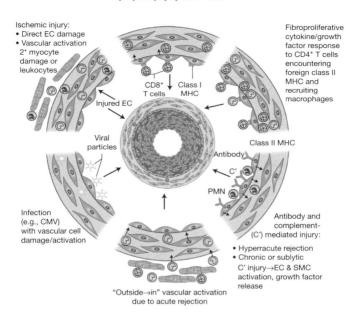

Fig. 7.4 Multiple mechanisms in the pathogenesis of transplantation-associated arteriosclerosis. Each of the depicted immune and nonimmune mechanisms may pertain to variable extents in individual patients. In addition to these mechanisms, the risk factors for usual atherogenesis (dyslipidemia, smoking, diabetes, hypertension, etc.) doubtless also apply when present. Also, superimposition of graft vascular disease on preexisting donor atherosclerosis can occur. *CMV,* cytomegalovirus; *EC,* endothelial cell; *MHC,* major histocompatibility complex; *PMN,* polymorphonuclear leukocytes; *SMC,* smooth muscle cells. (Adapted from Libby P. Transplantation-associated arteriosclerosis: potential mechanisms. In: Tilney N, Strom T, eds. *Transplantation Biology.* Philadelphia, PA: Lippincott-Raven Publishers; 1996: 577–586.)

rejection can be hyperacute, acute, or chronic. Preformed antibodies against donor determinants mediate hyperacute rejection, a process that occurs within minutes to hours after transplantation. This form of allograft rejection has become relatively rare due to the practice of prospective cross-matching in sensitized recipients. Acute rejection can be cellular or humoral. In acute cellular rejection, T cells directed against the donor myocardium trigger an inflammatory response that leads to myocyte necrosis and graft failure. Antibodies directed against the graft vasculature mediate acute humoral rejection.

This type of rejection can lead to local complement activation, vessel damage, and graft failure. Allograft vasculopathy also called "chronic rejection" results from immune and nonimmune responses against the graft vasculature and leads to diffuse and concentric narrowing of donor coronary arteries including smaller intramyocardial branches (Fig. 7.3). We prefer the term allograft vasculopathy to chronic rejection, as the major immunological mechanisms differ substantially. CD8+ T-cell–mediated myocardiocytolysis characterizes acute cellular parenchymal rejection. In contrast, CD4+ T cells likely dominate in the pathogenesis of proliferative lesions in the arterial intima of graft vasculopathy. Acute cellular and humoral rejection contribute to early transplant death, while allograft vasculopathy typically causes later transplant mortality.[24]

Transplant immunosuppression can be divided into induction and maintenance therapies (Table 7.1). Induction therapies, including antithymocyte globulin or basiliximab, may be given for a limited duration, shortly after transplant, to allow earlier reduction of steroid dosage or to delay introduction of calcineurin inhibitors (CNIs) in patients at risk for nephrotoxicity. Antithymocyte globulin or basiliximab may reduce the risk of acute rejection without substantially altering posttransplant survival or complications.[25] Maintenance immunosuppression consists of lifelong therapy with some combination of corticosteroids, CNIs (cyclosporine or tacrolimus), and antimetabolites (azathioprine or mycophenolate mofetil). Mammalian target of rapamycin (mTOR) inhibitors (everolimus and sirolimus) can be used in combination with low-dose CNI, or after withdrawal of CNI, to reduce progression of allograft vasculopathy or CNI-induced nephrotoxicity.[26] While these potent inhibitors of adaptive immune responses have greatly attenuated acute allograft rejection, they have not allayed the chronic inflammatory response that begets the allograft vascular disease that remains a major challenge to the longevity of transplanted hearts.

For reasons that remain unclear, self-antigens can occasionally trigger the immune response leading to myocarditis. Cardiac infiltration by inflammatory cells resulting in myocardial necrosis characterizes the myocardidites. Myocarditis can have many etiologies including viral (Coksackievirus B, parvovirus, and adenovirus being among the most common), pharmacologic (e.g. anthracyclines), hematologic (e.g. eosinophilic myocarditis), and autoimmune (e.g., giant cell myocarditis).[28]

Knowledge regarding the immunobiology of myocarditis emerged from two types of animal experiments: (1) viral myocarditis caused by infection of mice with Coxsackievirus B3 and (2) experimental autoimmune myocarditis caused by immunization of mice with cardiac myosin or a myocarditogenic peptide derived from cardiac α-myosin heavy chain, or forced expression

Table 7.1

Immunosuppressive therapy in cardiac transplantation

Drug	Mechanism of action	Indications	Potential side effects
Antithymocyte globulin (rabbit or horse)	Polyclonal antibodies that deplete T cells, modulate adhesion and cell-signaling molecules, interfere with dendritic cell function, induce B-cell apoptosis and regulatory and natural killer T-cell expansion	1) Prophylaxis of acute rejection 2) Treatment of severe acute cellular rejection	Neutropenia, thrombocytopenia, anaphylaxis, severe cytokine release syndrome, hyperkalemia, infection
Basiliximab	Anti-IL-2 receptor monoclonal antibody that prevents IL-2 mediated T-cell proliferation	Prophylaxis of acute rejection	Anaphylaxis
Corticosteroids	Inhibit crucial transcriptional regulators of inflammatory genes, including NF-κB and AP-1.	1) Prophylaxis of acute rejection 2) Treatment of acute cellular rejection	Volume retention, hypertension, hyperglycemia, obesity, mood and behavioral changes, infection, osteopenia, avascular necrosis, gastritis/perforation, myopathy, cataracts
Calcineurin Inhibitors (cyclosporine and tacrolimus)	Inhibit calcineurin leading to reduced IL-2 production and decreased T-cell proliferation	Prophylaxis of acute rejection	*Cyclosporine:* Renal dysfunction, hypertension, tremor, hirsutism, gingival hyperplasia, infection. *Tacrolimus:* Renal dysfunction, hypertension, tremor, hyperlipidemia, diabetes, infection

Continued on following page

Table 7.1

Immunosuppressive therapy in cardiac transplantation (Continued)

Drug	Mechanism of action	Indications	Potential side effects
Anti-metabolites (azathioprine, mycophenolate mofetil)	Inhibit de novo purine synthesis and thus limit T- and B-cell proliferation	Prophylaxis of acute rejection	*Azathioprine:* Leukopenia, infection, malignancy, teratogenic *Mycophenolate mofetil:* Neutropenia, pure red cell aplasia, infection, malignancy, teratogenic, progressive multifocal leukoencephalopathy
mTOR inhibitors (everolimus, sirolimus)	Inhibit mTOR, a key regulatory protein required for cytokine driven T-cell proliferation. Also inhibits antibody production.	Prophylaxis of acute rejection	Stomatitis, hypertriglyceridemia, proteinuria, renal dysfunction, diarrhea, rash, infection, noninfectious pneumonitis

AP-1, Activating protein-1; *IL-2,* interleukin-2; *NF-κB,* nuclear factor kappa-light-chain-enhancer of activated B cells. See [24] and [27] for further detail.

of ovalbumin in the myocardium in mice with ovalbumin responsive T cells.[28]

In viral myocarditis, myocardial injury results from a direct viral cytopathic effect as well as activation of the host cellular immune response. During acute infection, NK cells infiltrate the myocardium and play a critical role in the early host response by preventing viral replication. A second wave of infiltrating leukocytes, composed primarily of CD3+ T cells that colocalize with CD68+ macrophages, peaks 7–14 days after viral infection. They destroy infected myocytes to promote viral clearance, and the ensuing damage exposes cryptogenic intracellular antigens, such as myosin-derived peptides, that generate an autoimmune cardiac-specific response leading to chronic inflammation, fibrosis and progression to dilated cardiomyopathy.[29] Similarly in other forms of autoimmune myocarditis, unknown triggers, combined with specific host factors, activate the innate immune response leading to myocyte damage and exposure of cryptic antigens that are recognized by autoimmune T-cell clones leading to sustained activation of the adaptive immune response and progressive myocardial damage.[28]

The therapeutic approach to myocarditis has relied on immunosuppressive therapy as a way to target proinflammatory mediators of disease. The Myocarditis Treatment Trial failed to show a benefit of corticosteroids, in combination with cyclosporine or azathioprine, in patients with histologically proven lymphocytic myocarditis and left ventricular dysfunction compared to placebo.[30] The failure of immunosuppressive therapy in this study may have resulted from suppression of the beneficial effects of the innate immune response on viral replication.[29] Another study evaluated the effects of corticosteroids with azathioprine in patients with histologically proven myocarditis and chronic heart failure with no evidence of myocardial viral genomes. In this study, immunosuppression resulted in a significant improvement in left ventricular function and volumes compared to placebo.[31] Clinically, treatment of myocarditis does not routinely use immunosuppression, save for patients with giant cell myocarditis where registry data indicate that the use of immunosuppression improved mean survival from 3 to 12.3 months.[32] However, only 11% of patients survived without transplantation. Recently, the rising use of immune checkpoint inhibitors for the treatment of solid tumors has also given rise to T-cell–mediated myocarditis in < 1% of patients.[33] Despite treatment with high-dose immunosuppressive therapy, almost half of these patients suffer major adverse cardiovascular events including cardiovascular death, cardiogenic shock, cardiac arrest, and hemodynamically significant complete heart block.[34]

Another arm of innate immunity, the complement system, also participates in certain vasculitides. A large body of experimental work has implicated complement activation in ischemia-reperfusion injury. Yet, anticomplement strategies have not proven productive in the clinical management of either vasculitis or reperfusion injury in humans.[35]

A novel aspect of inflammation has emerged from studies of clonal hematopoiesis (Fig. 7.5).[36,37] With age, humans often host clones of myeloid cells, classical participants in innate immunity,

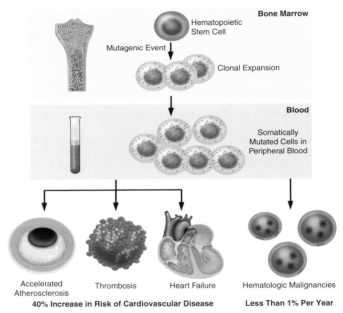

Fig. 7.5 Clonal hematopoiesis: a common, powerful, and recently recognized risk factor for atherothrombotic and heart failure events. Acquired mutations in bone marrow stem cells can give rise to a clone of circulating mutant leukocytes *(top panel)* in peripheral blood *(middle panel)*. Individuals who harbor these clones with somatic mutations in blood have a heightened risk of atherothrombotic and heart failure events *(lower panel, left)*. People with clonal hematopoiesis of indeterminate potential (CHIP) develop hematologic malignancy at a rate of 0.5%–1% per annum *(lower panel, right)*. CHIP portends a greater risk for cardiovascular events than for cancer. (From Libby P, Sidlow R, Lin AE, et al. Clonal hematopoiesis of indeterminate potential (CHIP) at the crossroads of aging, cardiovascular diseases and cancer. *J Am Coll Cardiol* 2019;74 (4):567–577.)

that bear mutations in genes implicated in driving acute leukemia. Over 10% of individuals over 70 will harbor such clones of mutant leukocytes. The development of acute leukemia generally requires successive accumulation in the same clone of two or three mutations in leukemia driver genes. Thus, most individuals with clonal hematopoiesis will never develop leukemia. Yet, these individuals have a striking enrichment in cardiovascular risk. This condition is called clonal hematopoiesis of indeterminate potential (CHIP). As in the case of monoclonal gammopathy of unknown significance (MGUS), most individuals with CHIP will never develop a hematologic malignancy.

Only a small subset of the forty-odd well-characterized driving mutations for leukemia cause CHIP and associate with enhanced cardiovascular risk.[37,38] The most common mutations that cause CHIP associate with enhanced inflammation in mice engineered to bear CHIP mutations.[37,39] Hence, CHIP represents a potent and common but only very recently recognized cardiovascular risk factor, totally independent of classical risk factors. As pharmacologic interventions exist that can target the pathways activated by CHIP mutations, management of CHIP may prove susceptible to antiinflammatory therapies in the future.

Central Hubs of Inflammatory Signaling (see Fig. 7.2)

Many of the triggers to innate immune responses delineated above activate central hubs of inflammatory signaling that represent potential therapeutic targets. A transcription factor known as nuclear factor kappa B (NF-κB), first recognized in B lymphocytes, orchestrates the expression of many proinflammatory cytokines and other inflammatory mediators.[40] Proinflammatory cytokines themselves activate this transcriptional control system providing an amplification mechanism. PAMPs and DAMPs through TLRs can also activate NF-κB. The details of NF-κB activation and signaling have undergone extensive analysis identifying numerous potential therapeutic targets. Inhibitors of the proteasome can augment concentrations of the inhibitor of NF-κB (IκB.) While experimental studies have shown efficacy of targeting NF-κB activation in muting experimental inflammation, drugs of practical utility in the treatment of cardiovascular disease have not emerged from this well-understood pathway. Indeed, as NF-κB activation may protect cells from apoptosis, survival of malignantly transformed cells might increase under circumstances of NF-κB inactivation, causing the unwanted effect of augmenting tumor growth.

Another intracellular multi-molecular structure, the inflammasome, consists of subunits that can sense various kinds of danger signals including certain PAMPs and DAMPs, especially crystalline structures such as silica, monosodium urate, or cholesterol monohydrate.[41] The danger-sensing moieties of inflammasomes ultimately activate an enzyme, caspase 1, that can process the inactive precursors of the proinflammatory cytokines IL-1β and IL-18 to their biologically active forms (Fig. 7.6). While various types of

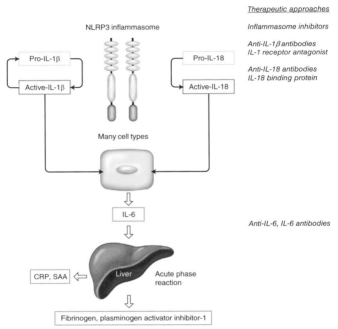

Fig. 7.6 The inflammasome interleukin (IL) IL-18, IL-1β, IL-6 pathway. The nod-like receptor family pyrin domain containing 3 *(NLRP3)* inflammasome, an intracellular supramolecuar structure senses various danger signals that ultimately activate the IL-1β convertase caspase-1. This converting enzyme processes the inactive precursors of the proinflammatory cytokines IL-1β and IL-18 to their biologically active mature forms. IL-1 can induce its own gene expression, an auto-induction amplification loop. IL-18 or IL-1β can induce the production of copious IL-6 from various cell types, thus amplifying pro-inflammatory signaling. IL-6 signals hepatocytes to boost synthesis of the acute phase reactants C-reactive protein, fibrinogen, and plasminogen activator inhibitor-1. Adapted from Ridker et al. *Eur Heart* J 41(23):2153–2163.

inflammasomes act as hubs of inflammatory signaling, the nod-like receptor family pyrin domain containing 3 (NLRP3) inflammasome has received particular attention because of its role in generating the primordial proinflammatory cytokine, IL-1β. Thus, targeting the inflammasome has given rise to new potential antiinflammatory strategies in development currently.

Another central hub in inflammatory signaling of relevance to cardiovascular disease, the Krüppel-like factors (KLFs) operate as transcription factors.[42] Activation of KLF2 by laminar shear stress transcriptionally regulates a cassette of genes implicated in protection against atherosclerosis and blood clot formation and stability.[43,44] Of direct relevance to cardiovascular pharmacology, the HMG-CoA reductase inhibitors, statins, also induce this transcription factor.[42] Thus, unlike the PCSK9 inhibitors, statins both lower LDL and can exert an independent antiinflammatory effect through the mediation of KLFs. Statins can also inhibit the prenylation of small G proteins involved in intracellular signaling. Thus, statins can have "pleiotropic" antiinflammatory effects that do not depend on LDL lowering through at least two sets of molecular mechanisms. This dual action of the statins, LDL lowering and an antiinflammatory action, may account for the marked success of this class of agents in forestalling cardiovascular disease both in primary and secondary prevention.

Epigenetic regulation can influence the transcription of genes involved in cardiovascular disease pathogenesis, including those implicated in inflammation.[45] Modifications of histones, proteins around which strands of DNA coil in nucleosomes, or of DNA itself mediate epigenetic control of gene transcription. Methylation and acetylation comprise the moieties that signal such epigenetic regulation. Various enzymes participate in the "writing" and "erasing" of these covalent modifications of chromatin components. "Readers" of these epigenetic modifications and provide links to components of transcriptional complexes that regulate the expression of genes.

In particular, one family of epigenetic "readers" has become a target of pharmacologic agents under evaluation as cardiovascular therapeutics that target in part inflammatory pathways. Bromodomain and extraterminal domain (BET) proteins bind to acetylated lysine residues in histones and promote the assembly of transcriptional complexes that enhance the expression of numerous genes involved in cardiovascular inflammation.[46] A recent clinical trial has evaluated the ability of an inhibitor of BET proteins to improve outcomes in diabetic patients with coronary artery disease.[47] This study did not show a significant reduction in major adverse cardiac events in diabetic individuals post acute coronary syndrome.

Mediators

The central hubs of inflammatory signaling delineated above influence the expression of a variety of mediators of inflammation in immunity implicated in cardiovascular disease (Fig. 7.2). A key event in most inflammatory processes and immune responses is the recruitment of leukocytes. A variety of endothelial surface molecules that mediate adhesive interactions with various classes of leukocytes participate in the recruitment of the inflammatory cells (Fig. 7.7). Molecules that bear homology to lectins known as the selectins cause leukocytes to associate with the surface of activated endothelial cells that express these adhesion molecules. Selectins cause a rolling interaction of the leukocytes. Members of the immunoglobulin superfamily such as intercellular adhesion molecule-1 (ICAM-1) or vascular cell adhesion molecule-1 (VCAM-1) mediate firmer and less transitory adhesion of leukocytes to the endothelial surface. The expression of leukocyte adhesion molecules can regulate the type of leukocyte recruited to a site of inflammation or immune response. For example, E-selectin interacts particularly with polymorphonuclear leukocytes implicated in acute inflammatory responses. VCAM-1 interacts with monocytes, the precursor of many tissue macrophages, and T lymphocytes that participate in more chronic adaptive immune responses in tissues.

Once bound to the endothelium, leukocytes receive signals that direct their migration to within tissues. Protein mediators of this directed migration or chemoattraction include a series of protein mediators known as chemokines.[48] Small molecules including certain lipid mediators may also promote the migration of leukocytes within tissues. Subsets of the numerous chemokine families can govern the type of leukocyte recruited. The chemokines provide a kind of "zip code" for signaling accumulation of acute versus chronic cellular mediators of inflammation and immunity.

Despite the molecular characterization of leukocyte adhesion molecules and chemoattractant cytokines and an abundance of in vitro and experimental animal data that demonstrates their function, inhibitors of these adhesive pathways have not borne fruit in terms of clinical application.[48] Leukocyte adhesion inhibitors have failed to improve ischemia reperfusion injury despite numerous preclinical studies suggesting efficacy. An inhibitor of the adhesion molecule P-selectin also failed to improve cardiovascular outcomes. Given the complexity and promise of potential specificity of interference in leukocyte accumulation pathways, targeting these mediators may yet prove beneficial in some circumstances.

Constituents of oxidized lipoproteins, notably oxidized phospholipids and reactive oxygen or reactive nitrogen species

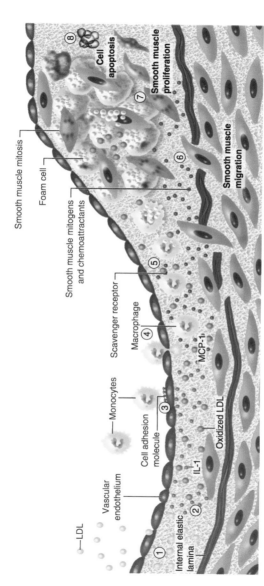

Fig. 7.7 See legend on next page

Smooth muscle mitosis

Foam cell

Smooth muscle mitogens and chemoattractants

Scavenger receptor

Macrophage

Monocytes

Cell adhesion molecule

Vascular endothelium

LDL

Internal elastic lamina

Cell apoptosis

Smooth muscle proliferation

Smooth muscle migration

MCP-1;

Oxidized LDL

IL-1

Fig. 7.7, Cont'd Local leukocyte and smooth muscle cell functions in the atherosclerotic plaque. (1) Accumulation of lipoprotein particles in the intima (yellow spheres). The modification of these lipoproteins is depicted by the darker color. Modifications include oxidation and glycation. (2) Oxidative stress, including products found in modified lipoproteins, can induce local cytokine elaboration (green spheres). (3) The cytokines thus induced increase expression of adhesion molecules (blue stalks on endothelial surface) for leukocytes that cause their attachment and chemoattractant molecules that direct their migration into the intima. (4) Blood monocytes, on entering the artery wall in response to chemoattractant cytokines such as monocyte chemoattractant protein 1 (MCP-1), encounter stimuli such as macrophage colony-stimulating factor that can augment their expression of scavenger receptors. (5) Scavenger receptors mediate the uptake of modified lipoprotein particles and promote the development of foam cells. Macrophage foam cells are a source of mediators, such as additional cytokines and effector molecules such as hypochlorous acid, superoxide anion (O_2^-), and matrix metalloproteinases. (6) Smooth muscle cells (SMCs) migrate into the intima from the media. (7) SMCs can then divide and elaborate extracellular matrix (ECM), promoting ECM accumulation in the growing atherosclerotic plaque. In this manner, the fatty streak can evolve into a fibrofatty lesion. (8) In later stages, calcification can occur (not depicted) and fibrosis continues, sometimes accompanied by SMC death (including programmed cell death or apoptosis), yielding a relatively acellular fibrous capsule surrounding a lipid-rich core that also may contain dying or dead cells and their detritus. IL, Interleukin; LDL, low-density lipoprotein. (From Libby P. The vascular biology of atherosclerosis. In: Zipes DP, Libby P, Bonow RO, Mann DL, Tomaselli GF, eds. Braunwald's Heart Disease, 11th ed. Philadelphia: Elsevier; 2018: 859–875.)

themselves, have undergone intensive investigation as potential targets in the treatment of atherosclerosis. Various classes of phospholipases that generate proinflammatory constituents of oxidized lipoproteins have undergone investigation as therapeutic targets. Rigorous clinical studies however have not substantiated improvement in cardiovascular outcomes with inhibitors of a soluble phospholipase (verasladib) or a lipoprotein associated phospholipase A_2 (LpPLA$_2$). Darapladib, an inhibitor of LpPLA$_2$, did not improve outcomes in individuals with either acute or chronic atherosclerotic cardiovascular disease in the SOLID and STABILITY trials.[49,50]

A variety of different classes of proteinases may participate in cardiovascular disease. An extensive preclinical literature supports roles for matrix metalloproteinases (MMPs) in remodeling of the extracellular matrix in both arteries and the myocardium.[51] Compensatory enlargement of arteries during atherogenesis likely involves the action of MMPs that degrade constituents of the arterial extracellular matrix such as elastin and interstitial collagen.[52] Penetration of medial smooth muscle cells into the intima to form an atheroma likewise requires lysis of extracellular matrix components mediated by MMPs. Arterial ectasia, giving rise to aortic aneurysms in the extreme, also involves degradation of extracellular matrix macromolecules. MMPs and various cathepsins implicated in elastin breakdown likely contribute to all of these situations that involve macrovascular remodeling.[53] These various families of proteinases generally depend on inflammatory mediators to augment their expression and activation. Thus, these proteases are central participants in inflammatory reactions.

Formation of microvessels, angiogenesis, also involves proteinase-mediated remodeling of the extracellular matrix. Remodeling of the ventricular myocardium following ischemic injury also involves breakdown of extracellular matrix constituents. A large literature implicates proteinases including the MMPs and certain cathepsins in the geometrical remodeling, repair, and healing of myocardial infarction. Despite the convincing preclinical data and experimental promise, no cardiovascular therapy that targets matrix-degrading proteinases has demonstrated efficacy in clinical trials.

Small molecule lipid mediators of inflammation, particularly the eicosanoids, have served successfully as targets for cardiovascular intervention. Most notably, aspirin, an inhibitor of cyclooxygenases, can improve cardiovascular outcomes in acute coronary syndromes and secondary prevention. Although the doses of aspirin that confer cardiovascular benefit may not quell systemic inflammation, they may act as antiinflammatory agents secondarily by inhibiting platelet activation. Platelets contain preformed proinflammatory mediators that can potentiate inflammatory processes locally upon their degranulation. Thus, low-dose aspirin may exert some of its benefit through an antiinflammatory action secondary to its inhibition of platelet activation. The selective cyclooxygenase-2 inhibitors have not only not shown an ability to improve cardiovascular outcomes but in some cases have shown signals of cardiovascular hazard.[54] Thus, aspirin treatment particularly in low doses appears to have achieved a "sweet spot" in inhibition of prostanoid production. Recent evidence from large-scale clinical trials, however, indicates that the bleeding risk counterbalances clinical benefit of low-dose aspirin in most primary prevention indications.[55,56]

Another class of small low-molecular-weight lipids can participate in cardiovascular inflammation—the leukotrienes, enzymes such as 5-lipoxygenase, and its activator FLAP—have undergone investigation in cardiovascular clinical trials. Despite the theoretical and experimental considerations that led to targeting of leukotrienes, inhibitors of the enzymes that govern the production of this class of mediators have not shown benefit in clinical trials.

The participation of adaptive immunity in atherosclerosis and certain forms of myocardial disease has received considerable experimental support buttressed by human observations. These considerations have led to several attempts to modulate adaptive immunity therapeutically in the context of cardiovascular disease.[57] Elimination of B cells with a therapeutic antibody that targets cluster of differentiation molecule (CD20) can benefit certain vasculitides. As natural antibodies secreted by B1 lymphocytes can mitigate experimental atherogenesis, a number of attempts to vaccinate with modified lipoproteins that elicit these natural antibodies are in various stages of clinical development.[58] The concept of a vaccine for atherosclerosis has considerable attraction. While one clinical trial that evaluated a biomarker, fluorodeoxyglucose uptake, did not show benefit (GLACIER), several teams are striving to implement vaccination strategies in the clinic that could prove beneficial in mitigating atherosclerotic complications.[59,60]

Another clever and intriguing approach to manipulating adaptive immunity involves the administration of low doses of the proinflammatory cytokine IL-2 to individuals at risk for cardiovascular complications. High doses of IL-2, used in treatment of certain malignancies, can trigger a capillary leak syndrome and have proven hazardous from a cardiovascular perspective. Yet, low doses of IL-2 can skew the adaptive immune response toward an activation of regulatory T cells that can mitigate inflammation, largely through the production of TGF-β. Pilot clinical studies evaluating this ingenious approach are currently underway.[57, 61]

Among the metabolites of arachidonic acid, several families of mediators of resolution of inflammation have emerged. These complex structures known as resolvins or maresins can mitigate

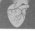

inflammation without impairing host defenses.[62] These classes of proresolving mediators are known as specific proresolving mediators, or SPMs. The elegant chemistry and assessment of protective functions in vivo have led to experiments that target atherosclerosis. Indeed, experimental evidence that SPMs can mitigate experimental atherosclerosis has emerged.[63,64] Whether achievable concentrations of these proresolving mediators will permit boosting of resolution of inflammatory processes in the cardiovascular system requires further study. The concept of promoting resolution without impairing host defenses or tumor surveillance or reducing defenses against infection has considerable appeal.

One place where targeted antiinflammatory therapy has shown clinical benefit in a rigorous and adequately powered clinical trial is targeting of the proinflammatory cytokine IL-1β. The Canakinumab Antiinflammatory Thrombosis Outcomes Study (CANTOS) targeted IL-1β with a monoclonal antibody, canakinumab, that very specifically inhibits IL-1β.[65] The study selected individuals who were in the stable phase following an acute coronary syndrome and who showed an indication of persistent inflammation despite receiving statins and other evidence based secondary prevention treatments, as indicated by an elevation in high sensitivity C-reactive protein (hs-CRP) above the approximate population median (2 mg/L). The median duration of treatment in the trial was 3.7 years. Administration of canakinumab 150 mg subcutaneously every 3 months yielded a statistically significant 15% reduction in relative risk of the primary composite endpoint of myocardial infarction, stroke, or cardiovascular death.[66] In an on-treatment analysis, individuals who achieved a greater than median response to canakinumab as judged by CRP reduction showed an over 30% decrease in cardiovascular and total mortality (Fig. 7.8).[67] Thus, CANTOS provided the first large-scale rigorous clinical trial evidence that targeting inflammation could provide a cardiovascular benefit.

Other studies targeting IL-1 and allied proinflammatory cytokines have shown evidence of benefit. The MRC IL-1 trial used anakinra, an inhibitor of the IL-1 receptor, that blocks responses to both the IL-1α and β isoforms, reduced the area under the curve of the hs-CRP response in patients undergoing acute coronary syndromes.[68] Anakinra administration has yielded positive signals in heart failure and experimentally as well.[69-71] Other studies have targeted the proinflammatory cytokine IL-6 in patients undergoing acute coronary syndromes and shown a decrease in the area under the curve of CRP particularly in those who underwent percutaneous intervention.[72-74] As there are numerous proinflammatory cytokines, their exploration as therapeutic targets in cardiovascular disease merits further investigation.[75] In CANTOS, as expected, there was a

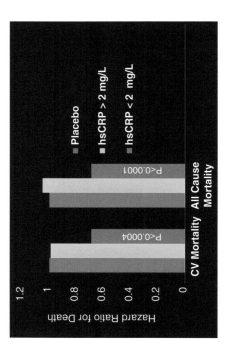

Fig. 7.8 Responders to canakinumab had mortality benefit in the on-treatment analysis from CANTOS. Multivariable adjusted hazard ratios (HR) for prespecified cardiovascular outcomes according to on-treatment high-sensitivity C-reactive protein (hsCRP) levels above or below 2 mg/L after drug initiation. HRs adjusted for age, gender, smoking, hypertension, diabetes, body mass index, baseline hsCRP, baseline low density lipoprotein-cholesterol. This on-treatment analysis underwent numerous sensitivity analyses to assess possible confounding that affirmed the conclusion. (Ridker PM, et al. Relationship of C-reactive protein reduction to cardiovascular event reduction following treatment with canakinumab: a secondary analysis from the CANTOS randomised controlled trial. *Lancet* 2018;391(10118):319–328.)

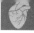

statistically significant albeit slight increase in infections, some of them fatal. While the type of infections and identification of those susceptible to infections during treatment with canakinumab should permit mitigation of this risk, this result illustrates the need to calibrate carefully antiinflammatory interventions when attempting to treat cardiovascular disease and carefully monitoring the benefit/risk ration. Although a slight increase in fatal infections occurred in CANTOS, a striking reduction in cancer mortality counterbalanced this risk.[76] This observation underscores the commonality of inflammatory mechanisms shared by cancer and cardiovascular disease.[2]

A large body of experimental literature and pilot clinical observations suggest that targeting the proinflammatory tumor necrosis alpha (TNF-α) could benefit individuals with heart failure. The large-scale clinical trials that evaluated this proposition did not show clinical benefit, and indeed suggested higher hazard rate of an anti-TNF strategy.[77] Thus, TNF neutralization, which has received wide acceptance in rheumatology and gastroenterology, does not appear a promising strategy for reducing cardiovascular risk. A prespecified secondary analysis of CANTOS did show a reduction in heart failure events and hospitalization for heart failure in patients receiving canakinumab.[78] Thus CANTOS also provided a proof of principle of the efficacy of anticytokine therapy in heart failure. Most therapies that have proven beneficial in treating patients with heart failure involve neurohumoral blockade. Hypotension and impaired renal function provide serious clinical limitations to ever increased neurohumoral blockade in our heart failure patients. Therefore, the concept of targeting inflammation that does not lower blood pressure or impair renal functions provides a therapy worthy of further exploration to complement the standard approaches of diuresis and blockade of the sympathetic nervous system and the renin-angiotensin-aldosterone system in patients with heart failure.

Conclusions, Challenges, and Future Perspective

The plethora of proinflammatory cytokines, in the context of the success of CANTOS, suggests that selective cytokine inhibition warrants further investigation.[79,80] Methotrexate, an antiinflammatory intervention that has revolutionized the treatment of rheumatoid arthritis and allied disorders, has an uncertain mechanism of antiinflammatory effect and did not show benefit in a large-scale cardiovascular outcomes trial, the cardiovascular inflammation reduction trial (CIRT).[81] This impeccably conducted trial yielded a null result despite a robust body of observational and preclinical data indicating its efficacy.[82] The population enrolled in CIRT did not have baseline elevation in inflammation as would be indicated by above median CRP, a distinct difference from CANTOS. Moreover, the low-dose weekly methotrexate employed in CIRT did not lower CRP or IL-6, again in contrast to the CANTOS findings.

Taken together, the results of CANTOS and CIRT point to the IL-1β pathway as an attractive target for further attempts to target inflammation in cardiovascular disease. The inflammasome activates pro-IL-1β to its active form. It also processes the precursor of IL-18 to the active cytokine. Some data suggest that the IL-1α isoform may also undergo activation by caspase-1, the enzyme component of the inflammasome that responds to the danger signals sensed by its other constituent proteins. IL-1β strongly induces IL-6. IL-6 signaling participates causally in cardiovascular disease as shown by recent concordant human genetic studies using Mendelian randomization approaches.[83,84] IL-6 can signal both through a classical pathway that involves activating the acute phase response in the hepatocyte through binding of the transmembrane form of the IL-6 receptor. IL-6 can also signal using a "trans" pathway by binding a soluble form of its receptor which can then activate extra hepatocyte cells bearing the coreceptor for IL-6, gp130 (see Fig. 7.9).

Strategies exist for neutralizing the cytokine IL-6 and its receptor, thus providing the ability to antagonize selectively classical or trans IL-6 signaling. Thus, IL-6 stands out as a logical candidate for further investigation as a target for antiinflammatory therapy in cardiovascular disease. As the acute-phase response boosts production of fibrinogen, the precursor of clots, and of plasminogen activator inhibitor-1 (PAI-1), a major inhibitor of endogenous fibrinolysis, inhibiting classical signaling of IL-6, and limiting the acute phase response would not only quell inflammation but might also reduce thrombus formation and favor fibrinolysis (Fig. 7.6).

IL-18 has multiple proinflammatory properties. In addition to its classical receptor, IL-18 can signal through a sodium-chloride co-transporter. Interference with IL-18 signaling can reduce experimental atherosclerosis. Thus, targeting IL-18 also merits consideration and further exploration of antiinflammatory strategies to treat cardiovascular disease. As the NLRP3 inflammasome generates both active IL-1β and active IL-18, targeting of the inflammasome could prove beneficial in cardiovascular disease as well. Although one might be concerned about upstream inhibition of IL-1β and IL-18 maturation, alternate pathways can also generate active forms of IL-1β. In contrast to CANTOS, which targeted the cytokine itself, inhibition of the inflammasome might theoretically interfere less with host defenses than canakinumab and avoid some of the unwanted infectious consequences of IL-1β inhibition.

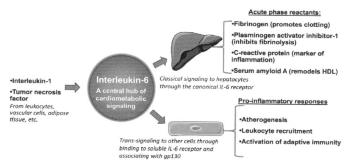

Fig. 7.9 **Interleukin-6: A central hub of cardiometabolic signaling.** Various stimuli, among them the proinflammatory cytokines interleukin (IL)-1 and tumor necrosis factor can stimulate the release of IL-6 from leukocytes, vascular cells, adipose tissue among other sources. IL-6 can bind to its canonical receptor on the surface of hepatocytes, leukocytes, and megakaryocytes. In response to IL-6, hepatocytes produce the products of the acute-phase response including those listed. In addition to this classical IL-6 signaling pathway, the alpha subunit of the transmembrane IL-6 receptor can undergo cleavage by the metalloproteinase ADAM-17 to produce a soluble form. When bound to IL-6 in the fluid phase of blood or in the extracellular space, the soluble receptor-ligand pair can associate with gp130 expressed on many cell types, and form a ternary complex that can elicit primarily proinflammatory responses. Thus, both canonical and "transsignaling" can promote aspects of cardiometabolic disease and atherothrombosis. *HDL,* High-density lipoprotein. (Libby P, Rocha VZ. All roads lead to IL-6: a central hub of cardiometabolic signaling. *Int J Cardiol* 2018;259:213–215.)

Several small molecule inhibitors of the inflammasome have begun clinical development. Mining the inflammasome-IL-1β, IL-18, to IL-6 to acute phase response pathways holds considerable promise for further exploration as antiinflammatory therapies in atherosclerosis (Fig. 7.2, 7.6, and 7.9).

As illustrated in CANTOS, using biomarkers for selective targeting of antiinflammatory therapies provides a scheme for targeting antiinflammatory therapies. As we strive to realize the promise of personalized medicine, the identification of subsets of individuals particularly likely to respond to a given intervention based on biomarker status could prove promising. The development of biomarkers of inflammation and their validation could also aid with pharmaceutical development.[85] The use of biomarkers could help select appropriate doses for clinical trials. Biomarker studies could also validate target engagement. Finally, the use of biomarkers and surrogate endpoints could provide early glimpses of clinical efficacy to aid the allocation of resources for large scale clinical trials to the most promising agents at doses likely to provide benefit.

The fundamental biology of inflammation and a wealth of experimental data have highlighted inflammation and the immune response as a potential series of therapeutic targets beyond the traditional pharmaceutical approaches to treating cardiovascular conditions. Multiple examples described above have demonstrated that interventions that have shown promise experimentally and in small-scale clinical investigations have often proved disappointing in appropriately powered randomized clinical trials. Accordingly, we must apply what we have learned while moving forward in expanding the results of CANTOS to identify further and ever safer approaches to targeting inflammation and immunity in cardiovascular disease. Given the wealth of the fundamental scientific underpinnings of this approach and the multitude of potential targets discussed in this chapter, it is likely that advances in therapeutics will realize the promise of targeted antiinflammatory therapies as a reality in cardiovascular therapeutics in the future.

References

Complete reference list available at www.expertconsult.com.

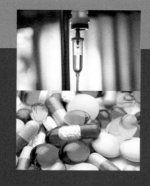

第8章
抗血栓药物

在心血管疾病的治疗中，抗血栓是久经考验的治疗及预防策略，这一地位深深根植于多种临床疾病的治疗之中。虽然抗血栓药物的不断进展及广泛使用降低了心血管事件的发生率及严重程度，但是临床医师仍要面对如出血等不良反应的挑战。本章致力于总结抗血栓药物的最佳循证依据、作用机制、特有性质、已批准的心血管疾病适应证、不良反应、潜在的药物相互作用及相关领域的研究进展。

血栓形成的基本因素及内容十分丰富，本章在内容上涵盖了动静脉血栓、血栓形成、血小板沉积、血小板反应能力、凝血酶的激活、全身和局部影响等，并提出了未来抗血栓治疗的可能靶点——血小板与中性粒细胞胞外诱捕网。

药物治疗的重要性将通过丰富多样的药物疗法、在特定临床情况下的用药指导或建议进行具体阐述，抗血栓药物包括作用于血小板的阿司匹林、脑康平和西洛他唑；血小板P2Y12受体拮抗剂，如噻氯匹定、氯吡格雷、普拉格雷和替格瑞洛；静脉注射用血小板GP Ⅱ b/ Ⅲ a受体拮抗剂，如阿昔单抗、替罗非班和依替巴肽；外周抗凝药物，如普通肝素和低分子肝素；间接、选择性凝血因子Ⅹa抑制剂，如合成五糖磺达肝素；直接凝血酶抑制剂，如水蛭素、比伐卢定和阿加曲班；口服直接凝血酶抑制剂，如达比加群、利伐沙班、阿哌沙班、依度沙班和贝曲沙班；维生素K拮抗剂，如华法林；直接口服抗凝药的逆转和替代，即靶向逆转药物，如依达赛珠单抗、凝血因子Ⅹa（重组）冻干粉注射剂等。

　　抗血栓是心血管疾病患者治疗的重要策略之一。科研人员在相关领域多年的深入研究和科技的快速进展为临床医师和患者提供了多种治疗选择。除了解抗血栓药物的药理学、临床用途和潜在的不良反应外，临床医师还必须了解抗血栓治疗最常见的并发症——出血的治疗方法。相信随着知识的不断积累，科研人员必将进一步打开新药研发的大门。

陈安天

Antithrombotic Drugs

RICHARD C. BECKER · SREEKANTH VEMULAPALLI ·
VLAD COTARLAN · MOHAMMED A. EFFAT

Introduction

Antithrombotic therapy represents a time-tested foundation for the
prevention and treatment of cardiovascular disease that is firmly
rooted in an understanding of the pathophysiology of common
clinical phenotypes, including acute coronary syndrome, acute
ischemic stroke, venous thromboembolic disease, stent thrombosis, heart chamber thrombosis, and mechanical device thrombosis.
In each case, one or more well-delineated abnormalities present
within the vasculature, circulating blood cells, plasma and its constituents associated with local conditions that affect laminar blood
flow, shear stress, and biochemical events is responsible for
impaired circulation and organ perfusion that can be either life-
threatening or life-altering.

The development and wide-scale availability of effective
antithrombotic drugs has substantially reduced the number and
severity of cardiovascular events; however, several challenges
remain, including cost, wide-scale availability, consistent and
evidence-based utilization by clinicians, and the potential for
adverse effects such as bleeding.

This chapter is dedicated to summarizing the best available
evidence on antithrombotic drugs, their mechanisms of action,
unique properties, approved indications for use in cardiovascular
disease, side effects, potential drug interactions, and advances in
the field that may pave the way for increasingly safe, effective,
and affordable agents.

Coagulation, Thrombosis, and Hemostasis

A chapter dedicated to cardiovascular drugs and antithrombotic
therapy would not be complete without a brief summary of the distinguishing characteristics of coagulation, thrombosis, and hemostasis. Coagulation is a series of biochemical events that can occur

in vitro and ex vivo if the conditions can support protease assembly, thrombin generation, and fibrin formation. By contrast, thrombosis occurs primarily on cellular surfaces within the circulatory system, requires platelets and derived particles, and is the end-result of localized injury or nonbiologic materials, impaired or nonlaminar blood flow, and systemic conditions that favor either platelet activation, coagulation protease assembly, or thrombin generation. Hemostasis is a complex, physiological state that requires vascular integrity and reparative capacity, distinct platelet populations with both autocrine and equally importantly paracrine system function, and regulatory pathways to limit clotting solely and specifically where and when needed to stem blood loss (Fig. 8.1).

Thrombosis

Arterial Thrombosis

The clinical expression of atherosclerotic vascular disease is determined by pathologic events leading to coronary thrombosis (or thromboembolism). There are two key factors: (1) the propensity of plaques to rupture, and (2) the thrombogenicity of exposed plaque components. Ischemic stroke differs with a much lower

TRADITIONAL PERSPECTIVE OF COAGULATION

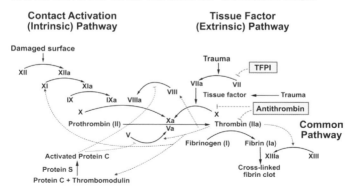

Fig. 8.1 A traditional and primarily biochemistry-based view of coagulation, including the contact activation and tissue factor pathways of initiation, point of convergence (common pathway) and multiple routes for pathway(s) cross talk. *TFPI,* Tissue factor pathway inhibitor.

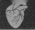

incidence of plaque rupture and more commonly thrombosis *in situ*, artery-to-artery embolism and cardioembolism.

Thrombogenesis

Pathologic events leading to coronary thrombosis (or thromboembolism) are the basis of clinical phenotypes. There are two key factors: (1) the propensity of plaques to rupture, and (2) the thrombogenicity of exposed plaque components.

The morphologic characteristics of plaques destined to rupture have been determined using necropsy and atherectomy tissue samples and show extracellular lipid and a lipid core occupying a large proportion of the overall plaque volume. The degree of cross-sectional narrowing of the vessel lumen is typically less than 50%.[1] In addition to a large lipid core, vulnerable plaques are characterized by a thin fibrous cap and high macrophage density.[2] Whereas individuals with atherosclerotic coronary artery disease (CAD) exhibit a diversity of plaque types, most have a preponderance of one specific type (vulnerable or nonvulnerable), and patients with recurring symptoms frequently lack capacity for healing of the fibrous cap.

Under normal physiologic conditions, cellular blood components interact with the vessel wall for the purpose of vascular repair. The exposure of circulating blood to disrupted or dysfunctional surfaces initiates a series of integrated steps that give rise to the rapid deposition of platelets, erythrocytes, leukocytes, and insoluble fibrin establishing a mechanical barrier to blood loss.

Thrombosis occurring within the arterial circulatory system is composed of platelets and fibrin in a tightly packed network. By contrast, venous thrombi consist of a more loosely woven network of erythrocytes, leukocytes, and fibrin. Overall, the site, size, and composition of thrombi forming within the heart and arterial circulatory system are determined by alterations in blood flow and:

- thrombogenicity of vascular endothelial and endocardial surfaces;
- concentration and reactivity of plasma cellular protein and glycoprotein components;
- full functional capability of vascular physiologic protective mechanisms.

Platelet Deposition

The role of platelets is to tether and attach to disrupted vascular surfaces and subsequently adhere firmly, activate, and aggregate to form a rapidly enlarging platelet mass. Under physiologic conditions this sequence of events represents the primary step in hemostasis. By contrast, pathologic thrombosis is characterized by a robust and poorly regulated response to vessel wall injury that escalates to the point of circulatory compromise and impaired perfusion.

The biology of platelet deposition involves several processes:

- platelet attachment to collagen or exposed surface adhesive proteins;
- platelet activation and intracellular signaling;
- the expression of platelet receptors for adhesive proteins;
- platelet aggregation; and platelet recruitment mediated by thrombin, thromboxane A_2, adenosine diphosphate, and other mediators.

Platelet Response Capacity

Platelets play an essential role in sensing and responding to perturbations in the blood and vasculature. Their reaction to environmental cues has both local and systemic consequences. As purveyors of the vascular space, they transmit information locally and systemically. Platelet function is tightly regulated within the vasculature, and several factors (e.g., nitric oxide [NO], prostacyclin, and adenosine diphosphase [ADPase] activity) present on the endothelial surface[3] maintain them in a normally resting state (Fig. 8.2). Platelets adhere to damaged, disrupted, dysfunctional or inflamed endothelial cells, exposed subendothelial tissue and nonphysiological shear flow.[4] Local generation of thrombin and other platelet activators augments intraplatelet signaling systems. Platelets themselves respond to these and other stimuli by secreting prothrombotic proteins from dense α-granules and by changing their shape through rearrangement of the cytoskeletal network. Secretion of prothrombotic proteins and signaling elicit a second wave of platelet activation and inside-out signaling to alter the configuration of integrins on the platelet surface and assume a high affinity state. Activation of integrin αIIbβ3 and subsequent binding of fibrinogen that bridges adjacent platelets is essential for platelet aggregation.[5]

Activation of Coagulation Proteases

Thrombin is generated rapidly in response to vascular injury. It also plays a central role in platelet recruitment and formation of an insoluble fibrin network. The thrombotic process is localized, amplified, and modulated by a series of biochemical reactions driven by the reversible binding of circulating proteins (coagulation proteases)

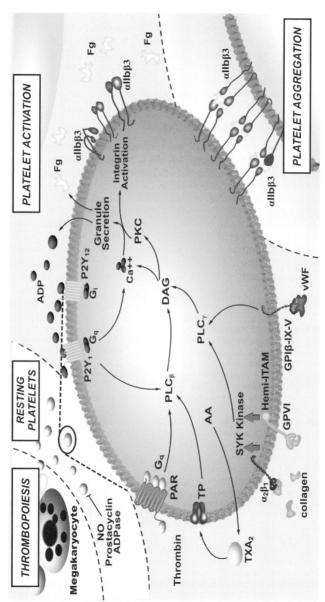

Fig. 8.2 See figure legend on next page.

to damaged vascular cells, elements of exposed subendothelial connective tissue (especially collagen), platelets (which express tissue factor (TF)-containing microparticles and receptor sites for coagulation proteases), and macrophages. These events lead to an assembly of enzyme complexes that increase local concentrations of procoagulant material; in this way, a relatively minor initiating stimulus can be greatly amplified to yield a thrombus (see Fig. 8.1).

Coagulation on Cellular Surfaces

A cell-based model of coagulation underscores the importance of TF-bearing cells and activated platelets serving as a scaffold for procoagulant proteins to assemble and ultimately form a localized fibrin clot.[6] In this integrated model system, coagulation occurs in three overlapping stages: 1) *initiation, amplification,* and *propagation* (Fig. 8.3). *Initiation* occurs primarily after exposure of the TF/VIIa complex at a site of vascular injury. This complex activates localized human Factor (F)X, which then combines with FVa to form the prothrombinase complex and generate a small amount of thrombin; 2) Thrombin then primes the system for rapid *amplification* by activating platelets, FXI, FVIII, and additional FV; 3) In

---

Fig. 8.2, cont'd   Schematic representation of contemporary platelet biogenesis and activation. Megakaryocytes derived from myeloid stem cells give rise to platelets. Several factors present or released from endothelial cells, including nitric oxide *(NO)*, prostacyclin, and ADPase, act to keep circulating platelets in a resting state. Platelets are initially activated by several triggers, including (but not limited to) adhesion to collagen via glycoprotein VI (GPVI) and the $\alpha 2\beta 1$ integrin, von Willebrand factor *(vWF)* binding to GPIb-IX-V complex, and generation of thrombin at or near the platelet surface that signals through protease-activated receptors *(PAR)*. These pathways elicit downstream activation of phospholipase C *(PLC)* isoforms to generate second messengers inositol 1, 4, 5-triphosphate (not shown) and 1,2-diacylglycerol *(DAG)*, which in turn, link to pathways that drive secretion of alpha granule contents including prothrombotic proteins fibrinogen *(Fg)* and vWF, as well as the secretion of dense granules to release a number of soluble platelet agonists such as ADP and serotonin. Activation is reinforced by secreted ADP acting on P2Y1 and $P2Y_{12}$ receptors, as well as the activation of the thromboxane receptor *(TP)* from thromboxane A2 *(TXA2)* generated from arachidonic acid *(AA)* released during the initial wave of platelet activation. Platelet aggregation occurs through Fg-mediated integrin $\alpha IIb\beta 3$ interactions with adjacent activated platelets. *ADP,* Adenosine diphosphate. (Modified from Becker RC, Sexton T, Smyth SA. Translational implications of platelets as vascular first responders. *Circ Res* 2018;122:506–522.)

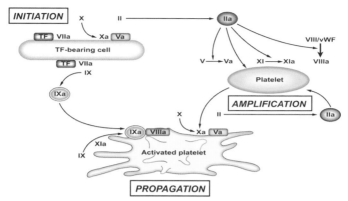

Fig. 8.3 The cell-based model of coagulation describes an interaction between procoagulant surfaces and proteases essential for coagulation. Coagulation occurs on the surface of tissue factor *(TF)*-bearing cells and activated platelets in three overlapping steps: (1) initiation of the pathway follows FVIIa binding to exposed TF, provoking the generation of a small amount of thrombin; (2) thrombin then activates other coagulation proteases and platelets, facilitating coagulation protease assembly in the priming phase of coagulation and; (3) the surface of activated platelets serves as the biological template for a burst of thrombin generation, with resulting thrombus propagation. *vWF,* von Willebrand factor. (Data from Hoffman M, Monroe III DM. A cell-based model of hemostasis. *Thromb Haemostasis* 2001;85:958–965.)

the *propagation* stage, activated FIX, generated through both FXIa and TF/VIIa, combines with FVIIIa to form the tenase complex and generate FX on the platelet surface. Subsequent formation of the prothrombinase complex provokes a burst of thrombin, converting fibrinogen to stable fibrin monomers, which then polymerize and are covalently stabilized by FXIIIa.

Contact and Intrinsic Pathway-Mediated Coagulation

The contact system includes FXII, FXI, kallikrein, and high-molecular-weight kininogen (HMWK) and participates actively in inflammation (FXII, kallikrein, HMWK) and coagulation (FXII, FXI). The contact system is activated following exposure of FXII to a number of anionic surfaces, generating activated FXII (FXIIa) that triggers the intrinsic pathway of coagulation, beginning with FXI and followed by factors IX and VIII. Although it was previously believed that all coagulation factors play a similar role in hemostasis and thrombosis, evidence points to differing functions for FXI and FXII.

CONTACT PATHWAY

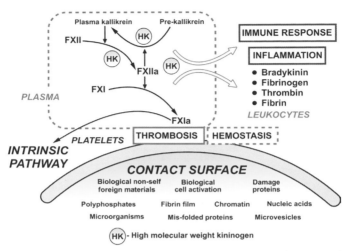

Fig. 8.4 The contact-based model of coagulation plays a fundamental role for the interface of coagulation, immunity and inflammation.

Specifically, the contact activation proteins contribute to pathologic thrombus formation without being actively involved in normal hemostasis (Fig. 8.4).

Human FXI

Human FXI is a 160-kDa serine protease glycoprotein that circulates as a homodimer of two identical 80 kDa polypeptides.[7] Each individual polypeptide consists of a 35-kDa C-terminal light chain containing the catalytic domain, and an N-terminal 45 kDa heavy chain carrying four approximately 90 amino acid tandem repeats termed apple domains. The apple domains of FXI facilitate binding to other proteins: A1 contains binding sites to HMWK and thrombin, A3 to FIX, heparin, and glycoprotein Ibα (GP1bα), and A4 to FXI and FXII.[8] Early observations revealed that FXI could be activated by thrombin as well as FXIIa and suggested that this route of bioamplification was favored in vivo over FXII-mediated activation.[9] Subsequent experiments revealed that FXI-mediated activation of thrombin was essential for continued thrombin generation in the presence of low levels of TF, but not when higher levels of TF were present. In addition, the GP1bα receptor on the surface of platelets contains binding sites for FXII, thrombin, and FXI, bringing these proteins into close proximity on the platelet surface and allowing FXI to be activated and subsequently activate FIX in the presence of calcium ions, amplifying coagulation and thrombin generation.[10]

The effect of FXI concentration on thrombin kinetics varies widely among individuals,[11] likely reflecting the several unique functional characteristics of the protease and mirroring the variable bleeding phenotype seen in FXI-deficient patients. Even with severe FXI deficiency, tenase complexes can form via the extrinsic TF/VIIa complex and, in turn, lead to the formation of prothrombinase complexes on the platelet surface. In most instances, decreasing FXI concentrations steadily slow the rate of thrombin generation without affecting the total amount of thrombin formed. In a cell-based model system, as little as 5% of normal plasma levels of FXI led to some thrombin generation, with a maximal amount of thrombin generated at 50% of normal FXI levels.

The in vivo evidence suggests strongly that FXI contributes to fibrin formation and platelet activation, stabilizing occlusive thrombi under high-flow conditions. This differs from its participation in hemostasis, in which FXI-driven fibrin formation is not needed to prevent blood loss following vascular injury in most tissues;[12] however, it likely participates with major breaches of vascular integrity as encountered during complex surgery and severe trauma.[13]

Human FXII

Human FXII is an 80-kDa glycoprotein consisting of an enzymatic light chain and a heavy chain comprised of several conserved domains that mediate binding to negatively charged surfaces and other proteins.[14] These domains include common structural elements found in several coagulant and fibrinolytic proteins, such as fibronectin type I and II, two epidermal growth factor (EGF)-like domains, and a kringle domain.[14]

FXII can be slowly autoactivated by binding to a negatively charged surface, such as kaolin or dextran sulfate, and initiate the contact activation pathway by activating FXI and the intrinsic pathway of coagulation or activating plasma prekallikrein and facilitating inflammatory responses.[15] A search for the primary (or dominant) activator in vivo has been challenging, as a number of negatively charged substances, such as polyphosphates, nucleic acids, sulfatides, fatty acids, protein aggregates, and activated platelets, have each been found to activate FXII in vitro.[16] The absence of FXII and FXI protect against polyphosphate-triggered thrombosis in animal models, suggesting that polyphosphate released from platelets activates the intrinsic pathway to exert its procoagulant effect. The distinct properties of proteins within the contact system has generated interest in drug development.[17-19]

Venous Thrombosis

Venous thrombi are characterized by layers of fibrin, platelets, red cells, and leukocytes and develop under conditions of stasis, lowered oxygen tension, oxidative stress, proinflammatory gene up-regulation, and impaired endothelial-cell regulatory capacity. Although the relative proportion of platelets is low, they play a pivotal role by releasing polyphosphates, microparticles, and proinflammatory mediators and by interacting with neutrophils to generate DNA–histone–granule constituent complexes.[20] These nuclear materials induce platelet adhesion, activation, and aggregation; the expression of factors V and Va and von Willebrand factor; prothrombinase assembly; and thrombin generation.

Artificial Nonbiological Surfaces and Prosthetic Materials

Several hundred years ago William Hewson made a landmark observation regarding the inherent thrombogenicity of artificial surfaces: he found that human blood remained in a fluid state for hours when contained within an isolated peripheral vein segment but clotted almost immediately when it was allowed to drain into a bowl.[21] Subsequent experiments with glass, rubber, polymers, and other materials suggested that the thrombogenic properties of artificial surfaces differed widely according to surface topography, critical surface tension, chemistry, and physical structure. It has become increasingly clear, however, that the *surface* and bulk *interior* of an artificial material may be substantially different because of nonhomogeneity, contamination, or environmental exposure. The relationship between surface chemistry, physical structure, platelet activation, and coagulation is dynamic and complex.

Systemic and Local Influences

Plasma Proteins

In general, positively charged surfaces favor thrombus formation whereas negatively charged surfaces are comparatively resistant to thrombus formation. Although these properties may reflect the normally negative charge of vascular endothelial cells, surface elements, circulating blood components, and plasma proteins likely play an important role as well.[22] Artificial surfaces with a net positive charge are highly adsorptive of plasma proteins (and blood cells), all of which have a negative charge of physiologic importance. The diffusive mobility and concentration of plasma proteins exceed those of platelets, which suggests that artificial surfaces are probably coated with proteins before platelets adhere and form a confluent monolayer. Electron microscopy has shown that a thin film of plasma components (primarily proteins) develops within several seconds on all artificial surfaces exposed to whole blood. As a result, it seems likely that the composition, concentration, and conformational characteristics of surface-bound protein molecules initially determine the thrombogenicity of the underlying artificial material.[23]

Fibrinogen, a prominent plasma protein readily available in high concentrations, is the first protein adsorbed to an artificial surface exposed to blood. Depending on the orientation of the molecules (either standing "on end" or horizontal in tightly packed layers), the surface concentration of fibrinogen may exceed that found normally in plasma by 100-fold,[24] and experimental evidence supports a direct role for surface-bound fibrinogen in determining relative thrombogenicity. The adsorption of other plasma proteins—including von Willebrand factor, fibronectin, and thrombospondin, as well as circulating coagulation factors—also contributes but predominantly in a secondary capacity.

The initial adsorption of plasma proteins to an artificial surface is often followed by a period of "prothrombosis," which may be followed by a relative state of thromboresistance. This metamorphosis, often referred to as "passivation," varies according to physical and chemical alterations of the surface proteins, their electrostatic potential, and perhaps most important an intrinsic capacity or inherent propensity to interact with platelets and coagulation factors.[25]

Platelets

Platelet adherence to artificial surfaces is an early event that follows the adsorption of plasma proteins.[26] The presence of fibrinogen in high concentrations facilitates platelet aggregation, but only after activation has taken place. Interestingly, despite the common occurrence of platelet adhesion and surface monolayer development, not all materials promote or support platelet aggregates. The process of platelet activation is determined, as with plasma proteins, by surface properties including physical characteristics, electrical charge, and surface chemistry. In vivo, surface conditions (shear stress and surface tension) exert an important effect on platelet behavior through erythrocytes—a rich source of adenosine diphosphate (ADP). High-shear states, in addition to promoting interactions between plasma protein and artificial surfaces, can damage erythrocyte membranes (lysis), causing the release of ADP, a potent platelet agonist.[27] The process of platelet deposition involves six steps: (1) platelet attachment, (2) platelet adhesion, (3) platelet activation, (4) the expression of platelet receptors for adhesive proteins, (5) platelet aggregation, and (6) platelet recruitment.

Coagulation

Artificial surfaces, particularly those carrying a negative charge, are capable of activating factors XII and XI and prekallikrein, initiating contact activation of the intrinsic coagulation pathway. Activation of the contact system is initiated by the binding of FXII to a negatively charged surface where "autoactivation" to an active serine protease occurs.[28] A small concentration of FXIIa leads to activation of its substrates—prekallikrein, FXI, and HMWK. Although prekallikrein and FXI can bind directly to artificial surfaces, activation of these enzymes does not occur in the absence of HMWK. In turn, adsorption of HMWK requires FXIIa-underscoring the importance of contact activation and its inhibition in the early stages of exposure of prosthetic materials to circulating blood.

Emerging Construct and Future Targets for Antithrombotic Therapy

Platelets and Neutrophil Extracellular Traps

In response to strong stimulation, neutrophils release neutrophil extracellular traps (NETs) that consist of DNA and histones in a process that involves histone citrullination by peptidylarginine deiminase-4, chromatin unwinding, breakdown of nuclear membranes, and cytolysis.[29] A key function of the extracellular chromatin material is to entrap and confine microbes to promote their destruction.

Platelets can trigger NET formation and may also bind to histones to form platelet-NET attachments (Fig. 8.5). Von Willebrand factor is believed to be a linker molecule for binding of NETs to areas of vascular injury (Fig. 8.6). Histones activate platelets through toll-like receptor (TLR)-dependent mechanisms to generate the release of polyphosphates,[30] which, in turn, amplify coagulation. Platelet–neutrophil interactions facilitate NET formation.

EMERGING PARADIGMS

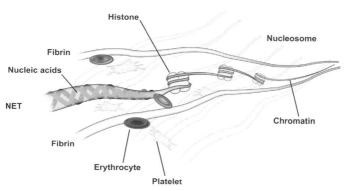

Fig. 8.5 Fundamental constructs for coagulation with the addition of several emerging paradigms that could serve as the basis for future targets of antithrombotic therapy. These include neutrophil extracellular traps of neutrophil extracellular traps *(NETs)* that consist of chromatin and nucleosomes. (Data from Wisler JW, Becker RC. Emerging paradigms in arterial thrombosis. *J Thromb Thrombolysis* 2014;37:4–11.)

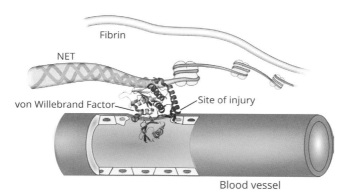

Fig. 8.6 Focused view of neutrophil extracellular traps *(NETs)* providing molecular and protein-based targets for innovative therapies, including polyphosphate/nucleic acid binders and von Willebrand factor inhibitors.

Cardiovascular Drug Therapy

The management of atherothrombotic vascular disease involving the coronary, cerebral, and peripheral vascular beds includes a broad array of antithrombotic agents. It is important for clinicians in the field of cardiology to be familiar with these commonly used agents, their mechanisms of action, pharmacology, adverse effects, drug interactions, and evidence-based use in patient care.

Platelet-Directed Therapies

The pivotal role of platelets in thrombosis provides a biology-based platform for targeted approaches to drug development, clinical trial testing, and employment in patient care (Table 8.1).

Aspirin

Aspirin has been available for over a century and represents a mainstay both in the prevention and treatment of atherosclerotic vascular events including stroke, myocardial infarction (MI), pulmonary arterial disease (PAD), and sudden death. Accordingly, a majority of patients with atherosclerotic vascular disease will receive aspirin.

Pharmacodynamics

Aspirin irreversibly acetylates cyclooxygenase (COX), impairing prostaglandin metabolism and thromboxane A_2 (TXA_2) synthesis. As a result, platelet aggregation in response to collagen, ADP, thrombin (in low concentrations), and TXA_2 is attenuated.[31] Because aspirin more selectively inhibits COX-1 activity (found predominantly in platelets) than COX-2 activity (expressed in tissues following an inflammatory stimulus), its ability to prevent platelet aggregation is seen at relatively low doses, compared with the drug's potential antiinflammatory effects, which require much higher doses.[32]

Pharmacokinetics

Aspirin is rapidly absorbed in the proximal gastrointestinal (GI) tract (stomach, duodenum), achieving peak serum levels within 15–20 minutes and platelet inhibition within 40–60 minutes of oral administration. Enteric-coated preparations are less well absorbed, causing an observed delay in peak serum levels and platelet

Table 8.1

Oral and parenteral platelet antagonists used in cardiovascular disease

Drug	Clopidogrel	Prasugrel	Ticagrelor	Cangrelor	Tirofiban	Eptifibatide	Abciximab	Voraxapar
Prodrug	Yes	Yes	No	No	No	No	No	No
Route	Oral	Oral	Oral	IV	IV	IV	IV	Oral
Mechanism of action	P2Y$_{12}$ inh	P2Y$_{12}$ inh	P2Y$_{12}$ inh	P2Y$_{12}$ inh	GPIIb/IIIa inh	GPIIb/IIIa inh	GPIIb/IIIa inh	PAR-1 inh
Onset of action	2–6 h	30 min	30 min	2 min	<15 min	<15 min	<10 min	1–2 h
Duration of action	3–10 d	7–10 d	3–5 d	1–2 h	4–8 h	4–8 h	24–48 h	2–3 wk
Withdrawal before surgery	5 d	7 d	5 d	1 h	8 h	8 h	>48 h	–
Loading dose	300–600 mg	60 mg	180 mg	30 µg/kg 4 µg/kg/min infusion	25 µg/kg 0.15 µg/kg/ min infusion	180 µg/kg 2 µg/kg/min infusion	0.25 mg/kg 0.125 µg/kg/ min infusion	–
Regular dose	75 mg OD	10 mg OD	90 mg BID					

BID, Twice Daily; *Inh,* inhibition; *IV,* intravenous; *OD,* once daily.

inhibition to 60 and 90 minutes, respectively. The antiplatelet effect occurs even before acetylsalicylic acid is detectable in peripheral blood, probably from platelet exposure in the portal circulation.

The plasma concentration of aspirin decays rapidly with a circulating half-life of approximately 20 minutes. Despite the drug's rapid clearance, platelet inhibition persists for the platelet's life span (7 ± 2 days) due to aspirin's irreversible inactivation of COX-1. Because 10% of circulating platelets of circulating platelets are replaced every 24 hours, platelet activity returns toward normal (≥50% activity) within 5 to 6 days of the last aspirin dose.[33]

Adverse Effects

The adverse-effect profile of aspirin in general and its associated risk for major hemorrhage (GI, urologic, intracranial) in particular are determined largely by: dose; duration of administration; associated structural (peptic ulcer disease, *Helicobacter pylori* infection) defects; hemostatic (inherited, acquired) abnormalities; concomitant use of other antithrombotic agents; and concomitant medical conditions or invasive procedures, including surgery. Enteric coating of aspirin may lessen dyspepsia, but it does not reduce the likelihood of adverse effects involving the GI tract. Patients with gastric erosions or peptic ulcer disease who require treatment with aspirin should concomitantly receive a proton pump inhibitor to minimize the risk of hemorrhage. An aspirin allergy, while not common, can occur with angioedema or overt anaphylaxis.

Clinical Experience

Aspirin's beneficial effect is determined by a disease, condition, or clinical scenario–based absolute risk of vascular events. Patients at low risk (healthy individuals without predisposing risk factors for vascular disease) derive minimal benefit (see next section on primary prevention), while those at high risk (acute coronary syndrome, prior MI or percutaneous coronary intervention [PCI] stroke) derive considerable benefit.[34] A risk-based approach to aspirin administration is recommended to avoid subjecting individuals who are unlikely to benefit from aspirin administration to its potential adverse effects.

Primary Prevention of Vascular Events

Aspirin has been used for the primary prevention of atherosclerotic coronary vascular disease (ASCVD) for decades; however, additional information afforded by randomized clinical trials has changed the paradigm for clinicians and patients.

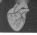

In the ASPREE (Aspirin and Cancer Prevention in the Elderly) study, 19,114 men and women greater than 70 years of age or older ($\geq$65 years in African Americans or Hispanic Americans) who did not have a history of cardiovascular disease, dementia or disability received either aspirin 100 mg or placebo daily. After a median of 4.7 years of follow-up, the composite rate of death, dementia or persistent physical disability did not differ between groups. The prespecified secondary endpoint of fatal and nonfatal MI, fatal or nonfatal stroke, including intracranial hemorrhage (ICH) or hospitalization for heart failure was 10.7 events per 1000 patient-years in the aspirin group and 11.3 events per 1000 person-years in the placebo group (hazard ratio [HR] 0.95; 95% CI, 0.83–1.08; P = ns). A major adverse cardiovascular event, defined as a composite of fatal coronary heart disease, nonfatal MI, or fatal or non-fatal stroke occurred in 7.8 per 1000 person-years and 8.8 per 1000 persons years, respectively (HR 0.89, 95% CI 0.77–1.03, P = ns). The major hemorrhage rate was 8.6 events per 1000 person-years and 6.2 events per 1000 person-years, respectively (HR 1.38; 95% CI 1.18–1.62; $P \leq 0.001$).[35]

In the ASCEND[36] study, 15,480 adults with diabetes mellitus without known cardiovascular disease were randomly assigned to either aspirin 100 mg daily or matching placebo. During a median follow-up of 7.4 years, serious vascular events occurred in 8.5% and 9.6% of patients, respectively (rate ratio [RR] 0.88; 95% CI, 0.79–0.97; P = 0.01). By contrast, major bleeding events occurred in 4.1% and 3.2% of patients, respectively (RR 1.29; 95% CI, 1.09–1.52; P = 0.003).

The benefit-to-risk ratio for aspirin at a dose of 75–100 mg daily becomes favorable with a 10-year ASCVD risk $\geq$10%; however, bleeding risk must be considered carefully (e.g., history of peptic ulcer disease, thrombocytopenia, heritable or acquired hemostatic disorders). Aspirin in the primary prevention of MI and stroke should also be considered in patients who have not achieved optimal control of ASCVD risk factors. Prophylactic aspirin in adults $\geq$70 years of age is not recommended. Last, the potential benefit of aspirin in persons $\leq$40 years of age has not been studied. There may be a role in high-risk settings, to include high calcium score as determined by coronary computed tomography (CT) angiography and uncontrolled risk factors (Table 8.2).[37]

Stable Cardiovascular Disease

In the COMPASS study, 27,395 participants with stable atherosclerotic vascular disease (coronary artery or peripheral artery) were randomly assigned to receive rivaroxaban 2.5 mg twice daily plus

Table 8.2

Aspirin for the primary prevention of cardiovascular disease		
COR	**LOE**	**Recommendations**
IIb	A	1. Low-dose aspirin (75–100 mg orally daily) might be considered for the primary prevention of ASCVD among select adults 40 to 70 years of age who are at higher ASCVD risk but not at increased bleeding risk (S4.6-1-S4.6-8).
III: Harm	B-R	2. Low-dose aspiring (75–100 mg orally daily) should not be administered on a routine basis for the primary prevention of ASCVD among adults >70 years of age (S4.6-9).
III: Harm	C-LD	3. Low-dose aspirin (75–100 mg orally daily) should not be administered for the primary prevention of ASCVD among adults of any age who are at increased risk of bleeding (S4.6-10).

ASCVD, Atherosclerotic coronary vascular disease; *COR,* class of recommendation; *LOE,* level of evidence.
Data from Arnett et.al. 2019 ACC/AHA Guideline of the Primary Prevention of Cardiovascular Disease. *Circulation* 2019 online.

aspirin 100 mg once daily, rivaroxaban 5 mg twice daily or aspirin 100 mg once daily. The primary outcome was a composite of cardiovascular death, stroke, or MI. The study was stopped for superiority of the rivaroxaban plus aspirin group after a mean follow-up of 23 months. The primary outcome occurred in fewer patients in the rivaroxaban plus aspirin group than in the aspirin alone group (4.1% versus 5.4%; HR 0.76; 95% CI 0.66–0.86; $P < 0.001$);[38] however, there was a higher rate of major bleeding (3.1% versus 1.9%; HR 1.70, 95% CI 1.40–2.05; $P < 0.001$). There was no difference in either intracranial or fatal bleeding between groups. All-cause death was lower in the rivaroxaban plus aspirin group when compared with the aspirin alone group. Participants receiving rivaroxaban alone did not benefit compared to those treated with aspirin alone, but major bleeding rates were higher.

Additional analysis of the COMPASS study revealed a particularly marked effect of combined rivaroxaban and aspirin for the prevention of primary and secondary stroke.[39] Ischemic/uncertain strokes were reduced by nearly half as was the occurrence of fatal and disabling stroke. Independent predictors of stroke included prior stroke, hypertension, increased systolic blood pressure at baseline, age, diabetes mellitus, and Asian ethnicity. Prior stroke was the strongest predictor of incident stroke with a HR of 3.63.

Secondary Prevention of Vascular Events

The Antiplatelet Trialists Collaboration,[40] based on a comprehensive evaluation of existing data, provides convincing evidence in support of aspirin's ability to prevent vascular events (vascular death, nonfatal MI, nonfatal stroke) in a wide variety of high-risk patients. Antiplatelet therapy (predominantly aspirin therapy) reduces nonfatal MI by approximately one-third, nonfatal stroke by one-third, and vascular death by one-quarter.

Aspirin Dosing

An updated meta-analysis of the Antiplatelet Trialists' Collaboration provides additional information on the differential effects of aspirin dosing.[40] Among 3570 patients in three trials directly comparing aspirin ($\geq$75 mg daily versus aspirin <75 mg daily) there were significant differences in vascular events (two trials compared 75–325 mg aspirin daily versus <75 mg daily and one trial compared 500–1500 mg aspirin daily versus <75 mg daily). Considering both direct and indirect comparisons of aspirin dose, the proportional reduction in vascular events was 19% with 500–1500 mg daily, 26% with 160–325 mg daily and 32% with 75–150 mg daily. The effect of antiplatelet drugs other than aspirin (versus control) were assessed in 166 trials that included 81,731 patients. Indirect comparisons provided no clear evidence of differences in reducing serious vascular events (χ^2 for heterogeneity between any aspirin regimen and other antiplatelet drugs = 10.8 ns). Most direct comparisons assessed the effects of replacing aspirin with another antiplatelet agent. While there remains interest in optimal dosing frequency for aspirin, particularly among individuals with diabetes mellitus, once-daily dosing is currently the standard of care.

Coronary Artery Bypass Grafting (CABG)

Aspirin Before CABG

In the ATACAS study,[41] 2100 patients scheduled to undergo CABG received either aspirin 100 mg or placebo preoperatively. The primary outcome was a composite of death and thrombotic complications (nonfatal MI, stroke, pulmonary embolism [PE], renal failure or bowel infarction) within 30 days of surgery. The primary outcome occurred in 19.3% and 20.4% of patients, respectively (RR 0.94; 95% CI 0.80 to 1.12; P = 0.55). Major hemorrhage rates did not differ between groups. There are several limitations to the study that require consideration. The investigators chose to use an enteric-coated aspirin preparation that is known to have delayed absorption and peak effect.[42] Patients participating in the

"Continuing *versus* Stopping Aspirin" study were given a 100-mg enteric-coated aspirin 1–2 hours prior to surgery. Based on the well-known pharmacokinetics of aspirin, there is a high likelihood that there was not sufficient time to reach maximum concentration (C_{max}) and maximum platelet inhibition prior to the start of the surgery. Once surgery begins and the patient is placed on cardio-pulmonary bypass, local concentrations and related pharmacody-namics effects, i.e., at coronary sites of plaque of newly placed bypass conduits, would be quite low. This study had a higher than expected rate of MI in both groups. The ATACAS investigators spec-ulate that this was the end-result of closer monitoring and increased troponin surveillance, i.e., higher detection rate. Could this actually be because aspirin was stopped in many patients at least 4 days prior to surgery, leading to a higher risk of complications? By stop-ping aspirin early, there could have also been patients who were excluded from participating in the study if they experienced a cor-onary event in the interim before CABG. This would have biased the outcomes. Perhaps there is a separate take-home message that applies to some high-risk patients: aspirin should not be stopped prior to CABG.

A number of clinical trials have been conducted to determine the effectiveness of antiplatelet therapy in preventing early (≤10 days) and late (6–12 months) saphenous vein graft occlusion. Ten of the trials investigated aspirin doses ranging from 100 mg to 975 mg daily. Several also evaluated patients receiving internal mammary artery coronary bypass grafts.[43] Considered collectively, and aided by the Antiplatelet Trialists' Collaboration overview, the data show improved saphenous vein graft patency with aspirin administration. Although a direct benefit on internal mammary bypass graft patency has not been established, treatment is recom-mended given the common coexistence of vascular disease (and the risk for thrombotic events).

Percutaneous Coronary Intervention

PCI, including plain old balloon angioplasty (POB), rotational atherectomy, and laser angioplasty, with or without stent place-ment, is associated with vascular injury, atheromatous plaque dis-ruption, platelet activation, and coronary thromboembolism. Several studies have documented reduced periprocedural compli-cations, including thrombus formation, abrupt closure, and MI, with antiplatelet therapy given prior to PCI (relative risk reduction [RRR], 60%).[44] The current recommendations for PCI include aspi-rin 81–325 mg prior to PCI and 81–325 mg daily after PCI for second-ary prevention of cardiovascular events. For patients unable to tolerate aspirin, pretreatment with clopidogrel (600 mg oral loading dose) followed by 75 mg daily is suggested.

Peripheral Artery Disease

Although proven to reduce cardiovascular mortality in CAD, there are modest data evaluating the efficacy of aspirin in patients with PAD. The 2002 Antiplatelet Trialists' meta-analysis demonstrated a significant 23% odds reduction in ischemic events when antiplatelet agents were compared to placebo. Two-thirds of the trials included in the meta-analysis evaluated agents other than aspirin. Since that time, three randomized, controlled trials have evaluated aspirin versus placebo in patients with PAD. Two of these studies enrolled asymptomatic patients with ABI ≤ 0.99 and 0.95, respectively, and failed to show a benefit from aspirin use. [45] The third trial, the Critical Leg Ischemia Prevention Study (CLIPS), enrolled patients with either symptomatic PAD or ABI <0.85 and demonstrated a risk reduction in cardiovascular and vascular ischemic events of 64% in patients randomized to aspirin.[46] By contrast, a 2009 meta-analysis of aspirin therapy in patients with PAD showed no significant change in cardiovascular events, all-cause mortality, or cardiovascular mortality.[47] The current recommendations from the AHA/ACC are as follows: antiplatelet therapy with aspirin alone (75–325 mg per day) or clopidogrel alone (75 mg per day) is recommended to reduce MI, stroke and vascular death in patients with symptomatic PAD (level IA).[48]

Left Ventricular Assist Device

Low-dose aspirin is *not* routinely discontinued prior to left ventricular assist device (LVAD) implantation; however, if it is, restarting is suggested postoperatively on day 2 or 3 and continued indefinitely unless bleeding occurs. The recommended aspirin dose for the HeartMate II is 81–325 mg daily, while a dose of 325 mg daily is recommended for the HeartWare LVAD.[49-51]

Aspirin Response Variability

Aspirin's ability to inhibit platelet aggregation is variable and influenced by the population studied, conditions, and the methodology employed.[52] Laboratory response can also be affected by concomitant administration of Ibuprofen and by acute illness.[53] Given that there appears to be little or no variability in the level of COX-1-dependent platelet aggregation among patients compliant with recommended doses of aspirin, much of the variability in aspirin response is believed to be due to biological variability and heritability of COX-1-independent ADP, collagen, and epinephrine responses.[54]

The COX-2 enzyme prevalent in inflammatory cells may play a role in aspirin response variability.[55] Specifically, pharmacogenomic analyses have shown associations between polymorphisms in PTGS2, the gene encoding COX-2, and the efficacy of aspirin-mediated reduction in thromboxane B_2 production.[55]

The most convincing data supporting genetic determination of aspirin response variability exists for the Pl^A polymorphism of the ITGB3 gene encoding GPIIIa. GPIIIa is pivotal for platelet binding of fibrinogen, von Willebrand factor, fibronectin, and vitronectin. Carriers of Pl^{A2} are more resistant to the antithrombotic effect of aspirin than carriers of Pl^{A1}, and multiple studies have suggested a heightened increased risk of MI, cerebral vascular events, and venous thrombosis. Despite several interesting observations, the findings of multiple studies on the effect of Pl^A polymorphisms have been divergent and several meta-analyses have drawn different conclusions.[56]

Clinical Impact of Aspirin Response Variability

Despite its proven benefit, aspirin does have inherent limitations, and the evidence compiled over several decades shows that patients receiving aspirin can still experience cardiovascular events. Although multiple studies and meta-analyses have documented increased risk of cardiovascular events in patients defined as in vitro nonresponders,[57,58] other studies have demonstrated no difference in clinical outcomes based on in vitro aspirin responsiveness or based on genetic polymorphisms associated with in vitro resistance. As a result, routine platelet function testing is not recommended.

Drug Therapy After Peripheral Artery Revascularization

In contrast to the data for aspirin administration in asymptomatic PAD, there are data supporting its use as adjuvant therapy following lower extremity bypass. In a meta-analysis, the Antiplatelet Trialists' Collaboration[40] demonstrated an odds reduction of 43% for the prevention of vascular occlusion with aspirin therapy compared to placebo. The analysis consisted primarily of patients who had undergone lower extremity bypass; however, two studies did assess the usefulness of aspirin as adjuvant therapy in patients undergoing lower extremity angioplasty. A subsequent randomized trial and two Cochrane systematic reviews support a more robust effect for aspirin in prosthetic grafts than in autologous conduits.[59]

Percutaneous transluminal angioplasty (PTA), often with stent insertion, is a common treatment approach for patients with aorto-iliac and superficial femoral artery obstructive disease. An early Cochrane review supported aspirin, 50–330 mg daily either with or without dipyridamole, initiated before femoro-politeal

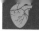

endovascular treatment, as an effective and safe strategy to reduce reocclusion at 6 and 12 months as compared to placebo or VKA.[60] The ACCF/AHA guidelines give aspirin a class I indication for patients undergoing lower extremity revascularization, either bypass grafting or endovascular intervention.

Based on the beneficial effect of dual antiplatelet therapy (DAPT) with aspirin and clopidogrel for preventing coronary stent thrombosis, there has been significant interest in the effect of DAPT after lower extremity PTA with stenting. Ticlopidine has been shown to reduce loss of vessel patency (odds ratio [OR] 0.53; 95% CI 0.33–0.85) and amputation (OR 0.29; 95% CI 0.08–1.01).[61] A strategy of aspirin plus clopidogrel for 24 hours *before* and 4 weeks *after* endovascular procedures has become a common approach to the reduction of acute and subacute thrombotic complications after endovascular procedures.

The clopidogrel and acetylsalicylic acid in bypass surgery for peripheral artery disease (CASPAR) trial randomized patients to either clopidogrel plus aspirin or placebo plus aspirin with a primary composite outcome of graft occlusion, revascularization, above ankle amputation or death. There was a nonsignificant difference in the primary endpoint in the overall population and venous graft subgroups; however, in the prosthetic graft subgroup, aspirin plus clopidogrel significantly reduced the primary endpoint (HR 0.65; 95% CI 0.45–0.95; $P = 0.025$) without an increase in severe bleeding.[62] As a result, the ACCF/AHA guidelines give DAPT a class IIb (may be considered) recommendation in patients previously revascularized who are at high risk for ischemic events.

Venous Thromboembolism

Becattini and colleagues reported a marked reduction in recurrent venous thromboembolism among 402 carefully selected patients with unprovoked events who were randomly assigned to either aspirin (100 mg daily) or placebo and were followed for 2 years (recurrence rate per year, 6.6% versus 11.2%; HR 0.58, 95% CI 0.36–0.93). The adverse-event profile accompanying aspirin treatment was acceptable to most patients and physicians. A majority of the recurrences of venous thromboembolism occurred in the absence of known risk factors; death attributed to PE was infrequent, and major or clinically relevant nonmajor bleeding was rare.

Contraindications to Aspirin

The major contraindications are aspirin intolerance, recent GI bleeding, active or recurring peptic ulcer, other potential sources of GI or genitourinary bleeding, and anaphylaxis. The risk of aspirin-induced GI bleeding is increased by alcohol, corticosteroid therapy, and nonsteroid antiinflammatory drugs (NSAIDs). Hemophilia (A, B, or C) is not an absolute contraindication to aspirin when there are strong cardiovascular indications; however, working closely with the patient and a hematology specialist is suggested.

Drug Interactions With Aspirin

Concurrent warfarin and aspirin therapy increases the risk of bleeding, especially with an aspirin dose above 75 mg daily. Among NSAIDs, those with dominant COX-1 activity (e.g., ibuprofen and naproxen), but not those with dominant COX-2 activity (e.g., diclofenac), may interfere with the cardioprotective effects of aspirin. Angiotensin-converting enzyme (ACE) inhibitors and aspirin have potentially opposing effects on renal hemodynamics, with aspirin inhibiting and ACE inhibitors promoting the formation of vasodilatory prostaglandins. Phenobarbital, phenytoin, and rifampin decrease the efficacy of aspirin through induction of the hepatic enzymes metabolizing aspirin. The effect of oral hypoglycemic agents and insulin may be enhanced by aspirin.

Aggrenox

Pharmacodynamics

The dipyridamole component of aggrenox and cilostazol, both phosphodiesterase inhibitors, is used predominantly in patients with peripheral vascular and cerebrovascular disease. Aggrenox is a combination platelet antagonist that includes aspirin (25 mg) and dipridamole (200 mg extended-release preparation). It is typically taken twice daily. Aspirin's mechanism of action has been discussed previously. Dipyridamole inhibits cyclic adenosine monophosphate (cAMP)-phosphodiesterase (PDE) and cyclic-3', 5'-GMP-PDE.[63] Dipyridamole inhibits platelet aggregation by two mechanisms. First, it attenuates adenosine uptake into platelets (as well as endothelial cells and erythrocytes). The resulting increase elicits a rise in cellular adenylate cyclase concentrations, resulting in elevated cAMP levels, which inhibit platelet activation to several stimuli, including ADP, collagen, and platelet-activating factor. Dipyridamole also inhibits PDE. The subsequent increase in cAMP elevates nitric oxide concentration, facilitating platelet inhibitory potential.[64]

Pharmacokinetics

The pharmacokinetic profile of aspirin has been summarized previously. Peak dipyridamole levels in plasma are achieved within several hours of oral administration (400 mg dose of Aggrenox).

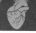

Extensive metabolism via conjugation with glucuronic acid occurs in the liver. There are no significant pharmacokinetic interactions between aspirin and dipyridamole coadministered as Aggrenox.

Adverse Effects

The European Stroke Prevention Study-2[65] (ESPS) reported that 79.9% of patients experienced at least one on-treatment adverse event. The most common side effects were GI complaints and headache. Dipyridamole has vasodilatory effects and should be used with caution in patients with severe CAD in whom episodes of angina pectoris may increase. Patients receiving Aggrenox should not be given adenosine for myocardial perfusion studies.

Administration in Older Patients

Plasma concentrations of dipyridamole are approximately 40% higher in patients greater than 65 years of age compared with younger individuals.

Clinical Experience

Aggrenox has not been studied in patients with ACS. The European Stroke Study (ESPS)-2[65,66] included 6602 patients with ischemic stroke (76% of the total population) or transient ischemic attack who were randomized to receive aggrenox, dipyridamole alone, aspirin alone, or placebo. Aggrenox reduced the risk of stroke by 22.1% compared with aspirin and by 24.4% compared with dipyridamole. Both differences were statistically significant ($P = 0.008$ and $P = 0.002$, respectively).

Aggrenox is not considered inter changeable with its individual components, particularly aspirin, which may be required in larger doses among patients with CAD. In addition, the vasodilatory effects of dipyridamole can cause coronary "steal" and angina pectoris. Accordingly, Aggrenox should be used cautiously, if at all, in the setting of advanced CAD.

Cilostazol

Pharmacodynamics

Cilostazol, a guinolinone derivative, and several of its metabolites inhibit phosphodiesterase III activity and suppress cAMP degradation with a resultant increase in cAMP in platelets and blood vessels, leading to inhibition of platelet aggregation and vasodilation, respectively.[66] Increasing cAMP concentrations within endothelial cells causes vasodilation, whereas elevated levels in platelets impair their ability to aggregate.

Pharmacokinetics

Cilostazol is well absorbed after oral administration, particularly when given with a high-fat meal. Metabolism occurs via the hepatic cytochrome P450 (CYP450) enzymes, and most of the metabolites are excreted in the urine (75% of overall clearance). One of the two active metabolites is responsible for more than 50% of PDE III inhibition. Pharmacokinetics are approximately dose proportional. Cilostazol and its active metabolites have apparent elimination half-lives of about 11 to 13 hours. Cilostazol and its active metabolites accumulate about twofold with chronic administration and reach steady state blood levels within a few days.

Adverse Effects

The most common adverse effect associated with cilostazol administration is headache. Other relatively frequent causes of drug discontinuation include palpitations and diarrhea. Several PDE III inhibitors have been associated with decreased survival in patients with class III/IV congestive heart failure. Cilostazol is contraindicated in patients with heart failure of any severity. Cilostazol and several of its metabolites are inhibitors of phosphodiesterase III. Several drugs with this pharmacologic effect have caused decreased survival compared to placebo in patients with class III–IV heart failure.

Use in Older Patients

The clearance of cilostazol (and its metabolites) has not been determined in patients older than age 65.

Use in Patients With Renal Insufficiency

Moderate-to-severe renal impairment increases cilostazol metabolite levels and alters protein binding of the parent compound. Patients with advanced renal insufficiency have not been studied.

Drug Interactions

Aspirin

Short-term (less than or equal to 4 days) coadministration of aspirin with Cilostazol increased the inhibition of ADP-induced ex vivo platelet aggregation by 22% to 37% when compared to either aspirin or Cilostazol alone. Short-term (less than or equal to 4 days) coadministration of aspirin with Cilostazol increased the inhibition of arachidonic acid-induced ex vivo platelet aggregation by 20% compared to Cilostazol alone and by 48% compared to aspirin alone.

Clinical Experience

Cilostazol is approved for the treatment of intermittent claudication. Across seven clinical trials, the improvement in walking distance (compared with placebo) was approximately 30 meters.[67] Although there is experience with cilostazol after coronary arterial stenting, its long-term administration to patients with CAD has not been studied. Short-term coadministration with aspirin reduced ADP-mediated platelet aggregation by 30% to 40% (compared with aspirin alone). The CILostazol-based triple antiplatelet therapy ON ischemic complication after drug-eluting stenT implantation trial (CILON-T) randomized 960 patients to DAPT with aspirin and clopidogrel versus aspirin and clopidogrel plus 6 months of cilostazol. While the addition of cilostazol resulted in a reduction in platelet reactivity at 6 months (201.7 ± 87.9 platelet reactivity units versus 255.7 ± 73.7 PRU, $P < 0.001$), there was no difference in the primary endpoint of cardiac death, nonfatal MI, ischemic stroke, or target lesion revascularization (8.5 versus 9.2%, $P = 0.74$).[68] Cilostazol should not be considered a substitute for aspirin or clopidogrel in patients with ACS who have concomitant peripheral artery disease.

Vorapaxar

Vorapaxar is a tricyclic himbacine-derived selective inhibitor of protease activated receptor (PAR-1). By inhibiting PAR-1, a thrombin receptor expressed on platelets, vorapaxar prevents thrombin-mediated platelet activation and aggregation.

Pharmacodynamics

Vorapaxar inhibits platelet aggregation through the reversible antagonism of PAR-1, also known as thrombin receptor. PARs are a family of G-protein coupled receptors highly expressed on platelets and activated by serine protease activity of thrombin to mediate thrombotic response. By blocking PAR-1 activation, vorapaxar inhibits thrombin-induced platelet aggregation and thrombin receptor agonist peptide (TRAP)-induced platelet aggregation. Vorapaxar does not inhibit platelet aggregation induced by other agonists such as ADP, collagen, or a thromboxane mimetic.

Pharmacokinetics

After oral administration, vorapaxar is rapidly absorbed and peak concentrations occur at a median tmax of 1 hour under fasting conditions. The mean absolute bioavailability is 100%. Vorapaxar is primarily eliminated as its metabolite M19 through the feces (91.5%), and partially eliminated in the urine (8.5%). It has an effective half-life of 3–4 days with an apparent terminal half-life of 8 days.

Adverse Effects

Hemorrhagic complications were observed in the two large phase III clinical trials of vorapaxar. In TRA-2P,[69] moderate or severe bleeding occurred in 4.2% of patients who received vorapaxar and 2.5% of those who received placebo (HR 1.66; 95% CI 1.43–1.93; $P < 0.001$). There was an increase in the rate of intracranial hemorrhage in the vorapaxar group (1.0% versus 0.5% in the placebo group, $P < 0.001$). In TRACER,[70 71] rates of moderate and severe bleeding were 7.2% in the vorapaxar group and 5.2% in the placebo group (HR 1.35; 95% CI 1.16–1.58; $P < 0.001$). Intracranial hemorrhage rates were 1.1% and 0.2%, respectively (HR 3.39; 95% CI 1.78–6.45; $P < 0.001$). The trial was stopped by the data and safety monitoring committee. Rates of nonhemorrhagic adverse events were similar in the two groups.

Clinical Experience

In the TRA-2P study,[69] 26,449 patients who had a history of MI, ischemic stroke, or PAD were randomized to receive vorapaxar (2.5 mg daily) or matching placebo and followed for a median of 30 months. The primary efficacy endpoint was the composite of death from cardiovascular causes, MI, or stroke. After 2 years, the data and safety monitoring board recommended discontinuation of the study treatment in patients with a history of stroke owing to the risk of intracranial hemorrhage. At 3 years, the primary endpoint had occurred in 1028 patients (9.3%) in the vorapaxar group and in 1176 patients (10.5%) in the placebo group (HR 0.87; 95% CI 0.80–0.94; $P < 0.001$). Cardiovascular death, MI, stroke, or recurrent ischemia leading to revascularization occurred in 1259 patients (11.2%) in the vorapaxar group and 1417 patients (12.4%) in the placebo group (HR 0.88; 95% CI 0.82–0.95; $P = 0.001$). Among the 3787 patients with PAD at study entry, there was no difference in the primary outcomes between treatment groups (11.3% and 11.9%, respectively; 0.94 [0.78, 1.14]; $P = 0.22$).

In the TRACER study,[70] vorapaxar was compared with placebo in 12,944 patients who had ACS without ST-segment elevation. The primary endpoint was a composite of death from cardiovascular causes, MI, stroke, recurrent ischemia with rehospitalization, or urgent coronary revascularization. Follow-up in the trial was terminated early after a safety review. After a median follow-up of 502 days (interquartile range, 349–667), the primary endpoint occurred in 1031 of 6473 patients receiving vorapaxar versus 1102 of 6471 patients receiving placebo (Kaplan-Meier 2-year rate, 18.5% versus 19.9%; HR 0.92; 95% CI 0.85–1.01; $P = 0.07$). A composite of death from cardiovascular causes, MI, or stroke occurred in

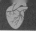

822 patients in the vorapaxar group versus 910 in the placebo group (14.7% and 16.4%, respectively; HR 0.89; 95% CI 0.81–0.98; $P = 0.02$). Among 936 patients with PAD at study entry, there were no differences in the primary outcome between groups (HR 0.85; 95% CI 0.67–1.08).

Vorapaxar is indicated for reducing the incidence of thrombotic cardiovascular events in patients with a history of MI or with peripheral artery disease.

Platelet P2Y$_{12}$ Receptor Antagonists

The density of P2Y$_{12}$ receptors on the platelet surface, coupled with its active role in the platelet activation and aggregation, makes it a highly attractive target for pharmacologic inhibition (Table 8.3).

Ticlopidine

Ticlopidine was the first oral platelet P2Y$_{12}$ receptor antagonist.

Pharmacodynamics

Ticlopidine hydrochloride, after oral ingestion, interferes with platelet membrane function by inhibiting ADP-induced platelet-fibrinogen binding and subsequent platelet-to-platelet interactions. The effect on platelet function is irreversible for the life of the platelet. Ticlopidine causes a time and dose-dependent inhibition of both platelet aggregation and release of platelet granule constituents.

Pharmacokinetics

After oral administration of a single 250 mg dose, ticlopidine is rapidly absorbed with peak plasma levels occurring at approximately 2 hours after dosing and is extensively metabolized. Absorption is greater than 80%. Administration after meals results in a 20% increase in the mean area under the concentration curve (AUC) of ticlopidine. The apparent half-life of ticlopidine after a single 250 mg dose is about 12.6 hours; with repeat dosing at 250 mg BID, the terminal elimination half-life rises to 4 to 5 days. Steady-state trough values in elderly patients (mean age 70 years) are about twice those in younger volunteer populations.

Ticlopidine is metabolized extensively by the liver; only trace amounts of intact drug are detected in the urine. Following an

Table 8.3

Major clinical trials of antiplatelet therapy in acute coronary syndrome

Trial acronym	Study description	Summary results
ACCOAST	NSTE-ACS patients; prasugrel pretreatment versus prasugrel at time of LHC but pre-PCI	No significant change in primary ischemic outcomes; significant increase in bleeding with pretreatment. Prasugrel recommended following angiography and before planned PCI; pretreatment discouraged
ATLANTIC	STE-ACS patients; ticagrelor prehospital versus ticagrelor at time of primary PCI	No change in primary outcomes related to vessel patency; pretreatment reduced post primary PCI stent thrombosis. Prehospital ticagrelor should not be routinely recommended
CHAMPION PHOENIX	Patients with stable angina or ACS undergoing PCI; aspirin plus cangrelor versus aspirin plus clopidogrel	Intravenous cangrelor reduced the rates of death, MI, ischemia-driven revascularization, and stent thrombosis in patients undergoing PCI
CURE	NSE-ACS/UA patients; clopidogrel versus placebo with aspirin	Clopidogrel led to a significant reduction in death from CV causes, nonfatal MI, and stroke
CURRENT-OASIS 7	NSTE and STE-ACS patients; evaluated standard versus higher doses of aspirin and clopidogrel	No benefit of higher doses of aspirin or clopidogrel in ACS
DAPT	Patients with previous PCI with DES; 12 Months versus 30 months DAPT	Prolonged DAPT reduced MI, stroke, and death; and significantly increased major, but not fatal, bleeding. DAPT duration can be extended in patients with low bleeding/high ischemic risk
PEGASUS-TIMI-54	Prior MI 1–3 years; aspirin versus aspirin plus ticagrelor 60 mg BID or 90 mg BID	Prolonged DAPT reduced CV death, MI and stroke; increased major, but not fatal bleeding. DAPT duration can be extended beyond 12 months in patients with low risk of bleeding

PLATO	NSTE-STE ACS patients; ticagrelor versus clopidogrel in addition to aspirin	Compared to clopidogrel, ticagrelor reduced CV death, non-fatal MI and stroke; Increase in nonfatal bleeding
TRILOGY-ACS	Patients with NSTE-ACS not undergoing PCI; prasugrel versus clopidogrel in addition to aspirin	No change in the primary endpoint of CV death, nonfatal MI, or stroke
TRITON TIMI 38	Patients with UA, NSTE-ACS undergoing PCI; prasugrel versus clopidogrel in addition to aspirin	Compared to clopidogrel, prasugrel reduced CV death, non-fatal MI, stroke and stent thrombosis in patients undergoing PCI if bleeding risk not excessive. Avoid in patients >75 years, weight <60 kg, and previous TIA

BID, Twice daily; *CV*, cardiovascular; *DAPT*, dual antiplatelet therapy; *ICH*, intracranial hemorrhage; *IDR*, ischemia driven revascularization; *LHC*, left heart catheterization; *MACE*, major adverse cardiovascular events; *MI*, myocardial infarction; *NSTE-ACS*, non ST elevation acute coronary syndrome; *PCI*, percutaneous coronary intervention; *PPCI*, primary percutaneous coronary intervention; *RCT*, randomized controlled trial; *STE-ACS*, ST elevation acute coronary syndrome; *TIA*, transient ischemic attack; *TIMI*, thrombolysis in myocardial infarction; *UA*, unstable angina.

oral dose of radioactive ticlopidine hydrochloride administered in solution, 60% of the radioactivity is recovered in the urine and 23% in the feces.

Adverse Effects

Ticlopidine is associated with a risk of life-threatening blood dyscrasias, including thrombotic thrombocytopenic purpura (TTP), neutropenia/agranulocytosis, and aplastic anemia. Hemorrhagic events most often effecting the GI tract can also occur.

Clinical Experience

Ticlopidine

Despite limited clinical use because of side effects such as neutropenia, agranulocytosis, and thrombotic thrombocytopenic purpura, ticlopidine has been proven effective in preventing MI, stroke, and transient ischemic attack (TIA) in patients with PAD. Specifically, in the randomized, double-blind Swedish Ticlopidine Multicentre Study (STIMS), ticlopidine reduced mortality by 29.1% as compared to placebo.[71] Ticlopidine may also be effective in reducing the progression of femoral atherosclerosis and be beneficial in maintaining patency of peripheral bypasses.[59] Among patients with a prior TIA or stroke, ticlopidine should be reserved for patients who are intolerant or allergic to aspirin therapy or who have failed aspirin therapy. Safer options are available.

Clopidogrel

Pharmacodynamics

Clopidogrel, a thienopyridine derivative, is a platelet antagonist that is several times more potent than ticlopidine but associated with fewer adverse effects (described below). The important role of ADP-mediated platelet activation and aggregation in atherothrombotic vascular disease has made the surface $P2Y_{12}$ receptor a favored target for drug development. Clopidogrel irreversibly inhibits the binding of ADP to its platelet receptor ($P2Y_{12}$) and the subsequent G-protein linked mobilization of intracellular calcium and activation of the glycoprotein (GP) IIb/IIIa complex.[72] At steady state, the average inhibition to ADP is between 40% and 60%.

Pharmacokinetics

Clopidogrel is rapidly absorbed following oral administration with peak plasma levels of the predominant circulating metabolite occurring approximately 60 minutes later. As a prodrug, it is extensively metabolized in the liver to an active compound with a plasma elimination half-life of 7.7 ± 2.3 hours. Dose-dependent inhibition of ADP-mediated platelet aggregation is observed several hours after a single oral dose of clopidogrel, with a more significant inhibition achieved with loading doses ($\geq$300 mg). A 600-mg oral loading dose achieves effective platelet inhibition in 2–3 hours. Repeated doses of 75 mg clopidogrel per day (without a loading dose) inhibit aggregation with steady state being reached between day 3 and day 7.

Adverse Effects and Safety

The available information suggests that clopidogrel offers safety advantages over ticlopidine, particularly with regard to bone marrow suppression and other hematologic abnormalities. Although Idiopathic thrombocytopenic purpura (ITP) and TTP have been reported with clopidogrel,[73] their occurrence is rare.

Clinical Experience

Peripheral Artery Disease

The well-documented benefit derived from platelet inhibition in patients with vascular disease, coupled with a concerning adverse-effect profile observed ticlopidine, fostered the rapid development of clopidogrel. The Clopidogrel versus Aspirin in Patients at Risk for Ischemic Events (CAPRIE) Study[74] randomized patients with atherosclerotic vascular disease, defined as recent stroke, MI, or PAD, to either clopidogrel 75 mg per day or aspirin 325 mg daily. Patients treated with clopidogrel (by intention-to-treat analysis) had a 5.32% annual risk of ischemic stroke, MI, or vascular death compared with 5.83% among aspirin-treated patients (RRR 8.7%; 95% CI 0.3–16.5; $P = 0.043$). There was no major difference in safety between treatment groups; however, a greater proportion of patients receiving aspirin had the study drug permanently discontinued because of GI hemorrhage, indigestion, nausea, or vomiting. Approximately 1 out of every 1000 patients treated with clopidogrel experienced neutropenia ($<1.2 \times 10^9$cells/L) (similar to aspirin treatment).

The trial design employed in CAPRIE was not configured to answer the important question of benefit and risk for dual platelet inhibition (aspirin plus clopidogrel). Accordingly, an additional study was undertaken. The CHARISMA (Clopidogrel for High Atherothrombotic Risk and Ischemic Stabilization, Management, and Avoidance) study[75] randomly assigned 15,603 patients with clinically evident cardiovascular disease or multiple risk factors to receive clopidogrel plus aspirin or low-dose aspirin plus placebo.

Patients were subsequently followed for a median of 28 months.[76] Respective rates for the principal secondary endpoint, which included hospitalization for ischemic events, were 16.7% and 17.9%, respectively (relative risk 0.92; 95% CI,0.86–0.995; $P = 0.04$). Rates of severe bleeding were 1.7% and 1.3%, respectively. Among patients with clinically evident atherothrombosis, the secondary endpoint occurred in 6.9% of patients receiving combination therapy versus 7.9% of those given aspirin alone (RR 0.88; 95% CI 0.77–0.998; $P = 0.046$). By contrast, patients with multiple risk factors (but no documented atherothrombotic disease) experienced a primary endpoint rate of 6.6% with combination therapy versus 5.5% with aspirin alone (RR 1.2; 95% CI 0.91–1.59; $P = 0.2$). The rate of death from cardiovascular causes was higher with combination therapy (3.9% versus 2.2%, $P = 0.01$).

On the basis of data from CHARISMA, one should conclude that the combination of clopidogrel plus aspirin is *not* more effective than aspirin alone in reducing the rate of MI, stroke, or death from cardiovascular causes among patients with *stable* cardiovascular disease or multiple cardiovascular risk factors. By contrast, benefit may be expected among individuals with symptomatic atherothrombotic disease.

Coronary Arterial Stenting

A multicenter, randomized, controlled trial, Clopidogrel Plus aspirin vs Ticlopidine Plus aspirin in Stent Patients Study (CLASSICS)[77,78] included 1020 patients undergoing PCI who received either aspirin (325 mg qd) plus ticlopidine (250 mg BID), aspirin plus clopidogrel (75 mg daily), or aspirin plus front-loaded clopidogrel (300 mg as an initial dose followed by 75 mg qd). Treatment was continued for 28 days after stent placement. Intravenous (IV) GPIIb/IIIa antagonists were *not* administered to patients enrolled in the trial. The primary safety endpoint was a composite of neutropenia, thrombocytopenia, bleeding, and drug discontinuation for adverse events (noncardiac). The secondary efficacy endpoint was a composite of MI, target vessel revascularization, and cardiovascular death. The primary endpoint was reached in 9.1% of ticlopidine-treated patients, 6.3% of clopidogrel-treated patients, and 2.9% of front-loaded clopidogrel-treated patients. Early drug discontinuation occurred in 8.2%, 5.1%, and 2.0% of patients, respectively. The most common adverse events prompting drug discontinuation were allergic reactions, GI distress, and skin rashes. The secondary cardiovascular endpoint was reached by 0.9%, 1.5%, and 1.3% of patients, respectively.

The importance of adequate platelet inhibition in patients undergoing PCI was confirmed in the PCI-CURE study.[78] A total of 2658 patients undergoing PCI were randomized to double-blind treatment with clopidogrel or placebo (aspirin alone) for, on average, 6 days before the procedure followed by 4 weeks of open-label thienopyridine (after which study drug was resumed for 8 months). The primary endpoint (cardiovascular death, MI, or urgent target vessel revascularization within 30 days) was reached in 4.5% of clopidogrel-treated patients and 6.4% of placebo-treated patients (30% relative risk reduction). Long-term administration of clopidogrel was associated with a lower rate of death, MI, or any revascularization with no increased bleeding complications.

Acute Coronary Syndrome (ACS)

Non-ST-Segment Elevation Myocardial Infarction (NSTEMI) and Unstable Angina

The benefit of therapy with aspirin and clopidogrel was investigated in the Clopidogrel in Unstable Angina to Prevent Recurrent Events (CURE) trial.[79] A total of 12,562 patients experiencing an ACS without ST-segment elevation received clopidogrel (300 mg immediately, 75 mg daily) plus aspirin (75–325 mg daily) or aspirin alone for 3–12 months. The composite of death, MI, or stroke occurred in 9.3% and 11.4 % of patients, respectively (RR reduction 20%). In hospital refractory ischemia, congestive heart failure, and revascularization procedures were also less frequent in clopidogrel-treated patients. There was a greater risk of major hemorrhage with combination therapy (3.7% versus 2.7%, RR 1.38); however, life-threatening bleeding and hemorrhagic stroke occurred at similar rates between groups.

Pre-PCI Treatment, Duration of Therapy, and Clinical Benefit

The CREDO (Clopidogrel for the Reduction of Events During Observation) trial[80] evaluated the long-term benefit (12 months) of treatment with clopidogrel after PCI as well as the potential benefit of initiating clopidogrel with a preprocedure loading dose (both in addition to aspirin therapy). A total of 2116 patients scheduled for elective PCI were randomly assigned to receive clopidogrel (300 mg) or placebo 3 to 24 hours before PCI. All patients received aspirin (325 mg). A majority of patients had either a recent MI or unstable angina as an indication for PCI. Thereafter, all patients received clopidogrel (75 mg daily) through day 28. From day 29 through 12 months, patients in the loading dose group received clopidogrel (75 mg daily) or placebo. Both groups continued to receive standard therapy including aspirin (81–325 mg daily). Pretreatment with clopidogrel was associated with a statistically nonsignificant 18.5% RRR for the combined endpoint of death, MI or target vessel revascularization at 28 days.

To better determine the optimal dosage for clopidogrel loading, the Antiplatelet therapy for Reduction of MYocardial Damage during Angioplasty (ARMYDA-2) trial randomized patients scheduled to undergo PCI to either a 300 mg or 600 mg loading dose of clopidogrel. The 600 mg loading dose was associated with a decrease in the primary endpoint of death, MI, or target vessel revascularization (4% versus 12%, $P = 0.041$) without a significant increase in bleeding.[81]

Duration of Dual Antiplatelet Therapy After PCI

In the DAPT study[82] patients were enrolled after they had undergone a coronary stent procedure in which a drug-eluting stent (DES) was placed. After 12 months of treatment with a thienopyridine drug (clopidogrel or prasugrel) and aspirin, patients were randomly assigned to continue receiving thienopyridine treatment or to receive placebo for another 18 months; all patients continued receiving aspirin. The coprimary efficacy endpoints were stent thrombosis and major adverse cardiovascular and cerebrovascular events (CVEs) (a composite of death, MI, or stroke) during the period from 12 to 30 months. The primary safety endpoint was moderate or severe bleeding. A total of 9961 patients were randomly assigned to continue thienopyridine treatment (most were receiving clopidogrel) or to receive placebo. Continued treatment with thienopyridine, as compared with placebo, reduced the rates of stent thrombosis (0.4% versus 1.4%, HR 0.29; 95% CI 0.17–0.48; $P < 0.001$) and major adverse cardiovascular and CVEs (4.3% versus 5.9%, HR 0.71; 95% CI 0.59–0.85; $P < 0.001$). The rate of MI was lower with thienopyridine treatment than with placebo (2.1% versus 4.1%, HR 0.47; $P < 0.001$). The rate of death from any cause was 2.0% in the group that continued thienopyridine therapy and 1.5% in the placebo group (HR 1.36; 95% CI 1.00–1.85; $P = 0.05$). The rate of moderate or severe bleeding was increased with continued thienopyridine treatment (2.5% versus 1.6%, $P = 0.001$). An elevated risk of stent thrombosis and MI was observed in both groups during the 3 months after discontinuation of thienopyridine treatment. DAPT beyond 1 year after placement of a drug-eluting stent, as compared with aspirin therapy alone, significantly reduced the risks of stent thrombosis and major adverse cardiovascular and CVEs but was associated with an increased risk of bleeding.

Clinical Decision-Making and Dual Antiplatelet Therapy

Complex PCI is associated with higher ischemic risk, which can be mitigated by long-term DAPT. However, concomitant high bleeding risk (HBR) may also be present, making it unclear whether short or long-term DAPT should be prioritized. A study by Costa and colleagues[83] investigated the effects of ischemic (by PCI complexity) and bleeding (by PRECISE-DAPT [PREdicting bleeding Complications in patients undergoing stent Implantation and SubsequEnt Dual AntiPlatelet Therapy] score) risks on clinical outcomes and on the impact of DAPT duration after coronary stenting. Complex PCI was defined as $\geq$ three stents implanted and/or $\geq$ three lesions treated, bifurcation stenting, and/or stent length >60 mm, and/or chronic total occlusion revascularization. Ischemic and bleeding outcomes in high ($\geq$25) or nonhigh (<25) PRECISE-DAPT strata were evaluated based on randomly allocated duration of DAPT. Among a total of 14,963 patients from eight randomized trials, 3118 underwent complex PCI and experienced a higher rate of ischemic, but not bleeding, events. Long-term DAPT in non-HBR patients reduced ischemic events in both complex (absolute risk difference: -3.86%; 95% CI -7.71 to $+0.06$) and noncomplex PCI strata (absolute risk difference: -1.14%; 95% CI -2.26 to -0.02), but not among HBR patients, regardless of complex PCI features. The bleeding risk according to the TIMI scale was increased by long-term DAPT only in HBR patients, regardless of PCI complexity.

ST-Segment Elevation Myocardial Infarction (STEMI)

The CLARITY-TIMI 28 trial[84] and the Clopidogrel and Metoprolol in Myocardial Infarction Trial/Second Chinese Cardiac Study (COM-MIT/CCS-2-Clopidogrel) trial suggested a role for clopidogrel in the treatment of ST-segment elevation MI (STEMI).[85] In the CLARITY-TIMI 28 study, addition of clopidogrel (300 mg loading dose, then 75 mg/day) to a regimen of aspirin plus thrombolysis before angiography improved infarct-related artery patency and reduced ischemic complications in patients who presented within 12 hours of onset of STEMI. The primary efficacy endpoint (a composite of infarct-related arterial occlusion [TIMI grade 0/1], death or recurrent MI before angiography) was reduced by 36% with clopidogrel, with the effect being driven predominantly by a reduction in arterial reocclusion. There was no increase in major bleeding or intracranial hemorrhage.

In the COMMIT trial, 45,852 patients with STEMI or bundle branch block (93%) and ST-segment depression (7%) were randomized to clopidogrel 75 mg daily or placebo in addition to aspirin 162 mg daily and usual care. Treatment with clopidogrel was associated with a 9% (95% CI 3%–14%) reduction in death, re-infarction, or stroke (2121 [9.2%] clopidogrel versus 2310 [10.1%] placebo, $P = 0.002$). This was accompanied by a 7% reduction in all-cause mortality (1726 [7.5%] versus 1845 [8.1%], $P = 0.03$). Similar to CLARITY-TIMI 28, there was no increase in overall bleeding, or bleeding among patients receiving fibrinolytic therapy.

Clopidogrel Pharmacodynamic Response Variability

High on-treatment platelet reactivity, defined as 1) platelet reactivity index >50% by vasodilator stimulated phosphoprotein phosphorylation (VASP –P) analysis; 2) >235 to 240 $P2Y_{12}$ reaction units by VerifyNow $P2Y_{12}$ assay; 3) >46% maximal 5 µmol/l ADP-induced aggregation; and 4) >468 arbitrary aggregation units/min in response to ADP by Multiplate analyzer[86] has been proposed to be a predictor of outcome following PCI. The Gauging Responsiveness with a VerifyNow assay-Impact on Thrombosis and Safety (GRAVITAS)[87,88] trial randomized 2214 patients with high on-treatment platelet reactivity (HPR) 12–24 hours after PCI with drug-eluting stents to high dose clopidogrel (600 mg initial dose, 150 mg daily thereafter) versus standard dose clopidogrel (no additional loading dose, 75 mg daily thereafter). Although high-dose clopidogrel provided a 22% absolute reduction in on-treatment platelet reactivity at 30 days (62% absolute reduction, 95% CI 59%–65% versus 40%, 95% CI 37%–43%; $P < 0.001$), at 6 months there was no significant difference in death from cardiovascular causes, nonfatal MI, or stent thrombosis. A secondary analysis of GRAVITAS determined the relationship between on-treatment platelet reactivity and cardiovascular outcomes. On-treatment reactivity of <208 P2Y12 reaction units was associated with a significantly lower risk of the primary endpoint at 60 days (HR 0.23; 95% CI 0.05–0.98; $P = 0.047$) even after adjustment for other predictors of outcome. Taken together, these data suggest that on-treatment platelet reactivity does correlate with the risk of adverse cardiac events; however, multiple randomized trials have failed to translate the initial observations to routine clinical practice that includes dose adjustment based on either platelet activity or genetic polymorphisms for the CYP 2C19 gene (see section on pharmacogenomics).

MitraClip Implantation and Transcutaneous Mitral Valve Replacement (TMVR)

The administration of periprocedural antiplatelet and anticoagulant agents for patients receiving MitraClip implantation is important for reducing the risk of stroke, systemic embolism, and device thrombosis. However, no evidence-based guidelines have yet addressed the choice or duration of antiplatelet and anticoagulant regimens; thus current choices remain contingent on the operators' experience and discretion. Many patients undergoing MitraClip or TMVR have coexisting morbidities such as atrial fibrillation requiring anticoagution. In the EVEREST trials, a regimen of aspirin 325 mg daily for 6–12 months was used. Clopidogrel at a dose of 75 mg daily was given for 1 month.[89]

Atrial Septal Defect / Patent Foramen Ovale (ASD/PFO) Percutaneous Closure

In patients undergoing ASD/PFO closure, a postprocedural antithrombotic therapy regimen typically includes a combination of aspirin 75–325 mg daily plus clopidogrel 75 mg daily for 1–3 months followed by aspirin monotherapy for an additional 3–5 months.[90,91]

Left Atrial Appendage (LAA) Closure

The patient population for whom left atrial appendage (LAA) closure (or exclusion) is recommended has a contraindication for long-term anticoagulation due to high risk of bleeding. A brief course of DAPT post procedure is generally administered followed by long-term aspirin monotherapy. The European Heart Rhythm Society consensus recommends using DAPT for up to 6 months after device implantation in patients with contraindications to OAC.[92] In patients with a prohibitive risk of bleeding, a single antiplatelet agent may be reasonable.

Prasugrel

Pharmacodynamics

Prasugrel, a third-generation thienopyridine $P2Y_{12}$ inhibitor, was approved by the US Food and Drug Administration (FDA) in July 2009 for patients with ACS undergoing PCI.

Pharmacokinetics

Prasugrel, a prodrug, undergoes rapid deesterification to an intermediate thiolactone, which is then converted to the active metabolite via a single CYP-dependent step. Maximal plasma concentrations of prasugrel's active metabolite are reached within 0.5 hours after oral administration. Inhibition of ADP binding to the platelet $P2Y_{12}$ receptor begins 15–30 minutes after administration of a 60 mg loading dose, and a maximal 60%–70% platelet inhibition is achieved at 2–4 hours.

During maintenance therapy with 10 mg daily dosing, there is a steady state of 50% platelet inhibition. After discontinuation of prasugrel, platelet aggregation returns to pretreatment levels within 7–10 days.

When compared to clopidogrel, administration of prasugrel results in earlier production and greater concentration of the equipotent active metabolites. Subsequently, prasugrel produces a more rapid onset and more consistent and greater level of platelet inhibition than clopidogrel in healthy subjects and patients with CAD.[93]

Safety

In the Trial to Assess Improvement in Therapeutic Outcomes by Optimizing Platelet Inhibition with Prasugrel–Thrombolysis in Myocardial Infarction (TRITON–TIMI) 38 (n = 13608), major bleeding was observed in 2.4% of patients treated with prasugrel and 1.8% of patients receiving clopidogrel (HR 1.32; 95% CI 1.03–1.68; $P = 0.03$). Prasugrel-treated patients experienced a higher incidence of life-threatening bleeding (1.4% versus 0.9%, $P = 0.01$) and fatal bleeding, including ICH (0.4% versus 0.1%, $P = 0.002$).[94] Bleeding risks were greatest in patient's ≥75 years old, those with a history of TIA or stroke, and those weighing <60 kg. As a result, prasugrel is *contraindicated* in patients with a history of TIA or stroke, and a dosage of 5 mg daily should be considered for patients <60 kg. In patient's ≥75 years of age, prasugrel is generally *not* recommended and should be used only after careful consideration of the potential risks and benefits.

Clinical Experience

Acute Coronary Syndrome

The benefit of prasugrel in patients with ACS was demonstrated in the TRITON-TIMI 38 trial. Moderate-to high-risk ACS patients scheduled to undergo PCI were randomized to either prasugrel (60 mg loading dose and 10 mg maintenance dose) or clopidogrel (300 mg loading dose and 75 mg maintenance dose) for 6–15 months. The primary endpoint of death from cardiovascular causes, nonfatal MI, or nonfatal stroke was observed in 9.9% of patients receiving prasugrel and 12.1% of patients receiving clopidogrel (HR 0.81; 95% CI 0.73–0.90; $P < 0.001$). There was also a decrease in the secondary endpoints of MI (7.4% versus 9.7%, $P < 0.001$), urgent target-vessel revascularization (2.5% versus 3.7%, $P < 0.001$), and stent thrombosis (1.1% versus 2.4%, $P < 0.001$) with prasugrel versus clopidogrel.[94]

Ticagrelor

Pharmacodynamics

Ticagrelor is a high-affinity ADP analogue that causes *reversible* inhibition of the P2Y$_{12}$ receptor. Unlike the thienopyridines, ticagrelor does *not* require metabolic activation or conversion for platelet inhibition; however, an active metabolite exerts an equally potent effect.

Pharmacokinetics

Ticagrelor is rapidly absorbed and undergoes enzymatic degradation to an active metabolite, which has similar pharmokinetics to the parent compound. Due to its rapid absorption, plasma concentrations of ticagrelor peak 1–3 hours after oral administration in a dose-dependent manor. This results in an average of 60%–80% inhibition of ADP-induced platelet aggregation 2–4 hours after a 180-mg loading dose. Plasma half-life is 6–13 hours, necessitating twice-daily administration.

As compared to clopidogrel, ticagrelor administration results in earlier, more robust, and more consistent and pronounced platelet inhibition. In patients with NSTEMI previously treated with clopidogrel, ticagrelor administration provided further platelet inhibition, regardless of the patient's level of responsiveness to clopidogrel.[95]

Adverse Effects

In the Study of Platelet Inhibition and Patient Outcomes (PLATO) (n = 18,624), ticagrelor plus aspirin versus clopidogrel plus aspirin was associated with a higher rate of major bleeding not related to CABG (4.5% versus 3.8%, $P = 0.03$). Fatal bleeding did not differ between groups. There was no significant difference in the rates of overall major bleeding between ticagrelor and clopidogrel (11.6% versus 11.2%, $P = 0.43$).[96] There was a numerically higher incidence of ICH among patients randomized to ticagrelor plus aspirin. Based on a comprehensive post hoc analysis of the US cohort of PLATO,[97] a boxed warning was included in FDA approval stating that the use of ticagrelor with maintenance doses of aspirin above 100 mg daily decreased its effectiveness. Thus, an aspirin dose of ≤100 mg daily is recommended.

Clinical Experience

Acute Coronary Syndrome

The benefits of ticagrelor in ACS were established in the PLATO trial. Patients were randomized to either ticagrelor (180 mg loading dose, 90 mg twice daily thereafter) or clopidogrel (300–600 mg loading dose, 75 mg daily thereafter). At 12 months, the primary composite endpoint of death from vascular causes, MI, or stroke occurred in 9.8% of the ticagrelor group and 11.7% of the clopidogrel group (HR 0.84; 95% CI 0.77–0.92; $P < 0.001$). Secondary endpoints, including MI (5.8% in the ticagrelor group versus 6.9% in the clopidogrel group, $P = 0.005$) and death from vascular causes (4.0% versus 5.1%, $P = 0.001$), were also reduced by ticagrelor.[98] As a result of these data, ticagrelor has a class I, level of evidence B, recommendation in patients undergoing PCI after ACS.

Long-Term Use of Ticagrelor

In the PEGASUS study,[99] 21,162 patients who had experienced a MI 1 to 3 years earlier were randomized to ticagrelor at a dose of 90 mg twice daily, ticagrelor at a dose of 60 mg twice daily, or placebo. All patients received low-dose aspirin and were followed for a median of 33 months. The primary efficacy endpoint was the composite of cardiovascular death, MI, or stroke. The primary safety endpoint was TIMI major bleeding. The two ticagrelor doses each reduced, as compared with placebo, the rate of the primary efficacy endpoint, with Kaplan–Meier rates at 3 years of 7.85% in the group that received 90 mg of ticagrelor twice daily, 7.77% in the group that received 60 mg of ticagrelor twice daily, and 9.04% in the placebo group (HR for 90 mg of ticagrelor versus placebo 0.85; 95% CI 0.75–0.96; $P = 0.008$; HR for 60 mg of ticagrelor versus placebo 0.84; 95% CI 0.74–0.95; $P = 0.004$). Rates of TIMI major bleeding were higher with ticagrelor (2.60% with 90 mg and 2.30% with 60 mg) than with placebo (1.06%) ($P < 0.001$ for each dose versus placebo); the rates of intracranial hemorrhage or fatal bleeding in the three groups were 0.63%, 0.71%, and 0.60%, respectively.

Peripheral Artery Disease

In the EUCLID trial,[100] 13,885 patients with symptomatic peripheral artery disease were randomized to receive monotherapy with ticagrelor (90 mg twice daily) or clopidogrel (75 mg once daily). Patients were eligible if they had an ABI of 0.80 or less or had undergone previous revascularization of the lower limbs. The primary efficacy endpoint was a composite of adjudicated cardiovascular death, MI, or ischemic stroke. The primary safety endpoint was major bleeding. The median follow-up was 30 months. The mean baseline ABI in all patients was 0.71, 76.6% of the patients had claudication, and 4.6% had critical limb ischemia. The primary efficacy endpoint occurred in 751 of 6930 patients (10.8%) receiving ticagrelor and in 740 of 6955 patients (10.6%) receiving clopidogrel (HR 1.02; 95% CI 0.92–1.13; $P = 0.65$). In each group, acute limb ischemia occurred in 1.7% of the patients (HR 1.03; 95% CI 0.79–1.33; $P = 0.85$) and major bleeding in 1.6% (HR 1.10; 95% CI 0.84–1.43; $P = 0.49$). The routine use of ticagrelor is not supported in the management of patients with PAD.

ST-Segment Elevation Myocardial Infarction

The efficacy of ticagrelor in the long-term post STEMI treated with fibrinolytic therapy remains uncertain. To evaluate the efficacy of ticagrelor when compared with clopidogrel in STEMI patients treated with fibrinolytic therapy, an international, multicenter, randomized, open-label with blinded endpoint adjudication trial enrolled 3799 patients (age <75 years) with STEMI receiving fibrinolytic therapy.[101] Patients were randomized to ticagrelor (180 mg loading dose, 90 mg twice daily thereafter) or clopidogrel (300–600 mg loading dose, 75 mg daily thereafter). The key outcomes were cardiovascular mortality, MI, or stroke, and the same composite outcome with the addition of severe recurrent ischemia, transient ischemic attack, or other arterial thrombotic events at 12 months. The combined outcome of cardiovascular mortality, MI, or stroke occurred in 129 of 1913 patients (6.7%) receiving ticagrelor and in 137 of 1886 patients (7.3%) receiving clopidogrel (HR 0.93; 95% CI 0.73–1.18; $P = 0.53$). The composite of cardiovascular mortality, MI, stroke, severe recurrent ischemia, transient ischemic attack, or other arterial thrombotic events occurred in 153 of 1,913 patients (8.0%) treated with ticagrelor and in 171 of 1886 patients (9.1%) receiving clopidogrel (HR 0.88; 95% CI 0.71–1.09; $P = 0.25$). The rates of major, fatal, and intracranial bleeding were similar between the ticagrelor and clopidogrel groups.

Platelet-Directed Therapies and Coronary Stent Thrombosis

Coronary stents improve outcomes in patients undergoing PCI, particularly those with ACS. However, stent thrombosis is a largely preventable and devastating complication associated with high rates of morbidity and mortality.[102] A majority of events occur between 0 and 30 days after PCI and the expected rate of thrombosis during this time is <1%. Late stent thrombosis, defined as thrombosis occurring greater than 30 days after PCI, occurs at a 0.2%–0.6% rate.[103] The overall incidence of stent thrombosis is lessening with time, operator experience, and stent materials and design.

While the most common cause of stent thrombosis is nonadherence to DAPT, contributing factors include increased platelet activation, thrombin generation, and inflammation associated with ACS. Drug eluting stents (DES) impair endothelial healing, helping to attenuate in-stent restenosis while also increasing the risk of thrombus formation. Examination of necropsy samples from patients who underwent DES insertion revealed that the ratio of nonendothelial cell covered stent struts to total struts was the best predictor of subsequent thrombosis. Despite the fact that bare-metal stents (BMS) are thought to develop an endothelial cell monolayer more completely than DES, there remains no discernable difference in the rates of stent thrombosis between DES and BMS within the first 12 months after PCI.[104]

Stent thrombosis typically presents as STEMI and is associated with significant morbidity and mortality. Accordingly, the American College of Cardiology (ACC) and the American Heart Association (AHA) have established guidelines regarding the use and length of antiplatelet therapy in patients with ACS following PCI (see Table 8.4). Aspirin should be continued indefinitely and a $P2Y_{12}$ inhibitor should be continued for at least 1 year unless the morbidity from bleeding risk outweighs the expected benefit.

On-Treatment Platelet Reactivity Testing

Although the mechanisms of clopidogrel dose-response variability are not yet completely elucidated, multiple lines of evidence strongly suggest that variable active metabolite generation is the primary explanation. Variable levels of active metabolite generation following clopidogrel administration may be explained by (1) variable intestinal absorption affected by an ABCB1 gene polymorphism, (2) functional variability in P450 activity due to drug-to-drug interactions, and (3) single nucleotide polymorphisms (SNPs) of specific CYP450 genes.[105] Coadministration of clopidogrel with proton pump inhibitors, lipophilic statins, and calcium channel blockers metabolized via CYP2C19 and CYP3A4 causes a diminished pharmacodynamics response to clopidogrel. Controversy remains, however, as to the clinical consequences of these interactions with respect to ischemic events.

High On-Treatment Platelet Reactivity and Post-PCI Events

The first prospective study demonstrating the link between HPR and ischemic events in patients treated with stents was the PRE-PARE POST-STENTING study. In this study by Gurbel et al., of 192 patients undergoing elective PCI and 300 mg loading dose of clopidogrel plus 75 mg daily maintenance dose, those patients with the highest quartile of on-treatment platelet reactivity had an OR of 2.7 for 6 month post-PCI ischemic events.[106] Although this study employed light transmittance aggregometry, subsequent studies have used the VerifyNow $P2Y_{12}$ assay, the VASP-phosphorylation assay, and the Multiplate analyzer to demonstrate that on-treatment

Table 8.4.

2014 AHA/ACC guideline recommendations for antithrombotic therapy in ACS

Recommendations	Dosing and special considerations	COR	LOE
Non-enteric-coated aspirin to all patients promptly after presentation	162–325 mg	I	A
Aspirin maintenance dose continued indefinitely	81–325 mg/d*	I	A
For patients who are not able to take aspirin: Clopidogrel loading dose followed by daily maintenance or ticagrelor loading dose followed by daily maintenance	300 mg or 600 mg loading dose, then 75 mg/d 180 mg loading dose, then 90 mg BID	I	B
P2Y$_{12}$ inhibitor therapy (clopidogrel, prasugrel, or ticagrelor) loading and continued for at least 12 months post-PCI	300 mg or 600 mg loading dose, then 75 mg/d 180 mg loading dose, then 90 mg BID 60 mg loading dose, then 10 mg daily	I	B
Ticagrelor in preference to clopidogrel for patients treated with an early invasive or ischemia-guided strategy	180 mg loading dose, then 90 mg BID	IIa	B
GPIIb/IIIa inhibitor in patients treated with an early invasive strategy and DAPT with intermediate/high-risk features (e.g. positive troponin)	Preferred options are eptifibatide or tirofiban	IIb	B
SQ enoxaparin for duration of hospitalization or until PCI is performed	1 mg/kg SQ every 12 hours (reduce dose to 1 mg/kg/d SQ in patients with CrCl <30 mL/min) Initial 30 mg IV loading dose in selected patients	I	A
SQ fondaparinux for the duration of hospitalization or until PCI is performed	2.5 mg SQ daily	I	B

Continued on following page

Table 8.4.

2014 AHA/ACC guideline recommendations for antithrombotic therapy in ACS (Continued)

Recommendations	Dosing and special considerations	COR	LOE
Administer additional anticoagulant with anti-IIa activity if PCI is performed while patient is on fondaparinux	N/A	I	B
IV UFH for 48 hours or until PCI is performed	Initial loading dose 60 IU/kg (max 4000 IU) with initial infusion 12 IU/kg/h (max 1000 IU/h) Adjusted to therapeutic aPTT range	I	B
IV fibrinolytic treatment not recommended in patients with NSTE-ACS	N/A	III: Harm	A

aPTT, Activated partial thromboplastin time; *BID*, twice daily; *COR*, class of recommendation; *CrCl*, creatinine clearance; *DAPT*, dual antiplatelet therapy; *GP*, glycoprotein; *IV*, intravenous; *LOE*, level of evidence; *max*, maximum; *N/A*, not available; *NSTE-ACS*, non ST elevation acute coronary syndromes; *PCI*, percutaneous coronary intervention; *SQ*, subcutaneous; *UFH*, unfractionated heparin.
Amsterdam EA, et al. 2014 AHA/ACC guideline for the management of patients with non–ST-elevation acute coronary syndromes: A report of the American College of Cardiology/American Heart Association task force on practice guidelines. *J Am Coll Cardiol* 2014;64:e139–e228.

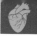

platelet reactivity is an independent risk factor for ischemic events after PCI.[107]

In order for platelet reactivity testing to be clinically useful, optimal cutpoints or "thresholds" must be established. In a majority of prior studies, cutpoints have been determined with receiver-operating characteristic (ROC) curve analysis in patients undergoing elective PCI. Despite the use of different ischemic endpoints (CV death, MI, stent thrombosis, and urgent revascularization), studies have suggested that the optimal cutpoint for VASP-PRI testing is between 48% and 53%.[108] Similar studies using the VerifyNow $P2Y_{12}$ assay have demonstrated that a cutoff value below 240 $P2Y_{12}$ reaction units (PRU) is prognostic for thrombotic events (CV death, stent thrombosis, and nonfatal MI). While the negative predictive value for these cutoffs is high, the positive predictive value is low for all assays, likely because on-treatment platelet reactivity is not the only determinant of post-PCI ischemic events. The consistency of the platelet reactivity cutoffs determined by multiple studies suggests that there may be a threshold level of platelet reactivity below which ischemic events may be prevented.[109] Given the bleeding risk associated with dual antiplatelet therapy after PCI, there may be a therapeutic window for $P2Y_{12}$ receptor antagonist therapy associated with both a reduction in thrombotic events and a low rate of bleeding. Although there have been no large studies that have established a "cutpoint" for gauging bleeding risk, several observational studies have reported an association between low platelet reactivity on clopidogrel and increased in-hospital bleeding after PCI.[110]

Pharmacogenomics and $P2Y_{12}$ Inhibitor Therapy

Studies examining in vitro metabolism of clopidogrel and clinical outcomes have noted significant unfavorable variability in the production of its active metabolite related to genetic variation in patients. As a result, the FDA added a "boxed warning" to clopidogrel suggesting methods for testing for genetic differences and suggesting potential alternative drug therapies. No recommendations were made suggesting specific clinical scenarios in which genetic testing should be undertaken.[104,111]

Although genetic variation in the generation of clopidogrel's active metabolite is a function of heterogeneity in intestinal absorption, hepatic CYP metabolism, and $P2Y_{12}$ receptor structure, it appears that variation in the CYP2C19 appears to be the most consistent determinant of differences in response to clopidogrel.[105] Twenty-five SNPs lie within the CYP2C19 gene, of which the most clinically relevant variants are CYP2C19*2, CYP2C19*3, and

CYP2C19*17. Of these variants, the first two account for greater than 90% of cases of poor metabolism and the third is responsible for a gain of function that results in increased metabolism. Because of the differential prevalence of certain SNPs within the nonwhite population, the prevalence of the poor metabolizer genotypes ranges from 20%–30% in white individuals, from 30%–45% in African Americans, and up to 50%–65% in East Asians.[112]

The genetic variability in response seen with clopidogrel does not seem to extend to the newer $P2Y_{12}$ agents, prasugrel and ticagrelor. Prasugrel undergoes metabolism to its active metabolite via rapid deesterification to an intermediate, thiolactone, which is then converted to active metabolite via a single CYP-dependent step that is more uniform, rapid, and complete than clopidogrel metabolism.[113] As a result, prasugrel metabolism is not subject to variation in CYP2C19.[114] Similarly, ticagrelor does not require CYP-dependent metabolism, and is thought to provide more consistent inhibition of $P2Y_{12}$ receptors regardless of variation in CYP2C19.[115] Multiple meta-analysis have correlated CYP2C19 genotype and clinical outcomes in post-PCI patients treated with clopidogrel. In pooling several studies of between 8000 and 12,000 high-risk patients, these meta-analyses reported that adverse cardiac outcomes increased by 30% and there was a twofold-higher risk of stent thrombosis per reduced function variant.[116] The risk of adverse outcomes and stent thrombosis increased in a step-wise fashion with an increasing number of reduced-function alleles. The risk may be particularly high in Asian populations where CYP2C19 polymorphisms are prevalent.

TAILOR-PCI is the largest genotype-based cardiovascular clinical trial randomizing participants to conventional DAPT or prospective genotyping-guided DAPT. Enrolled patients completed surveys before and 6 months after randomization.[117] A total of 1327 patients completed baseline surveys of whom 28%, 29%, and 43% were from Korea, Canada, and the US, respectively. Most patients (77%) valued identifying pharmacogenetic variants; however, fewer Korean (44%) as compared with Canadian (91%) and American (89%) patients identified pharmacogenetics as being important ($P < 0.001$). After adjusting for age, sex, and country, those who were confident in their ability to understand genetic information were significantly more likely to value identifying pharmacogenetic variants (OR 30.0; 95% CI 20.5–43.8). Only 21% of Koreans, as opposed to 86% and 77% of patients in Canada and the United States, respectively, were confident in their ability to understand genetic information ($P < 0.001$).

After clinical genotyping, each institution recommended alternative antiplatelet therapy (prasugrel, ticagrelor) in PCI patients with a loss-of-function allele. Major adverse cardiovascular events (defined as MI, stroke, or death) within 12 months of PCI were compared between patients with a loss-of-function allele prescribed clopidogrel versus alternative therapy. Risk was also compared between patients without a loss-of-function allele and loss-of-function allele carriers prescribed alternative therapy. Cox regression was performed, adjusting for group differences with inverse probability of treatment weights. Among 1815 patients, 572 (31.5%) had a loss-of-function allele. The risk for major adverse cardiovascular events was significantly higher in patients with a loss-of-function allele prescribed clopidogrel versus alternative therapy (23.4 versus 8.7 per 100 patient-years; adjusted HR 2.26; 95% CI 1.18–4.32; $P = 0.013$). Similar results were observed among 1210 patients with acute coronary syndromes at the time of PCI (adjusted HR 2.87; 95% CI 1.35–6.09; $P = 0.013$). There was no difference in major adverse cardiovascular events between patients without a loss-of-function allele and loss-of-function allele carriers prescribed alternative therapy (adjusted HR 1.14; 95% CI 0.69–1.88; $P = 0.60$).

What Is the Role of Platelet Function Testing in Routine Clinical Practice?

To establish the clinical utility of platelet function testing several criteria must be met. First, there must be a reproducible and standardized assay to measure genotype or platelet function. Second, studies must consistently link specific genotypes or platelet function measures with clinical outcomes. Third, recommendations for modification of pharmacotherapy must be established, and these management strategies must be validated in appropriately powered randomized trials to demonstrate their efficacy and safety.

In the TRIGGER-PCI trial, patients with stable CAD and high on-treatment platelet reactivity (HTPR) (>208 PRUs by the VerifyNow test) after elective PCI with at least one DES were randomly assigned to either prasugrel 10 mg daily or clopidogrel 75 mg daily. Platelet reactivity of the patients on the study drug was reassessed at 3 and 6 months. The study was stopped prematurely for futility because of a lower than expected incidence of the primary endpoint.[118] In 212 patients assigned to prasugrel, PRU decreased from 245 (225–273 median [interquartile range]) at baseline to 80 (42–124) at 3 months, whereas in 211 patients assigned to clopidogrel, PRU decreased from 249 (225–277) to 241 (194–275) ($P < 0.001$ versus prasugrel). The primary efficacy endpoint of cardiac death or MI at 6 months occurred in no patient on prasugrel versus one patient who was on clopidogrel. The primary safety endpoint of noncoronary artery bypass graft TIMI major bleeding at 6 months occurred in three patients (1.4%) on prasugrel versus one patient (0.5%) on clopidogrel.

The ARCTIC investigators randomly assigned 2440 patients scheduled for PCI to a strategy of platelet-function monitoring, with drug adjustment in patients who had a poor response to antiplatelet therapy, or to a conventional strategy without monitoring and drug adjustment. The primary endpoint was the composite of death, MI, stent thrombosis, stroke, or urgent revascularization 1 year after stent implantation. For patients in the monitoring group, the VerifyNow P2Y$_{12}$ and aspirin point-of-care assays were used in the catheterization laboratory before stent implantation and in the outpatient clinic 2 to 4 weeks later.[119] In the monitoring group, high platelet reactivity in patients taking clopidogrel (34.5% of patients) or aspirin (7.6%) led to the administration of an additional bolus of clopidogrel, prasugrel, or aspirin along with glycoprotein IIb/IIIa inhibitors during the procedure. The primary endpoint occurred in 34.6% of the patients in the monitoring group, as compared with 31.1% of those in the conventional-treatment group (HR 1.13; 95% CI 0.98 to 1.29; $P = 0.10$). The main secondary endpoint, stent thrombosis or any urgent revascularization, occurred in 4.9% of the patients in the monitoring group and 4.6% of patients in the conventional-treatment group (HR 1.06; 95% CI 0.74 to 1.52; $P = 0.77$). The rate of major bleeding events did not differ significantly between groups.

The ANTARCTIC investigators conducted a multicenter,[120] open-label, blinded-endpoint, randomized controlled superiority study in patients aged 75 years or older who had undergone PCI for ACS to prasugrel 5 mg daily with dose or drug adjustment in case of inadequate response (monitoring group; n = 442) or oral prasugrel 5 mg daily with no monitoring or treatment adjustment (conventional group; n = 435). Platelet function testing was performed 14 days after randomization and repeated 14 days after treatment adjustment in patients in the monitoring group. The primary endpoint was a composite of cardiovascular death, MI, stroke, stent thrombosis, urgent revascularization, and Bleeding Academic Research Consortium-defined bleeding complications (types 2, 3, or 5) at 12 months' follow-up. The primary endpoint occurred in 120 (28%) patients in the monitoring group compared with 123 (28%) patients in the conventional group (HR 1.003; 95% CI 0.78–1.29; $P = 0.98$). Rates of bleeding events did not differ significantly between groups.

Deescalation of Therapy Employing Platelet Function Tests

The (TROPICAL-ACS) trial[121] randomized patients with successful PCI to standard treatment with prasugrel for 12 months (control group; n = 1306) or a step-down regimen (1 week prasugrel followed by 1-week clopidogrel and platelet-function test-guided maintenance therapy with clopidogrel or prasugrel from day 14 after hospital discharge; guided deescalation group; n = 1304). The primary endpoint was net clinical benefit (cardiovascular death, MI, stroke or bleeding grade 2 or higher according to Bleeding Academic Research Consortium [BARC]) criteria) 1 year after randomization (noninferiority hypothesis; margin of 30%). The primary endpoint occurred in 95 patients (7%) in the guided deescalation group and in 118 patients (9%) in the control group ($P_{noninferiority}$ = 0.0004; HR 0.81; 95% CI 0.62–1.06; $P_{superiority}$ = 0.12). Despite early deescalation, there was no increase in the combined risk of cardiovascular death, MI, or stroke in the deescalation group (32 patients [3%]) versus in the control group (42 patients [3%]; $P_{noninferiority}$ = 0.0115). There were 64 BARC 2 or higher bleeding events (5%) in the deescalation group versus 79 events (6%) in the control group (HR 0.82; 95% CI 0.59–1.13; P = 0.23).

Periprocedural Management of Antiplatelet Therapy

It is estimated that up to 5% of patients will require surgery within the first year after stent implantation and that up to a third of all cases of stent thrombosis occur in the perioperative setting, often as a result of discontinuation of DAPT.[122]

The risk of ischemic events in the periprocedural period varies with the anatomic location of the implanted stent and the time elapsed since stent placement. As always, ischemic risk must be balanced with bleeding risk, which varies by the type and anatomic location of the procedure being performed (Fig. 8.7). The periprocedural approach to patients with CAD and prior stent placement are summarized in Tables 8.5 and 8.6.

Periprocedural Management of Antiplatelet Therapy and Coronary Artery Bypass Grafting

Perioperative management of antiplatelet therapy in the setting of urgent coronary artery bypass grafting (CABG) can be challenging. An assessment of ischemic/thrombotic risk must be gauged in the context of bleeding risk (Table 8.7). The BRIDGE trial randomized 210 patients with ACS or recent coronary stent on thienopyridine to either receiving cangrelor or placebo while awaiting CABG surgery.[123] Cangrelor administered at a dose of 0.75 µg/kg/min was associated with a greater proportion of patients with low levels of

MANAGEMENT OF PLATELET DIRECTED THERAPY

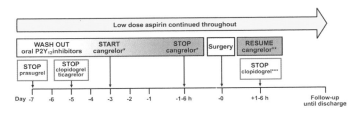

Fig. 8.7 An approach to optimal management of platelet-directed therapy in patients undergoing surgery. Clopidogrel and ticagrelor should be discontinued for 5 days and prasugrel for 7 days. Start cangrelor at bridging dose regimen 3–4 days after prasugrel discontinuation and 2–3 days of clopidogrel and ticagrelor discontinuation and discontinue 1–6 hours before surgery. After surgery, prasugrel and ticagrelor administration should be discouraged and clopidogrel should be resumed with a loading dose as soon as oral administration is possible, and the risk of severe bleeding is acceptable. If the use of oral $P2Y_{12}$ inhibiting therapy is not possible, postsurgery bridging might be considered. (Data from Rossini R, et al. A multidisciplinary approach on the perioperative antithrombotic management of patients with coronary stents undergoing surgery: surgery after stenting 2. *JACC: Cardiovascular Inter 2018*;11:417–434.)

platelet reactivity (primary endpoint) during the treatment period as compared to placebo (PRU <240, 98.8% versus 19.0%; RR = 5.2; 95% CI 3.3–8.1; $P < 0.001$). Excessive CABG-related bleeding occurred in 11.8% versus 10.4% of patients in the cangrelor and placebo groups, respectively (RR = 1.1; 95% CI 0.5–2.5; $P = 0.763$). There were no significant differences in major bleeding prior to CABG. Although this trial was not powered to assess clinical endpoints such as stent thrombosis or mortality, it does suggest that bridging therapy with cangrelor may be useful in patients on thienopyridines at high risk for coronary events while awaiting CABG.

Periprocedural Management of Antiplatelet Therapy and GI Procedures

As for any procedure, management of antiplatelet therapy periendoscopy is dependent on accurate assessment of the risk of bleeding and the risk of adverse coronary events. There is significant variation in the reported rates of cardiopulmonary complications

Text continues on p. 60

Table 8.5

The balance of risk for stent thrombosis and surgical risk for bleeding

Hemorrhagic risk	Type of surgery	Antiplatelet/ anticoagulant drug	Thrombotic risk		
			Low	Intermediate	High
Low	Hernioplasty Plastic surgery of incisional hernias Cholecystectomy Appendectomy Colectomy Gastric resection Intestinal resection Breast surgery	ASA	Continue	Elective surgery: postpone Nondeferrable surgery: continue	Elective surgery: postpone Nondeferrable surgery: continue
		P2Y$_{12}$ receptor inhibitors	Discontinue 5 days before for clopidogrel/ ticagrelor, 7 days before for prasugrel Resume within 24–72 h (with a loading dose)	Elective surgery: postpone Nondeferrable surgery: continue	Elective surgery: postpone Nondeferrable surgery: continue
		NOAC		Discontinue at least 24–96 h before[a] Resume within 48–72 h[b]	
Intermediate	Hemorrhoidectomy Splenectomy Gastrectomy Obesity surgery Rectal resection Thyroidectomy	ASA	Continue	Elective surgery: postpone Nondeferrable surgery: continue	Elective surgery: postpone Nondeferrable surgery: continue
		P2Y$_{12}$ receptor inhibitors	Discontinue 5 days before for clopidogrel/ticagrelor, 7 days before for prasugrel	Elective surgery: postpone	Elective surgery: postpone

Continued on following page

Table 8.5

The balance of risk for stent thrombosis and surgical risk for bleeding (Continued)

Hemorrhagic risk	Type of surgery	Antiplatelet/ anticoagulant drug	Thrombotic risk		
			Low	Intermediate	High
		NOAC	Resume within 24–72 h (with a loading dose)	Nondeferrable surgery: Discontinue 5 days before for clopidogrel/ ticagrelor, 7 days before for prasugrel Resume within 24–72 h[c] (with a loading dose) Discontinue at least 24–96 h before[a] Resume within 48–72 h[b]	Nondeferrable surgery: Discontinue 5 days before for clopidogrel/ ticagrelor, 7 days before for prasugrel Resume within 24–72 h[c] (with a loading dose) Consider. bridge therapy[c]
High	Hepatic resection Duodenocefalopancreasectomy	ASA	Discontinue	Elective surgery: postpone Nondeferrable surgery: continue Elective surgery: postpone	Elective surgery: postpone Nondeferrable surgery: continue Elective surgery: postpone
		P2Y$_{12}$ receptor inhibitors	Discontinue 5 days before for clopidogrel/ticagrelor,		

		Nondeferrable surgery:	Nondeferrable surgery:
NOAC	7 days before for prasugrel Resume within 24–72 h (with a loading dose)	Discontinue 5 days before for clopidogrel/ ticagrelor, 7 days before for prasugrel Resume within 24–72 h[c] (with a loading dose) Discontinue at least 48–96 h before[a] Resume within 48–72 h[b]	Discontinue 5 days before for clopidogrel/ticagrelor, 7 days before for prasugrel Resume within 24–72 h[c] (with a loading dose) Consider bridge therapy[c]

Use of P2Y$_{12}$ receptor inhibitors is to be considered in association with aspirin (ASA).

[a]Evaluate creatinine clearance and type of non-vitamin K antagonist oral anticoagulant (NOAC).

[b]As soon as possible, once adequate hemostasis has been achieved (consider bridge therapy in patients in whom resumption of full-dose anticoagulation may carry a bleeding risk that could outweigh the risk of cardioembolism).

[c]Collegial discussion of risk, even with family or patient.

From Rossini R, et al. A multidisciplinary approach on the perioperative antithrombotic management of patients with coronary stents undergoing surgery: surgery after stenting 2. *JACC: Cardiovascular Inter 2018;11:417–434.*

Table 8.6

Thrombotic risk in patients with coronary artery stents undergoing surgery

Surgery to PCI Time	PCI patients with clinical* or angiographic* increased ischemic risk characteristics					PCI patients without clinical* or angiographic* increased ischemic risk characteristics				
	POBA	BMS	First-Generation DES	Second-Generation DES†	BVS	POBA	BMS	First-Generation DES	Second-Generation DES†	BVS
<1 month	High	High	High	High	High	High (<2 weeks) intermediate	High	High	High	High
1–3 months	Intermediate	High	High	High	High	Low	Intermediate	High	Intermediate	High
4–6 months	Intermediate	High	High	Intermediate/ high	High	Low	Low/ intermediate	Intermediate	Low/ intermediate	High
6–12 months	Intermediate	Intermediate	Intermediate	Intermediate	High	Low	Low	Intermediate	Low	High
>12 months	Low	Low	Low	Low	Undetermined	Undetermined Low	Low	Low	Low	Undetermined

BMS, bare-metal stent(s); BVS, bioresorbable vascular scaffold; PCI, percutaneous coronary intervention; POBA, plain old balloon angioplasty.
From Rossini R, et al. A multidisciplinary approach on the perioperative antithrombotic management of patients with coronary stents undergoing surgery: surgery after stenting 2. JACC: Cardiovascular Inter 2018;11:417–434.

Table 8.7

Balance of risk for stent thrombosis and bleeding in cardiac surgery

Hemorrhagic risk	Type of surgery	Antiplatelet/ anticoagulant drug	Thrombotic risk		
			Low	Intermediate	High
Low	-	ASA	-	-	-
		P2Y$_{12}$ receptor inhibitors	-	-	-
		NOAC	-	-	-
Intermediate	Valve repair Valve replacement OPCAB	ASA	Continue	Elective surgery: postpone Nondeferrable surgery: continue	Elective surgery: postpone Nondeferrable surgery: continue
	CABG	P2Y$_{12}$ receptor inhibitors	Discontinue 5 days before for clopidogrel/ ticagrelor, 7 days before for prasugrel	Elective surgery: postpone	Elective surgery: postpone Nondeferrable surgery:
	Minithoracotomy		Resume within 24–72 h (with a loading dose)	Nondeferrable surgery:	• Discontinue 5 days before for clopidogrel/ ticagrelor, 7 days before for prasugrel
	TA-TAVI			• Discontinue 5 days before for clopidogrel/ ticagrelor, 7 days before for prasugrel	

Continued on following page

Table 8.7

Balance of risk for stent thrombosis and bleeding in cardiac surgery (Continued)

Hemorrhagic risk	Type of surgery	Antiplatelet/ anticoagulant drug	Thrombotic risk		
			Low	Intermediate	High
	TAo-TAVI				• Resume within 24–72 h[a] (with a loading dose) Consider bridge therapy[b]
				• Resume within 24–72 hours[a] (with a loading dose)	
		NOAC		Discontinue at least 24–96 h before[c] Resume within 48–72 h[d]	
High risk	Reintervention Endocarditis	ASA	Continue	Elective surgery: postpone Nondeferrable surgery: continue	Elective surgery: postpone Nondeferrable surgery: continue
	CABG in PCI failure Aortic dissection Aortic surgery with expected CEC time >120 min	P2Y$_{12}$ receptor inhibitors	Discontinue 5 days before for clopidogrel/ ticagrelor, 7 days before for prasugrel Resume within 24–72 h (with a loading dose)	Elective surgery: postpone	Elective surgery: postpone Nondeferrable surgery: • Discontinue 5 days before for clopidogrel/ ticagrelor,
				Nondeferrable surgery:	

	• Discontinue 5 days before for clopidogrel/ticagrelor, 7 days before for prasugrel	7 days before for prasugrel
	• Resume within 24–72 h[a] (with a loading dose)	• Resume within 24–72 h[a] (with a loading dose) Consider bridge therapy[b]
NOAC	Discontinue at least 48–96 h before[c] Resume within 48–72 h[d]	

Use of P2Y$_{12}$ receptor inhibitors is to be considered in association with aspirin (ASA). *CABG*, Coronary artery bypass graft; *NOAC*, non-vitamin K antagonist oral anticoagulant; *OPCAB*, off-pump coronary artery bypass; *PCI*, percutaneous coronary intervention; *TA-TAVI*, transapical-transcatheter aortic valve implantation; *TAo-TAVI*, transaortic-transcatheter aortic valve implantation.

[a]Point-of-care hemostatic testing, if available, may reduce resuming time.
[b]Collegial discussion of risk, even with family or patient.
[c]Evaluate creatinine clearance and type of NOAC.
[d]As soon as possible, once adequate hemostasis has been achieved (consider bridge therapy in patients in whom resumption of full-dose anticoagulation may carry a bleeding risk that could outweigh the risk of cardioembolism).
From Rossini R, et al. A multidisciplinary approach on the perioperative antithrombotic management of patients with coronary stents undergoing surgery: surgery after stenting 2. *JACC: Cardiovascular Inter 2018;11:417–434.*

associated with endoscopy. In a prospective survey of 14,149 gastros-copies, the 30-day complication rate was 0.2%. Eleven patients were diagnosed with pneumonia, resulting in 8 deaths, 3 patients with fatal pulmonary emboli, and 19 patients (14 deaths) with acute MI.[124] Although not optimally defined, the mechanism of cardiopulmonary complications associated with endoscopy may be related to vagal stimulation (via air insufflation of a hollow viscus), catecholamine release secondary to dehydration, anxiety, or pain, and changes in serum electrolytes secondary to colonic purgative solutions.

Johnson and colleagues performed a retrospective longitudinal analysis to assess the diagnosis, procedure, and prescription drug codes in a United States commercial claims database.[125] Data from patients at increased risk (n = 82,025; defined as patients with pulmonary comorbidities or cardiovascular disease requiring antithrombotic medications) were compared with data from 398,663 average-risk patients. In a 1:1 matched analysis, 51,932 patients at increased risk undergoing colonoscopy were compared with 51,932 matched (on the basis of age, sex, and comorbidities) patients at increased risk who did not undergo colonoscopy. Cardiac, pulmonary, and neurovascular events 1–30 days after colonoscopy were determined (Fig. 8.8).

Thirty days after outpatient colonoscopy, non-GI adverse events (AEs) were significantly higher in patients taking antithrombotic medications (7.3%; OR 10.75; 95% CI 10.13–11.42) or those with pulmonary comorbidities (1.8%; OR 2.44; 95% CI 2.27–2.62) versus average-risk patients (0.7%) and in patients 60–69 years old (OR 2.21; 95% CI 2.01–2.42) or 70 years or older (OR 6.45; 95% CI 5.89–7.06), compared with patients younger than 50 years. The 30-day incidence of non-GI AEs in patients at increased risk who underwent colonoscopy was also significantly higher than in matched patients at increased risk who did not undergo colonoscopy in the anticoagulant group (OR 2.31; 95% CI 2.01–2.65) and in the chronic obstructive pulmonary disease group (OR 1.33;95% CI 1.13–1.56).

Taking into account the risk of bleeding associated with endoscopy in patients receiving DAPT and the risk of cardiovascular events associated with cessation of antiplatelet therapy, clinicians must employ a thoughtful approach based on ischemic/thrombotic and bleeding risk.[126] In most instances, antiplatelet therapy can be continued unless the risk and potential impact of bleeding is very high (e.g., neurosurgery, major trauma with active bleeding).

Intravenous Platelet GPIIb/IIIa Receptor Antagonists

The evolution of GPIIb/IIIa receptor antagonist began with murine monoclonal antibodies and more recently has focused on small

GASTROINTESTINAL RISK

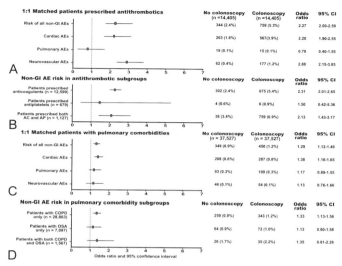

Fig. 8.8 Increased risk for postprocedural non-gastrointestinal (GI) adverse events (AEs) in patients with colonoscopy versus 1:1 matched patients without colonoscopy. (A and B) Risk of overall non-GI, cardiac, pulmonary, and neurovascular adverse events in patients prescribed antithrombotic medications for cardiovascular conditions, comparing 14,405 patients with colonoscopy versus 14,405 matched patients without colonoscopy. (C and D) AE risk in 1:1 matched groups of patients with pulmonary comorbidities, comparing 37,527 patients with colonoscopy versus 37,527 patients without colonoscopy. (Data from Johnson DA, et al. Increased post-procedural non-gastrointestinal adverse events after outpatient colonoscopy in high-risk patients. *Clin Gastroenterol Hepatol* 2017;15:883–891.)

peptide or nonpeptide molecules that have structural similarities to fibrinogen. There are currently three IV GPIIb/IIIa receptor antagonists: abciximab, tirofiban, and eptifibatide (Table 8.8).

Abciximab

Pharmacodynamics

Abciximab is the Fab fragment of the chimeric human-murine monoclonal antibody c7E3. IV administration of abciximab, in doses ranging from 0.15 mg/kg to 0.3 mg/kg, produces a rapid

Table 8.8

Drug-specific characteristics for glycoprotein (GP)-IIb/IIIa receptor antagonists			
Characteristic	Abciximab	Eptifibatide	Tirofiban
Type	Antibody	Peptide	Nonpeptide
Molecular weight, daltons	≈ 50,000	≈ 800	≈ 500
Platelet-bound half-life	Long	Short	Short
Plasma half-life	Short (min)	Extended (2 h)	Extended (2 h)
Drug/GPIIb/IIIa receptor ratio	1.5–2.0	250–2500	>250
50% return of platelet function	12 h	≈ 4 h	≈ 4 h
Route of clearance	RES	Renal/ hepatic	Renal
Dose adjustment required with renal insufficiency	No	Yes	Yes

RES, reticuloendothelial system.

dose-dependent inhibition of platelet aggregation in response to ADP. At the highest dose, 80% of platelet GPIIb/IIIa receptors are occupied within 2 hours and platelet aggregation, even with 20 μM ADP, is completely inhibited. Sustained inhibition is achieved with prolonged infusions (12–24 hours) and low-level receptor blockade is present for up to 10 days following cessation of the infusion: however, platelet inhibition during infusions beyond 24 hours has not been well characterized. Platelet aggregation in response to 5 μM ADP returns to ≥50% of baseline within 24 hours of drug cessation.

Pharmacokinetics

Following an IV bolus, free plasma concentrations of abciximab decrease rapidly with an initial half-life of less than 10 minutes and a second-phase half-life of 30 minutes, representing rapid binding to the platelet GPIIb/IIIa receptor. Abciximab remains in the circulation for 10–14 days in a dynamic, platelet-bound state.

Clinical Experience

In the EPIC trial,[127] 2100 patients undergoing either balloon coronary angioplasty or atherectomy at high risk for ischemic/thrombotic complications received a bolus of abciximab (0.25 mg/kg) followed by a 12-hour continuous infusion (10 μg/min). This treatment reduced the occurrence of death, MI, or the need for an urgent intervention (repeat angioplasty, stent placement, balloon pump insertion, or bypass grafting) by 35%. At 6 months,[128] the absolute difference in patients with a major ischemic event or elective revascularization was 8.1% comparing patients who received abciximab (bolus plus infusion) with those given placebo (35.1% versus 27.0%; 23% reduction). At 3 years,[129] the composite endpoint occurred in: (1) 41.1% of those receiving an abciximab bolus plus infusion; (2) 47.4% of those receiving an abciximab bolus only; and (3) 47.2% of those receiving placebo.

The Evaluation in PTCA to Improve Long-term Outcome with Abciximab GPIIb/IIIa Blockade (EPILOG) study[130] included 2792 patients undergoing elective or urgent percutaneous coronary revascularization who received either abciximab with standard, weight-adjusted unfractionated heparin (UFH) (initial bolus 100 U/kg, target activated clotting time [ACT] $\geq$300 seconds) or placebo with standard-dose, weight-adjusted heparin. At 30 days, the composite event rate was observed in both high-risk and low-risk patients.

The c7E3 Fab Antiplatelet Therapy in Unstable Refractory Angina (CAPTURE) study[131] was designed to investigate whether abciximab, given during the 18–24 hours before coronary angioplasty, could improve outcome in patients with refractory (myocardial ischemia despite nitrates, heparin, and aspirin) unstable angina. A total of 1265 patients were randomly assigned to abciximab or placebo. By 30 days, the primary endpoint (death, MI, urgent revascularization) occurred in 11.3% of abciximab-treated patients and in 15.9% of placebo-treated patients (n = 0.012). The rate of MI was lower *before* and *during* coronary interventions in those given abciximab.

Patients participating in the Global Use of Strategies to Open Occluded Arteries (GUSTO) IV-ACS trial[132] had chest pain and either ST-segment depression or elevated troponin levels. They were randomized to receive placebo, abciximab for 24 hours, or abciximab for 48 hours with recommended avoidance of revascularization during the initial 48 hours. Neither abciximab group fared better than placebo with respect to death or MI at 30 days. In addition, early mortality rates were higher with a prolonged abciximab infusion, suggesting a prothrombotic (or other adverse) effect.

In the GUSTO V study,[133,134] 16,588 patients with acute STEMI received either reteplase (standard dose) or half-dose reteplase plus abciximab. Although the 30-day mortality rates did not differ significantly, there were fewer nonfatal ischemic complications of MI with reteplase plus abciximab compared with reteplase alone. Intracranial hemorrhage rates did not differ between treatments; however, moderate-to-severe bleeding was more likely with combined therapy, and patients >75 years of age were at increased risk for hemorrhagic stroke (OR 1.91).

Tirofiban

Pharmacodynamics

Tirofiban, a tyrosine derivative with a molecular weight of 495 kDa, is a nonpeptide inhibitor (peptidomimetic) of the platelet GPIIb/IIIa receptor. Tirofiban, like other nonpeptides, mimics the geometric, stereotactic, and charge characteristics of the RDG (Arg-Gly-Asp) sequence (of fibrinogen), thus interfering with platelet aggregation.

Clinical Experience

The Randomized Efficacy Study of Tirofiban Outcomes and Restenosis (RESTORE) trial[135] was a randomized double-blind, placebo-controlled trial of tirofiban in patients with ACS undergoing PCI. Patients (n = 2139) received tirofiban as a 10 µg/kg IV bolus over a 3-minute period and a continuous infusion of 0.15 µg/kg/min over 36 hours. All patients received UFH and aspirin. The primary composite endpoint (death, MI, angioplasty, failure requiring bypass surgery or unplanned stent placement, recurrent ischemia requiring repeat angioplasty) at 30 days was reduced, from 12.2% in the placebo group to 10.3% in the tirofiban group (16% relative reduction).

The Platelet Receptor Inhibition in Ischemic Syndrome Management (PRISM) trial[136] included 3231 patients with non–ST-segment elevation ACS. All patients received aspirin and were randomized to treatment with either UFH or tirofiban, given as a loading dose of 0.6 µg/kg/min over 30 minutes followed by a maintenance infusion of 0.15 µg/kg/min for 48 hours (angiography/revascularization was discouraged during the infusion period). The primary composite endpoint (death, MI, refractory ischemia) at 48 hours was 5.6% in tirofiban-treated patients and 3.8% in placebo (aspirin/heparin)-treated patients (risk reduction 33%). Benefit was maintained but overall was more modest at 7 and 30 days.

The PRISM in Patients Limited by Unstable Singes and Symptoms (PLUS) trial[137] included 1915 patients with non–ST-segment elevation ACS who were treated with aspirin and UFH and subsequently randomized to either tirofiban (0.4 µg/kg/min x 30 min; then 0.1 µg/kg/min for a minimum of 48 hours and a maximum of 108 hours) or placebo (unfractionated heparin). Angiography and revascularization were performed at the discretion of the treating physician. Tirofiban treated patients had a lower composite event rate of 7 days than the placebo group, 12.9% versus 17.9%, with a risk reduction of 34%. The benefit was mainly due to a reduced incidence of MI (47% risk reduction) and refractory ischemia (30% risk reduction). The benefit was maintained at 30 days (22% risk reduction in composite event rate) and at 6 months.

The trial originally included a tirofiban-alone arm (no heparin) that was dropped because of excess mortality at 7 days.

The importance of early PCI among patients with non–ST-segment elevation ACS was underscored in the Treat Angina With Aggrastat and Determine Cost of Therapy With an Invasive or Conservative Strategy (TACTICS)— TIMI 18 trial[138] as was the benefit of aggressive pharmacologic therapy (GPIIb/IIIa receptor antagonist) in combination with PCI for patients at greatest risk for adverse ischemic outcomes (prior MI, ST-segment changes, elevated cardiac biomarkers).

Eptifibatide

Pharmacodynamics

Eptifibatide (Integrilin®) is a nonimmunogenic cyclic heptapeptide with an active pharmacophore that is derived from the structure of barbourin, a platelet GPIIb/IIIa inhibitor from the venom of the southeastern pigmy rattlesnake. In a pilot study of PCI, patients were randomized to one of four eptifibatide dosing schedules: 180 µg/kg bolus, 1 µg/kg/min infusion; 135 µg/kg bolus, 0.5 µg/kg/min infusion; 90 µg/kg bolus, 0.75 µg/kg/min infusion; and 135 µg/kg bolus, 0.75 µg/kg/min infusion.[139] All patients received aspirin and UFH and were continued on the study drug for 18–24 hours. The two highest bolus doses produced >80% inhibition of ADP-mediated platelet aggregation within 15 minutes of administration in a majority of patients (>75%). A constant infusion of 0.75 µg/kg/min maintained the antiplatelet effect, whereas an infusion of 0.50 µg/kg/min allowed gradual recovery of platelet function. In all dosing groups, platelet-function returned to >50% of baseline within 4 hours of terminating the infusion.

Pharmacokinetics

The plasma half-life of eptifibatide is 10–15 minutes, and clearance is predominantly renal (75%) and, to a lesser degree, hepatic (25%). The antiplatelet effect has a rapid onset of action and is rapidly reversible.

Clinical Experience

The Integrilin to Minimize Platelet Aggregation and Coronary Thrombosis (IMPACT-II) trial[140] enrolled 4010 patients undergoing elective, urgent, or emergent PCI. Patients were assigned to either placebo, a bolus of 135 µg/kg eptifibatide followed by an infusion of 0.5 µg/kg/min for 20 to 24 hours, or 135 µg/kg bolus with a 0.75-µg/kg/min infusion. By 30 days, the composite endpoint (death, MI, unplanned revascularization, stent placement for abrupt closure) occurred in 11.4%, 9.2%, and 9.9% of patients, respectively. Although the benefit of treatment was maintained at 6 months, the differences between groups were not statistically significant.

The IMPACT-AMI Study[141] was designed to determine the effect of eptifibatide on coronary arterial patency when used adjunctively with Alteplase (tPA). A total of 132 patients with MI received tPA, heparin, and aspirin, and were randomized to receive a bolus dose, followed by a continuous infusion of one of six eptifibatide doses or placebo. The doses ranged from 36–180 µg/kg (bolus) and 0.2–0.75 µg/kg/min (infusion). Study drug was started within 24 hours. The highest-dose eptifibatide groups had more complete reperfusion (TIMI grade 3 flow) and shorter mean time to ST-segment recovery than placebo-treated patients. The composite clinical event rate (death, reinfarction, revascularization, heart failure, hypertension or stroke) was relatively high in all groups: 44.8% in eptifibatide-treated patients and 41.8% in placebo-treated patients.

The Platelet Glycoprotein IIb/IIIa in Unstable Angina Receptor Suppression Using Integrilin Therapy (PURSUIT) trial[142] included patients with non–ST-segment elevation ACS with symptoms within 24 hours and electrocardiographic changes within 12 hours (of ischemia). A total of 10,948 patients were randomized to eptifibatide: 180 µg/kg bolus plus 1.3 µg/kg/min infusion, or 180 µg/kg bolus plus 2.0 µg/kg/min infusion or placebo for up to 3 days (in addition to UFH [in most patients] and aspirin). The 30-day event rate of death or nonfatal MI was 14.2% with eptifibatide and 15.7% with placebo (1.5% absolute reduction). A reduction in MI or death (composite) with eptifibatide was observed at later time points.

The Enhanced Suppression of the Platelet GPIIb/IIIa Receptor with Integrilin Trial (ESPRIT) was designed to test the hypothesis that a minimum threshold of 80% GPIIb/IIIa receptor blockade was required for benefit.[143] A total of 2064 patients received either eptifibatide (180 µg/kg boluses [x 2] 10 minutes apart plus a continuous infusion of 2.0 µg/kg/min for 18 to 24 hours) or placebo prior to PCI. The trial was terminated early for efficacy, as patients receiving eptifibatide had a 4.0% absolute reduction in death, MI, urgent target vessel revascularization, or "bailout" GPIIb/IIIa antagonist use within 48 hours compared with placebo. Major events were significantly lower at 30 days as well. The Early versus Delayed, Provisional Eptifibatide in Acute Coronary Syndromes (EARLY–ACS) trial randomized NSTEMI/UA patients to a strategy of early, routine administration of eptifibatide versus delayed, provisional administration in 9492 patients. The primary composite endpoint of death, MI, recurrent ischemia requiring urgent revascularization, or thrombotic complication during PCI occurred at similar rates in both groups; however, there was significantly higher bleeding and transfusion requirements in the "early" group.[144]

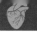

By contrast, ISAR-REACT 2 randomized 2022 NSTEMI patients scheduled to undergo PCI to either abciximab or placebo on top of a background therapy of 600 mg of oral clopidogrel loading. They demonstrated a reduction in the primary composite endpoint of 30 day death, MI, or urgent revascularization with abciximab (RR = 0.75; 95% CI 0.58–0.97; P = 0.3) without an increase in major or minor bleeding.[145] GP IIb/IIIa inhibitors are given a class I recommendation (should perform) for upstream administration at the time of PCI in those NSTEMI/UA patients who were not adequately pretreated with thienopyridines and in whom ongoing ischemia or high risk features exist, and a class IIb recommendation (reasonable to perform) in addition to thienopyridines for intermediate risk patients undergoing coronary angiography with intent to perform PCI.

Agent-Specific Pharmacologic Properties

Although considered collectively as GPIIb/IIIa receptor antagonists, abciximab, tirofiban, and eptifibatide differ at several levels, including their molecular weight, binding characteristics, route of clearance, plasma half-life, platelet-bound and biologic half-life, potential reversibility approved indications, and use in clinical practice. The duration of platelet inhibition following drug discontinuation and the potential for reversing the pharmacologic effect are particularly important properties in cases of emergent surgery and major hemorrhagic complications. In general, a return of platelet function toward a physiologic state ($\leq$50% inhibition) occurs within 4 hours following the cessation of tirofiban and eptifibatide. In contrast, 12 hours are required for abciximab. Some of the delayed return of physiologic platelet function following abciximab termination may be counterbalanced by its low free plasma concentrations and drug-to-receptor ratio. These properties are responsible for the rapid return of hemostatic potential following platelet transfusions (and may also limit platelet inhibiting potential with marked mobilization of GPIIb/IIIa receptors from platelet storage pools). In contrast, the high plasma concentrations observed with the small-molecule inhibitors limit the effectiveness of platelet transfusions. Fibrinogen supplementation (fresh frozen plasma [FFP], cryoprecipitate) is the more logical choice for restoration of hemostatic potential, given the competitive nature of binding and relative availability of platelet GPIIb/IIIa receptors.[146]

Cangrelor

Cangrelor is a rapid-acting, reversible, potent, competitive inhibitor of the P2Y$_{12}$ receptor.

Pharmacodynamics

Given intravenously, cangrelor acts within 20 minutes to achieve 85% inhibition of ADP-induced platelet aggregation. By whole blood impedance aggregometry there is 98% inhibition of platelet aggregation.

Pharmacokinetics

Cangrelor is rapidly deactivated in circulation by dephosphorylation to its primary metabolite, which has negligible antiplatelet activity. It is excreted in urine (58%) and feces (35%) with an average half-life of 3–6 minutes.

Adverse Events

In the CHAMPION-PLATFORM study, there was no significant difference in the rate of blood transfusion (1.0% in the cangrelor group and 0.6% in the placebo group, $P = 0.13$); however, bleeding at femoral artery access sites was more common among patients receiving cangrelor than placebo.

Clinical Experience

In CHAMION-PLATFORM, 5362 patients who had not been treated with clopidogrel were randomly assigned to receive either cangrelor or placebo at the time of PCI, followed by 600 mg of clopidogrel. The primary endpoint was a composite of death, MI, or ischemia-driven revascularization at 48 hours. Enrollment was stopped when an interim analysis concluded that the trial would be unlikely to show superiority for the primary endpoint.[147] The primary endpoint occurred in 185 of 2654 patients receiving cangrelor (7.0%) and in 210 of 2641 patients receiving placebo (8.0%) (OR in the cangrelor group 0.87; 95% CI 0.71–1.07; $P = 0.17$) (by a modified intention-to-treat population adjusted for missing data). In the cangrelor group, two prespecified secondary endpoints were significantly reduced at 48 hours: the rate of stent thrombosis, from 0.6% to 0.2% (OR 0.31; 95% CI 0.11 to 0.85; $P = 0.02$), and the rate of death from any cause, from 0.7% to 0.2% (OR 0.33; 95% CI 0.13–0.83; $P = 0.02$). The rates of adverse events related to the study treatment were low in both groups, though transient dyspnea occurred significantly more frequently with cangrelor than with clopidogrel (1.2% versus 0.3%).

In a subsequent trial, PHOENIX,[148] 11,145 patients who were undergoing either urgent or elective PCI and were receiving guideline-recommended therapy were randomly assigned to receive a bolus dose followed by an infusion of cangrelor, or to receive a loading dose of 600 mg or 300 mg of clopidogrel. The primary efficacy endpoint was a composite of death, MI, ischemia-driven revascularization, or stent thrombosis at 48 hours after randomization; the key secondary endpoint was stent thrombosis at 48 hours. The primary safety endpoint was severe bleeding at 48 hours. The rate of the primary efficacy endpoint was 4.7% in the cangrelor group and 5.9% in the clopidogrel group (adjusted

OR with cangrelor 0.78; 95% CI 0.66–0.93; $P = 0.005$). The rate of the primary safety endpoint was 0.16% in the cangrelor group and 0.11% in the clopidogrel group (OR 1.50; 95% CI 0.53–4.22; $P = 0.44$). Stent thrombosis developed in 0.8% of the patients in the cangrelor group and in 1.4% in the clopidogrel group (OR 0.62; 95% CI 0.43–0.90; $P = 0.01$).

Transition to an Oral P2Y$_{12}$ Receptor Antagonist

When planning to transition from cangrelor to an oral P2Y$_{12}$ receptor antagonist, it is important for the clinician to know that cangrelor occupies the platelet P2Y$_{12}$ binding site, precluding the binding and pharmacodynamic effect of clopidogrel and prasugrel. Accordingly, these oral agents should be administered *after* cessation of cangrelor. By contrast, the binding site for ticagrelor is distinct allowing it to be administered during cangrelor administration.

Bleeding Complications Associated With Platelet-Directed Therapy

Clinical Impact

The contribution of platelets to the clinical expression of atherosclerotic vascular disease and the well-documented benefit derived from their pharmacologic attenuation provides a strong rationale for use in routine clinical practice. It is not uncommon for more than one platelet antagonist to be administered concomitantly. Accordingly, the impact on hemostasis and the overall risk of bleeding must be weighed against benefit.

A meta-analysis of 50 randomized clinical trials,[149] including a total of 338,191 patients with coronary and or peripheral artery disease, found a very low risk of hemorrhagic stroke (0.2%) with aspirin (up to 325 mg daily), thienopyridines, and IV GPIIb/IIIa receptor antagonists. The risk of major hemorrhage was greater, ranging from 1.7% with aspirin to 3.6% in those receiving IV GPIIb/IIIa receptor antagonists. The incidence of combined major and minor hemorrhagic events was 3.6% for low-intensity aspirin (<100 mg daily), 9.1% for moderate-intensity aspirin (100–325 mg daily), and 8.5% for clopidogrel.

Bleeding and Clinical Outcomes

In the PLATO trial, spontaneous ischemic events (MI or stroke) were determined in relationship to spontaneous major bleeding events (PLATO major, TIMI major, GUSTO severe) with a focus on risk of mortality using time-dependent Cox proportional hazards models. The comparison was performed using ratio of HRs for mortality increase after ischemic versus bleeding events.[150] A total of

822 patients (4.4%) had ≥ 1 spontaneous ischemic event; 485 patients (2.6%), ≥ 1 spontaneous PLATO major bleed, 282 (1.5%), ≥ 1 spontaneous TIMI major bleed; and 207 (1.1%), ≥ 1 spontaneous severe GUSTO bleed. In patients who had both events, bleeding occurred first in most patients. Overall, major bleeding events were associated with increased short- and long-term mortality. The association was similar to the increase associated with spontaneous ischemic events: ratio of HRs (95% CIs) for short- and long-term mortality after spontaneous ischemic versus bleeding events: 1.46 (0.98–2.19) and 0.92 (0.52–1.62) (PLATO major); 1.26 (0.80–1.96) and 1.19 (0.58–2.24) (TIMI major); and 0.72 (0.47–1.10) and 0.83 (0.38–1.79) (GUSTO severe) (all $P > 0.05$).

Management of Bleeding Complications

The initial management of bleeding is dictated by its severity and clinical impact. Minor bleeding may only require close observation and local measures, while more serious or life-threatening hemorrhage may dictate aggressive supportive measures, a change in or cessation of antithrombotic medication, blood replacement products or repletion of platelets, and prohemostatic substrate. There are currently no reversal agents for platelet antagonists. The risk of thrombosis must be carefully considered as should reinitiation of platelet-directed therapy once hemostasis has been achieved.[151a]

Supporting Data for Attenuating P2Y$_{12}$ Antagonist Pharmacodynamic Effects

In the Antagonize P2Y$_{12}$ Treatment Inhibitors by Transfusion of Platelets in an Urgent or Delayed Timing After Acute Coronary Syndrome or Percutaneous Coronary Intervention Presentation-Acute Coronary Syndrome (APTITUDE-ACS)[151b] study patients presenting with ACS or for elective PCI who received loading doses of clopidogrel (600 mg, n = 13 or 900 mg, n = 12), prasugrel 60 mg (n = 10), or ticagrelor 180 mg (n = 10) were included. Platelet aggregation was assessed ex vivo by mixing platelet-rich plasma from blood sampling performed at baseline in increasing proportions with platelet-rich plasma sampled 4 hours after loading dose. The percentage restoration of residual platelet aggregation achieved was significantly decreased with increasing potency of P2Y$_{12}$ receptor inhibitors (RI) (83.9% $\pm$ 11%, 73% $\pm$ 14%, 66.3% $\pm$ 15%, 40.9% $\pm$ 19% for clopidogrel 600 mg, clopidogrel 900 mg, prasugrel, and ticagrelor, respectively; P for trend < 0.0001). In the APTITUDE-Coronary Artery Bypass Graft (APTITUDE-CABG) study, vasodilator-stimulated phosphoprotein-platelet reactivity index, a specific marker of the P2Y$_{12}$ RI drug-effect, was assessed before and after in vivo prothrombin (PT) administered for excessive bleeding in patients undergoing cardiac surgery while on a maintenance dose of aspirin and clopidogrel (n=45), prasugrel (n=6), or ticagrelor (n=3). When compared with baseline, there was a significant relative increase of 23.1% in platelet activation after platelet transfusion (42.2% $\pm$ 23.6% versus 56.6% $\pm$ 18.2%, P = 0.0008). The overall effect was modest with increasing potency of P2Y$_{12}$ inhibition.

The Challenge of Attenuating Ticagrelor's Pharmacodynamic Effect

The dynamic equilibrium of ticagrelor plasma concentrations and platelet binding creates a unique scenario when attempting to attenuate its pharmacodynamics effect. Comparatively high plasma levels translate to binding and inhibiting transfused platelets.[152a] Several other approaches have been tested. PRI-VASP was determined before and after in vitro platelet supplementation of platelet poor (PP) and platelet-rich plasma (PRP) at increasing concentrations from 79 whole blood samples of patients treated with ticagrelor, prasugrel, or clopidogrel. Compared to prasugrel- and clopidogrel-treated patients, the PRI-VASP of ticagrelor-treated patients showed no significant increase after in vitro administration of PP. PRI-VASP was performed in ticagrelor-treated samples after in vitro addition of centrifuged PRP platelets resuspended in PP buffer; PP with human serum or human serum alone. PP with human serum or human serum alone were able to significantly increase PRI-VASP in samples of ticagrelor-treated patients (11.7% $\pm$ 10.9% $\rightarrow$ 61.3% $\pm$ 10.9%, P = 0.006; 11.7% $\pm$ 10.9% $\rightarrow$ 54.1% $\pm$ 2.7%, P < 0.001). This effect could also be shown using human albumin (18.9% $\pm$ 5.1% $\rightarrow$ 80 g/L human albumin: 48.1% $\pm$ 8.3%, P < 0.001), suggesting that serum protein binding of ticagrelor effectively reduces its availability to bind and inhibit platelets.[152b]

A randomized, double-blind, placebo-controlled, phase I trial evaluated IV PB2452, a monoclonal antibody fragment that binds ticagrelor with high affinity, as a ticagrelor reversal agent. Platelet function was determined in healthy volunteers before and after 48 hours of ticagrelor pretreatment and again after the administration of PB2452 or placebo. Platelet function was assessed with the use of light transmission aggregometry, a point-of-care P2Y$_{12}$ platelet-reactivity test, and a vasodilator-stimulated phosphoprotein assay. Of the 64 volunteers who underwent randomization, 48 were assigned to receive PB2452 and 16 to receive placebo. After 48 hours of ticagrelor pretreatment, platelet aggregation was suppressed by approximately 80%. PB2452 administered as an initial IV bolus followed by a prolonged infusion (8, 12, or 16 hours) was associated with a significantly greater increase in platelet function than placebo, as measured by multiple assays. Ticagrelor reversal occurred within 5 minutes after the initiation of PB2452 and was sustained for more than 20 hours. There was no evidence of a rebound in platelet activity after drug cessation.[153]

Summary of Recommendations in Patients With ACS

Platelet antagonists play a pivotal role in the contemporary management of patients with ACS. A summary of drugs, clinical use, and supportive data derived from clinical trials is provided in Tables 8.9 and 8.10.

Table 8.9

Medical and antithrombotic therapy in the management of acute coronary syndrome: comparisons for American College of Cardiology/American Heart Association and European Society of Cardiology		
Nitrates	**ACC/AHA**	**ESC**
β-blockers aspirin	Sublingual nitroglycerin (I-C) or intravenous nitroglycerin for patients with hypertension, heart failure, or persistent symptoms (M3) Initiation of β-blockers within 24 h (I-A)	Sublingual or intravenous nitroglycerin (I-C) Early initiation of β-blockers (I-B)
GPIIb/IIIa inhibitors	Loading dose of aspirin 162–325 mg, maintenance dose of 81 mg/day indefinitely (I-A) Considered for initial therapy in patients undergoing early invasive strategy (IIb-B)	Loading dose of aspirin 150–300 mg, maintenance dose of 75–100 mg/day indefinitely (I-A) Considered during PCI for bailout situations (IIa-C)

Table 8.9

Medical and antithrombotic therapy in the management of acute coronary syndrome: comparisons for American College of Cardiology/American Heart Association and European Society of Cardiology (Continued)

Nitrates	ACC/AHA	ESC
Parenteral anticoagulation	Administered at time of PCI for high-risk patients, treated with unfractionated heparin and pretreated with clopidogrel (IIa-B) Recommended use of unfractionated heparin (I-B), enoxaparin (I-A), or fondaparinux (I-B) irrespective of treatment strategy	Fondaparinux recommended as having most favorable efficacy- safety profile irrespective of management strategy (I-B)
P2Y$_{12}$ inhibitors	Bivalirudin in patients undergoing early invasive strategy until PCI (I-B) Clopidogrel or ticagrelor, or prasugrel (for PCI patients), for up to 12 months (II-B)	Ticagrelor (I-B), prasugrel (I-B), or clopidogrel (I-B) for up to 12 months Cangrelor may be considered (IIb—A)

From Alame AJ, et al. Comparison of the American College of Cardiology/American Heart Association and the European Society of Cardiology Guidelines for the management of patients with non–ST-segment elevation acute coronary syndromes. *Coron Artery Dis* 2017;28:294–300.

Table 8.10

Guideline-directed therapy for special patient populations with acute coronary syndrome

	ACC/AHA	ESC
Elderly patients	Guideline-directed medical therapy, early invasive strategy, and revascularization for patients >75 years (I-A) Recommend coronary artery bypass graft surgery over percutaneous coronary intervention, especially in	Recommend an invasive strategy and revascularization according to current evidence (IIa-A)

Continued on following page

Table 8.10

Guideline-directed therapy for special patient populations with acute coronary syndrome (Continued)

	ACC/AHA	ESC
	patients with diabetes mellitus or three-vessel coronary artery disease (I-B)	
Patients with diabetes	Same treatment as for patients without diabetes mellitus (I-A) mellitus	Recommend invasive to noninvasive management, drug-eluting to bare metal stents, and coronary artery bypass graft surgery to percutaneous coronary intervention (I-A)
Patients with chronic kidney disease	Recommend an invasive strategy (IIa-B)	Recommend coronary artery bypass graft surgery over percutaneous coronary intervention if life expectancy >1 year, and percutaneous coronary intervention over coronary artery bypass graft surgery if life expectancy <1 year (IIa-B)

From Alame AJ, et.al. Comparison of the American College of Cardiology/American Heart Association and the European Society of Cardiology Guidelines for the management of patients with non–ST-segment elevation acute coronary syndromes. *Coron Artery Dis* 2017;28:294–300.

Anticoagulants

The participation of coagulation proteases, particularly FXa and FIIa (thrombin), in several phases of cell-based coagulation form a biology-centered use of pharmacologic therapy in patients with cardiovascular disease. Among hospitalized patients, the anti-thrombin (AT) drugs (UFH, low-molecular-weight heparins [LMWH], pentasaccharide) and direct thrombin inhibitors (DTIs) are used frequently, often in combination with platelet antagonists (Tables 8.11 and 8.12).

Table 8.11

Pharmacokinetic characteristics of parenteral anticoagulants

	Unfractionated heparin	Enoxaparin	Dalteparin	Fondaparinux	Bivalirudin	Argatroban
Target	AT	AT	AT	AT	Thrombin	Thrombin
Bioavailability	unpredictable	90%–92% (post-SQ)	87% (SQ)	100% (SQ)	40%–80%	100% IV
Vd	40–70 mL/min (same as blood volume)	4.3 L	3–4 L	7–11 L	0.24 L/Kg	0.174 L/kg
Protein binding	>90%	<UFH	<UFH	≥ 94% specifically to ATIII	No plasma proteins; just thrombin	55% 20% albumin 35% α-acid glycoprotein
Time to peak activity (hours)	Rapid after bolus, 4–6 h after infusion	3–5 h (SQ) (pk anti-Xa activity)	2–4 h(SQ) (pk anti-Xa activity)	2–3 h (SQ) (pk steady-state concentration)	2 min after bolus; 4 min after 15 min infusion (pk plasma concentrations)	3–4 h after infusion (pk plasma concentrations)
Half-life (hours)	1.0–1.5 (infusion)	5.0 (prolonged in severe RI, and with repeated dosing)	3–5 (prolonged in RI)	17 (young) 21 (elderly)	0.5 (prolonged in moderate–severe RI)	0.5–1.0

Continued on following page

Table 8.11

Pharmacokinetic characteristics of parenteral anticoagulants (Continued)

	Unfractionated heparin	Enoxaparin	Dalteparin	Fondaparinux	Bivalirudin	Argatroban
Elimination	Primarily by reticuloendothelial system. Small fraction excreted in urine.	80% Renal	Renal	Renal	Renal and proteolytic cleavage	Hepatic hydroxylation; 16% renal excretion as unchanged drug 14% biliary excretion as unchanged drug
CYP metabolism	No	No	No	No	No	Yes
CYP isoenzymes	No	No	No	No	No	CYP 3A4/5; Minimal believed to contribute significantly

anti-Xa, Anti-factor Xa; CI, continuous infusion; CYP, cytochrome P; pk, peak; RI, renal insufficiency; SQ, subcutaneous.
From DeWald TA, Becker RC. The pharmacology of novel oral anticoagulants. J Thromb Thrombolysis 2014;37:217–233.

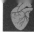

Table 8.12

Labeled indications for parenteral anticoagulants

Anticoagulant	Labeled indication(s)
UFH	Prophylaxis and treatment of venous thrombosis and its extension
	Prophylaxis and treatment of PE
	Prophylaxis and treatment of peripheral artery embolism
	Treatment of acute and chronic consumptive coagulopathies
	Atrial fibrillation with embolization
	Prevention of clotting in arterial and cardiac surgery
	May be used as an anticoagulant in blood transfusions, extracorporeal circulation, and dialysis procedures
	Prevention of postoperative DVT and PE in patients undergoing major abdominal surgery who are at risk of developing thromboembolic disease
Enoxaparin	Prophylaxis of DVT in acutely ill medical patients with severely restricted mobility, abdominal surgery, hip replacement surgery, or knee replacement surgery
	Treatment of acute DVT with or without PE
	Prophylaxis of ischemic complications in the setting of unstable angina or NSTEMI
	Treatment of acute STEMI managed medically or with percutaneous coronary intervention PCI
Dalteparin	Prophylaxis of ischemic complications of unstable angina or NSTEMI
	Prophylaxis of DVT in acutely ill medical patients with severely restricted mobility, abdominal surgery, or hip replacement surgery
	Extended treatment of symptomatic venous thromboembolism to reduce recurrence in patients with cancer
Fondaparinux	Treatment of DVT or PE (in conjunction with warfarin)
	Prophylaxis of DVT or PE after orthopedic surgery, including hip replacement, hip fracture, or knee replacement surgery
	Prophylaxis of DVT or PE after abdominal surgery in patients who are at risk for thromboembolic complications

Continued on following page

Table 8.12

Labeled indications for parenteral anticoagulants (Continued)

Anticoagulant	Labeled indication(s)
Argatroban	Prophylaxis or treatment of thrombosis in adult patients with HIT
	Use as an anticoagulant during PCI in adult patients with or at risk for HIT
Bivalirudin	Use as an anticoagulant in patients with unstable angina undergoing PCI
	Use as an anticoagulant in patients undergoing PCI with provision use of glycoprotein IIb/IIIa inhibitor
	Use as an anticoagulant in patients with or at risk of HIT or HITTS undergoing PCI

DVT, Deep vein thrombosis; *HIT*, heparin-induced thrombocytopenia; *HITTS*, heparin-induced thrombocytopenia and thrombosis syndrome; *NSTEMI*, non ST segment elevation myocardial infarction; *PCI*, percutaneous coronary intervention; *PE*, pulmonary embolism; *STEMI*, ST segment elevation myocardial infarction; *UFH*, unfractionated heparin.
From DeWald TA. Anticoagulants: pharmacokinetics, mechanisms of action, and indications. *Neurosurg Clin N Am* 2018;29:503–513.

Parenteral Anticoagulant Drugs

Heparins

Unfractionated Heparin

UFH achieves a rapid anticoagulant effect. UFH is a heterogeneous mixture of sulfated glycosaminoglycans of variable lengths and molecular weights. The anticoagulant effects and pharmacologic properties vary with the size of the molecules. UFH exerts its anticoagulant effects in three well-characterized and distinct ways. The major anticoagulant effect is the result of its high affinity for AT and the conformational change in AT that occurs from the binding of heparin and AT, inactivating FIXa, FXa, FXIa, and FXIIa. Thrombin and FXa are highly sensitive to inhibition by the heparin/AT complex. Inhibition of thrombin by UFH requires its binding to AT that occurs at a unique pentasaccharide sequence of the molecule and simultaneous binding of heparin to thrombin by 13 additional saccharide units. One-third of UFH molecules contain the high-affinity pentasaccharide required for its anticoagulant activity. The second mechanism of UFH's anticoagulant effect is inactivation of thrombin by heparin cofactor II.[154] The third mechanism that may not be clinically relevant at expected drug concentrations is through modulation of FXa generation achieved by UFH binding to factor IXa.

Low-Molecular-Weight Heparins

LMWHs are derived from UFH by chemical depolymerization. The overall process creates fragments that are approximately one-third the molecular weight of UFH.[155] LMWHs have a major role in catalyzing AT-mediated inhibition of coagulation factors; however, 50% to 75% of LMWH chains are too short to catalyze thrombin inhibition. These short chains do promote FXa inhibition, and accordingly LMWHs are comparatively more selective inhibitors of FXa than UFH. Other favorable features of LMWHs from UFH include reduced protein binding that improves their pharmacokinetic properties and results in a more predictable anticoagulant response and reduced interaction with platelets, which reduces the likelihood of heparin-induced thrombocytopenia (HIT).

Direct Thrombin Inhibitors

DTIs interact directly with thrombin and do not require AT (or heparin cofactor II) to achieve an anticoagulant effect. They specifically and reversibly inhibit free and clot-bound thrombin by binding to the active site of thrombin. *Argatroban* is a univalent direct thrombin inhibitor, binding only to the catalytic (active) site of thrombin as a competitive inhibitor of thrombin. *Bivalirudin* is a bivalent thrombin inhibitor, binding to both the catalytic (active) site and the substrate recognition (exosite 1) site of thrombin molecule.[156] Inhibition of thrombin attenuates formation of fibrin, reduces thrombin generation, and may limit platelet activation and aggregation. The direct oral thrombin inhibitor dabigatran will be discussed in a separate section.

Direct FXa Inhibitors

Fondaparinux, the first of a class of selective inhibitors of FXa, is a chemically synthesized sulfated pentasaccharide that specifically targets AT. After binding to AT, a permanent conformational change occurs in the molecule that causes an increased affinity for FXa. Fondaparinux does *not* inhibit thrombin directly, but inactivation of FXa by AT provides strong inhibition of thrombin generation.

Clinical Experience: General Use

In the hospital setting, common clinical indications for anticoagulants include prophylaxis of venous thromboembolism in acutely ill medical patients; prophylaxis of venous thromboembolism after surgical procedures, such as knee or hip replacement; thrombosis prophylaxis in patients with ACS; the treatment of acute venous and arterial thromboembolism; and periprocedural anticoagulation during coronary or other vascular interventions.

Unfractionated Heparin

UFH is a heterogeneous, negatively charged mucopolysaccharide consisting of approximately 18–50 saccharide units (molecular weight 5000–30,000 daltons).

Pharmacodynamics

UFH binds to AT and exerts its anticoagulant effects primarily through inhibition of thrombin and FXa.

Pharmacokinetics

Following IV administration, UFH binds to several plasma proteins, endothelial cells, and macrophages, explaining the wide variability in anticoagulant effect seen for a given dose. It is cleared from the circulation through both a rapid saturable mechanism and a slower first-order mechanism. The primary site of metabolism is within the reticular endothelial system. As a result, there is a dose-dependent half-life ranging from 60 minutes after a dose of 100 U/kg to 180 minutes for a dose of 400 U/kg.[157] A metabolite, uro-heparin, with minimal anticoagulant properties is cleared renally.

Adverse Effects

Bleeding and HIT are the most common and feared complications of UFH administration. Other adverse effects include hypersensitivity reactions, adrenal hemorrhage with shock, and osteopenia (with long-term administration).

Clinical Experience

Clinical trials have been conducted to compare the benefits of UFH and aspirin among patients with unstable angina and NSTEMI. The first trial, performed by Theroux and colleagues,[158] compared aspirin (325 mg twice daily), heparin (5000 U bolus, 1000 U per hour by IV infusion), their combination, and placebo in 479 patients. This is the only large-scale study that compared heparin (alone) and aspirin (alone), as well as their combination. Refractory angina occurred in 8.5%, 16.5%, and 10.7% of patients, respectively (0.47 relative risk for heparin compared with aspirin [95% CI 0.21–1.05; $P = 0.06$]). MI occurred in 0.9%, 3.3%, and 1.6% of patients, respectively (0.25 RR; 95% CI 0.03–2.271; $P = 0.18$), and any event was observed in 9.3%, 16.5%, and 11.5% of patients, respectively (0.52 RR, 95% CI 0.24–1.14; $P = 0.10$). Serious bleeding, defined as a fall in hemoglobin concentration of 2 g or more, or the need for a transfusion, occurred in 1.7%, 1.7%, and 3.3% of patients, respectively. Most of these events followed cardiac catheterization.

Many subsequent trials investigated the potential advantages of combination therapy (heparin plus aspirin) compared with aspirin monotherapy. Although outcomes with these treatments were not statistically different, consistent trends observed across each study favored combined pharmacotherapy and its ability to reduce death or MI (combined endpoint). A pooled analysis of the Antithrombotic Therapy in Acute Coronary Syndromes (ATACS) trial, the Research Group on Instability in Coronary Artery Disease in Southeast Sweden (RISC) study, and the Theroux trial yielded a relative risk of 0.44 (95% CI 0.21–0.93) for death/MI, in favor of combination therapy.[159-161]

HIT Therapy

Lepirudin, argatroban, and bivalirudin can be used in the management of HIT. In patients with suspected or proven HIT who require

PCI, argatroban (direct thrombin inhibitor, 240 µg/kg bolus followed by 20 µg/kg/min infusion) can be used during the intervention, with or without a GPIIb/IIIa antagonist.[162] Bivalirudin is licensed for use when HIT or heparin induced thrombocytopenia and thrombosis syndrome (HITTS) complicates PCI.

Clinical Experience

Acute Myocardial Infarction

In acute MI STEMI, UFH can be administered with thrombolytic therapy or during primary PCI. In ACS, UFH can be administered and is most beneficial in the setting of an elevated troponin value (Table 8.13). Other anticoagulant options and specific dosing recommendations are summarized in Tables 8.13 and 8.14, respectively.

Table 8.13

2014 ACC/AHA guideline recommendations for parenteral anticoagulants in non–ST-segment elevation acute coronary syndrome (NSTE-ACS)		
Recommendation	Class of recommendation	Level of evidence
SQ enoxaparin for duration of hospitalization or until PCI is performed	I	A
Bivalirudin until diagnostic angiography or PCI is performed in patients with early invasive strategy only	I	B
SQ fondaparinux for the duration of hospitalization or until PCI is performed	I	B
Administer additional anticoagulant with anti-IIa activity if PCI is performed while patient is on fondaparinux	I	B
IV UFH for 48 hours or until PCI is performed	I	B
IV fibrinolytic treatment not recommended in patients with NSTE-ACS	III	A

IV, Intravenous; *NSTE-ACS*, non–ST-segment elevation acute coronary syndrome; *PCI*, percutaneous coronary intervention; *SQ*, subcutaneous; *UFH*, unfractionated heparin.
From Amsterdam EA et al. 2014 AHA/ACC Guideline for the management of patients with non–ST-elevation acute coronary syndromes: a report of the American College of Cardiology/American Heart Association task force on practice guidelines. *J Am Coll Cardiol* 2014;64:e139–e228.

Table 8.14

Dosing of parenteral anticoagulant drugs in NSTE-ACS

Anticoagulant	Upstream therapy for NSTE-ACS	During PCI (if upstream therapy given for NSTE-ACS)	During PCI (no upstream therapy given or elective PCI)
Bivalirudin	0.1 mg/kg IV bolus, 0.25 mg/kg/h IV infusion	0.5 mg/kg IV bolus, increase infusion to 1.75 mg/kg/h If UFH was given, discontinue UFH, wait for 30 minutes, then give 0.75 mg/kg IV bolus, 1.75 mg/kg/h IV infusion	0.75 mg/kg IV bolus, 1.75 mg/kg/h IV infusion
Unfractionated heparin (UFH)	Loading dose of 60 U/kg (max 4000 U) as IV bolus Maintenance IV infusion of 12 U/kg/h (max 1,000 U/h) to maintain aPTT at 1.5–2.0 times control (approximately 50–70 seconds)	IV GPIIb/IIIa planned: IV bolus doses with target ACT 200–250 seconds No IV GP IIb/IIIa planned: IV bolus doses with target ACT 250–300 seconds for HemoTec; 300–350 seconds for Hemochron	IV GPIIb/IIIa planned: 50–70 U/kg IV bolus with target ACT 200–250 seconds No IV GPIIb/IIIa planned: 70–100 U/kg IV bolus to achieve target ACT of 250–300 seconds for HemoTec; 300–350 seconds for Hemochron
Enoxaparin	Loading dose of 30 mg IV may be given in selected patients Maintenance of 1 mg/kg SQ every 12 hours Extend dosing interval to 1 mg/kg SQ every 24 hours if estimated CrCl <30 mL/min	Last SQ dose within 8 hours: no additional therapy Last SQ dose 8–12 hours prior or if <2 therapeutic SQ doses administered: 0.3 mg/kg IV bolus	0.5–0.75 mg/kg IV bolus

8 — Antithrombotic Drugs

Continued on following page

Table 8.14

Dosing of parenteral anticoagulant drugs in NSTE-ACS (Continued)

Anticoagulant	Upstream therapy for NSTE-ACS	During PCI (if upstream therapy given for NSTE-ACS)	During PCI (no upstream therapy given or elective PCI)
Fondaparinux	2.5 mg SQ once daily Avoid for CrCl <30 mL/min	Use another agent with anti-IIa activity considering whether GPIIb/IIIa planned	N/A (use other agent if no prior exposure to fondaparinux)

ACT, Activated clotting time; *aPTT*, activated partial thromboplastin time; *CrCl*, creatinine clearance: *GP*, glycoprotein; *IV*, intravenous; *NSTE-ACS*, non–ST-segment acute coronary syndrome; *PCI*, percutaneous coronary intervention; *SQ*, subcutaneous.
From Amsterdam EA et al. 2014 AHA/ACC guideline for the management of patients with non–ST-elevation acute coronary syndromes: a report of the American College of Cardiology/American Heart Association task force on practice guidelines. *J Am Coll Cardiol* 2014;64:e139–e228.

Elective PCI

In elective PCI, a standard regimen is 70–100 IU/kg, with additional weight-adjusted boluses to achieve and maintain an ACT of 200–250 seconds.[163] If a GPIIb/IIIa antagonist is coadministered, the initial heparin dosage is reduced to 70 IU/kg (bolus), followed by additional bolus doses as needed to maintain an ACT of 200 seconds. Heparin should be discontinued immediately after PCI.

Extracorporeal Membrane Oxygenation

Mechanical circulatory support (MCS) has been critical for cardiac surgery and postcardiotomy cardiogenic shock. CPB provides heart-lung support during open heart surgeries while extracorporeal membrane oxygenation (ECMO) can provide short-term partial or total cardiac support for postcardiotomy syndrome and a wide spectrum of severe cardiogenic shock patients. In addition to full cardiac support, ECMO provides oxygenation through an artificial lung. Blood exposure to the large surface of the ECMO circuits disrupts normal hemostasis like other MCS devices but also induces a strong inflammatory response similar to cardiopulmonary bypass (CPB). In the absence of HIT, anticoagulation with UFH is necessary to prevent clotting of the ECMO circuit with a goal activated partial thromboplastin time (aPTT) 1.5–2.0 times the upper limit of normal. As with other MCS devices that require anticoagulation, thrombotic and bleeding complications are common and occur in up to 50% of ECMO supported patients. Anticoagulation can be held during ECMO support if life-threatening bleeding occurs.[164]

Left Ventricular Device Thrombosis

The diagnosis of LVAD thrombosis is made by clinical exam and history, laboratory results, pump parameters, and echocardiographic imaging including ramp studies. Standard treatment for suspected or confirmed pump thrombosis is anticoagulation with IV UFH and the addition of antiplatelet therapy. Direct thrombin inhibitors, primarily bivalirudin, have been used as an alternative anticoagulant to UFH, but are more expensive and not clearly proven to be superior to UFH. Bivalirudin can be used in patients with HIT. DAPT with aspirin plus clopidogrel or dipyridamole can be considered to enhance antiplatelet effect.[165] Pump exchange is usually performed for confirmed LVAD thrombosis not responsive to medical treatment especially in patients with hemodynamic compromise and end organ hypoperfusion. Heart transplantation is another option if a donor heart is available. Thrombolytic therapy is *not* recommended for either suspected or confirmed pump thrombosis in patients who are candidates for pump exchange due to high risk for intracranial hemorrhage. Clinical experience with direct thrombin inhibitors, GPIIb/IIIa inhibitors, and thrombolytics has been summarized in comprehensive reviews.[166,167]

Transcatheter Valve and Structural Heart Interventions

Structural heart procedures are often associated with a significant risk of both thromboembolic and bleeding complications; hence in such context, the delicate balance between the thrombotic and bleeding risks must be carefully weighed. Although such procedures have been exceedingly associated with successful outcomes, the incidence of thromboembolic complications, particularly CVEs, has been generating ongoing concerns.[168] To date, the effectiveness of antiplatelet therapy and its optimal regimen before and after percutaneous valvular and structural heart interventions remain a subject of investigation.

Transcatheter Aortic Valve Replacement (TAVR)

In the Placement of Aortic Transcatheter Valves (PARTNER) Trial, the incidence of stroke was higher in the TAVR group compared with surgical replacement at 1-year follow-up (5.1% versus 2.4%, $P = 0.07$). Evaluation of the clinical impact of valve thrombosis and the role of oral anticoagulation therein, especially that of novel oral anticoagulant agents, requires additional investigations.

Current guidelines recommend the use of DAPT with aspirin and clopidogrel for 3–6 months in patients undergoing TAVR (Table 8.15).[169,170] However, no evidence for clear benefit of DAPT over single antiplatelet therapy has yet been seen from clinical trials; and as such, it may be reasonable to adopt a strategy of a single antiplatelet therapy except for patients with concomitant atrial fibrillation.

Indirect, Selective FXa Inhibitors

Synthetic Pentasaccharide: Fondaparinux

Fondaparinux is a synthetic pentasaccharide that requires AT for selective FXa binding. Unlike heparin compounds, fondaparinux does not inhibit thrombin directly, nor does it interact with platelets (or platelet derived proteins). After subcutaneous (SQ) administration in healthy volunteers fondaparinux is nearly 100% bioavailable and the absorption is rapid (C_{max} within 2 hours).[171] Clearance occurs by renal mechanisms with a terminal half-life of 17 +/- 3 hours (slightly longer in elderly volunteers). Overall, drug clearance is 25% lower in patients with mild renal impairment (creatinine clearance [CrCl] 50–80 mL/min; approximately 40% lower with

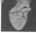

Table 8.15

Recommendations for antithrombotic drugs during and after TAVR		
TAVR	American College of Cardiology (ACC)/ American Heart Association (AHA)/ Society of Thoracic Surgeons (STS)	European Society of Cardiology (ESC)
Procedural	Unfractionated heparin (ACT >300 seconds)	
Postprocedural	Aspirin 75–100 mg/day indefinitely; Clopidogrel 75 mg/day for 6 months; if VKA indicated, no clopidogrel	Aspirin or clopidogrel indefinitely; Aspirin and clopidogrel early after TAVI; if VKA indicated, no antiplatelet therapy

ACT, Activated clotting time; *TAVR,* transcatheter aortic valve replacement; *VKA,* vitamin K antagonist.
Data from Nishimura RA, et al. 2017 AHA/ACC Focused update of the 2014 AHA/ACC guideline for the management of patients with valvular heart disease: a report of the American College of Cardiology/American Heart Association task force on clinical practice guidelines. *J Am Coll Cardiol* 2017;70:252–289.

moderate renal impairment [CrCl 30–50 mL/min], and 55% lower in the setting of severe renal impairment [CrCl <30 mL/min]).

Clinical Experience

Fondaparinux is approved for the prophylaxis of deep venous thrombosis in patients undergoing abdominal surgery, traumatic hip surgery, hip replacement, and knee replacement.

The Organization to Assess Strategies in Acute Ischemic Syndromes (OASIS)-5 Study[172] assigned 20,078 patients with ACS to receive fondaparinux (2.5 mg daily SQ) or enoxaparin (1 mg per kilogram of body weight twice daily SQ) for a mean of 6 days and evaluated death, MI, or refractory ischemia at 9 days (the primary outcome measure), as well as major bleeding and a combination of the two. The numbers of patients with primary outcome events were similar in the two groups (fondaparinux, 5.8%, versus enoxaparin, 5.7%; HR in the fondaparinux group, 1.01; 95% CI 0.90–1.13), satisfying the noninferiority criteria. The rate of major bleeding at 9 days was markedly lower with fondaprinux than with enoxaparin (2.2% versus 4.1%; HR 0.52; $P < 0.001$). A composite of the primary outcome measure and major bleeding at 9 days favored fondaparinux (7.3% versus 9%; HR 0.81;$P < 0.001$). Fondaparinux was associated with a significant reduction in the number of patients with fatal bleeding and TIMI major bleeding. Regardless of treatment, patients who had major bleeding during hospitalization had significantly higher rates of death, reinfarction, or stroke at 30 days and at 180 days than did patients without major or minor bleeding. These higher event rates associated with bleeding persisted after adjustments were made for a number of clinical characteristics often associated with bleeding. Accordingly, almost the entire difference in mortality between fondaparinux and enoxaparin-treated patients could be attributed to the lower rate of bleeding associated with fondaparinux.

In a subgroup analysis, benefits and risks were consistently in favor of fondaprinux. Rates of bleeding were consistently lower with fondaprinux, regardless of whether UFH was administered before randomization. The proportions of patients undergoing PCI (39.5% in the fondaparinux group and 39.5% in the enoxaparin group) and coronary arterial bypass grafting (15.3% and 14.5%, respectively) were similar in the two groups. Rates of the combination of death, MI, and refractory ischemia were similar at 9 days, at 30 days, and at the end of the study. An increase in guiding catheter thrombus formation was observed with fondaprinux (0.9% versus 0.4%); however, rates of other complications, including pseudoaneurysm formation, large hematomas, major bleeding, and complications involving the vascular access site, were all less common with fondaparinux than with enoxaparin. Collectively, the rate of death, MI, stroke, major bleeding, or any procedural complication at 9 days was 16.6% with fondaparinux as compared with 20.6% with enoxaparin (RR 0.81; 95% CI 0.73–0.90; $P < 0.001$)

The OASIS-6 study[173] was a randomized double-blind comparison of fondaparinux 2.5 mg once daily versus placebo for up to 8 days in 12,092 patients with STEMI. The composite of death or reinfarction at 30 days served as the primary outcome measure, with secondary assessments at 9 days and at final follow-up (3–6 months). Death or reinfarction at 30 days was significantly reduced from 11.2% in the control group to 9.7% among patients receiving fondaparinux; in a comparison of patients receiving fondaparinux versus those given UFH, fondaprinux was found to be superior in preventing death or reinfarction at 30 days (HR 0.82; 95% CI 0.66–1.02; $P = 0.08$) and at study end (HR 0.77; 95% CI 0.64–0.93; $P = 0.008$). Significant benefit was observed among patients receiving fibrinolytic therapy (HR 0.83; 95% CI 0.73–0.94; $P = 0.003$), but not in those undergoing primary PCI. The use of a single fixed dose (2.5 mg once daily SQ) of fondaparinux without monitoring or dose adjustment for weight across a broad range of creatinine levels, coupled with simplicity, safety, and efficacy in ACS, may facilitate its use.

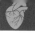

Low-Molecular-Weight Heparin

Low-molecular-weight heparin (LMWH) is prepared by the depoly-merization of porcine UFH. A variety of processes are used, giving distinctive products whose molecular weights range from 4000 to 6500 Da. Like UFH, approximately one-third of LMWH polysaccha-ride chains contain the pentasaccharide-binding site for antithrom-bin. The LMWH-AT complex (consisting of a predominance of shorter-chain polysaccharides) has relatively weak AT activity but retains the ability to inactivate FXa. The ratio of anti-Xa activity to anti-IIa (antithrombin) activity varies from 2:1 to 4:1. Similar to UFH, LMWH does not inhibit thrombin bound to fibrin.

Pharmacokinetics

When LMWH is given in either fixed or weight-adjusted doses by the SQ route, greater than 90% of the dose is absorbed. By contrast to UFH, LMWH has minimal binding to cells or plasma proteins, resulting in persistence of free drug in the circulation and a longer half-life. While the half-life of UFH averages about 90 minutes, the half-life of LMWH averages about 180 minutes (the half-lives of three LMWHs range from 90 to 260 minutes).

Safety

Thrombocytopenia is infrequently observed with LMWH adminis-tration, but antibodies directed against complexes of LMWH and platelet factor 4 have been detected in some patients. On rare occa-sion, the full-blown syndrome of HIT occurs. Equally rare is necrosis at the site of skin injections with LMWH, which may represent a form of local HIT.

Clinical Experience

The original experience with LMWH[174] included 205 patients with unstable angina who were randomized to either aspirin (200 mg daily), aspirin (200 mg daily) plus UFH (5000 U bolus, 400 U/kg per day infusion), or high-dose nadroparin (214 IU/kg twice daily by SQ injection) plus aspirin (200 mg daily). Patients underwent continuous ST-segment monitoring during the first 48 hours of treat-ment. Overall, 73% of patients receiving LMWH were free from ischemic events, compared with 39% of those receiving UFH and 40% of patients given aspirin alone. There were fewer silent ische-mic events in the LMWH group (18%) compared with those receiv-ing UFH (29%) or aspirin alone (34%). Recurrent angina occurred in 9%, 26%, and 19% of patients, respectively, and MIs were not observed in LMWH-treated patients (compared with 1% in the UFH and 6% in the aspirin alone groups). Major bleeding occurred infrequently in all treatment groups.

A larger study, FRagmin during InStability in Coronary artery disease (FRISC)-1,[175] included 1506 patients with unstable angina and NSTEMI randomized to LMWH (dalteparin, 120 IU/kg body weight subcutaneous [SQ] [maximum 10,000 IU] twice daily for 6 days, then 7500 IU once daily for 35–45 days) or placebo. All patients received aspirin (300 mg first dose, 75 mg daily thereafter). Accordingly, FRISC I investigated the combination of LMWH plus aspirin versus aspirin alone. The risk of death or MI was reduced by 63% at day 6. The probability of death, MI, and need for revascularization remained lower in the LMWH-treated patients at 40 days; however, modest differences between groups was observed beyond the treatment period.

In the FRIC study,[176] 1482 patients with unstable angina and NSTEMI were assigned either twice-daily weight-adjusted SQ injections of LMWH (dalteparin 120 IU/kg) or dose-adjusted (target APTT 1.5 times the control) IV UFH for 6 days (acute treatment phase). Patients randomized to UFH received a continuous infusion for at least 48 hours and were given the option of either continuing the infusion or changing to a SQ regimen (12,500 U every 12 hours). In the double-blind comparison that took place from days 6 to 45 (prolonged treatment phase), patients received either LMWH (dalteparin, 7500 IU SQ once daily) or placebo. Aspirin (75–165 mg/day) was initiated in all patients as early as possible after hospital admission and continued throughout the study. During the first 6 days, the rate of death, recurrent angina, and MI was 7.6% in the UFH-treated patients and 9.3% in the LMWH-treated patients (RR 1.18; 95% CI 0.84–1.66). Revascularization was required in 5.3% and 4.8% (CI 0.57–1.35) of patients, respectively. Between days 6 and 45, the composite endpoint was reached in 12.3% of patients in both the LMWH and placebo groups.

The Efficacy and Safety of subcutaneous Enoxaparin in Non-Q Wave Coronary Events (ESSENCE) trial[177] randomly assigned 3171 patients with angina at rest or NSTEMI either LMWH (Enoxaparin, 1 mg/kg SQ twice daily) or IV UFH (target aPTT 55–85 seconds). Therapy was continued for a minimum of 48 hours (maximum 8 days). All patients received aspirin (100–325 mg daily). The median duration of therapy for both groups was 2.6 days. At 14 days, the risk of death, recurrent angina, or MI was 16.6% among patients receiving LMWH and 19.8% for patients given UFH (16% risk reduction). A similar risk reduction (15%) for the composite outcome was observed at 30 days. The benefit of LMWH treatment was maintained at 1 year.[178]

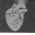
The TIMI IIB Study, compared enoxaparin and UFH in 3910 patients with unstable angina and NSTEMI.[179] The trial design had several unique features compared with ESSENCE. First, enoxaparin therapy was initiated with a 30-mg IV bolus, followed by 1.0 mg/kg SQ twice daily. Second, UFH treatment was given according to a weight-adjusted dosing strategy (70 U/kg bolus, followed by 15 U/kg/h infusion to a target APTT 1.5–2.5 times control). Lastly, there was an out-of-hospital treatment phase comparing enoxaparin and placebo for approximately 6 weeks (patients ≥65 kg received <60 mg SQ BID; those <65 kg received 45 mg SQ BID for a total of 43 days). Treatment with enoxaparin was associated with a significant reduction in the composite outcome of death, MI or urgent revascularization compared with UFH at day 14 (14.2% versus 16.7%; RRR 15%, $P = 0.03$). Continued treatment beyond the initial hospital phase did not provide added benefit (17.3% versus 19.7%, RRR 12%, $P = 0.051$).

A meta-analyses of the ESSENCE and TIMI IIB trials, totaling 7081 patients with non–ST-segment elevation ACS, revealed a 20% reduction in the risk of any ischemic event[180] favoring enoxaparin over UFH. The differences were statistically significant at 48 hours and 43 days. The combined endpoint of death or MI was reduced by 20% at 48 hours ($P = 0.02$) and 18% at 43 days ($P = 0.02$). A significant treatment benefit for enoxaparin on the rate of death, nonfatal MI or urgent revascularization was observed at one year (HR 0.88, $P = 0.008$, absolute difference 2.5%). A progressively greater treatment benefit was observed as the level of patient risk increased.

Combined Pharmacology and Coronary Interventional Strategies

The FRagmin and fast revascularization during InStability in Coronary artery disease (FRISC II)[181] included 2267 patients with unstable coronary disease who received 5 days of dalteparin (120 IU/kg SQ q12h) and were then randomized to either an invasive or conservative treatment strategy. In a separate randomization, patients received either dalteparin (5000–7500 IU SQ q12h) or placebo injections for 3 months. By 30 days there was a significant reduction in death or MI favoring dalteparin-treated patients (3.1% versus 5.9%, $P = 0.002$). The benefit decayed over the next 2 months. An invasive strategy (coronary angiography and revascularization) was associated with a significant reduction in death or MI at 6 months compared with ischemia-driven revascularization (9.4% versus 12.1%, $P = 0.03$). The mortality rates were 1.9% and 2.9%, respectively (FRISC II Investigators, 1999). At 24-month follow-up, there were reductions in mortality (3.7% versus 12.7%, RR 0.72,

$P = 0.005$) and the composite endpoint of death or MI (12.1% versus 16.3%, RR 0.74, $P = 0.003$) in the invasive compared with the non-invasive group. The need for repeat hospitalizations and late revascularization procedures was lower in patients who underwent an early invasive strategy.

The Randomized Intervention Trial of unstable Angina (RITA) study randomized 1810 patients with non–ST segment elevation ACS who received enoxaparin (1 mg/kg SQ twice daily for 2 to 8 days) and aspirin to either an early intervention or conservative strategy.[182] At 4 months, 9.6% of patients randomized to an early intervention had either died, experienced an MI, or experienced refractory angina compared with 14.5% in the conservative group (RR 0.66; 95% CI 0.51, 0.85; $P = 0.001$). Death or MI was similar in both treatment groups at 1 year (7.6% versus 8.3%, respectively, RR 0.91; 95% CI 0.67, 1.25; $P = 0.58$). Fewer patients undergoing early intervention experienced symptoms of angina or required antianginal medications.

In the Superior Yield of the New Strategy of Enoxaparin, Revascularization and GPIIb/IIIa Inhibitors (SYNERGY) trial,[183] 10,027 high-risk non–ST-segment elevation ACS patients were randomized to UFH or enoxaparin. Overall, 92% of patients underwent coronary angiography, 47% had PCI (in-hospital), and 57% received GPIIb/IIIa antagonists. The primary endpoint of death or nonfatal MI at 3 days occurred in 14.5% of patients assigned to UFH and 14.0% of those given enoxaparin (OR 0.956; 95% CI 0.869–1.063), fulfilling the noninferiority criteria. There were no differences in ischemic events during PCI between the antithrombins. Major bleeding was modestly increased with enoxaparin. Transfusion rates did not differ and there was a relationship between advancing age, reduced CrCl, and risk of hemorrhage.

In the Enoxaparin and Thrombolysis Reperfusion for Acute Myocardial Infarction Treatment (ExTRACT)-TIMI 25 study,[184] 20,506 patients with STEMI who were scheduled to undergo fibrinolysis received enoxaparin throughout the index hospitalization or UFH for at least 48 hours. The primary efficacy endpoint, death or nonfatal recurrent MI through day 30, occurred in 12% of patients in the UFH group and 9.9% of those in the enoxaparin group (17% reduction in RR, $P < 0.001$). Nonfatal reinfarction occurred in 4.5% of patients receiving UFH and 3% of those who were given enoxaparin (33% reduction in RR, $P < 0.001$). A nonstatistically significant reduction in death occurred (7.5% versus 6.9%, respectively, $P = 0.11$). Major bleeding occurred in 1.4% and 2.1% of patients, respectively. The composite of death, nonfatal reinfarction, or nonfatal intracranial hemorrhage (a measure of net clinical benefit) occurred in 12.2% of patients administered heparin and 10.1% of those given enoxaparin ($P < 0.001$).

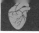

In the Acute Myocardial Infarction Treated with Primary Angioplasty and Intravenous Enoxaparin or Unfractionated Heparin to Lower Ischemic and Bleeding Events at Short and Long-term Follow-up (ATOLL)[185] trial, 910 patients were randomized to treatment with enoxaparin or UFH before PCI. There was a nonsignificant reduction in the major endpoint of 30-day incidence of death, complication of MI, procedure failure, or major bleeding in the enoxaparin group (28% versus 34%; RR = 0.83; 95% CI 0.68–1.01; $P = 0.06$). However, treatment with enoxaparin was associated with a significant reduction in the main secondary endpoint, death, recurrent ACS, or urgent revascularization (30 [7%] versus 52 [11%] patients; RR = 0.59; 95% CI 0.38–0.91; $P = 0.015$).

LMWH and Platelet GPIIb/IIIa Receptor Antagonist Combination Therapy

The available information, derived from clinical trials of PCI, suggest that anti-Xa activity >0.5 IU/mL is associated with a low incidence of ischemic/thrombotic and hemorrhagic events.[186] The potential benefit of enoxaparin (1 mg/kg every 12 hours) and the platelet GPIIb/IIIa receptor antagonist, tirofiban (10 mg/kg bolus, 0.1 mg/kg/min for a minimum of 48 hours), compared with weight-adjusted UFH and tirofiban, was investigated in the A to Z trial[187]—a prospective, open-label, randomized study of 3987 patients with non–ST-segment elevation ACS. Death, recurrent MI, or refractory ischemia at 7 days occurred in 8.4% of enoxaparin-treated patients and 9.4% of those receiving UFH (HR 0.88) (criteria for noninferiority satisfied). The RRs were of larger magnitude (favoring enoxaparin) among patients at highest risk and those treated conservatively. Major bleeding was more common in patients receiving enoxaparin (0.9% versus 0.4% with UFH; one excess major hemorrhagic event for every 200 patients treated); however, transfusion rates were low overall (0.9%) and did not differ between groups.

A meta-analysis of clinical trials comparing enoxaparin and UFH for the treatment of ACS was conducted by Murphy and colleagues. A total of 12 trials including 49,088 patients was analyzed and revealed a numerical reduction in the net clinical endpoint of death or MI, or major bleeding by 30 days favoring enoxaparin (12.5% versus 13.5%, OR 0.9, $P = 0.051$). Death or MI was significantly reduced with enoxaparin as compared to UFH (9.8% versus 11.4%, OR = 0.84, $P < 0.001$), but major bleeding occurred more frequently with enoxaparin (4.3% versus 3.4%, OR = 1.25, $P = 0.019$). The net clinical endpoint was significantly lower with enoxaparin in trials of STEMI (OR = 0.84, $P = 0.015$), but there was no significant difference in NSTEACS trials. (OR = 0.97).[188]

In the Acute Catheterization and Urgent Triage Strategy (ACUITY) trial,[189] 13819 patients with ACS randomly received either bivalirudin plus a GPIIb/IIIa receptor antagonist, heparin (heparin or enoxaparin) plus a GPIIb/IIIa receptor antagonist, or bivalirudin alone. The primary outcome, which consisted of all-cause mortality, MI, or unplanned revascularization for ischemia at 30 days, did not differ significantly between groups. Bivalirudin alone was associated with a 50% reduction in major bleeding complications.

Influence of Renal Function

FXa inhibition pharmacokinetics were studied in 445 patients receiving enoxaparin (1.0–1.25 mg/kg SQ q 12 hours).[190] The mean apparent clearance, distribution volume, and plasma half-life were 0.733 L/h, 5.24 L, and 5 hours, respectively. CrCl emerged as the most important factor affecting apparent clearance, area under the curve, and anti-Xa activity. Clearance was reduced by 22% in patients with CrCl $\leq$40 mL/min (compared to patients with normal renal function [CrCl >80 mL/min]). These patients had higher peak and trough anti-Xa activity and were also more likely to experience major hemorrhagic events. Renal performance may not influence pharmacokinetics following single-dose IV administration of enoxaparin.

Direct Thrombin Inhibitors

The pivotal role of thrombin in all phases of coagulation, cellular proliferation, and cellular interactions involved centrally in inflammatory processes provides an attractive target for pharmacologic inhibition. The development of DTIs has evolved rapidly to include both IV and oral preparations.

Hirudin

Hirudin is extracted from the parapharyngeal gland of the medicinal leech *hirudo medicinalis*. Several derivatives and recombinant preparations have been developed including the most widely used agent lepirudin. Hirudin binds to both the catalytic and fibrinogen-binding sites of thrombin and thus is considered a bivalent inhibitor.

Pharmokinetics

The plasma half-life of hirudin is 50–65 minutes, with a biologic half-life of 2 hours. The properties of heparins, hirudin, and bivalirudin are highlighted in Table 8.11. The predominant renal clearance of hirudin must be emphasized for safe clinical use.

Hirudin forms a tight complex with thrombin, inhibiting the conversion of fibrinogen to fibrin as well as thrombin-induced platelet aggregation.[191] These actions are independent of the presence of antithrombin, and also affect thrombin bound to fibrin. On the downside, the ability of thrombin to complex with thrombomodulin, activating protein C, is also inhibited. Hirudin does not bind to platelet factor 4, nor does it elicit antibodies that can cause platelet and endothelial cell activation; thus, it can be safely administered to patients with HIT. Hirudin does have weak immunogenicity, so that diminished (or rarely increased) responsiveness after repeated dosing is possible.

Clinical Experience

In the GUSTO IIb trial,[192] patients with non–ST-segment elevation ACS received either UFH or hirudin (0.1 mg/kg IV bolus, 0.1 mg/kg/h infusion). At 24 hours the risk of death or nonfatal MI was reduced in hirudin-treated patients (1.3% versus 2.1%, $P = 0.001$). The primary endpoint of death or nonfatal MI at 30 days was reached in 8.9% and 9.8% of patients, respectively (OR 0.89, $P = 0.06$). The risk of moderate bleeding was increased with hirudin treatment (8.8% versus 7.7%, $P = 0.03$).

The Organization to Asses Strategies for Ischemic Syndromes (OASIS-1)-1 study[193] included 909 patients with unstable angina or suspected MI without ST segment elevation who were randomized to receive UFH (5000 U bolus, 1000–1200 U/h infusion), low-dose hirudin (0.2 mg/kg bolus, 0.1 mg/kg/h infusion), or moderate-dose hirudin (0.4 mg/kg bolus, 0.15 mg/kg/h infusion). Doses of UFH and hirudin were titrated to a target APTT of 60–100 seconds. Hirudin, compared to UFH, reduced the composite incidence of cardiovascular death, MI, or refractory angina at 7 days (OR 0.57; 95% CI 0.32, 1.02) and a composite of death, MI, or refractory/severe angina requiring revascularization at 7 days (OR 0.49; 95% CI 0.27, 0.86). Overall event rates were lowest in the moderate-dose hirudin group.

The favorable results in OASIS-1 prompted a large phase III trial, OASIS-2,[194] which randomized 10,141 patients with non–ST-segment elevation ACS to a 72-hour infusion of either moderate-dose hirudin (as defined in OASIS–1) or UFH. The primary outcome (composite of death or MI at 7 and 35 days) was reported in 3.6% and 4.2% of patients (OR 0.87; 95% CI 0.75, 1.01), respectively. Although statistically significant differences between groups were not observed. the combined OASIS-1 and OASIS-2 experience revealed a significant reduction in the likelihood of death or MI at 35 days among hirudin-treated patients (OR 0.86; 95% CI 0.74–0.99).

Hirudin is almost exclusively excreted through the kidneys, and as a result, renal function must be considered carefully prior to administration. A majority of clinical trials excluded patients with a creatine of 2.0 mg/dl or greater. It is important to acknowledge that even in the setting of mild renal impairment (CrCl 50–80 mL/min), excessive levels of systemic anticoagulation (and accompanying risk for hemorrhage) can occur with nonmodified dosing. If hirudin is administered to patients with renal insufficiency, frequent APTT monitoring is highly recommended.

Bivalirudin

Bivalirudin is a 20-amino-acid-long synthetic peptide with thrombin-specific anticoagulant properties. Bivalirudin reversibly binds thrombin, free as well as clot bound, at the catalytic site and the anion-binding exosite, thereby preventing the formation and activation of fibrin, FXIIIa, and other coagulation factors.

Pharmacodynamics

Bivalirudin is an intravenous, direct, and reversible inhibitor of thrombin that acts through binding both to the catalytic and anion-binding exosite. It prolongs the thrombin, aPTT, and PT in a concentration-dependent manner.

Pharmacokinetics

Following a 1-mg/kg IV bolus, peak concentration is achieved rapidly, with a plasma half-life of 25 minutes among patients with normal renal function. Drug elimination is reduced by 20% in the setting of moderate renal impairment, 50% in several renal impairment, and 80% in dialysis-dependent patients. The drugs pharmacokinetic characteristics translate to half-lives of 34 minutes, 57 minutes, and 3.5 hours, respectively.

Clinical Experience

Bivalirudin is FDA approved for use in patients with non–ST-segment elevation ACS undergoing PCI. The basis for approval stems from several large-scale clinical trials.[195] Among 4312 patients with new-onset, severe, accelerating or rest angina undergoing PCI, a 22% reduction in death, MI, or urgent revascularization at 7 days was observed in those given bivalirudin compared with UFH (6.2% versus 7.9%, $P = 0.03$). The absolute and relative differences were maintained at 90 days. A marked reduction (62%) in bleeding complications among bivalirudin-treated patients was also reported.

In the Randomized Evaluation in Percutaneous coronary intervention Linking Angiomax to reduced Clinical Events (REPLACE-1) trial,[196] 1020 patients received either bivalirudin (0.75 mg/kg bolus, 1.75 mg/kg/h infusion) or UFH. Prior treatment with aspirin and a thienopyridine was encouraged in anticipation of stenting. A platelet GPIIb/IIIa receptor antagonist was administered to 71% of patients. Bivalirduin was associated with a 19% reduction in the clinical endpoint of death, MI, urgent revascularization, and bleeding complications (minor, major, transfusions) at 48 hours.

REPLACE-2[197] randomized 6010 patients undergoing urgent or elective PCI to bivalirudin plus provisional GPIIb/IIIa receptor antagonist (abciximab or eptifibatide) administration or UFH plus a GPIIb/IIIa receptor antagonist. Aspirin and clopidogrel pretreatment were recommended. Approximately 45% of patients had either unstable angina or MI (within the prior 7 days). The composite of death, MI, and urgent revascularization at 30 days occurred in 7.1% of heparin and 7.6% of bivalirudin-treated patients (OR 0.917; 95% CI 0.772, 1.089; $P = 0.32$). Major bleeding was documented in 4.1% and 2.4% of patients, respectively ($P = 0.001$). Minor bleeding (25.7% versus 13.4%, $P = 0.001$) and thrombocytopenia ($<100,000/mm^3$) (1.7% versus 0.7%, $P < 0.001$) were also less common with bivalirudin treatment. GPIIb/IIIa receptor antagonist therapy was given to 7.2% of patients randomized to bivalirudin.

Bivalirudin in STEMI

The HORIZONS-AMI[198] trial examined the use of bivalirudin in 3600 patients with STEMI. Patients were randomized to either heparin 60 U/kg IV, subsequently titrated to ACT of 200–250 seconds plus a GPIIb/IIIa inhibitor (abciximab or eptifibatide), or to bivalirudin monotherapy (0.75 mg/kg bolus; infusion 1.75 mg/kg/h) stopped at the end of the procedure plus provisional GPIIb/IIIa inhibitors for large thrombus or refractory no-flow. Net adverse clinical events, the primary endpoint, were 9.2% in the bivalirudin group and 12.1% in the UFH-GPIIb/IIIa group ($P \leq 0.0001$ for noninferiority, and $P = 0.006$ for superiority). In addition to the observed decrease in net adverse clinical events, there was a corresponding decrease in major bleeding with bivalirudin (4.9% versus 8.3%, $P = \leq 0.001$ for noninferiority and $P \leq 0.0001$ for superiority).

Impact of Renal Insufficiency

Patients with moderate and severe renal impairment have reductions in bivalirudin clearance; however, analysis of data derived from 4312 patients with unstable angina showed increased bleeding risk for both bivalirudin and UFH-treated patients with progressive degrees of renal insufficiency. The incidence of major bleeding was, however, consistently less for bivalirudin than UFH at all levels of renal impairment.

The overall data suggest that a bivalirudin dose adjustment is indicated for patients with moderate or severe renal impairment. In a retrospective study of 73 patients with renal dysfunction treated with bivalirudin for HIT with or without ACS, the average bivalirudin dose (mg/kg/h) achieving a therapeutic aPTT was 0.07 ± 0.04, 0.15 ± 0.08, and 0.16 ± 0.07 mg/kg/h for patients with estimated glomerular filtration rate (eGFR) (by Cockcroft-Gault) between 15–30, 31–60, and >60 mL/min, respectively. When renal function was calculated by modification of diet in renal disease (MDRD), the average bivalirudin dose achieving a therapeutic APTT was 0.07 ± 0.04, 0.12 ± 0.07, and 0.20 ± 0.07 mg/kg/h for patients with an eGFR between 15–30, 31–60, and >60 mL/min, respectively. Taken together, these data further suggest the bivalirudin dose adjustment should be considered in patients with moderate to severe renal insufficiency.[199]

Alternatively, the encouraging results from REPLACE-2 may provide an opportunity for reducing hemorrhagic risk in patients with renal insufficiency by virtue of the short infusion length for bivalirudin administration and provisional use of GPIIb/IIIa receptor antagonists (which may themselves increase the risk of hemorrhage in this high risk patient subset). The use of bivalirudin among individuals with and those at risk for HIT who require PCI is favored (over argatroban) by many interventional cardiologists based on experience in the angioplasty suite and comparative analyses among patients with ACS.

Argatroban

Argatroban is a synthetic direct thrombin inhibitor derived from L-arginine that acts through binding reversely to the active site of thrombin. There was a linear relationship between argatroban plasma levels and prolongations of the thrombin time, aPTT, and PT.

Pharmacokinetics

Peak concentrations of Argatroban are reached rapidly after IV injection, with a plasma half-life ranging between 39 and 51 minutes. Metabolism occurs in the liver by hydroxylation and aromotization via CYP3A4/5.

Clinical Experience

Argatroban is approved for use among patients with HIT, including those with current HIT, previous HIT, and/or those with heparin-dependent antibodies.

Comparative Benefits of Direct Thrombin Inhibitors

A meta-analysis of clinical trials was performed to obtain additional information and precise estimates of DTIs in the management of ACS.[200] A total of 11 randomized trials including 35,970 patients were identified. Compared with UFH, DTIs were associated with a lower risk of death or MI at the end of treatment (up to 7 days) (4.3% versus 5.1%; OR 0.85; 95% CI 0.77 0.94; $P = 0.001$) and at 30 days (7.4% versus 8.2%; OR 0.91; 95% CI 0.84, 0.99; $P = 0.02$). There were seven trials, including 30,154 patients with either an ACS (unstable angina or NSTEMI) or undergoing PCI. In those with ACS, treatment with a direct thrombin inhibitor was associated with a reduction in death or MI compared to UFH (3.7% versus 4.6%; OR 0.80; 95% CI 0.70, 0.92). Similar reductions were observed in PCI trials (3.0% versus 3.8%; OR 0.79; 95% CI 0.59, 1.06). There was a statistically insignificant increased rate of major bleeding with DTIs in trials of ACS (1.6% versus 1.4%; OR 1.11; 95% CI 0.93, 1.34), but there was a significant difference in PCI trials (3.7% versus 7.6%; OR 0.46; 95% CI 0.36, 0.59). There were no differences in the rates of intracranial hemorrhage.

The risk reduction in death or MI at the end of treatment was similar in trials comparing hirudin or bivalirudin with UFH, but there was a slight excess with univalent inhibitors (4.7% versus 3.5%; OR 1.35; 95% CI 0.89, 2.05). When major bleeding outcomes were analyzed by agent, hirudin was associated with an excess of major bleeding compared with UFH (1.7% versus 1.3%; OR 1.28; 95% CI 1.06, 1.55), whereas both bivalirudin (4.2% versus 9.0%; OR 0.55; 95% CI 0.34, 0.56) and univalent inhibitors (0.7% versus 1.3%; OR 0.55; 95% CI 0.25, 1.20) were associated with lower rates of major bleeding.

Dosing Strategies: An Opportunity for Improved Safety

In a prospective observational analysis of 30,136 patients with non–ST-segment elevation ACS, 42% received an initial dose of either UFH, LMWH or a LMWH or a GPIIb/IIIa receptor antagonist outside the recommended range of dosing. Patient characteristics associated with excess drug dosing including older age, female sex, low body weight, renal insufficiency, diabetes mellitus, and congestive heart failure. Excess antithrombotic drug dosing was associated with major bleeding complication, increased hospital length, and higher mortality.[201]

Bleeding and Outcomes in ACS

Although bleeding has always been considered an important safety concern for patients with ACS or undergoing PCI, only recently have the long-term effects of bleeding on mortality been explored. In a meta-analysis of four multicenter, randomized clinical trials of patients with NSTEMI demonstrated increases in 30-day mortality with increasing bleeding severity (HR for 30 day mortality by mild, moderate, or severe bleeding 1.6 [1.3–1.9], 2.7 [2.3–3.4], and 10.6 [8.3–13.6]).[202] Six-month mortality by mild, moderate, and severe bleeding was also increased (HR by mild, moderate, or severe bleeding 1.4 [1.2–1.6], 2.1 [1.8–2.4], and 7.5 [6.1–9.3]). Subsequently, a study by Eikelboom et al. analyzing aggregate data from other ACS trials confirmed a dose-related association between bleeding and death in ACS patients.[203] Although the exact contribution of bleeding to overall mortality in ACS remains undefined, the OASIS-5 trial, which investigated fondaparinux versus enoxaparin in ACS demonstrated a reduction in bleeding associated with fondaparinux. More importantly, this reduction in bleeding was associated with reduced overall mortality. The authors subsequently concluded that bleeding is an important predictor of outcomes in ACS. Although not fully understood, several mechanisms have been proposed to explain the association of bleeding with mortality in ACS. Certainly, the hemodynamic effects associated with massive bleeding might result in higher mortality. Likewise, mass effect from intracranial bleeding would be expected to cause higher rates of morbidity and mortality. Even lesser levels of bleeding, however, have been shown to increase levels of neurohormones, such as norepinephrine, angiotensin, endothelin-1, and vasopressin, in order to maintain blood pressure. These neurohormones have been associated with cardiac events.

In addition to the neurohormonal activation associated with bleeding, measures taken as a result of bleeding, including discontinuation of antiplatelet and anticoagulant therapy, may paradoxically increase mortality. In the GRACE registry of ACS patients, those with bleeding complications more frequently had antithrombotic therapy, including aspirin, thienopyridines, and heparin, discontinued. Discontinuation of aspirin, thienopyridines, or UFH in the setting of major bleeding resulted in higher in-hospital mortality rates.[204] Given that patients with ACS and those undergoing PCI are in a heightened state of platelet activation and thrombosis, withholding antithrombotic therapy may result in activation of the coagulation system and potential stent thrombosis.

Reversal and Replacement Therapy for Parenteral Anticoagulants

The approach to major or life-threatening hemorrhage among patients receiving parenteral anticoagulants requires an understanding of drug pharmacology, mechanism(s) or action, and potential risks of reversal or replacement therapy. For unfractionated heparin, protamine sulfate (12.5–50 mg IV) is the drug of choice (1 mg protamine sulfate will neutralize 100 units of UFH). For LMWH, protamine sulfate (0.5–1.0 mg for every 1 mg of LMWH given within the past 8 hours) is recommended. It is important to recognize that protamine sulfate will neutralize approximately 40%–50% of LMWH-specifically the factor IIa effect. Prothrombin complex concentrate (PCC) can be given for refractory bleeding. While andexanet alfa was designed as a universal FX anticoagulant reversal agent, potentially including fondaparinux, the current FDA labeling does not include either LMWH or very low MWH reversal.

The approach to parenteral direct thrombin inhibitors, in addition to supportive measures, includes PCC and recombinant FVII for refractory bleeding. The use of idarucizumab, a reversal agent specifically designed to reverse dabigatran's anticoagulant effect, is not recommended and would not be expected to have an effect.

Oral Anticoagulant Drugs

Common indications for oral anticoagulant medications include stroke prophylaxis in patients with atrial flutter or atrial fibrillation, thrombosis prophylaxis in patients with mechanical heart valves, treatment and secondary prevention of venous thromboembolism, and thromboembolism prophylaxis in specific patient populations including those with a known heritable or acquired thrombophilias.

Pharmacokinetics and Drug Disposition

The pharmacokinetic characteristics of oral anticoagulant drugs are presented in Tables 8.16 and 8.17. Their optimal use
Text continues on p. 105

Table 8.16

Pharmacokinetic characteristics of oral anticoagulants

	Dabigatran	Rivaroxaban	Apixaban	Edoxaban	Betrixaban	Warfarin
Target	FIIa	FXa	FXa	FXa	FXa	Vitamin K–dependent factors II, VII, IX, and X
Bioavailability	6.5% (absolute)	66% (20 mg dose) increases with food	50% (absolute)	60% (absolute)	34%	80%–100%
Vd	50–70 L	50 L	21 L	>107 L (Vd$_{ss}$)	32 L/kg	8–10 L
Protein binding	35%	>90%	87%	40%–59%	60%	95%–97%
Time to C$_{max}$ (hours)	1–2	2–4	1–4	1–2	3–4	1–2
Half-life (hours)	12–17	5–9	8–15	10–14	19–27	7 d, effective half-life 20–60 hours
Hepatic metabolism/ biotransformation	Up to 20% glucuronidation (phase II)	66% undergoes metabolic degradation	30%–35% O-demethylation and hydroxylation major sites (phase I)	Minimal; primarily through conjugation, oxidation by CYP 3A4 and hydrolysis (phase I)	Major biotransformation pathway; via hydrolysis	Major; extensive

Renal excretion Biliary excretion	80% unchanged ~20%	66% (33% direct excretion as unchanged, 33% excreted after metabolic degradation) 28% feces (7% unchanged)	25%–30% 30%–35%	40%–50% 50%	11% Biliary secretion primary route of excretion (via hepatic P-gp) as unchanged drug; 85% recovered in feces.	>90% inactive metabolites
CYP metabolism	No conjugation	30%	15%	Yes (% NR)	Minimal <1% (hydrolysis)	Yes
CYP isoenzymes	No	Yes (CYP3A4/5, CYP2J2) Major	Yes CYP3A4/5 Minor (minimal role of CYP1A2, 2C8, 2C9, 2C19, and 2J2)	Yes CYP3A4	< 1% via CYP 1A1, 1A2, 2B6, 2C9, 2C19, 2D6, and 3A4.	Yes 2C9, 2C19, 2C8, 2C18, 1A2, and 3A4 (genetic polymorphism of 2C9 results in variability in response)
Drug transporters	Substrate P-gp (dabigatran etexilate)	Substrate P-gp Substrate ABCG2 (BCRP)	Substrate P-gp Substrate ABCG2 (BCRP)	Substrate P-gp Substrate ABCB1 (MDR1)	Substrate P-gp NR	Substrate and inhibitor of hepatic P-gp ABCB1 (MDR1)

ABCB1 (MDR1), ATP-binding cassette subfamily B member 1 (multidrug resistance protein 1); *ABCG2 (BCRP)*, ATP-binding cassette subfamily G member 2 (breast cancer resistance protein); *CYP*, cytochrome P; *FIIa*, factor IIa; *FXa*, factor Xa; *NR*, not reported; *P-gp*, permeability glycoprotein; *Vd$_{ss}$*, volume of distribution at steady state.

From DeWald TA, Becker RC. The pharmacology of novel oral anticoagulants. *J Thromb Thrombolysis* 2014;37:217–233.

Table 8.17

Summary of pharmacokinetic properties and characteristics for oral direct thrombin and factor Xa inhibitors

Dabigatran: Vd is 60–70 L consistent with moderate tissue distribution. Limited data available on extremes of body weight. Patients weighing 50 kg had notably higher trough concentrations compared to those weighing 100 kg in RE-LY. No current recommendations for dose modification based on body weight

Rivaroxaban: Vd is 50 L, with moderate tissue distribution. Extremes in body weight (50 or 120 kg) did not (25%) influence exposure; no dosage adjustment recommended

Apixaban: Vd is 21 L, small with limited distribution, primarily to blood. Extremes in weight (B50 and C120 kg) have a modest effect on apixaban exposure and do not alter the apixaban plasma concentration and anti-Xa activity relationship. Dose reduction is recommended only if weight is B 60 kg and pt is either C 80 years old or serum creatinine C 1.5 mg/dL

Dabigatran has low oral bioavailability (6%–7%). High doses (150 mg) are administered to overcome low-bioavailability Tartaric acid present in dabigatran etexilate enhances absorption and minimizes variations in acidic environment Rivaroxaban has dose dependent oral bioavailability (80%–100%) at 10 mg, 66 % at 20 mg

Oral bioavailability of apixaban is 50% for doses up to 10 mg

Coadministration of dabigatran etexilate with food has no effect on the extent of dabigatran absorption; it may be administered with or without meals

Rivaroxaban coadministration with a meal moderately improves bioavailability of the 15 and 20 mg doses; must be administered with a meal. Medications that alter gastric pH do not modify the PK of rivaroxaban, but gastric site of release is important for adequate drug exposure

Apixaban displays prolonged absorption; food does not affect bioavailability. Absorption occurs throughout the GI tract

Absorption (bowel): Until absorbed and bioconverted to dabigatran, dabigatran etexilate is a substrate for P-gp efflux transporter and should not be coadministered with inducers of P-gp

Rivaroxaban is a substrate for efflux transporters P-gp and BCRP/ABCG2. Coadministration of inhibitors or inducers of these transporters may result in changes in rivaroxaban exposure

Apixaban is a substrate for efflux transporters P-gp (minimal) and BCRP/ABCG2

Liver: Dabigatran undergoes hepatic phase II glucuronidation; up to 20% hepatic biotransformation. No significant CYP role, no interaction with drug transporters once bioconverted to parent compound. Large interpatient variability when administered in the presence of moderate hepatic impairment

Rivaroxaban undergoes moderate hepatic biotransformation. Cautious use in patients with moderate hepatic impairment, contraindicated with

Table 8.17

Summary of pharmacokinetic properties and characteristics for oral direct thrombin and factor Xa inhibitors (Continued)

moderate hepatic impairment and coagulopathy. Rivaroxaban is a substrate for CYP 3A4/5, CYP 2J2, and efflux transporters P-gp and BCRP/ABCG2. Avoid coadministration of rivaroxaban with combined P-gp and strong CYP 3A4 inhibitors. Affinity for influx (uptake transporters is unknown)

Hepatic biotransformation appears responsible for approximately one third of apixaban drug elimination. No clear understanding of the impact of moderate hepatic impairment; severe hepatic impairment not studied. Apixaban is a substrate for CYP 3A4, P-gp, and BCRP/ABCG2. Coadministration of apixaban with strong dual inducers of CYP 3A4 and P-gp is not recommended. Dose reduction is needed if administered with strong dual inhibitors

Kidney: Dabigatran: Important role of renal function for elimination. Dose reduction is necessary when CrCl is B 30 mL/min.

Limited clinical outcome data in this population. No recommendations for use when CrCl is 15 mL/min or in setting of HD. No anticipated interactions with efflux transporters (P-gp) at the kidney

Rivaroxaban: Important role of renal function for elimination of drug. Dose reduction is recommended when CrCl is 15–50 mL/min. Potential interactions with efflux transporters P-gp and BCRP/ABCG2 at kidney of unknown clinical consequence

Apixaban: Renal excretion accounts for elimination of approximately one-third of a dose. Recommendations include dose reduction if serum creatinine is C 1.5 mg/dL AND pt is either C 80 years age or B 60 kg body weight. Potential interactions with efflux transporters (P-gp and BCRP/ABCG2) at kidney of unknown clinical consequence.

BCRP/ABCG2, ATP-binding cassette subfamily G member 2 (breast cancer resistance protein; *CrCL*, creatinine clearance; *CYP*, cytochrome P; *GI*, gastrointestinal; *P-gp*, permeability glycoprotein; *Vd*, volume of distribution.
From DeWald, Becker RC. The pharmacology of novel oral anticoagulants. *J Thromb Thrombolysis* 2014;37:217–233.

incorporates a balance of desired and undesirable medication effects. The magnitudes of both the desired response and toxicity are functions of drug concentration at the site or sites of action.[205] A thorough understanding of medication-specific pharmacokinetic features and potential interactions is essential for optimal prescribing and patient outcome. Medication-specific differences in anticoagulant absorption, distribution, metabolism, and elimination as well as disease-specific or condition-specific variations in these fundamental processes govern safe and effective use in clinical practice. Specifically, differences in bioavailability, distribution (including protein binding), metabolism (including CYP450), and route of elimination may significantly influence drug response. Membrane transporters have become recognized determinants of the pharmacokinetic disposition of many drugs. A growing number of membrane transporters have been characterized, with a clinically translatable focus on their expression in the epithelial tissue of intestine, liver, kidney, and blood-brain barrier and how they modulate bioavailability and anticoagulant activity. The full impact of the growing number of transporters (both efflux and uptake) is unknown at present; however, the role of efflux transporters, specifically permeability glycoprotein (P-gp), is routinely evaluated and documented for many medications in preclinical studies.[206] All oral anticoagulants presented in this review demonstrate that P-gp interactions to some extent have an impact on drug disposition, notably by interaction with other P-gp modulators. Drug substrates for both CYP450 3A4 isoenzyme and P-gp are more likely involved in major drug interactions than drugs that are substrates for only one system. Pertinent drug interactions related to P-gp and CYP450 are summarized in Table 8.18.

The bioavailability of the oral anticoagulants varies widely. For some drugs, the bioavailability changes with coadministration of food. For example, the bioavailability of rivaroxaban (20-mg dose) is 66%.[207] Coadministration of rivaroxaban with food increases the bioavailability of a 20-mg dose, as measured by mean AUC by 39% and C_{max} by 76%. Accordingly, the 15-mg and 20-mg dosage strengths of rivaroxaban should be taken with food (typically the largest meal of the day), and current recommendations suggest administration with the evening meal. The bioavailability of the 10-mg dosage strength is 80% to 100% and does not require food to achieve sufficient concentrations for effective anticoagulation. As such, use of 10-mg rivaroxaban daily for reduction of risk of recurrent deep vein thrombosis (DVT) and/or PE in patients with continued risk, or for prophylaxis of DVT after hip or knee replacement, may be taken with or without food. By contrast, coadministration of food reduces the bioavailability of betrixaban. The oral bioavailability of betrixaban is 34%; however, consuming a high-fat meal prior to betrixaban administration results in a reduction in both the AUC and C_{max} by 50%, and a reduction in AUC and C_{max} of 70% and 61%, respectively, for a low-fat meal. At this time, labeled administration recommendations are that betrixaban be taken at the same time each day with food.[208]

The volume of distribution (Vd) varies considerably across the oral anticoagulants. This parameter is a function of drug lipophilicity/tissue affinity, plasma and tissue protein binding affinity, and the presence of active drug transporters on barrier tissues (kidney and liver). The differences in Vd explain the extent of tissue distribution of different anticoagulants; however, insufficient

Table 8.18

Potential drug-to-drug interactions for oral anticoagulant drugs

Medication	Interactions [a]	Management
Apixaban	Strong dual CYP3A4 and P-gp inducers (e.g., rifampin, carbamazepine, phenytoin, and St. John's wort) Strong dual CYP3A4 and P-gp inhibitors (e.g., ketoconazole, itraconazole, ritonavir, and clarithromycin)	Avoid concomitant use In patients taking 5 mg twice daily of apixaban, reduce dose to 2.5 mg twice daily. In patients taking 2.5 mg twice daily, avoid concomitant use.
Betrixaban	P-gp inhibitors (e.g., amiodarone, azithromycin, verapamil, ketoconazole, and clarithromycin)	Reduce dose of betrixaban in patients receiving a P-gp inhibitor. Avoid concomitant use of betrixaban and P-gp inhibitor in patients with severe renal dysfunction (CrCL 15–29 mL/min).
Dabigatran	P-gp inducers (e.g., rifampin) P-gp inhibitors (e.g., ketoconazole and dronedarone)	Avoid concomitant use • For indication of stroke prophylaxis in AF: In patients with moderate renal impairment (CrCl 30–50 mL/min), reduce dabigatran dose to 75 mg twice daily. Avoid in patients with severe renal impairment (CrCl 15–30 mL/min). • For indication of treatment and reduction in the risk of recurrence of DVT and PE; avoid concomitant use of dabigatran and P-gp inhibitors in patients with CrCl <50 mL/min. • For indication of prophylaxis of DVT and PE after hip replacement surgery: in patients with CrCl >50 mL/min taking P-gp inhibitors, such as dronedarone or ketoconazole, consider separating the administration timing of dabigatran and the P-gp inhibitor by several hours. Avoid concomitant use of dabigatran and P-gp inhibitors in patients with CrCl <50 mL/min.

Continued on following page

Table 8.18

Potential drug-to-drug interactions for oral anticoagulant drugs (Continued)

Medication	Interactions [a]	Management
Edoxaban	P-gp inducers (e.g., rifampin)	Avoid concomitant use.
Rivaroxaban	• Strong dual CYP3A4 and P-gp inducers (e.g., carbamazepine, phenytoin, rifampin, and St. John's wort)	Avoid concomitant use.
	Strong dual CYP3A4 and P-gp inhibitors (e.g., ketoconazole, ritonavir)	Avoid concomitant administration.
	• Moderate dual CYP3A4 and P-gp inhibitors (e.g., erythromycin) in patients with renal impairment (CrCl 15 mL/min to <80 mL/min)	Rivaroxaban should not be used in patients with CrCl 15 mL/min to <80 mL/min concomitantly with combined P-gp and moderate CYP3A4 inhibitors unless the potential benefit justifies the potential risk.
Warfarin	Medications highly probable of warfarin potentiation (e.g., ciprofloxacin, cotrimoxazole, erythromycin, fluconazole, isoniazid, metronidazole, miconazole, voriconazole, amiodarone, clofibrate, diltiazem, fenofibrate, propafenone, propranolol, sulfinpyrazone, phenylbutazone, piroxicam, citalopram, entacapone, sertraline, cimetidine, omeprazole, anabolic steroids, zileuton)	Avoid if possible. If concomitant therapy must be used, increase the frequency of monitoring and adjust the warfarin dose based on the INR results.
	Medications highly probable of warfarin inhibition (e.g., griseofulvin, nafcillin, ribavirin, rifampin, cholestyramine, mesalamine, barbiturates, carbamazepine, and mercaptopurine)	Avoid if possible. If concomitant therapy must be used, increase the frequency of monitoring and adjust the warfarin dose based on the INR results.

AF, Atrial fibrillation; CrCl, creatinine clearance; DVT, deep vein thrombosis; INR, international normalized ratio; PE, pulmonary embolism; P-gp, permeability glycoprotein.
From DeWald TA, Becker RC. The pharmacology of novel oral anticoagulants. J Thromb Thrombolysis 2014;37:217–233.

information is available at this time to estimate the clinical impact of this difference with respect to patient outcomes.

Finally, drug elimination represents a clinically important variable for consideration when initiating and monitoring anticoagulant therapy. Drug elimination is the process of irreversible removal of drug from the body by all routes of elimination, including biotransformation (metabolism) and drug excretion. Enzymes involved in biotransformation are located primarily in the liver where common routes of metabolism include oxidation, reduction, hydrolysis, and conjugation.

The CYP450 system is a family of enzymes responsible for most drug metabolism oxidation reactions. Many isoenzymes within this family exist and their role in the metabolism of medications is well established. Although hepatic disease or impairment may result in loss of function that reduces metabolism or elimination of drugs, it is difficult to know when these changes are clinically important, and recommendations regarding modification of dosing in the setting of hepatic impairment are nonspecific and difficult to apply.[209] Understanding the primary route of metabolism and elimination may assist in the selection of preferred anticoagulant therapy.

In addition to metabolism and biotransformation, drugs are eliminated by excretion into bile or into urine. The processes by which a drug is excreted by the kidneys may include any combination of glomerular filtration, active tubular secretion, or tubular reabsorption. In the presence of renal disease, both glomerular filtration and renal tubular secretion can decrease, impairing the renal clearance of drugs and their metabolites. The degree to which impairment in these processes prolongs the presence or half-life of a drug, potentially extending the pharmacodynamics effect, is dependent on the proportion of drug excreted by the renal route of elimination and the extent of renal impairment. Knowledge of anticoagulant-specific reliance on the renal route of elimination can guide preferred treatment choices and tailor individualized monitoring plans.

Oral Direct Thrombin Inhibitors

Detailed Summary of Pharmacokinetics and Pharmacodynamics

Dabigatran

Dabigatran has low oral bioavailability estimated to be 6%–7%. To overcome this potential barrier, high doses of its prodrug, dabigatran etexilate, are given. The chemical characteristics of the prodrug (less basic and less hydrophilic) facilitates intestinal absorption. In addition, to promote an acidic environment required for dabigatran etexilate absorption, the drug is packaged in capsules containing tartaric acid. Dabigatran is layered onto seal-coated spherical tartaric acid starter cores. While this feature improves drug dissolution and limits any role of variation in individual gastric pH, it may be the source of dyspepsia associated with dabigatran therapy. Removal of the drug pellets from the capsule shell results in a 75% increase in dabigatran etexilate bioavailability, compared to the intact capsule formulation. Modification of this delivery system (chewing, breaking, or opening the capsule) is not recommended. During and following absorption, dabigatran etexilate is converted to its active metabolite, dabigatran, by hydrolysis in the enterocytes, portal vein, and liver leaving minimal prodrug or intermediates detectable in plasma.[210] Dabigatran is not a substrate of any drug transporter investigated; however, dabigatran etexilate is a substrate with moderate affinity for P-gp transport system. Although minimal drug interactions are expected, the potential for clinically relevant drug interactions of dabigatran exists only during the absorption phase when administered with other modulators of P-gp activity. Coadministration of dabigatran with both inducers (rifampin) of P-gp and inhibitors of P-gp (ketoconazole, amiodarone, verapamil, quinidine) results in considerable changes in dabigatran exposure, C_{max} and AUC. A population pharmacokinetic analysis of the Randomized Evaluation of Long-Term Anticoagulation Therapy (RE-LY) trial demonstrated concomitant administration of proton pump inhibitors, amiodarone, and verapamil significantly affected oral bioavailability of dabigatran, however the result was only a moderate effect (23%) on change in steady state exposure (increased or decreased).[211] It is recommended that coadministration of dabigatran with rifampin should be avoided. Current US labeling for dabigatran recommends reducing the dose of dabigatran when coadministered with systemic ketoconazole, and to avoid its use completely in patients with severe renal impairment receiving inhibitors of P-gp.

Rivaroxaban

Rivaroxaban is administered as a film-coated tablet with a bioavailability that is dose-dependent. The effect of food on rivaroxaban absorption was evaluated in healthy male subjects.[212] In two interaction studies, subjects received either two 5 mg tablets (fasted and fed) and four 5 mg tablets (fasted), or one 20 mg tablet (fasted and fed). In this study, C_{max} and AUC were increased, and interindividual variability decreased at higher doses of rivaroxaban in the presence of food.[213] In general, administration of medication with food prolongs residence time in the stomach secondary to reduced gastric motility after a meal, and possibly increases both solubility and dissolution. In the case of rivaroxaban, the improved rate and extent of absorption observed with food is likely attributable to lipophilicity and improved solubility from its baseline nearly insoluble form. Medications that alter gastric pH do not modify the pharmacokinetics of rivaroxaban; however gastric site of drug release is important for rivaroxaban absorption. Rivaroxaban exposure is reduced when the drug is released in the proximal small intestine, and even further reduced if released in the distal small intestine or ascending colon. Alternative strategies for oral administration (feeding tubes) of rivaroxaban that deliver drug to any site beyond the stomach should be avoided. Rivaroxaban is a substrate for P-gp and the ATP-binding cassette transporter protein, breast cancer resistant protein (BCRP), gene symbol ABCG2.[214] Like P-gp, BCRP is a transporter protein with localized tissue distribution on the apical surface of epithelial cells, found at relatively high levels in the blood–brain barrier, placenta, liver, gut, and kidney, and is increasingly recognized for the ability to modulate absorption, distribution, metabolism, and elimination of xenobiotics in these tissues. Existing interaction studies involving BCRP drug interactions have focused primarily on the multidrug resistance (MDR) effects in oncology; however, naturally occurring flavonoids have demonstrated inhibition of BCRP-mediated transport, particularly chrysin and biochanin A, found commonly in food sources of broccoli, celery, chili peppers, and soy products.[215] While inhibitors or inducers of this transporter protein (BCRP) may result in changes in rivaroxaban exposure, the overall clinical impact is unknown. Drug interaction studies evaluating the concomitant use of rivaroxaban with drugs that are combined P-gp and CYP 3A4 inhibitors have demonstrated an increase in rivaroxaban exposure. The pharmacodynamic effects (FXa inhibition and PT prolongation) of this exposure may increase bleeding risk, and concomitant administration of ketoconazole, itraconazole, lopinavir/ritonavir, ritonavir, indinavir/ ritonavir, and conivaptan is not recommended.

Apixaban

Apixaban has been studied in PK/PD studies and multiple clinical trials.[216] Existing pharmacokinetic studies of apixaban have demonstrated good oral bioavailability, with 50% of a dose absorbed in humans. Food does not affect the bioavailability of apixaban. After oral administration, apixaban is absorbed throughout the GI tract, with approximately half of the drug absorbed in the distal small bowel and ascending colon. In human liver and hepatocytes, apixaban demonstrates insignificant metabolic clearance.

The primary metabolite identified is formed by CYP 3A4 in human liver microsomes, but there are nonactive circulating metabolites. Apixaban has low potential to inhibit or induce CYP, or to form reactive metabolites, and the drug interaction potential is accordingly low. Apixaban is a substrate of the transport proteins P-gp and BCRP (ABCG2). The identification of apixaban as a substrate for P-gp is consistent with observed changes in apixaban AUC and C_{max} when coadministered with strong inhibitors (ketoconazole) and inducers (rifampin) of both P-gp and CYP 3A4. Current recommendations include a reduction in apixaban dose when coadministered with drugs that are strong dual inhibitors of CYP 3A4 and P-gp: ketoconazole, itraconazole, ritonavir, clarithromycin.

Edoxaban

The pharmacokinetics of edoxaban in healthy volunteers have been described in single- and multiple-dose administration studies.[217] Edoxaban tablets and powder for oral solution have been evaluated and demonstrated similar bioavailability. Coadministration of edoxaban with food results in a modest but clinically insignificant effect of food on edoxaban pharmacokinetics. The absolute bioavailability of edoxaban following a single oral dose is 60%. Edoxaban is a substrate for CYP 3A4 and also P-gp.[218] Simulations based on PK/PD models support halving the prescribed dose of edoxaban for those patients taking strong inhibitors of P-gp, including ketoconazole, erythromycin, azithromycin, quinidine, verapamil, and dronedarone. In an exposure–response analysis of edoxaban administration to patients with nonvalvular atrial fibrillation (NVAF), coadministration of edoxaban with strong inhibitors of P-gp increased edoxaban exposure. In this analysis, the incidence of bleeding events increased significantly with increasing edoxaban exposure, which was best characterized by edoxaban minimum concentrations at steady state (Cmin,ss).

Absorption of drugs from the intestinal lumen is a complex process influenced by physiochemical properties of the medications, as well as physiological factors in the GI tract. Existing data suggest the presence of uptake and efflux transporters in the GI tract play an important role in drug absorption, display genetic variability, and should be considered in drug-to-drug interactions. In total, these factors may contribute to individual variation in drug absorption and, potentially, response.

Betrixaban

Betrixaban is an oral anticoagulant that exerts its action by preventing thrombin generation without having a direct effect on platelet aggregation. Betrixaban presents a rapid absorption at a dose of 80 mg. Its peak plasma concentration is registered within 3–4 hours after oral administration in healthy humans. The oral bioavailability is 34% and it can be reduced with consumption of high-fat food. Betrixaban is an orally active inhibitor of coagulation FXa (activated FX) with anticoagulant activity. Betrixaban is primarily excreted unchanged in the bile and has a half-life of about 19 hours.

Dabigatran

Pharmacodynamics. Dabigatran etexilate is a prodrug that undergoes conversion to dabigatran, a small molecule direct-thrombin inhibitor capable of reversibly binding thrombin. GI absorption of the prodrug is dependent on a low pH, and peak plasma concentrations are achieved between 2 and 3 hours after ingestion.

Pharmacokinetics

The half-life of dabigatran is 12–17 hours and is 80% renally excreted. Because prodrug and drug metabolism is independent of CYP450, the drug is considered relatively safe in moderate liver disease but must be used with caution in patients with significant renal dysfunction.[210]

Clinical Experience

Venous thromboembolism. In the RE-Cover trial[219a] a randomized, double-blind, noninferiority trial involving patients with acute venous thromboembolism who were initially given parenteral anticoagulation therapy for a median of 9 days (interquartile range, 8–11), we compared oral dabigatran, administered at a dose of 150 mg twice daily, with warfarin that was dose-adjusted to achieve an international normalized ratio (INR) of 2.0–3.0. The primary outcome was the 6-month incidence of recurrent symptomatic, objectively confirmed venous thromboembolism and related deaths. Safety endpoints included bleeding events, acute coronary syndromes, other adverse events, and results of liver function tests. A total of 30 of the 1274 patients randomly assigned to receive dabigatran (2.4%), as compared with 27 of the 1265 patients randomly assigned to warfarin (2.1%), had recurrent venous thromboembolism; the difference in risk was 0.4 percentage points (95% CI −0.8–1.5; $P < 0.001$ for the prespecified noninferiority margin). The HR with dabigatran was 1.10 (95% CI 0.65–1.84). Major bleeding episodes occurred in 20 patients assigned to dabigatran (1.6%) and in 24 patients assigned to warfarin (1.9%) (HR with dabigatran 0.82; 95% CI 0.45–1.48), and episodes of any bleeding were observed in 205 patients assigned to dabigatran (16.1%) and 277 patients assigned to warfarin (21.9%; HR with dabigatran 0.71;

95% CI 0.59–0.85). The numbers of deaths, acute coronary syndromes, and abnormal liver function tests were similar in the two groups. Adverse events leading to discontinuation of the study drug occurred in 9.0% of patients assigned to dabigatran and in 6.8% of patients assigned to warfarin ($P = 0.05$). For the treatment of acute venous thromboembolism, a fixed dose of dabigatran is as effective as warfarin and has a safety profile that is similar to that of warfarin.

In two double-blind, randomized trials (RE-MEDY and RE-SONATE studies[219a,219b]), dabigatran at a dose of 150 mg twice daily with warfarin (active-control study) was compared with placebo (placebo-control study) in patients with venous thromboembolism who had completed at least 3 initial months of therapy. In the active-control study, recurrent venous thromboembolism occurred in 26 of 1430 patients in the dabigatran group (1.8%) and 18 of 1426 patients in the warfarin group (1.3%) (HR with dabigatran 1.44; 95% CI 0.78– 2.64; $P = 0.01$ for noninferiority). Major bleeding occurred in 13 patients in the dabigatran group (0.9%) and 25 patients in the warfarin group (1.8%) (HR 0.52; 95% CI 0.27–1.02). Major or clinically relevant bleeding was less frequent with dabigatran (HR 0.54; 95% CI 0.41–0.71). Acute coronary syndromes occurred in 13 patients in the dabigatran group (0.9%) and 3 patients in the warfarin group (0.2%) ($P = 0.02$). In the placebo-control study, recurrent venous thromboembolism occurred in 3 of 681 patients in the dabigatran group (0.4%) and 37 of 662 patients in the placebo group (5.6%) (HR 0.08; 95% CI 0.02–0.25; $P < 0.001$). Major bleeding occurred in two patients in the dabigatran group (0.3%) and zero patients in the placebo group. Major or clinically relevant bleeding occurred in 36 patients in the dabigatran group (5.3%) and 12 patients in the placebo group (1.8%) (HR 2.92; 95% CI 1.52 –5.60). Acute coronary syndromes occurred in one patient each in the dabigatran and placebo groups.

Atrial Fibrillation

In the RE-LY study, a total of 18,113 patients with nonvalvular AF and a mean CHADS$_2$ score of 2.1 were randomized to either of two doses of dabigatran (110 mg twice daily or 150 mg twice daily) versus open-label warfarin for the secondary prevention of stroke and thromboembolism. The trial had a 1.69% event rate of stroke or systemic embolism in the warfarin arm versus 1.53% in the 110 mg BID dabigatran arm ($P < 0.001$ for noninferiority) and 1.11% in the 150 mg BID dabigatran arm ($P < 0.001$) for superiority. The rate of major bleeding, defined as a reduction in hemoglobin of at least 20 g/L, transfusion of 2 units of blood, or symptomatic bleeding in a critical area or organ, was lower in the 110 mg dabigatran arm (2.71% versus 3.36% per year with warfarin, $P = 0.003$) and similar to warfarin in the 150 mg BID dabigatran arm (3.11% versus 3.36% per year with warfarin, $P = 0.31$).[220]

Several subgroup analyses of RELY have been published. An analysis of 1270 patients undergoing cardioversion showed low stroke rates (0.8% for 110 mg BID, 0.3% for 150 mg BID, and 0.6% for warfarin, respectively).[221] Transesophageal echocardiograms (TEEs) performed in conjunction with cardioversion showed a similarly low incidence of atrial thrombi (1.8% for 110 mg BID, 0.3% for 150 mg BID, and 0.6% for warfarin). Dabigatran has been FDA-approved in both a 150-mg dose and, based solely on pharmacodynamics studies, a 75-mg dose for use in patients with CrCl of 15–30 mL/min.

Ablation

In RE-CIRCUIT,[222] patients scheduled for catheter ablation (CA) for paroxysmal or persistent atrial fibrillation were randomly assigned to receive either dabigatran (150 mg twice daily) or warfarin (target INR, 2.0–3.0). Ablation was performed after 4–8 weeks of uninterrupted anticoagulation, which was then continued for 8 weeks after ablation. The primary endpoint was the incidence of major bleeding events during and up to 8 weeks after ablation; secondary endpoints included thromboembolic and other bleeding events. The trial enrolled 704 patients, and 635 patients underwent ablation. The incidence of major bleeding events during and up to 8 weeks after ablation was lower with dabigatran than with warfarin (5 patients [1.6%] versus 22 patients [6.9%]; absolute risk difference −5.3 percentage points; 95% CI −8.4 to −2.2; $P < 0.001$). Dabigatran was associated with fewer periprocedural pericardial tamponade events and access site hematomas than warfarin. One thromboembolic event occurred in the warfarin group.

Bleeding With Dabigatran in AF

Although treatment with dabigatran 110 mg, but not 150 mg, was associated with a significant reduction in the primary safety endpoint of major bleeding, both doses were associated with fewer intracranial bleeds than warfarin (warfarin 0.76% per year versus dabigatran 110 mg BID: 0.23% per year [RR 0.30; 95% CI 0.19–0.45], and dabigatran 150 mg BID: 0.32% per year [RR 0.41; 95% CI 0.28–0.60]).[223] Dabigatran 150 mg BID was associated with a significant increase in GI bleeding (1.56%) as compared to warfarin (1.07% per year; RR 1.48; 95% CI 1.18–1.85) and dabigatran 110 mg BID (1.15% per year: RR 1.36; 95% CI 1.09–1.70).[223] Renal insufficiency and combined administration with aspirin

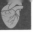

increased bleeding risk, though this was independent of antico-agulant and dose.[224]

Rivaroxaban

Pharmacodynamics. Rivaroxaban exerts its anticoagulant effect by direct, reversible binding to FXa.

Pharmacokinetics

Oral administration results in 60%–80% bioavailability, and peak plasma concentrations occur at about 3 hours. In patients with normal renal and hepatic function, rivaroxaban's plasma half-life is between 5 and 9 hours.[225]

Clinical Experience

Venous thromboembolism. In the EINSTEIN DVT study,[226] oral rivaroxaban alone (15 mg twice daily for 3 weeks, followed by 20 mg once daily) was compared with SQ enoxaparin followed by a vitamin K antagonist (either warfarin or acenocoumarol) for 3, 6, or 12 months in patients with acute, symptomatic DVT. In parallel, a double-blind, randomized, event-driven superiority study was undertaken that compared rivaroxaban alone (20 mg once daily) with placebo for an additional 6 or 12 months in patients who had completed 6–12 months of treatment for venous thromboembolism. The primary efficacy outcome for both studies was recurrent venous thromboembolism. The principal safety outcome was major bleeding or clinically relevant nonmajor bleeding in the initial-treatment study and major bleeding in the continued-treatment study.[226] The study of rivaroxaban for acute DVT included 3449 patients: 1731 given rivaroxaban and 1718 given enoxaparin plus a vitamin K antagonist. Rivaroxaban had noninferior efficacy with respect to the primary outcome (36 events [2.1%] versus 51 events with enoxaparin-vitamin K antagonist [3.0%]; HR 0.68; 95% CI 0.44–1.04; $P < 0.001$). The principal safety outcome occurred in 8.1% of the patients in each group. In the continued-treatment study, which included 602 patients in the rivaroxaban group and 594 in the placebo group, rivaroxaban had superior efficacy (8 events [1.3%] versus 42 with placebo [7.1%]; HR 0.18; 95% CI 0.09–0.39; $P < 0.001$). Four patients in the rivaroxaban group had nonfatal major bleeding (0.7%), versus none in the placebo group ($P = 0.11$).

In the EINSTEIN PE study,[227] 4832 patients who had acute symptomatic PE with or without DVT were randomly assigned to receive rivaroxaban (15 mg twice daily for 3 weeks, followed by 20 mg once daily) or standard therapy with enoxaparin followed by an adjusted-dose vitamin K antagonist for 3, 6, or 12 months. The primary efficacy outcome was symptomatic recurrent venous

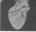

thromboembolism. The principal safety outcome was major or clinically relevant nonmajor bleeding.

Rivaroxaban was noninferior to standard therapy (noninferiority margin, 2.0; $P = 0.003$) for the primary efficacy outcome, with 50 events in the rivaroxaban group (2.1%) versus 44 events in the standard-therapy group (1.8%) (HR 1.12; 95% CI 0.75–1.68). The principal safety outcome occurred in 10.3% of patients in the rivaroxaban group and 11.4% of those in the standard-therapy group (HR 0.90; 95% CI 0.76–1.07; $P = 0.23$). Major bleeding was observed in 26 patients (1.1%) in the rivaroxaban group and 52 patients (2.2%) in the standard-therapy group (HR 0.49; 95% CI 0.31–0.79; $P = 0.003$). Rates of other adverse events were similar in the two groups.

A fixed-dose regimen of rivaroxaban alone was noninferior to standard therapy for the initial and long-term treatment of PE and had a potentially improved benefit-risk profile.

Atrial Fibrillation

In the Rivaroxaban Once Daily Oral Direct FXa Inhibition Compared with Vitamin K Antagonism for Prevention of Stroke and Embolism Trial in Atrial Fibrillation (ROCKET-AF) trial,[228] 14,264 patients with nonvalvular AF were randomly assigned to either fixed-dose rivaroxaban (20 mg daily or 15 mg daily in patients with a CrCl of 30–49 mL/min) or dose-adjusted warfarin. In the per-protocol analysis, the primary endpoint of stroke or systemic embolism occurred in 188 patients on rivaroxaban (1.7% per year) and 241 patients on warfarin (2.2% per year, HR for the rivaroxaban group = 0.79, 95% CI 0.66–0.96, $P < 0.001$ for noninferiority). Major and nonmajor clinical bleeding occurred in 1475 patients receiving rivaroxaban (14.5% per year, HR 1.03; 95% CI 0.96–1.11; $P = 0.44$). There was a significant reduction in intracranial hemorrhage (0.5% versus 0.7%, $P = 0.02$) and fatal bleeding (0.2% versus 0.5%, $P = 0.003$) in the rivaroxaban group. In contrast, major GI bleeding was more common in the rivaroxaban group (224 events, 3.2%) when compared with warfarin (154 events, 2.2%, $P < 0.001$). On the basis of these data, the FDA approved rivaroxaban for stroke and thromboembolic prophylaxis in nonvalvular AF.

Atrial Fibrillation and PCI

In the PIONEER-AF-PCI trial,[229] 2124 participants with NVAF who had undergone PCI with stenting were randomized to receive, in a 1:1:1 ratio, low-dose rivaroxaban (15 mg once daily) plus a $P2Y_{12}$ inhibitor for 12 months (group 1), very-low-dose rivaroxaban (2.5 mg twice daily) plus DAPT for 1, 6, or 12 months (group 2), or standard therapy with a dose-adjusted vitamin K antagonist (once daily) plus DAPT for 1, 6, or 12 months (group 3). The primary safety outcome was clinically significant bleeding (a composite of major bleeding or minor bleeding according to TIMI criteria or bleeding requiring medical attention). The rates of clinically significant bleeding were lower in the two groups receiving rivaroxaban than in the group receiving standard therapy (16.8% in group 1, 18.0% in group 2, and 26.7% in group 3; HR for group 1 versus group 3, 0.59; 95% CI 0.47–0.76; $P < 0.001$; HR for group 2 versus group 3, 0.63; 95% CI 0.50–0.80; $P < 0.001$). The rates of death from cardiovascular causes, MI, or stroke were similar in the three groups (Kaplan-Meier estimates, 6.5% in group 1, 5.6% in group 2, and 6.0% in group 3; P values for all comparisons were nonsignificant). In participants with atrial fibrillation undergoing PCI, the administration of either low-dose rivaroxaban plus a $P2Y_{12}$ inhibitor for 12 months or very-low-dose rivaroxaban plus DAPT for 1, 6, or 12 months was associated with a lower rate of clinically significant bleeding than was standard therapy with a vitamin K antagonist plus DAPT for 1, 6, or 12 months.

Heart Failure

The COMMANDER HF randomized clinical trial[230] evaluated the effects of adding low-dose rivaroxaban to antiplatelet therapy in patients with recent worsening of chronic HF with reduced ejection fraction, CAD, and sinus rhythm. The trial randomized 5022 patients postdischarge from a hospital or outpatient clinic after treatment for worsening HF. Patients were required to be receiving standard care for HF and CAD and were excluded for a medical condition requiring anticoagulation or a bleeding history. Patients were randomized in a 1:1 ratio. Although the primary endpoint of all-cause mortality, MI, or stroke did not differ between rivaroxaban and placebo, there were numerical advantages favoring rivaroxaban for MI and stroke. Accordingly, a post hoc analysis of the COMMANDER HF placebo-controlled trial in patients with CAD and worsening HF was undertaken. Patients were randomly assigned to receive 2.5 mg of rivaroxaban given orally twice daily or placebo in addition to their standard therapy. For this post hoc analysis, a thromboembolic composite was defined as either (1) MI, ischemic stroke, sudden/unwitnessed death, symptomatic PE, or symptomatic DVT or (2) all of the previous components except sudden/unwitnessed deaths because not all of these are caused by thromboembolic events. Of 5022 patients, 3872 (77.1%) were men, and the overall mean (SD) age was 66.4 (10.2) years. Over a median (interquartile range) follow-up of 19.6 (11.7–30.8) months, fewer patients assigned to rivaroxaban compared with placebo had a thromboembolic event including sudden/unwitnessed deaths: 328 (13.1%)

versus 390 (15.5%) (HR 0.83; 95% CI 0.72–0.96; $P = 0.01$). When sudden/unwitnessed deaths were excluded, the results analyzing thromboembolic events were similar: 153 (6.1%) versus 190 patients (7.6%) with an event (HR 0.80; 95% CI 0.64–0.98; $P = 0.04$).[231]

Stable Cardiovascular Disease

In the COMPASS study, 27,395 participants with stable atherosclerotic vascular disease (coronary artery or peripheral artery) were randomly assigned to receive rivaroxaban 2.5 mg twice daily plus aspirin 100 mg once daily, and 5 mg twice daily or aspirin 100 mg once daily. The primary outcome was a composite of cardiovascular death, stroke, or MI. The study was stopped for superiority of the rivaroxaban plus aspirin group after a mean follow-up of 23 months. The primary outcome occurred in fewer patients in the rivaroxaban plus aspirin group than in the aspirin alone group (4.1% versus 5.4%; HR 0.76; 95% CI 0.66–0.86; $P < 0.001$),[38] but, there was a higher rate of major bleeding (3.1% versus 1.9%; HR 1.70; 95% CI 1.40–2.05; $P < 0.001$). There was no difference in either intracranial or fatal bleeding between groups. All-cause death was lower in the rivaroxaban plus aspirin group when compared with aspirin alone. Participants receiving rivaroxaban alone did not experience fewer events than aspirin alone, but major bleeding rates were higher.

Additional analysis of the COMPASS study revealed a particularly marked effect of combined rivaroxaban and aspirin for the prevention of primary and secondary stroke.[39] Ischemic/uncertain strokes were reduced by nearly half, as were the occurrence of fatal and disabling stroke. Independent predictors of stroke were prior stroke, hypertension, elevated systolic blood pressure at baseline, age, diabetes mellitus, and Asian ethnicity. Prior stroke was the strongest predictor of incident stroke with a HR of 3.63.

Ablation

VENTURE-AF was a prospective randomized trial of uninterrupted rivaroxaban and vitamin K antagonists (VKAs) in patients with NVAF undergoing CA. Patients (n = 248) were assigned to uninterrupted rivaroxaban (20 mg once daily) or to an uninterrupted VKA prior to CA and for 4 weeks afterwards. The primary endpoint was major bleeding events after CA. Secondary endpoints included thromboembolic events (composite of stroke, systemic embolism, MI, and vascular death) and other bleeding or procedure-attributable events. Patients were 59.5 ± 10 years of age, 71% male, 74% paroxysmal AF, and had a CHA2DS2-VASc score of 1.6. The average total heparin dose used to manage ACT during the procedure was slightly higher (13,871 versus 10,964 units; $P <$ 0.001) and the mean ACT level attained slightly lower (302 versus 332 units; $P < 0.001$) in rivaroxaban and VKA arms, respectively. The incidence of major bleeding was low (0.4%; one major bleeding event). Similarly, thromboembolic events were low (0.8%; one ischemic stroke and one vascular death). All events occurred in the VKA arm and all after CA. The number of any adjudicated events (26 versus 25), any bleeding events (21 versus 18), and any other procedure-attributable events (5 versus 5) were similar.[232]

Rivaroxaban-Associated Bleeding

The management of bleeding complications among patients receiving rivaroxaban has been investigated. In a rabbit bleeding model, recombinant activated factor VII and PCC partially improved coagulation laboratory parameters but did not reduce rivaroxaban associated bleeding.[233] Unlike dabigatran, rivaroxaban is 95% plasma protein bound, so hemodialysis is not expected to be useful. Activated charcoal may be useful if given within 8 hours of oral ingestion. In a randomized, placebo-controlled, double-blind trial of PCC in 12 healthy male volunteers on rivaroxaban, PCC immediately and completely reversed the prothrombin time and endogenous thrombin potential; however, no clinically relevant bleeding complications occurred during treatment.[234] See reversal and replacement section below.

Apixaban

Apixaban is a direct oral anticoagulant that binds the active site of FXa.

Pharmacodynamics

Apixaban is a potent, direct, oral, reversible, and highly selective inhibitor of FXa (inhibitory constant = 0.08 nM) that does not require AT for antithrombotic activity. Apixaban inhibits free and clot-bound FXa, as well as prothrombinase activity, which inhibits clot growth. By inhibiting FXa, apixaban decreases thrombin generation and thrombus development. It has no direct effect on platelet aggregation, but indirectly inhibits platelet aggregation induced by thrombin.

Pharmacokinetics

Apixaban has an oral bioavailability of 50%. Peak plasma drug concentrations are achieved at ~3 hours after administration and the half-life is 9–14 hours. Like rivaroxaban, metabolism is dependent on CYP450 activity.[235] Apixaban exposure increases dose proportionally for oral doses up to 10 mg. Elimination occurs via multiple pathways including metabolism, biliary excretion, and direct intestinal excretion, with approximately 27% of total apixaban clearance occurring via renal excretion. The pharmacokinetics of apixaban are consistent across a broad range of patients, and apixaban has limited clinically relevant interactions with most commonly prescribed medications, allowing for fixed dosages without the need for therapeutic drug monitoring.[236]

Clinical Experience

Venous thromboembolism. In the AMPLIFY study,[237] 5395 patients with acute venous thromboembolism were randomized to apixaban (at a dose of 10 mg twice daily for 7 days, followed by 5 mg twice daily for 6 months) or conventional therapy (SQ enoxaparin, followed by warfarin). The primary efficacy outcome was recurrent symptomatic venous thromboembolism or death related to venous thromboembolism. The principal safety outcomes were major bleeding alone and major bleeding plus clinically relevant nonmajor bleeding. The primary efficacy outcome occurred in 59 of 2609 patients (2.3%) in the apixaban group, as compared with 71 of 2635 (2.7%) in the conventional therapy group (RR 0.84; 95% CI 0.60–1.18; difference in risk [apixaban minus conventional therapy], -0.4 percentage points; 95% CI -1.3–0.4). Apixaban was noninferior to conventional therapy ($P < 0.001$) for predefined upper limits of the 95% CIs for both RR (<1.80) and difference in risk (<3.5 percentage points). Major bleeding occurred in 0.6% of patients who received apixaban and in 1.8% of those who received conventional therapy (RR 0.31; 95% CI 0.17–0.55; $P < 0.001$ for superiority).

Atrial Fibrillation

In a double-blind study,[238] 5599 patients with atrial fibrillation who were at increased risk for stroke, but in whom vitamin K antagonist therapy was considered unsuitable by their primary provider, were randomly assigned to receive apixaban (at a dose of 5 mg twice daily) or aspirin (81–324 mg per day). The primary outcome was the occurrence of stroke or systemic embolism. The data and safety monitoring board recommended early termination of the study because of a clear benefit in favor of apixaban. There were 51 primary outcome events (1.6% per year) among patients assigned to apixaban and 113 (3.7% per year) among those assigned to aspirin (HR with apixaban 0.45; 95% CI 0.32–0.62; $P < 0.001$). The rates of death were 3.5% per year in the apixaban group and 4.4% per year in the aspirin group (HR 0.79; 95% CI 0.62–1.02; $P = 0.07$).

The ARISTOTLE trial[239] randomized 18,201 patients with AF and at least one other risk factor for stroke to either warfarin or apixaban 5 mg twice daily. The rate of the primary outcome, ischemic or hemorrhagic stroke or systemic embolism, was 1.27% per year in the apixaban group and 1.60% per year in the warfarin group (HR with apixaban 0.79, 95% CI 0.66–0.95, $P < 0.001$ for noninferiority; $P = 0.01$ for superiority).

Atrial Fibrillation and PCI

The AUGUSTUS trial[240] was a two-by-two factorial, randomized, controlled trial that compared a vitamin K antagonist to apixaban, and aspirin to placebo, on a background of a $P2Y_{12}$ inhibitor in a population of patients with atrial fibrillation and either ACS or PCI (or both). Inclusion criteria were: 1) age ≥ 18 years; 2) previous atrial fibrillation with planned use of an oral anticoagulant; and 3) planned use of a $P2Y_{12}$ inhibitor for ≥ 6 months. Exclusion criteria were: 1) severe renal insufficiency; 2) history of intracranial hemorrhage; 3) other indications for anticoagulation; 4) coagulopathies; and 5) recent or planned coronary artery bypass surgery. Randomization of 4614 patients was performed within 14 days of ACS or PCI, with the median time at 6 days. In 92.6%, clopidogrel was the $P2Y_{12}$ inhibitor used. Median percentage of time in therapeutic range for those assigned to a vitamin K antagonist was 59%. No significant interaction was found between the two randomization factors for death or ischemic events ($P = 0.28$ for interaction). At 6 months, 154 patients (6.7%) who had been assigned to receive apixaban had died or had experienced an ischemic event, including MI, definite or probable stent thrombosis, stroke, or urgent revascularization as compared with 163 (7.1%) who had been assigned to receive a VKA. In the antiplatelet-regimen comparison, 149 patients (6.5%) who had been assigned to receive aspirin died or had an ischemic event, as compared with 168 (7.3%) who had been assigned to receive placebo. This difference was not significant, but more ischemic events occurred in the placebo group.

Ablation

In AXAFA-AFNET continuous apixaban (5 mg BID) was prospectively compared to VKA (INR 2–3) in atrial fibrillation patients at risk of stroke.[241] Primary outcome was a composite of death, stroke, or bleeding (Bleeding Academic Research Consortium 2–5). Overall, 674 patients (median age 64 years, 33% female, 42% nonparoxysmal atrial fibrillation) were randomized and 633 received study drug. The primary outcome was observed in 22/318 patients randomized to apixaban, and in 23/315 randomized to VKA (difference -0.38% [90% CI -4.0%, 3.3%], noninferiority $P = 0.0002$ at the prespecified absolute margin of 0.075), including two (0.3%)

deaths, two (0.3%) strokes, and 24 (3.8%) ISTH major bleeds. Acute small brain lesions were detected by MRI in a similar number of patients in each arm (apixaban 44/162 [27.2%]; VKA 40/161 [24.8%]; $P=0.64$). Cognitive function increased at the end of follow-up ($P=0.005$) without differences between study groups.

Apixaban-Associated Bleeding

In the AMPLIFY trial,[237] the composite outcome of major bleeding and clinically relevant nonmajor bleeding occurred in 4.3% of the patients in the apixaban group, as compared with 9.7% of those in the conventional-therapy group (RR 0.44; 95% CI 0.36–0.55; $P < 0.001$). In AVEROUS,[238] there were 44 cases of major bleeding (1.4% per year) in the apixaban group and 39 (1.2% per year) in the aspirin group (HR with apixaban 1.13; 95% CI 0.74–1.75; $P = 0.57$); there were 11 cases of intracranial bleeding with apixaban and 13 with aspirin. The rate of major bleeding was 2.13% per year for apixaban and 3.09% per year for warfarin (HR 0.69; 95% CI 0.60–0.80; $P < 0.001$) in the ARISTOTLE.[240,242] Major or clinically relevant nonmajor bleeding was noted in 10.5% of the patients receiving apixaban, as compared with 14.7% of those receiving a vitamin K antagonist (HR 0.69; 95% CI 0.58–0.81; $P < 0.001$ for both noninferiority and superiority) in the AUGUSTUS trial, and in 16.1% of the patients receiving aspirin, as compared with 9.0% of those receiving placebo (HR 1.89; 95% CI 1.59–2.24; $P < 0.001$).[240] The percentage of patients with a primary bleeding outcome event was highest among those receiving a vitamin K antagonist and aspirin (18.7%) and lowest among those receiving apixaban and placebo (7.3%).

Edoxaban

Edoxaban, a once-daily nonvitamin K antagonist oral anticoagulant, is a direct, selective, reversible inhibitor of FXa. In healthy subjects, single oral doses of edoxaban result in peak plasma concentrations within 1–2 hours of administration, followed by a biphasic decline. Exposure is approximately dose proportional for once daily doses of 15–150 mg. Edoxaban is predominantly absorbed from the upper GI tract, and oral bioavailability is approximately 62%. Food does not affect total exposure to edoxaban. The terminal elimination half-life in healthy subjects ranges from 10 to 14 hours, with minimal accumulation upon repeat once daily dosing up to doses of 120 mg.[243] The steady state Vd is approximately 107 L, and total clearance is approximately 22 L/h; renal clearance accounts for approximately 50% of total clearance, while metabolism and biliary secretion account for the remaining 50%. Intrinsic factors, such as age, sex, and race, do not affect edoxaban pharmacokinetics after renal function is taken into account. Oral administration of edoxaban results in rapid changes in anticoagulatory biomarkers, with peak effects on anticoagulation markers (such as anti-FXa), the prothrombin time, and the aPTT occurring within 1–2 hours of dosing.[244]

Drug interaction studies were nonetheless performed to investigate the effects of CYP3A4 inhibitors on the pharmacokinetics of edoxaban. Additionally, the effects of other drugs that could be dosed concomitantly with edoxaban were evaluated. Since edoxaban is a substrate of the efflux transporter P-gp, several drug interaction studies were conducted with P-gp inhibitors, substrates, and inducers.

Venous thromboembolism. In the Hokusai-VTE study,[245] patients with acute venous thromboembolism, who had initially received heparin, were randomly assigned to receive edoxaban at a dose of 60 mg once daily, or 30 mg once daily (in patients with CrCl of 30–50 mL/min or a body weight below 60 kg), or to receive warfarin. Patients received the study drug for 3 to 12 months. The primary efficacy outcome was recurrent symptomatic venous thromboembolism. The principal safety outcome was major or clinically relevant nonmajor bleeding. A total of 4921 patients presented with DVT and 3319 with a PE. Among patients receiving warfarin, the time in the therapeutic range was 63.5%. Edoxaban was noninferior to warfarin for the primary efficacy outcome, which occurred in 130 patients in the edoxaban group (3.2%) and 146 patients in the warfarin group (3.5%) (HR 0.89; 95% CI 0.70–1.13; $P < 0.001$ for noninferiority).

Atrial Fibrillation

The ENGAGE study[246] compared two once-daily regimens of edoxaban with warfarin in 21,105 patients with moderate-to-high-risk atrial fibrillation (median follow-up, 2.8 years). The primary efficacy endpoint was stroke or systemic embolism. The principal safety endpoint was major bleeding. The annualized rate of the primary endpoint during treatment was 1.5% with warfarin (median time in the therapeutic range, 68.4%) and 1.18% with high-dose edoxaban (HR 0.79; 97.5% CI 0.63–0.99; $P < 0.001$ for noninferiority) and 1.61% with low-dose edoxaban (HR 1.07; 97.5% CI 0.87–1.31; $P = 0.005$ for noninferiority). In the intention-to-treat analysis, there was a trend favoring high-dose edoxaban versus warfarin (HR 0.87; 97.5% CI 0.73–1.04; $P = 0.08$) and an unfavorable trend with low-dose edoxaban versus warfarin (HR 1.13; 97.5% CI 0.96–1.34; $P = 0.10$). The annualized rates of death from cardiovascular causes were 3.17% versus 2.74% (HR 0.86; 95% CI 0.77–0.97; $P = 0.01$), and 2.71% (HR 0.85; 95% CI 0.76–0.96; $P = 0.008$), and the corresponding rates of the key secondary endpoint (a composite of stroke, systemic embolism, or death

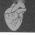

from cardiovascular causes) were 4.43% versus 3.85% (HR 0.87; 95% CI 0.78–0.96; $P = 0.005$), and 4.23% (HR 0.95; 95% CI 0.86–1.05; $P = 0.32$).

Edoxaban-Associated Bleeding

In the Hokusai-VTE study,[245] the safety outcome occurred in 349 patients (8.5%) in the edoxaban group and 423 patients (10.3%) in the warfarin group (HR 0.81; 95% CI 0.71–0.94; $P = 0.004$ for superiority). In the ENGAGE study,[246] rates of adverse events were similar in the two groups. The annualized rate of major bleeding was 3.43% with warfarin versus 2.75% with high-dose edoxaban (HR 0.80; 95% CI 0.71–0.91; $P < 0.001$) and 1.61% with low-dose edoxaban (HR 0.47; 95% CI 0.41–0.55; $P < 0.001$).

Betrixaban

Betrixaban is an oral anticoagulant that exerts its action by preventing thrombin generation without having a direct effect on platelet aggregation. Betrixaban presents a rapid absorption at a dose of 80 mg. Its peak plasma concentration is registered within 3–4 hours after oral administration in healthy humans.

Pharmacodynamics

Betrixaban is an oral, selective FXa inhibitor that binds the active site of FXa and inhibits free FXa. Direct FXa inhibition decreases prothrombinase activity and, therefore, thrombin generation. Betrixaban dosed at 40–80 mg daily has no clinically relevant effect on activated partial thrombin time, prothrombin time, or INR.[247]

Pharmacokinetics

Betrixaban has a half-life of 19–27 hours,[248] which is longer than values for the rest of the agents in its class. Betrixaban has a quick onset of action, and the time it takes for the drug to reach maximum plasma concentration is 3–4 hours; thus, a patient is fully anticoagulated relatively quickly after therapy initiation. Betrixaban is about 35% bioavailable. There is no published information on how crushing or chewing can affect bioavailability, and the package insert suggests that betrixaban should be administered with food. Furthermore, betrixaban is about 60% protein bound. Unlike other FXa inhibitors, betrixaban does not undergo extensive hepatic metabolism. Because the CYP450 isozyme system does not play a major role in the metabolism of betrixaban, drug interactions through this pathway are not a major concern. On the other hand, betrixaban is a substrate of P-gp; therefore, decreased or increased levels should be expected when betrixaban is administered with strong P-gp inducers or inhibitors, respectively.

Clinical Experience

Betrixaban is indicated for prophylaxis of VTE in adults hospitalized for acute medical illness who are at risk for thromboembolic
complications owing to moderate or severe restricted mobility
and other risk factors for VTE. Dose modifications are recommended for patients with severe renal disease (CrCl $\geq$15 to
<30 mL/min).

APEX was a randomized, double-blind, multinational clinical
trial comparing extended duration betrixaban (35–42 days) to
short duration of enoxaparin (6–14 days) in the prevention of
VTE in an acutely medically ill hospitalized population with risk
factors for VTE.[249] The trial randomized 7513 patients to either
betrixaban or enoxaparin treatment. Patients receiving betrixaban
took an initial dose of 160 mg orally on day 1, then 80 mg once
daily for 35 to 42 days, and received a placebo injection once daily
for 6 to 14 days. Patients in the enoxaparin arm received 40 mg
subcutaneously once daily for 6 to 14 days and took a placebo pill
orally once daily for 35 to 42 days. A total of 7441 patients partic-
ipated with a composite outcome comprised of either the occurrence of asymptomatic or symptomatic proximal DVT, nonfatal
PE, or VTE-related death. Fewer events were observed in patients
receiving betrixaban (4.4%) compared with those taking enoxaparin (6%) (RR 0.75; 95% CI 0.61, 0.91). At 35–42 days, extended
betrixaban reduced the risk of VTE (4.27% versus 7.95%, $P=0.042$)
without causing excess major bleeding (1.14% versus 3.13%,
$P=0.07$). Both VTE (3.32% versus 8.33%, $P=0.013$) and major
bleeding (0.00% versus 3.26%, $P=0.003$) were decreased in the
full-dose stratum. Patients who received betrixaban had more
nonmajor bleeding than enoxaparin (overall population: 2.56%
versus 0.28%, $P=0.011$; full-dose stratum: 3.32% versus 0.36%,
$P=0.010$). Mortality was similar at the end of study (overall population: 13.39% versus 16.19%, $P=0.30$; full-dose stratum: 13.65%
versus 16.30%, $P=0.39$).[250]

Betrixaban-Associated Bleeding

The most common adverse reactions ($\geq$5%) with betrixaban in the
Apex Trial were related to bleeding. Overall, 54% of patients receiving betrixaban experienced at least one adverse reaction compared with 52% taking enoxaparin. The frequency of patients
reporting serious adverse reactions was similar between betrixaban
(18%) and enoxaparin (17%). The most frequent reason for treatment discontinuation was bleeding, with an incidence rate for all
bleeding episodes of 2.4% and 1.2% for betrixaban and enoxaparin,
respectively. The incidence rate for major bleeding episodes was
0.67% and 0.57% for betrixaban and enoxaparin, respectively.

Drug Interactions

The dose of betrixaban should be reduced if it is coadministered with P-gp inhibitors, owing to increased bleeding risk. Betrixaban should be avoided in patients with severe renal impairment receiving concomitant P-gp inhibitors.

Vitamin K Antagonists

Warfarin

Warfarin, while available in an IV form, is predominantly administered orally.

Pharmacodynamics

Warfarin exerts its anticoagulant activity through inhibition of the synthesis of vitamin K–dependent coagulation factors II, VII, IX, and X-specifically, their carboxylation. Carboxylation of the N-terminal region of coagulation proteins II, VII, IX, and X is required for their biological activity and reduced vitamin K is required as a cofactor for the carboxylation step.

Pharmacokinetics

Warfarin interferes with clotting factor synthesis by inhibition of the C1 subunit of vitamin K epoxide reductase enzyme complex, reducing the regeneration of vitamin K_1 epoxide. Warfarin (and other coumarin derivatives) inhibit the reductase enzymes responsible for vitamin K recycling, indirectly slowing the rate of synthesis of clotting functionally active factors.[251] Therapeutic doses of warfarin reduce the total amount of active vitamin K–dependent clotting factors produced by the liver by 30% to 50%.

Clinical Experience

Dosing. A standard approach to initiating warfarin is to begin with 5 mg/day for 3 days, checking the INR daily and titrating the dose accordingly until it is in the lower threshold of anticoagulation (INR 2.0) is surpassed. Lower starting doses are preferred in older adults, those with increased risk of bleeding, concomitant liver disease, and in the presence of concomitant medications known to increase warfarin response. Genetic variations in hepatic enzymes explain lower dose requirements for persons of Asian descent[252] and higher doses for black and some Jewish populations.[253] In patients transitioning from parenteral anticoagulation, warfarin should be initiated 4–5 days before heparin (UFH, LMWH) is discontinued to allow for the inactivation of all circulating vitamin K–dependent coagulation factors; the heparin can be discontinued once the INR has been in the therapeutic range for 2 days.

Therapeutic INR Range

The INR, representing a prothrombin time according to an international reference thromboplastin, is recommended for warfarin management. In fact, the INR was developed solely for this purpose-acknowledging the complexity of warfarin and a need to obtain consistency across laboratories and for clinicians worldwide. An INR range of 2.0 to 3.0 is recommended for patients who have *DVT, PE,* those at risk of thromboembolism, including AF. Patients with *prosthetic heart valves* require a greater intensity of anticoagulation, and the recommended INR range is 2.0 to 3.5, with lower values for those with bioprosthetic valves and mechanical valves in the aortic position.[254] Once the steady-state warfarin requirement is known, the INR can be checked once every 4–6 weeks. Importantly, variation in INR control and variation in warfarin requirements may be influenced in individual patients by dietary changes, comorbid illness, changes in medication or doses, activity, and alcohol intake.

Self-Monitoring and Self-Guided Warfarin Therapy

Selected patients who can both self-monitor, using a home point-of-care coagulation device and self-guide according to a clinician-developed dosing algorithm have less thromboembolic events and lower mortality than those who only self-monitor.[255] Patient selection, education, communication, and a follow-up strategy are keys to safety and efficacy.

Pharmocogenetic-Guided Dosing

Bleeding risks are highest within the first 3 months of initiating warfarin therapy. In the CoumaGen-II study of VKORC genotype-guided warfarin dosing, the prior analysis of VKORC gave the genetically appropriate first dose. The result was 10% absolute reduction in the out-of-range INRs, 66% lower rate of DVT, and a reduction in serious adverse events at 90 days from 9.4% in controls to 4.5%. These data support a pharmacogenetic-based approach, if available and if rapid and affordable, prior to the initiation of warfarin.[256]

Dose Modifications

The dose of warfarin should be reduced in the presence of congestive heart failure; liver damage from any source, including alcohol;

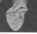

renal impairment (which increases the fraction of free drug in the plasma); and malnutrition (which leads to vitamin K deficiency). Thyrotoxicosis enhances the catabolism of vitamin K, reducing the dose of warfarin needed, whereas myxedema has the opposite effect. In older adults, the dose should be reduced because the response to warfarin increases with age. A variable intake of dietary vitamin K (e.g., green vegetables such as broccoli) increases INR variability. Patients should receive education and suggestions for maintaining a consistent amount of vitamin K in their food.

Drug Interactions With Warfarin

Warfarin interacts with many drugs through varying mechanisms. It is inhibited by drugs such as barbiturates or phenytoin that accelerate warfarin degradation in the liver. Potentiating drugs include allopurinol and amiodarone, and cephalosporin antibiotics that inhibit the generation of vitamin K. Drugs that decrease warfarin degradation and increase the anticoagulant effect include a variety of antibiotics such as metronidazole *(Flagyl)* and cotrimoxazole *(Bactrim)*. Antiplatelet drugs such as aspirin, clopidogrel, and NSAIDs may potentiate the risk of bleeding. Clinicians should avoid combination therapy unless there is a strong indication.

Contraindications

Contraindications include a recent ischemic stroke with a high-risk for hemorrhagic conversion, hemorrhagic stroke, uncontrolled systemic hypertension, and hepatic cirrhosis with impaired synthetic capacity. If anticoagulation is essential, the risk-benefit ratio must be evaluated carefully. Older age is not in itself a contraindication to anticoagulation.

Pregnancy and Warfarin

Warfarin is contraindicated in the first trimester because of its teratogenicity, and 2 weeks before birth because of the risk of fetal bleeding.

Warfarin-Associated Bleeding Risk

The most common complication is bleeding with increased risk of intracranial hemorrhage, especially in older adults.[257] A serious complication is *warfarin-associated skin necrosis*. The cause likely involves depletion in protein C, a natural anticoagulant. The best approach to prevention is to start with lower doses of warfarin while the patient is concomitantly on heparin; this is particularly important in patients with known protein C deficiency.

Mitral Stenosis or Regurgitation

In patients with mitral valve disease, the risk of thromboembolism is greatest in those with AF, marked left atrial (LA) enlargement, or previous embolic episodes; anticoagulation should be considered. By contrast, anticoagulation is not indicated in patients with mitral stenosis in sinus rhythm. *Percutaneous mechanical LA appendage closure* with the Watchman device is widely used in patients who are not good candidates for long-term anticoagulation. In a comparison with warfarin in AF patients and a CHADS$_2$ score of 1 or more,[258] the Watchman was noninferior to warfarin therapy for the prevention of stroke, systemic embolism, and cardiovascular death.

Heart Failure and Cardiomyopathy

Routine anticoagulation in patients with HF (whether HFpEF or HFrEF) is not recommended in the absence of AF or other specific indication.[259] A number of trials failed to show a benefit for warfarin anticoagulation in patients with LV systolic dysfunction or HFrEF in sinus rhythm.[260,261] Long-term anticoagulation with Coumadin with target INR 2–3 or a novel oral anticoagulant has a class I indication for patients with chronic HF with permanent or paroxysmal AF and one additional risk factor for cardio-embolic stroke (HTN, DM, previous stroke/TIA, age >75 years). Chronic anticoagulation is reasonable (class II indication) for patients with chronic HF and permanent or paroxysmal AF but without any additional risk factor.[259]

Other cardiomyopathies associated with increased thromboembolic risk are amyloid and LV noncompaction (LVNC). Anticoagulation is recommended in patients with amyloid CMP and AF in the absence of any other risk factor and should be considered even in the absence of AF especially in those with AL type.[262] Similarly, anticoagulation should be considered in patients with LVNC with AF without additional risk factors and in those with LVEF <40%.

Ventricular Assist Devices

All durable LVADs require long term anticoagulation with warfarin to prevent pump thrombosis. Warfarin is typically started after removal of chest tubes, but timing may vary depending on clinical setting and/or surgeon clinical judgement.[50] A retrospective non-controlled study of 418 HM2 patients reported similar risk for thrombotic events with reduced postoperative bleeding in patients who receive warfarin without heparin bridging and concluded that IV heparin for transition to warfarin may not be necessary in patients with low thrombotic risk.[263] This approach needs to be investigated and is not currently recommended.

Heart Transplant

Due to availability of donors and longer time, many currently transplanted patients have LVADs implanted. Warfarin is typically reversed with IV vitamin K (2.5–10 mg) depending on INR. Oral vitamin K is a safer option due to small risk of anaphylaxis reported with IV route and can be used when transplantation is not expected within 24–48 hours. Other options to quickly reverse anticoagulation include FFP or PCC. Kcentra contains inactive forms of factors II, VII, IX, X and is frequently used in the operating room for quick reversal of VKAs. In the absence of bleeding, aspirin 81 mg daily is started within the first few days post heart transplant to prevent coronary artery vasculopathy, although the evidence for primary prevention is limited and based on retrospective data.

Prosthetic Heart Valves

Warfarin is recommended in patients with mechanical prosthetic heart valves, typically titrated to an INR of 2.5 to 3.5 (Table 8.19). In patients with bioprosthetic mitral valves, the risk of thromboembolism is highest in the first 6–12 weeks, when warfarin is recommended. Thereafter, aspirin may be given, or antithrombotic therapy may be discontinued if there are no other indications. There is firm evidence supporting continued warfarin administration when mitral bioprosthetic valves are combined with AF, a large left atrium, or LV failure. In patients with bioprosthetic aortic valves the risk is low, and aspirin for 6–12 weeks is appropriate.[264,265]

Table 8.19

Antithrombotic therapy for patients with prosthetic heart valves				
	Mechanical		**Bioprosthetic**	
	Aortic position	**Mitral position**	**Aortic position**	**Mitral position**
Warfarin	++	++	+[a]	++ [a]
Aspirin	−	−	+	+
Combination therapy	+[b]	++	−	−

[a]Anticoagulant therapy is recommended for the first 3 postoperative months. Long-term treatment is reserved for patients with concomitant risk factors, prior thromboembolism, or documented left atrial thrombus.

[b]Aspirin (75–100 mg/d) in patients with prostheses other than bileaflet and those with atrial fibrillation, poor left ventricular function, or prior cardioembolic stroke.

Peripheral Artery Disease

A number of trials have been conducted to determine the utility of oral anticoagulants in patients with peripheral artery disease. The Warfarin Antiplatelet Vascular Evaluation (WAVE) trial investigators conducted a meta-analysis of nine trials involving 4889 patients and found that, compared to aspirin, oral anticoagulant therapy did not change mortality (OR = 1.04; 95% CI 0.55–1.29) or graft occlusion (OR = 0.91; 95% CI 0.77–1.06), but did increase major bleeding (OR = 2.13; 95% CI 1.27–3.57).[266] The current data do not support routine anticoagulant therapy in patients with PAD.[267 268]

Anticoagulant Management in Patients With Atrial Fibrillation and PCI

Among the most challenging scenarios for clinicians is the management of antithrombotic therapy in patients with atrial fibrillation who require PCI. The emergence of data from randomized trials as summarized previously offers guidance (Figs. 8.9 and 8.10).

Treatment of VKA-Associated Bleeding

Management of bleeding while on VKA is dictated by both the severity of bleeding, the intensity of anticoagulation as gauged by the INR, and the risk of thromboembolism associated with either cessation of drug treatment or reversal of anticoagulation. While minor bleeding associated with an elevated INR can be managed with temporary cessation of warfarin and administration of oral vitamin K, serious bleeding usually requires administration of IV vitamin K supplemented with FFP, PCC, or recombinant factor VIIa as needed. For life-threatening bleeding, immediate normalization of the INR is required. Although FFP can be used for this purpose, the use of factor concentrates is preferred because the volume of FFP required to correct the INR may be considerable and require hours to infuse.[269] Yasaka et al. found that a dose of 500 IU of PCC was optimal for rapid reversal of an INR <5 but that higher doses may be needed for higher INRs.[270] Finally, although not specifically approved for INR reversal, recombinant factor VIIa has been shown effective in reversing excessively prolonged INRs and bleeding in patients on warfarin at varying doses. Unfortunately, both PCCs and recombinant factor VIIa carry a risk of thromboembolic events,[271] which must be considered prior to use.

Four-factor PCC is the replacement agent of choice for warfarin-associated, acute, life-threatening hemorrhage and is dosed according to the baseline INR. A dose of 25–50 units/kg and maximum doses of 2500, 3500, and 5000 units for INR values of 2.0–3.9, 4.0–5.9, and greater than 6.0, respectively.

ATRIAL FIBRILLATION
and
PERCUTANEOUS CORONARY INTERVENTION

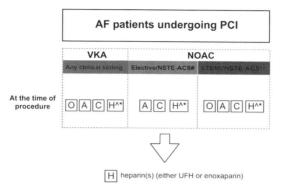

Fig. 8.9 A general approach to patients with atrial fibrillation *(AF)* on an oral anticoagulant undergoing a percutaneous coronary intervention *(PCI)*. *A, C, H, NOAC,* non-vitamin K antagonist oral anticoagulant; *NSTE-ACS,* non ST elevation acute coronary syndrome; *O, STEM,* ST-segment elevation myocardial infarction; *VKA,* vitamin K antagonist. (Data from 2018 Joint European consensus document on the management of antithrombotic therapy in atrial fibrillation patients presenting with acute coronary syndrome and/or undergoing percutaneous cardiovascular interventions. *Europace* 2019;21:192–193.)

Reversal and Replacement of Direct Oral Anticoagulant Drugs

Targeted Reversal Drugs

Idarucizumab

Idarucizumab is a humanized monoclonal antibody fragment (FAB, molecular weight is 47.8 kDa) that tightly binds and irreversibly inhibits dabigatran in a 1:1 ratio. The affinity of idarucizumab to dabigatran is 350 times the affinity of dabigatran to thrombin. In vitro and in vivo animal studies revealed an immediate and complete reversal of dabigatran's anticoagulant activity at equimolar concentrations after single bolus dose of idarucizumab. The drug did not interact with other thrombin substrates, coagulation factors or impact platelet activity.[272] In addition and despite its molecular

ATRIAL FIBRILLATION, PERCUTANEOUS CORONARY INTERVENTION, and ACUTE CORONARY SYNDROME

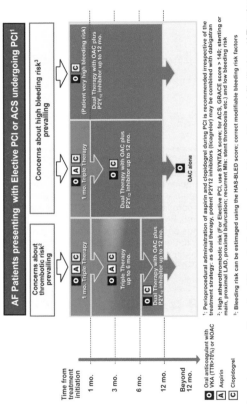

Fig. 8.10 A comprehensive perspective of antithrombotic therapy in patients with atrial fibrillation (AF) undergoing percutaneous coronary intervention (PCI). The risk of thrombosis and bleeding are factored into decision-making at multiple time points of a highly dynamic landscape. *ACS*, Acute coronary syndrome; *LAD*, left anterior descending artery; *MIs*, myocardial infarctions; *NOAC*, non-vitamin K antagonist oral anticoagulant; *VKA*, vitamin K antagonist; *TTR*, time in therapeutic range. (From 2018 Joint European consensus document on the management of antithrombotic therapy in atrial fibrillation patients presenting with acute coronary syndrome and/or undergoing percutaneous cardiovascular interventions. *Europace* 2019;21:192–193 with permission.)

structure idarucizumab does not possess thrombin-like activity and, unlike nonspecific reversal agents, has not, in the studies performed to date, caused an "over correction" as assessed by thrombin generation parameters. Idarucizumab is 100 times larger than dabigatran and the Vd of the former or idarucizumab-dabigatran complex is significantly lower than dabigatran alone. The half-life is 45 minutes in healthy volunteers, and elimination occurs primarily by a renal route. The efficacy and safety in patients with advanced chronic kidney disease are unknown.

No serious adverse events were reported among healthy volunteers in a double blinded placebo controlled phase II trial.[273] The median serum dabigatran concentrations in this study were similar to levels reported in the RE-LY trial. An infusion (over 5 minutes) of 1, 2, and 4 g resulted in a reduction of dilute thrombin time by 74%, 94%, and 98%, respectively. Similar responses were observed as determined by aPTT, ecarin clotting time and thrombin time measurements. Reversal was maintained over 72 hours with 2 g or higher doses of idarucizumab. Serum dabigatran concentrations remained elevated albeit inactive and in a bound state to the FAB fragment. Minor adverse reactions included skin irritation and erythema at the site of drug administration, dizziness, asthenia and flu-like symptoms. Idarucizumab vials contain sorbitol, and there is a potential risk of adverse events, including hypoglycemia, vomiting, and metabolic acidosis, in patients with hereditary fructose intolerance.

The safety and efficacy of idarucizumab as a reversal agent specifically for dabigatran were demonstrated in the Reversal Effects of Idarucizumab on Active Dabigatran (RE-VERSE AD) trial of 503 patients, 301 of whom had serious or life-threatening hemorrhage.[274,275] The median maximum percentage reversal of dabigatran, on the basis of either the diluted thrombin time or the ecarin clotting time, was 100%. Nearly half of the study patients had GI bleeding, and one-third presented with ICH. The median time to the cessation of bleeding was 2.5 hours. At 90 days in RE-VERSE AD, thromboembolic events had occurred in 6.3% of the patients reversed for hemorrhage. Over 90% of these complications occurred in patients who did *not* have reinitiation of anticoagulant therapy. There were no serious adverse safety signals (Tables 8.20 and 8.21).

Andexanet Alfa

Andexanet alfa is a recombinant modified FX molecule (FX decoy) that possesses a specific binding site for FX/Xa inhibitors. It lacks the membrane binding g-carboxyglutamate domains and catalytic site, and therefore does not exert a procoagulant effect.[276] The drug can reverse the anticoagulant activity of direct FXa inhibitors in a

Table 8.20

Approach to patients taking dabigatran with severe or life-threatening hemorrhage or an emergent need for surgery or an invasive procedure

CRITERIA FOR USE: if patient meets the following criteria, administration of idarucizumab is appropriate for the reversal of dabigatran

1. Currently taking dabigatran
2. Last dose was administered within 12 hours, or 24 hours in patients with CrCl <60 mL/min
3. Laboratory result of at least **ONE** of the following:
   a. aPTT >40 seconds
   b. Thrombin time (TT) >65 seconds
   c. Ecarin Clotting Time (ECT) that is elevated
4. Major or life-threatening bleeding
   a. Major bleeding is defined as:
      i. Bleeding with reduction in hemoglobin of at least 2 g/dL or leading to 2 units of blood/packed cells
      ii. Symptomatic bleeding in a critical area or organ (intracranial, intraocular, intraspinal or intramuscularly with compartment syndrome, retroperitoneal, intraarticular, or pericardial bleeding
   b. Life-threatening bleeding is defined as:
      i. Symptomatic intracranial bleeding
      ii. Bleeding with hypotension requiring use of IV inotropic agents
      iii. Bleeding requiring surgical intervention

Emergent surgery/procedure that cannot be delayed for at least 8 hours.

Table 8.21

Recommended dosing for idarucizumab	
Drug	**Potential reversal agent/therapy**
Dabigatran	Idarucizumab 5 g IV (administered as two separate infusions of 2.5 g over 5 to 10 minutes, total administration should be completed within 15 minutes)

Redosing:

a. The prescribing information for idarucizumab allows for redosing with 5 g 12–24 hours after initial dose if the patient has clinically relevant bleeding or need for second surgery/procedure with elevated coagulation parameters. There is no clinical data to support redosing at this time.
b. Redosing at physician's discretion if the following criteria are met:
c. 12–24 hours after first 5 g dose
   AND
   ii. Clinically relevant bleeding OR require a second emergency surgery/ urgent procedure; AND
   iii. Reelevation of coagulation parameters (aPTT and TT)

aPTT, Activated partial thromboplastin time; *IV,* intravenous; *TT,* thrombin time.

dose-dependent manner. Andexanet alfa also retains its ability to bind AT and is designed to reverse antithrombin-mediated indirect FXa inhibitors, including LMWHs and fondaparinux. Additional studies will be required before the current labeling is expanded.

Several randomized, double-blind, placebo-controlled trials in healthy volunteers investigated the efficacy and safety of various andexanet alfa doses in reversal of direct and indirect FXa inhibitors. ANNEXA-A and ANNEXA-R trials included older healthy volunteers after treatment with apixaban or rivaroxaban, respectively. AntiFXa activity of apixaban and rivaroxaban was immediately reversed after a bolus injection of 400 mg and 800 mg, respectively. Thrombin generation increased to normal without a rebound effect in the andexanet alfa arm. There were no thrombotic events in these trials. Reversal was maintained for 2 hours after a bolus injection and for a longer duration with a continuous infusion of 4 mg/min for rivaroxaban and 8 mg/min for apixaban.[277]

The ANNEXA-4 trial evaluated 352 patients[278] who had acute major bleeding within 18 hours after administration of a FXa inhibitor. The patients received a bolus of andexanet, followed by a 2-hour infusion. The coprimary outcomes were the percent change in antiFXa activity after andexanet treatment and the percentage of patients with excellent or good hemostatic efficacy at 12 hours after the end of the infusion, with hemostatic efficacy adjudicated on the basis of prespecified criteria. Efficacy was assessed in the subgroup of patients with confirmed major bleeding and baseline antiFXa activity of at least 75 ng/mL (or $\geq$0.25 IU/mL for those receiving enoxaparin). Patients had a mean age of 77 years, and most had substantial cardiovascular disease. Bleeding was predominantly intracranial (in 227 patients [64%]) or GI (in 90 patients [26%]). In patients who had received apixaban, the median antiFXa activity decreased from 149.7 ng/mL at baseline to 11.1 ng/mL after the andexanet bolus (92% reduction; 95% CI 91–93); in patients who had received rivaroxaban, the median value decreased from 211.8 ng/mL to 14.2 ng/mL (92% reduction, 95% CI 88–94). Excellent or good hemostasis occurred in 204 of 249 patients (82%) who could be evaluated. Within 30 days, death occurred in 49 patients (14%) and a thrombotic event in 34 (10%) (Tables 8.22 and 8.23).

Achieving Good Hemostasis

An ability to achieve good hemostasis is the goal of reversal or replacement therapy (Fig. 8.11). In addition, we will emphasize that the management of patients receiving anticoagulant therapy in whom major or life-threatening bleeding occurs must be

Table 8.22

Management for the use of andexanet alfa (Andexxa®) for acute bleed or trauma in patients taking factor Xa inhibitors

WARNINGS

1. No contraindications
2. Black Box Warning for thromboembolic and ischemic risk. May resume anticoagulant therapy as soon as medically appropriate
3. Infusion reactions

   APPROVED INDICATIONS FOR ANDEXANET ALFA

   Factor Xa Inhibitor Reversal: Andexanet alfa (Andexxa®) can be considered in patients with major/life-threatening bleeding or requiring emergency surgery/urgent procedure who are anticoagulated with factor Xa inhibitors

   a. FDA approved factor Xa reversal: rivaroxaban, apixaban
   b. Off label-factor Xa reversal: edoxaban, betrixaban, enoxaparin, fondaparinux

   CRITERIA FOR USE: if the patient meets the following criteria, administration of andexanet alfa is appropriate for the reversal of factor Xa inhibitors

4. Currently taking a factor Xa inhibitor
5. No previous reversal agent used
   a. Andexanet alfa should be used as the only reversal agent. It should not be given if the patient has already received Kcentra or other factor products
6. Time of last anticoagulant dose:
   a. Rivaroxaban: Last dose administered within 18 hours or 24 hours in patients with creatine clearance (CrCl) <50 mL/min
   b. Apixaban: Last dose administered within 18 hours or 24 hours in patients with SCr >1.5 g/dL
   c. Edoxaban: Last dose administered within 18 hours or 24 hours in patients with a CrCl <50 mL/min
   d. Betrixaban: Last dose administered within 18 hours or 24 hours in patients with a CrCl <30 mL/min
   e. Enoxaparin: Last dose administered within 18 hours or 24 hours in patients with a CrCl below 30 mL/min
   f. Fondaparinux: Last dose administered within 24 hours
7. Laboratory result of at least ONE of the following:
   a. PT GREATER than 16 seconds
   b. Anti-Xa GREATER than 0.5 units/mL
8. Major or life threatening bleeding
   a. Major bleeding is defined as:
      i. Bleeding with reduction in hemoglobin of at least 2 g/dL or leading to 2 units of blood/packed cells
      ii. Symptomatic bleeding in a critical area or organ (intracranial, intraocular, intraspinal or intramuscularly with compartment syndrome, retroperitoneal, intraarticular, or pericardial bleeding
   b. Life-threatening bleeding is defined as:
      i. Symptomatic intracranial bleeding
      ii. Bleeding with hypotension requiring use of intravenous inotropic agents
      iii. Bleeding requiring surgical intervention

Table 8.23

Recommended dosing for andexanet			
FXa inhibitor	**FXa inhibitor last dose**	**<8 hours or unknown time since last dose**	**≥8 hours**
Rivaroxaban	≤10 mg	Low dose	Low dose
Rivaroxaban	>10 mg/Unknown	High dose	
Apixaban	≤5 mg	Low dose	
Apixaban	>5 mg/Unknown	High dose	
ᵃEdoxaban		High dose	Unknown
ᵃEnoxaparin			

Dose	**Initial IV bolus**	**Follow-on IV infusion**
Low Dose	400 mg at target rate of 3 0 mg/min	4 mg/min for up to 120 minutes
High dose	800 mg at target rate of 30 mg/min	8 mg/min for up to 120 minutes

Off-label use:

a. Reversal of enoxaparin, fondaparinux, betrixaban, and edoxaban
   i. Must meet criteria listed above
b. Use should be determined by clinical pharmacist and attending physician
   i. Off-label use should be retroactively communicated to DPD and pharmacy manager on call due to time sensitive nature of administration
c. Limited dosing recommendations
   i. ANNEXA-4 used dosing similar to rivaroxaban for reversal of edoxaban and enoxaparin (high dose)
   ii. Betrixaban and low dose fondaparinux (2.5 mg) are prophylactic doses of anticoagulation and should be reversed with caution given the high thrombotic risk associated with andexanet alfa
   iii. Dose should be based on clinical judgement of attending physician and clinical pharmacist

REDOSING:

d. The prescribing information for andexanet alfa (Andexxa®) does not recommend redosing
e. Lack of commercially available anti-Xa monitoring calibrated to rivaroxaban, apixaban, and other oral factor Xa inhibitor makes monitoring of reversal effect inaccurate below

No current recommendations for dosing for fondaparinux or betrixaban reversal.
DPD, IV, intravenous.

ᵃEdoxaban and enoxaparin dosing from clinical trials (off-label use)

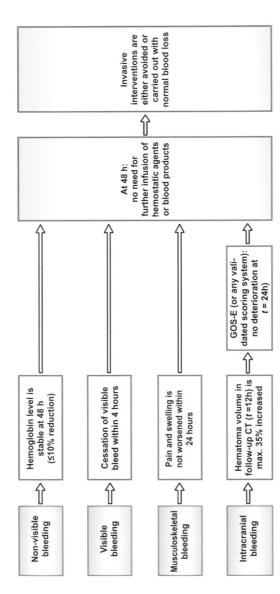

Fig. 8.11 A definition of achieving good hemostasis among patients with anticoagulant-associated major bleeding who receive reversal agents. *CT, computerized tomography; GOS-E,* Glasgow Outcome Scale Extended. (Data from Abdoellakhan RA, et al. Method agreement analysis and interobserver reliability of the ISTH proposed definitions for effective hemostasis in management of major bleeding. *J Thromb Haemost 2019;17:499–506.*)

APPROACH TO BLEEDING

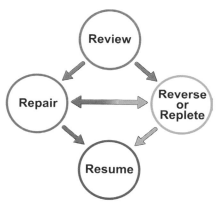

Fig. 8.12 The four key steps for managing DOAC-associated bleeding in clinical practice. (Data from EMCREG.)

multidimensional to achieve favorable outcomes (Fig. 8.12).[279] In addition, there must be a step-wise approach that includes initial stabilization and supportive care (Fig. 8.13) as well as a decision tree for resumption of anticoagulant therapy (Fig. 8.14).

Conclusions

Antithrombotic therapy is a mainstay in the management of patients with cardiovascular disease. Intensive investigation and exceptional progress over the past several decades have provided many therapeutic options that include platelet-directed antagonists and anticoagulants. Clinicians must always follow the best available evidence when making decisions on behalf of their patients. Management guidelines and frequent updates as new data emerge will remain a key component to optimal patient care. In addition to understanding the pharmacology, clinical use and potential adverse effects, clinicians must equally understand the approach to treatment for major or life-threatening hemorrhage, the most common complication of antithrombotic therapy. The future of antithrombotic therapy will be defined by optimal use and discernment by informed clinicians and patients and, as in the past, an increasing knowledge of biology and pathophysiology will open the door to new drug development (Table 8.24).

MANAGE DOAC BLEEDING

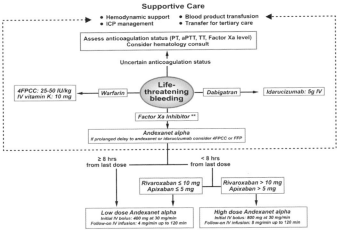

Fig. 8.13 Managing life-threatening bleeding in anticoagulated patients requires a comprehensive, multidisciplinary approach to achieve an optimal outcome. Life-threatening bleeding includes intracranial and other sites with excessive blood loss. The use of andexanet is FDA-approved for the reversal of rivaroxaban and apixaban. *aPTT,* Activated partial thromboplastin time; *DOAC,* direct oral anticoagulant; *FDA,* US Food and Drug Administration; *FFP,* fresh frozen plasma; *4FPCC,* 4-factor prothrombin complex concentrate; *ICP,* intracranial pressure; *IV,* intravenous; *PT,* prothrombin time; *TT,* thrombin time. (Data from Emergency Medicing Cardiac Research and Education Group [EMCREG].)

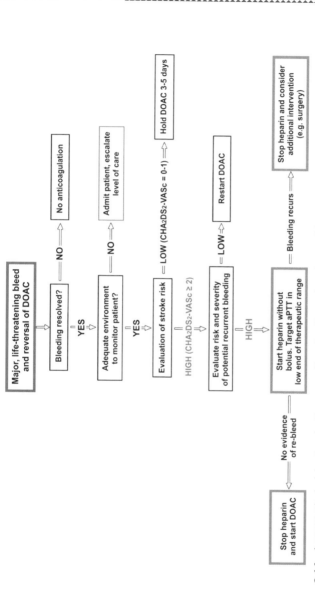

Fig. 8.14 A pragmatic decision tree for the resumption of anticoagulant therapy following reversal. Each decision should be made according to risk, benefit and patient values and preferences. *aPTT,* Activated partial thromboplastin time; *CHA2DS2-VASc,* congestive heart failure, coronary artery disease, age, diabetes, stroke, vascular disease-risk core for future stroke; *DOAC,* direct oral anticoagulant. (Data from EMCREG.)

Table 8.24

Future targets for antithrombotic drug development			
	Mechanism(s) of action	Source(s)	Role in primary hemostasis
Cell-free nucleic acids	Increase in auto-activation of factors XI and XII; cofactor for auto-activation of factor VII-activating protease	Apoptotic or necrotic cells	None reported
Histones	Direct activation of platelets via TLR2 and 4	Apoptotic or necrotic cells; released from inflammatory cells	None reported
DNA-histone complexes	Stimulate endothelial activation via increases in intracellular calcium and subsequent release of prothrombotic constituent proteins; direct activation of platelets; inhibition of tissue factor pathway inhibitor; stimulate factor XII-mediated thrombin generation	Apoptotic or necrotic cells; released from inflammatory cells	None reported
Polyphosphates	Increased thrombin-mediated factor V activation; activation of factors XI and XII; delayed fibrinolysis through	Released from platelets following activation with thrombin, ADP, and collagen	None reported

Table 8.24

Future targets for antithrombotic drug development (Continued)			
	Mechanism(s) of action	Source(s)	Role in primary hemostasis
	activation of thrombin-activatable fibrinolysis inhibitor		
Microvesicles	PS-bearing MV: Facilitation of formation of prothrombotic complexes Tf-bearing MV: Formation of Tf-factor Vila complexes	PS-bearing MV: Released from platelets and erythrocytes Tf-bearing MV: Released from monocytes, platelets, neutrophils, endothelial cells, and smooth muscle cells	None reported

ADP, Adenosine diphosphate; *MV,* microvesicles, *PS,* phosphatidylserine; *Tf,* tissue factor; *TLR,* Toll-like receptor.

References

Complete reference list available at www.expertconsult.com.

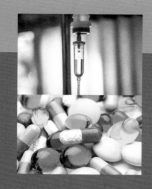

**第9章
抗心律失常药物**

在过去的几十年中，抗心律失常药物并没有发生实质性的变化。但最近提出了新的针对离子通道的潜在治疗靶点。同时，即便有一些试验药物因意外停止了试验，仍有新的药物不断被研发。目前大多数指南仍然主张将抗心律失常药物作为心房颤动和室性心动过速的一线治疗。另外，历史上的抗心律失常药物被赋予了治疗遗传性心律失常的新用途。因此，抗心律失常药物仍然非常重要。

抗心律失常药物主要分为Ⅰ、Ⅱ、Ⅲ、Ⅳ和Ⅴ共五类。Ⅰ类钠通道阻滞剂可进一步分为ⅠA类，包括奎尼丁、普鲁卡因胺、丙吡胺和阿马林；ⅠB类，包括利多卡因和美西律；ⅠC类，包括氟卡尼和普罗帕酮；ⅠD类*为雷诺嗪（*VauhganWilliams分类法中并无ⅠD类，因雷诺嗪作用机制与上述ⅠA类、ⅠB类、ⅠC类药物不同，故置于此处）。Ⅱ类为β肾上腺素受体拮抗剂。Ⅲ类复极化阻滞剂可分为混合作用型和单纯作用型两种，混合作用型包括胺碘酮、索他洛尔和决奈达隆；单纯作用型包括伊布利特、多非利特和Vernakalant。Ⅳ类则为钙通道阻滞剂。Ⅴ类为腺苷。其他药物包括伊伐布雷定、静脉镁制剂等。本章详细讨论了各药物的药代动力学、使用剂量、不良反应及药物相互作用等，同时涵盖了吸入型药物，并讲解了抗心律失常药物的新进展。更有意义的是，本章总结了室上性心动过速、心房颤动、心房扑动、室性心动过速、尖端扭转型室性心动过速等不同心律失常情况的药物选择。

目前因多种药物选择的复杂性、不良反应和致心律失常问题，使得心导管射频消融术等有创干预策略更受青睐。现有的抗心律失常药物的吸入剂型可能会为临床提供不良反应更少的新方法，但需要注意的是，新型抗心律失常药物的研究仍有限，新一代抗心律失常药物能否成功应用于临床还有待观察。

陈安天

Antiarrhythmic Drugs

ATUL VERMA

Overview of New Developments

Antiarrhythmic drugs have not changed substantially over the last several decades. Even when newer agents have been developed, the potential for proarrhythmia and increased mortality continue to plague their broader implementation. Recently, novel ion channel targets have been proposed and newer agents are being researched, but even some experimental agents have halted trials in phase II because of unexpected toxicity. Furthermore, as interventional therapies have progressed, such as implantable defibrillators and ablation, the urgency for new pharmacologic antiarrhythmic therapy has decreased. Most guidelines still advocate for antiarrhythmics remaining first-line therapy for both atrial fibrillation (AF) and ventricular tachycardia (VT). Furthermore, historical antiarrhythmics have now found new purpose for the treatment of various inherited arrhythmia disorders. Therefore, it is still important to understand this eclectic group of pharmacotherapies.

Antiarrhythmic Drugs

Antiarrhythmic drugs are used to suppress arrhythmias with the hopes of alleviating significant symptoms or possibly to affect survival. Prophylactic treatment of arrhythmias has been questioned since the publication of the Cardiac Arrhythmia Suppression Trial[1] and by a meta-analysis of nearly 100,000 patients with acute myocardial infarction (AMI) treated with antiarrhythmic drugs.[2] These studies showed that suppression of ventricular ectopy can actually increase mortality. Therefore, antiarrhythmic drugs should only be used when the suppression of arrhythmia outweighs the adverse effects of the drug. There are very few instances where antiarrhythmic drugs may actually reduce mortality and/or sudden death. β-blockers following myocardial infarction (MI) or in the setting of heart failure reduce mortality.[3] The only antiarrhythmic agent that appears to prevent sudden cardiac death (SCD) is amiodarone, and possibly dofetilide.[4,5] Amiodarone acts on multiple ionic channels and is therefore effective against a wide spectrum of arrhythmias. However, even amiodarone is inferior to implantable cardioverter defibrillators (ICDs) for sudden-death prevention in the patients at highest risk.[6]

Classification. There are five established classes of antiarrhythmic action (Table 9.1). The original Vaughan Williams classification with four classes now incorporates ionic mechanisms and receptors as the basis of the more complex Sicilian Gambit system for antiarrhythmic drug classification (Fig. 9.1).[7] Recently, a modernized, expanded classification scheme was developed for which the traditional Vaughan Williams classification remains the basis,

Table 9.1

Antiarrhythmic drug classes			
Class	Channel effects	Repolarization time	Drug examples
IA	Sodium block effect ++	Prolongs	Quinidine Disopyramide Procainamide Ajmaline
IB	Sodium block effect +	Shortens	Lidocaine Phenytoin Mexiletine
IC	Sodium block effect +++	Unchanged	Flecainide Propafenone
ID	Sodium block effect +	Prolongs	Ranolazine
II	β-Adrenergic block I_f, a pacemaker current; indirect Ca^{++} channel block;	Unchanged	β-blockers (excluding sotalol that also has class III effects)
III	Repolarizing K^+ currents	Markedly prolongs	Amiodarone Sotalol Ibutilide Dofetilide Vernakalant
IV	AV nodal Ca^{2+} block	Unchanged	Verapamil Diltiazem
V	K^+ channel opener (hyperpolarization)	Unchanged	Adenosine
Unclassified			Ivabradine

AV, Atrioventricular; += inhibitory effect; ++= markedly inhibitory effect; +++= major inhibitory effect.

CLASSES OF ANTIARRYTHMIC DRUGS

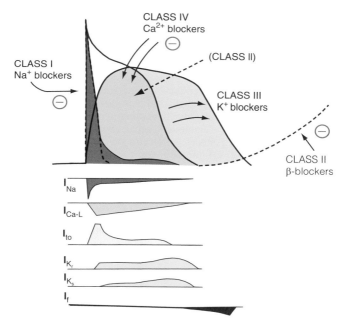

Fig. 9.1 The classical four types of antiarrhythmic agents. Class I agents decrease phase zero of the rapid depolarization of the action potential (rapid sodium channel). Class II agents, β-blocking drugs, have complex actions including inhibition of spontaneous depolarization (phase 4) and indirect closure of calcium channels, which are less likely to be in the "open" state when not phosphorylated by cyclic adenosine monophosphate. Class III agents block the outward potassium channels to prolong the action potential duration and hence refractoriness. Class IV agents, verapamil and diltiazem, and the indirect calcium antagonist, adenosine, all inhibit the inward calcium channel, which is most prominent in nodal tissue, particularly the atrioventricular node. Most antiarrhythmic drugs have more than one action. In the *lower panel* are shown the major currents on which antiarrhythmics act, according to the Sicilian gambit. *Ca-L*, long-lasting calcium; *I*, current; I_f, inward funny current; K_r, rapid component of repolarizing potassium current; K_s, slow component; *Na*, sodium; t_o, transient outward. (Figure © L.H. Opie, 2012.)

but the scheme also identifies new potential targets for emerging (or yet to emerge) drugs.[8] A quick reference table is provided summarizing some of the more common antiarrhythmic medications (Table 9.2).

Class IA: Quinidine, Procainamide, Disopyramide, and Ajmaline

The class IA agents inhibit the fast sodium channel with depression of phase 0 of the action potential and have intermediate kinetics, which is to say that they associate and dissociate from the sodium channels at an intermediate rate (between the rapid IB agents and the slow IC agents). These agents also block repolarizing potassium currents (a mild class III effect), which can prolong action potential duration and result in QT prolongation (Table 9.3). Torsades de pointes is therefore the major adverse effect. These agents can be used for treatment of either ventricular or atrial arrhythmias. With atrial flutters, however, they may slow down the atrial rate sufficiently to allow 1:1 conduction to the ventricle thereby accelerating the ventricular rate substantially (Fig. 9.2). There are no large-scale outcome trials to suggest that quinidine or other class I agents decrease mortality; rather there is indirect evidence that suggests increased mortality.

Quinidine

Historically, quinidine was the first antiarrhythmic drug used. It has been used for the treatment of both ventricular and atrial arrhythmias. It can also be used in the treatment of Brugada syndrome. Today, because of limited availability in some countries as well as its proarrhythmic potential, quinidine is not used as often, although its application to Brugada syndrome has led to a very small resurgence of interest in the drug.

Pharmacokinetics. Quinidine is a substrate of the cytochrome P450 enzymes and P-glycoprotein. In particular, it is a strong inhibitor of CYP2D6 (strong), and a less strong inhibitor of CYP3A4 and P-glycoprotein. These affects result in the numerous drug interactions of quinidine.

Clinical use. Quinidine is not often used today but can be used for the treatment of both atrial and ventricular arrhythmias. Quinidine has also been shown to be effective in management of ventricular fibrillation (VF) in the setting of Brugada syndrome. Brugada syndrome results from loss-of-function mutations in the SCN5A gene (and others), which code for the sodium channel. This impairs the inward sodium current and results in an unopposed I_{to} (transient outward potassium current) activity, which can set up

Table 9.2

Quick reference for common antiarrhythmic drugs

Agent	Dose	Pharmacokinetics and metabolism	Side effects and contraindications	Interactions and precautions
Lidocaine (class IB)	IV 75–200 mg; then 2–4 mg/min for 24–30 h. (No oral use)	Effect of single bolus lasts only few min, then $T_{1/2}$ approximately 2 h. Rapid hepatic metabolism. Level 1.4–5 μg/mL; toxic >9 mcg/mL.	Reduce dose by half if liver blood flow low (shock, β-blockade, cirrhosis, cimetidine, severe heart failure). High-dose CNS effects.	β-blockers decrease hepatic blood flow and increase blood levels. Cimetidine (decreased hepatic metabolism of lidocaine).
Mexiletine (class IB)	[a]IV 100–250 mg at 12.5 mg/min, then 2 mg/kg/h for 3.5 h, then 0.5 mg/kg/h. Oral 100–400 mg 8-hourly; loading dose 400 mg.	$T_{1/2}$ 10–17 h. Level 1–2 μg/mL. Hepatic metabolism, inactive metabolites.	CNS, GI side effects. Bradycardia, hypotension especially during cotherapy.	Enzyme inducers; disopyramide and β-blockade; increases the theophylline levels.
Phenytoin (class IB)	IV 10–15 mg/kg over 1 h. Oral 1 g; 500 mg for 2 days; then 400–600 mg daily.	$T_{1/2}$ 24 h. Level 10–18 μg/mL. Hepatic metabolism. Hepatic or renal disease requires reduced doses.	Hypotension, vertigo, dysarthria, lethargy, gingivitis, macrocytic anemia, lupus, pulmonary infiltrates.	Hepatic enzyme inducers[b].
Flecainide (class IC)	[a]IV 1–2 mg/kg over 10 min, then 0.15–0.25 mg/kg/h. Oral 50–400 mg 2 times daily. Hospitalize.	$T_{1/2}$ 13–19 h. Hepatic 2/3; 1/3 renal excretion unchanged. Keep trough level below 1 μg/mL.	QRS prolongation. Proarrhythmia. Depressed LV function. CNS side effects. Increased incidence of death postinfarct.	Many, especially added inhibition of conduction and nodal tissue.

Continued on following page

Table 9.2

Quick reference for common antiarrhythmic drugs (Continued)

Agent	Dose	Pharmacokinetics and metabolism	Side effects and contraindications	Interactions and precautions
Propafenone (class IC)	IV 2 mg/kg then 2 mg/min. Oral 150–300 mg 3 times daily.	$T_{1/2}$ variable 2–10 h, up to 32 h in nonmetabolizers. Level 0.2–3 µg/mL. Variable hepatic metabolism (P-450 deficiency slows).	QRS prolongation. Modest negative inotropic effect. GI side effects. Proarrhythmia.	Digoxin level increased. Hepatic inducers.
Ibutilide (class III)	IV infusion: 1 mg over 10 min, (under 60 kg: 0.1 mg/kg). If needed, repeat after 10 min.	Initial distribution $T_{1/2}$ is 1.5 minutes. Elimination $T_{1/2}$ averages 6 h (range 2–12 h). Efficacy is usually within 40 min.	Nausea, headache, hypotension, bundle branch block, AV nodal block, bradycardia, torsades de pointes, sustained monomorphic VT, tachycardia, ventricular extrasystoles. Avoid concurrent therapy with class I or III agents. Care with amiodarone or sotalol. C/I: previous torsades de pointes, decompensated heart failure.	Interactions with Class IA and other class III antiarrhythmic drugs that prolong the QT interval (e.g. antipsychotics, antidepressants, macrolide antibiotics, and some antihistamines). Check QT (see Fig. 9.4). Correct hypokalemia and hypomagnesemia.
Dofetilide (class III)	Dose 250 µg twice daily, maximum 500 µg twice	Oral peak plasma concentration in	Torsades de pointes in 3% of patients which can be	Increased blood levels with ketoconazole,

Drug	Dosage	Pharmacokinetics	Side effects/contraindications	Interactions/precautions
	daily if normal renal and cardiac function. If LV dysfunction, 250 µg twice daily. Check QT 2–3 h after dose, if QTc is 15% or >500 ms, reduce dose. If QTc >500 ms, stop.	2.5 hours and a steady state within 48 h. 50% excreted by kidneys unchanged.	function, bradycardia, or base-line QT↑. Avoid with other drugs increasing QT. C/I: previous torsades, creatinine clearance <20 mL/min.	verapamil, cimetidine, or inhibitors of cytochrome CYP3 A4, including macrolide antibiotics, protease inhibitors such as ritonavir. Other precautions as previously.
Sotalol (class III)	80–640 mg daily, occasionally higher in two divided doses.	$T_{1/2}$ 12 h. Not metabolized. Hydrophilic. Renal loss.	Myocardial depression, sinus bradycardia, AV block. Torsades if hypokalemic.	Added risk of torsades with IA agents or diuretics. Decrease dose in renal failure.
Amiodarone (class III)	Oral loading dose 600–1200 mg daily; maintenance 50–400 mg daily. IV 150 mg over 10 min, then 360 mg over 6 h, then 540 mg over remaining 24 h, then 0.5 mg/min.	$T_{1/2}$ 25–110 days. Level 1–2.5 µg/mL. Hepatic metabolism. Lipid soluble with extensive distribution in body. Excretion by skin, biliary tract, lachrymal glands.	Complex dose-dependent side effects including pulmonary fibrosis. QT prolongation. Torsades uncommon.	Class IA agents predispose to torsades. β-blockers predispose to nodal depression, yet give better therapeutic effects.

AF, Atrial fibrillation; AV, atrioventricular; BP, blood pressure; C/I, contraindication; ECG, electrocardiogram; GI, gastrointestinal; IV, intravenous; LV, left ventricular; SVT, supraventricular tachycardia; $T_{1/2}$, plasma half-life; VT, ventricular tachycardia; WPW, Wolff-Parkinson-White.

[a]Not licensed for intravenous use in the United States.

[b]Enzyme hepatic inducers are barbiturates, phenytoin, and rifampin, which induce hepatic enzymes, thereby decreasing blood levels of the drug.

Table 9.3

Effects and side effects of some ventricular antiarrhythmic agents on electrophysiology and hemodynamics

Agent	Sinus node	Sinus rate	A-His	PR	AV block	H-P	WPW	QRS	QT	Serious hemodynamic effects	Risk of torsades	Risk of monomorphic VT
Lidocaine	0	0	0/↓	0	0	0	↓/0	0	0	Toxic doses	0	0
Phenytoin	0	0	↑/0	0	Lessens	0	↓/0	0	↑	IV hypotension	0, +	0, +
Flecainide	0/↓	0	↓↓↓	↑	Avoid	↓↓	↓A/R	↑	↑ (via QRS)	LV ↓↓	0	+++
Propafenone	0/↓	0	↓↓	↑	Avoid	↓↓	↓A/R	↑	0	LV ↓	0	+++
Sotalol	↓↓	↓↓	→	↑	Avoid	0	A/R	0	↑	IV use	++	0, +
Amiodarone	↓	↓↑	→	0/↑	Avoid	0/↓	A/R	0	↑↑	IV use	+/−	0, +

A, antegrade; *A-His*, Atria-His conduction; *AV*, atrioventricular; *H-P*, His-Purkinje conduction; *IV*, intravenous; *LV*, left ventricular; *PR*, PR interval; *R*, retrograde; *VT*, ventricular tachycardia; *WPW*, Wolff-Parkinson-White syndrome accessory pathways.

Atrial rate very fast

Sinus Node

Atrioventricular Node

AV node blocking rapid inputs

Ventricular rate slowed

Left Bundle Branch

Right Bundle Branch

AV node has decremental properties that allow it to block conduction to ventricle (2:1, 3:1) when atrial rates are very high

Atrial rate slowed by IC drug

Sinus Node

Atrioventricular Node

AV node no longer blocking inputs

Ventricular rate increased

Left Bundle Branch

Right Bundle Branch

Atrial rate slows, which now permits AV node to conduct 1:1 to the ventricle with increase in ventricular rate

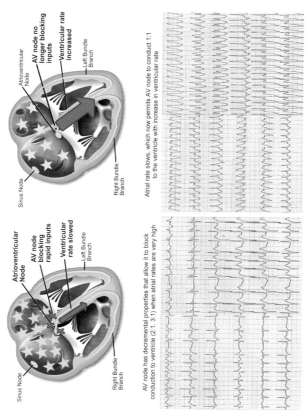

Fig. 9.2 See legend on next page

reentry in ventricular cells. Quinidine can inhibit I_{to}, thereby reducing the risk of VF in the setting of Brugada.[9]

Dose. For atrial and ventricular arrhythmias, quinidine sulfate intermediate release can be started at 200 mg every 6 hours and cautiously titrated upward. Extended release can be started at 300 mg every 8–12 hours and titrated to effect. The maximum dose is 600 mg every 8–12 hours for the intermediate release formulation. A 267 mg dose of quinidine gluconate is equal to 200 mg of quinidine sulfate. For Brugada, quinidine sulfate can be administered at 500 mg BID or TID. The dose of quinidine should be reduced if the QRS complex widens to 130% of its pretreatment duration, the QTc interval widens to 130% of its pretreatment duration and is >500 milliseconds, P waves disappear, or the patient develops significant tachycardia, symptomatic bradycardia, or hypotension. Quinidine titration should occur in a monitored setting.

Side effects. The major side effect of quinidine is ventricular proarrhythmia and sudden death, in particular torsades de pointes. This often occurs in association with QT prolongation (Fig. 9.3). In the setting of torsades, intravenous (IV) magnesium and alkalization of urine can help to reduce the effects of the quinidine. Gastrointestinal (GI) intolerance, namely nausea and diarrhea, are also common. At high doses, neurological side effects can occur. Heart block at the level of the sinus or AV node can also occur as can hypotension. Skin rash occurs in 5%–10% of patients and hepatotoxicity can also rarely occur.

Drug interactions and combination. Since quinidine inhibits CYP2D6 (strong), CYP3A4 (weak) and P-glycoprotein, drugs metabolized with these enzymes can be affected. Furthermore, any drug that affects the QT interval can also interact with quinidine. The number of culprit drugs interacting with quinidine is too numerous to list here but should always be checked when a patient is put on this drug.

Fig. 9.2, Cont'd   Conversion to 1:1 flutter by class IC agents. The atrioventricular (AV) node has decremental properties, which means that as more rapid atrial conduction enters the AV node, it slows conduction to cause AV block (3:1, 2:1), which helps to control (slow) the ventricular response. However, in the absence of an AV nodal blocker, class IC agents can slow the atrial rate sufficiently that the AV node now allows for 1:1 conduction, which can increase the ventricular rate. Class IC agents may also increase conduction velocity through the AV node. The result is a very rapid ventricular rate that can even degenerate to ventricular tachycardia/fibrillation and can be life-threatening. Therefore, administration of an IC agent should always be accompanied by an AV nodal blocker such as a β-blocker.

CLASS IA and III AGENTS: TORSADES DE POINTES

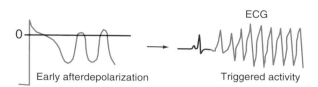

CLASS IC AGENTS: WIDE COMPLEX VT

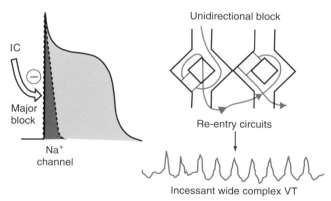

Fig. 9.3   Major proarrhythmic mechanisms. *Top*: Class IA and class III agents widen the action potential duration and in the presence of an early after-depolarization can give rise to triggered activity known as *torsades de pointes*. Note major role of QT prolongation. *Bottom*: Class IC agents have as their major proarrhythmic mechanism a powerful inhibition of the sodium channel, particularly in conduction tissue. Increasing heterogeneity together with unidirectional block sets the stage for reentry circuits and monomorphic wide-complex ventricular tachycardia *(VT)*. *ECG*, Electrocardiogram. (Figure © L.H. Opie, 2012.)

Procainamide

Like quinidine, procainamide is useful for the treatment of both atrial and ventricular arrhythmias. While IV procainamide can be maintained as an infusion for medium-term arrhythmia management, and oral forms are available for longer-term, outpatient management, most use of procainamide is for the acute conversion of AF, VT, or preexcited AF.

Pharmacokinetics. Procainamide has a very short half-life (2–5.5 hours), which means that oral dosing requires frequent dosing, making long-term compliance challenging. Even sustained-release formulas require dosing every 6–12 hours. For the IV preparation, a single bolus dose can be useful for acute termination of AF, VT, preexcited AF, or flutter. Maintenance infusions can be used, but procainamide is acetylated by the liver to N-acetyl-procainamide (NAPA), which also has active antiarrhythmic properties. Both procainamide and NAPA can accumulate in patients with renal and/or hepatic dysfunction and, therefore, increase the proarrhythmic potential. Both procainamide and NAPA levels may need to be monitored, which has made maintenance infusions of procainamide unpopular.

Clinical use. Procainamide can be used for the treatment of both atrial and ventricular arrhythmias. It is particularly useful for acute medical conversion in the emergency department. In the setting of preexcited atrial fibrillation, procainamide can prolong the refractoriness of both the AV node but also the accessory pathway. This avoids the potential for preferential and more rapid conduction through the pathway alone—possibly inducing VF—which can occur with administration of selective AV nodal blockers alone (Fig. 9.4). In regions where other IV sodium blockers are not available (like IV flecainide or ajmaline), IV procainamide is useful for drug testing to evoke the characteristic electrocardiogram (ECG) findings for Brugada syndrome for patients in whom the diagnosis is being considered but whose baseline ECG findings may be equivocal or absent. IV procainamide is also used in electrophysiology studies to evaluate for the presence of latent AV block by observing for prolongation in the HV interval to >100 milliseconds.

Dose. For acute conversion of atrial and ventricular arrhythmias, or for Brugada and His-ventricular interval (HV) testing, IV procainamide should be given at a dose of 10–17 mg/kg at a rate of 20–50 mg/minute. For a typical adult, this usually means a dose of about 1 g IV over 20 minutes. Maintenance infusion can be given at 1–6 mg/minute. For oral preparations, the sustained release can be given at 500–750 mg every 6 hours. Renal impairment requires dose reduction of 25%–50% with creatinine clearance <50 mL/min and 50%–75% with creatinine clearance <10 mL/minute. Hepatic dysfunction also requires dose reduction of 25%–50%.

Side effects. Like all other antiarrhythmics, procainamide has a risk of proarrhythmia, particularly heart block and QT prolongation. Monitoring for both prolongation in PR interval and QT interval is required. One of the major limitations of procainamide is the development of a drug-induced lupus erythematosus-like

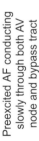

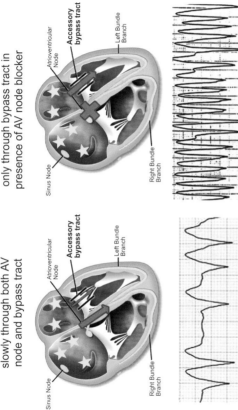

Fig. 9.4 Exacerbation of preexcited atrial fibrillation by lone atrioventricular (AV) nodal blockade. In atrial fibrillation *(AF)* that is conducting down both the AV node and an antegrade accessory pathway, the AF will often be wide because of the delta wave due to the preexcitation. The arrhythmia is typically wide and very irregular. Selective AV nodal blockers, like β-blockers and calcium channel blockers, should be avoided. They block the AV node allowing the AF to conduct exclusively through the usually very rapidly conducting pathway. This can dramatically increase the ventricular rate of the arrhythmia and even precipitate ventricular fibrillation, which is life-threatening. Therefore, in the presence of a wide-complex tachycardia (especially if it is irregular), selective AV nodal blocking agents should be avoided. Electrical cardioversion is typically best, but agents that block both the AV node and pathway may also be used, e.g., IV amiodarone, IV procainamide.

syndrome, which occurs in 20%–30% of patients. Patients will develop a positive antinuclear antibody (ANA) titer and/or symptoms of lupus. Development of either rising titers or symptoms should lead to drug discontinuation. Another important side effect is the development of blood dyscrasias. Agranulocytosis, neutropenia, hypoplastic anemia, and thrombocytopenia can all occur in 0.5%–1% of patients and can be fatal. Weekly blood monitoring is required for the first 3 months and then periodically thereafter. Blood counts may return back to normal within 1 month if the drug is discontinued. Finally, if IV procainamide is administered too quickly (faster than recommended rate), hypotension is a significant risk.

Drug interactions and combination. Any drug that affects the QT interval will interact with procainamide and should be avoided (Fig. 9.5).

Disopyramide

Disopyramide is a class IA drug and was approved for treatment of ventricular and atrial arrhythmias. However, it is not a very potent antiarrhythmic for either the ventricle or atrium. Its main therapeutic property is its profound negative inotropic effect. It can inhibit ventricular contraction by 40%–90% in low to high doses respectively and should therefore be completely avoided in patients with heart failure. The negative inotropy can be useful for patients with hypertrophic obstructive cardiomyopathy, particularly for reduction in outflow gradients. Disopyramide is more effective than both β-blockers and verapamil for outflow tract gradient reduction[10] and is often used prior to consideration of invasive therapy such as septal myectomy or alcohol ablation. Disopyramide may also be helpful for treatment of AF in patients with hypertrophic obstructive cardiomyopathy and does not seem to increase the risk of sudden death.[10] The main side effects are anticholinergic including dry mouth, prostatism, constipation, and urinary retention. Coadministration with pyridostigmine can alleviate the anticholinergic effects without impairing the antiarrhythmic effect.[11] Hypoglycemia can rarely occur. QT prolongation and widening of the QRS can occur.

Ajmaline

Ajmaline is another class IA antiarrhythmic that is not available in all jurisdictions worldwide (used predominantly in Europe). It has a very short half-life and is only used for IV administration. It blocks both sodium ion channels but also the hERG potassium channel. While it can be used for acute treatment of preexcited AF and some ventricular arrhythmias, it is predominantly used

LONG QT WITH RISK OF TORSADE

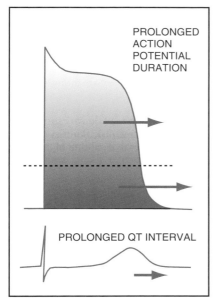

PROLONGED
ACTION
POTENTIAL
DURATION

PROLONGED QT INTERVAL

- *DISOPYRAMIDE*
  QUINIDINE
- *IBUTILIDE*
  DOFETILIDE
- *SOTALOL*
  (AMIODARONE)
- *TRICYCLICS*
  HALOPERIDOL
- *ANTIPSYCHOTICS*
- *PHENOTHIAZINES*
- *IV ERYTHROMYCIN*
  QUINOLONES (SOME)
- *ANTIHISTAMINICS*
  - *astemizole*
  - *terfenadine*
  - *KETOCONAZOLE*
- *Prolonged QTU:*
  Low K^+, Mg^{2+}
  (THIAZIDES)

Fig. 9.5 Therapeutic agents, including antiarrhythmics that may cause QT prolongation. Hypokalemia causes QTU, not QT, prolongation. Some antiarrhythmic agents act at least in part chiefly by prolonging the action potential duration, such as amiodarone and sotalol. QT prolongation is therefore an integral part of their therapeutic benefit. On the other hand, QT or QTU prolongation, especially in the presence of hypokalemia or hypomagnesemia or when there is cotherapy with one of the other agents prolonging the QT interval, may precipitate torsades de pointes. *IV*, Intravenous. (Figure © L.H. Opie, 2012.)

for electrophysiology testing. It is particularly useful for test for Brugada syndrome. In individuals where Brugada is suspected but the baseline ECG is either normal or equivocal, an IV ajmaline challenge may bring out the typical Brugada ECG pattern with ST segment elevation in V1–V3. It can be given as 1 mg/kg administered at 1 mg/sec or over 10 minutes. It can also be used to provoke HV lengthening (>100 milliseconds) to look for latent AV block.

Class IB: Lidocaine and Mexilitine

As a group, class IB agents inhibit the fast sodium current (typical class I effect; see Fig. 9.1) while shortening the action potential duration (APD) in nondiseased tissue. They also have rapid kinetics, which means they associate and dissociate from the sodium channels rapidly. The former is the more powerful effect, whereas the latter mitigates any QT prolongation. Class IB agents act selectively on diseased or ischemic tissue, where they are thought to promote conduction block, thereby interrupting reentry circuits. They have a particular affinity for binding with inactivated sodium channels with rapid onset-offset kinetics, which may be why such drugs are more selective for sodium channels in ventricular tissue versus atrial tissue. There are also differences in the β subunit of the rapid sodium channels in atrial versus ventricular tissue, which may affect binding of the class IB agents.[12]

Lidocaine

Lidocaine (Xylocaine, Xylocard) has become a standard IV agent for suppression of serious ventricular arrhythmias associated with AMI, cardiac surgery, or other ventricular storm. Lidocaine acts preferentially on the ischemic myocardium and is more effective in the presence of a high external potassium concentration. Therefore, hypokalemia must be corrected for maximum efficacy (also for other class I agents). This is an IV drug and therefore has no role in the control of chronic recurrent ventricular arrhythmias. The concept of prophylactic lidocaine to prevent VT and VF in AMI has long been outdated and is therefore no longer done.[2,13] Lidocaine has no value in treating supraventricular tachyarrhythmias.

Pharmacokinetics. The bulk of an IV dose of lidocaine is rapidly deethylated by liver microsomes (see Table 9.2). The two critical factors governing lidocaine metabolism and hence its efficacy are liver blood flow (decreased in old age and by heart failure, β-blockade, and cimetidine) and liver microsomal activity (enzyme inducers). Because lidocaine is so rapidly distributed within minutes after an initial IV loading dose, a second loading dose is often required followed by a continuous infusion (Fig. 9.6). Lidocaine metabolites circulate in high concentrations and may contribute to toxic and therapeutic actions. After prolonged infusions, the half-life may be longer (up to 24 hours) because of redistribution from poorly perfused tissues.

Clinical use. Lidocaine should not be used for prophylactic treatment of ventricular arrhythmias post-MI. Evidence from more than 20 randomized trials and 4 meta-analyses have shown that lidocaine reduces VF but adversely affects mortality rates, presumably because of bradyarrhythmias and asystole.[2] Lidocaine can be

LIDOCAINE KINETICS

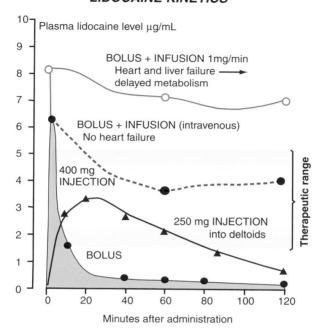

Fig. 9.6 Lidocaine kinetics. To achieve and to maintain an adequate blood level of lidocaine requires an initial bolus followed by an infusion. Often, a second bolus is required to get a steady state in addition to the infusion. Heart failure and liver failure delay metabolism of lidocaine which can increase the blood level and the accompanying danger of toxic effects. (Figure © L.H. Opie, 2012.)

used when tachyarrhythmias or very frequent premature ventricular contractions seriously interfere with hemodynamic status in patients with AMI (especially when already β-blocked). It can also be used to treat sustained ventricular arrhythmias and/or ventricular storm in patients presenting with refractory VT/VF (causing repeated implantable cardioverter defibrillator [ICD] shocks), especially during or after cardiac surgery or in the setting of ischemic cardiomyopathy. However, the efficacy of lidocaine alone is relatively low (15%–20%), but it can also be easily combined with other antiarrhythmic therapy, namely IV amiodarone and β-blockade.

Dose. A constant infusion would take 5–9 hours to achieve therapeutic levels (1.4–5 μg/mL), so standard therapy includes a loading dose of 75–100 mg intravenously, followed after 30 minutes by a second loading dose, or 400 mg intramuscularly. Thereafter lidocaine is infused at 2–4 mg/minute for 24–30 hours, aiming at 3 mg/minute, which prevents VF but may cause serious side effects in approximately 15% of patients, in half of whom the lidocaine dose may have to be reduced. Poor liver blood flow (low cardiac output or β-blockade), liver disease, or cimetidine or halothane therapy calls for halved dosage. The dose should also be decreased for older adult patients in whom toxicity develops more frequently and after 12–24 hours of infusion.

Side effects. Lidocaine is generally free of hemodynamic side effects, even in patients with congestive heart failure (CHF), and it seldom impairs nodal function or conduction (Table 9.3). The higher infusion rate of 3–4 mg/minute may result in neurologic toxicity such as drowsiness, numbness, speech disturbances, and dizziness, especially in patients older than 60 years of age. Minor adverse neural reactions can occur in approximately half the patients, even with 2–3 mg/minute of lidocaine. Occasionally there is sinoatrial (SA) arrest, but usually with coadministration of other drugs that potentially depress nodal function.

Drug interactions and combination. In patients receiving cimetidine, propranolol, or halothane, the hepatic clearance of lidocaine is reduced, and toxicity may occur more readily, so that the dose should be reduced. With hepatic enzyme inducers (barbiturates, phenytoin, and rifampin), the dose needs to be increased. Combination of lidocaine with early β-blockade is generally acceptable, because β-blockade can reduce liver blood flow and can rarely potentiate lidocaine-associated side effects (Tables 9.2, 9.4). Often, however, lidocaine IV is coadministered with IV amiodarone and β-blockade for the treatment of refractory ventricular arrhythmias/ventricular storm.

Lidocaine failure for VT and VF. If lidocaine apparently fails, consider other problems, especially concomitant hypokalemia, hypomagnesemia, severe ongoing ischemia, or other reversible underlying factors. There may have been a technical error in dosing—often people forget to bolus twice before starting the infusion. Lidocaine can also be used in combination with IV amiodarone and β-blockade for refractory ventricular arrhythmias. There is very little data comparing lidocaine with amiodarone IV. In a retrospective analysis of AMI patients, 6% developed sustained VT and VF, and of those who survived 3 hours, amiodarone, but not lidocaine, was associated with an increased risk of death.[7] However, the worse outcome of amiodarone-treated patients was likely due to selection of sicker patients as opposed to an effect of the drug itself.

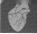

Table 9.4

Interactions (kinetic and dynamic) of antiarrhythmic drugs

Drug	Interaction with	Result
Lidocaine	β-blockers, cimetidine, halothane, enzyme inducers[a]	Reduced liver blood flow (increased blood levels) Decreased blood levels
Flecainide	Major kinetic interaction with amiodarone Added negative inotropic effects (β-blockers, quinidine, disopyramide) Added AV conduction depression (quinidine, procainamide)	Increase of blood F levels; half-dose As previously Conduction block
Propafenone	As for flecainide (but amiodarone interaction not reported); digoxin; warfarin	Enhanced SA, AV, and myocardial depression; digoxin level increased; anticoagulant effect enhanced
Sotalol	Diuretics, Class IA agents, amiodarone, tricyclics, phenothiazines (see Fig. 9.4)	Risk of torsades; avoid hypokalemia
Amiodarone	As for sotalol digoxin phenytoin flecainide warfarin	Risk of torsades Increased digoxin levels Double interaction, see text Increased flecainide levels Increased warfarin effect
Ibutilide	All agents increasing QT	Risk of torsades
Dofetilide	All agents increasing QT Liver interactions with verapamil, cimetidine, ketoconazole, trimethoprim	Risk of torsades Increased dofetilide blood level, more risk of torsades
Verapamil Diltiazem	β-blockers, excess digoxin, myocardial depressants, quinidine	Increased myocardial or nodal depression
Adenosine	Dipyridamole Methylxanthines (caffeine, theophylline)	Adenosine catabolism inhibited; much increased half-life; reduce A dose Inhibit receptor; decreased drug effects

AV, Atrioventricular; *IV,* intravenous; *SA,* sinoatrial.

[a]Enzyme inducers = hepatic enzyme inducers (i.e., barbiturates, phenytoin, rifampin).

Mexiletine (Mexetil)

Often considered an "oral form" of lidocaine, mexiletine can be useful for chronic management of ventricular arrhythmias (Table 9.2). It is typically not effective for treatment of acute ventricular arrhythmias (for which IV lidocaine is preferred), but patients on lidocaine can be transferred to oral mexiletine by giving the first dose as soon as the lidocaine infusion is stopped. Mexiletine is not useful for treatment of any atrial arrhythmias. Like lidocaine, the utility of mexiletine is reduced in the setting of hypokalemia and hypomagnesemia, therefore these electrolyte disorders should be corrected while on mexiletine.

Pharmacokinetics. Mexiletine is predominantly metabolized by CYP1A2 and CYP2D6. Therefore, medications that either inhibit or induce these enzymes can significantly alter the effects of mexiletine (see the "Drug interactions and combinations" section).

Clinical use. Mexiletine is most commonly used for chronic management of ventricular arrhythmias, especially in patients with cardiomyopathy and recurrent VT/VF. As monotherapy, mexiletine is often not very effective, so it is most commonly combined with oral amiodarone when amiodarone monotherapy has failed. It may be used as an alternative to amiodarone in those patients who have developed amiodarone toxicity. In long QT syndrome type III (LQTS 3), there is a mutation in the SCN5A subunit of the sodium channel that causes a gain in function and delays repolarization, therefore prolonging action potential duration and QT interval. Mexiletine has been used in patients with this subtype of LQTS to block the sodium current and regularize the QT interval and prevent torsades de pointes.

Dose. The drug may be started at 100–200 mg PO every 8 hours and can be titrated up in 50–100 mg intervals to a maximum dose of 300 mg every 8 hours. For LQTS 3, for pediatric patients, it is recommended to use 6–8 mg/kg/day in two or three divided doses for 2–3 days, then increase to 2–5 mg/kg/dose every 8–12 hours; continue to increase by 1–2 mg/kg/dose every 2–3 days until desired effect. The maximum daily dose is 15 mg/kg/day or 1200 mg/day whichever is less.

Side effects. The major dose-limiting side effect of mexiletine is GI intolerance—namely nausea, vomiting, and diarrhea, which can occur in about 30%–40% of patients. Many of these GI intolerances can be mitigated by taking the medication with food or by administering a concomitant proton pump inhibitor antacid. Neurological side effects include dizziness, tremor, ataxia, paresthesia, and blurred vision. These symptoms can occur in 10%–20% of patients. Rare but important side effects include blood dyscrasias such as marked leukopenia or thrombocytopenia. Truncal erythema, facial swelling, and pustules can develop rarely. Particularly in the Japanese, a marked hypersensitivity can occur with fever, rash, eosinophilia, and elevated liver enzymes.

Drug interactions and combination. Drugs that inhibit or induce CYP1A2 and CYP2D6 can significantly alter the effects of mexiletine. In particular, there are several protease inhibitors (used in the treatment of human immunodeficiency viruses [HIV]), which may interact with mexiletine. Interestingly, tobacco, heroin, and cannabis can all lower the levels of mexiletine. Selective serotonin reuptake inhibitors (SSRIs) can decrease metabolism of mexiletine (increasing drug levels) except for sertraline.

Phenytoin (Diphenylhydantoin)

Phenytoin (Dilantin, Epanutin) is now much less used. It may be effective against the ventricular arrhythmias occurring after congenital heart surgery. Occasionally in patients with epilepsy and arrhythmias a dual antiarrhythmic and antiepileptic action is useful. See Table 9.3 for effects.

Class IC: Flecainide and Propafenone

Class IC agents have acquired a particularly bad reputation as a result of the proarrhythmic effects seen in the Cardiac Arrhythmia Suppression Trial (CAST)[1] (flecainide) and the Cardiac Arrest Study Hamburg (CASH) study (propafenone).[13] As such, these drugs should absolutely be avoided in patients with coronary ischemia or structural heart disease (Fig. 9.3). Nonetheless, when carefully chosen, they fulfill a niche not provided by other drugs. As a group they have three major electrophysiologic (EP) effects (Table 9.3). First, they are powerful inhibitors of the fast sodium channel, causing a marked depression of the upstroke of the cardiac action potential, which may also explain their marked inhibitory effect on His-Purkinje conduction with QRS widening. In addition, they may variably prolong the APD by delaying inactivation of the slow sodium channel[14] and inhibition of the rapid repolarizing current (I_{Kr}).[15] In contrast to other class I agents, the IC's have very slow kinetics and dissociate slowly from the sodium channels during diastole, resulting in increased effect at a more rapid rate—so-called "use-dependence."[14] This characteristic may explain their excellent antiarrhythmic efficacy, especially against supraventricular arrhythmias. However, use-dependence may also contribute to the proarrhythmic activity of these drugs, especially in the diseased myocardium, resulting in incessant VT (Fig. 9.3). Some advocate performing exercise stress testing upon initiation of the drug to look for QRS widening that may not present at rest. If the QRS widens by 25% or more, the drug dose may need to be reduced or discontinued. However, absence of demonstrating use-dependence on exercise stress testing does not preclude the possibility of proarrhythmia from the drug. This class of drugs can also have significant negative chronotropic activity and should be avoided in patients with severe sinus node dysfunction or AV block. However, the drugs do not significantly prolong the QT interval (Table 9.3). Class IC agents are all potent antiarrhythmics used largely in the control of paroxysmal supraventricular tachyarrhythmias, especially AF, and ventricular arrhythmias resistant to other drugs. By inhibiting the ryanodine receptor open state and minimizing prolonged outward calcium movement, they are also effective in the unusual condition of catecholaminergic polymorphic VT.[16] Flecainide may also be useful in LQTS 3 characterized by the SCN5A:DeltaKPQ mutation in which the sodium channel repetitively opens prolonging the APD.[17]

Flecainide

Pharmacokinetics. Flecainide is metabolized by CYP2D6, which is inhibited by the SSRIs, therefore causing a significant interaction. Metabolites of flecainide are excreted mostly in the urine, so patients with impaired renal function need very close monitoring. For pharmacokinetics, side effects, and drug interactions, see Tables 9.2 to 9.4.

Clinical use. Indications are (1) paroxysmal supraventricular tachycardia (PSVT) including paroxysmal atrial flutter or fibrillation and Wolff-Parkinson-White (WPW) arrhythmias, and always only in patients without structural heart disease; (2) life-threatening sustained VT in which benefit outweighs proarrhythmic risks; (3) catecholaminergic polymorphic VT, by blocking open RyR2 channels;[16] and (4) LQTS 3 with the SCN5A:DeltaKPQ mutation.[19] Flecainide is especially useful for maintenance of sinus rhythm after cardioversion of AF[20] (Fig. 9.7) and for control of premature ventricular beats in patients with structurally normal hearts. Finally, IV flecainide is used in some jurisdictions (mainly Europe) for drug testing to evoke the typical Brugada ECG changes in patients with normal or equivocal resting ECGs; it can also be used to induce HV prolongation, which could be an indicator of latent AV block. Flecainide is *contraindicated* in patients with coronary ischemia, structural heart disease, and in patients with right bundle branch block and left anterior hemiblock unless a pacemaker is implanted. It is also contraindicated in the sick sinus syndrome and when the left ventricle is depressed and in the postinfarct state. Specifically, for AF, flecainide IV is superior to IV amiodarone for acute conversion at 8 hours (but not at 24 hours).[21] Oral flecainide is superior to

RECURRENT/PERSISTENT A FIB

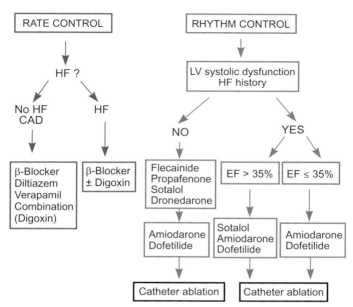

Fig. 9.7 Algorithm for drug therapy for rate control or rhythm control.
The presented algorithm is modified from recommendations of Canadian
Cardiovascular Society. *A fib*, Atrial fibrillation; *CAD*, coronary artery dis-
ease; *EF*, ejection fraction; *HF*, heart failure; *LV*, left ventricular.

placebo but similar to sotalol and propafenone for maintenance of
sinus rhythm with 65% of patients responding in the short term and
49% in the long term.[22] It is better tolerated than both quinidine and
propafenone. The PITAGORA trial demonstrated that flecainide
was noninferior to oral amiodarone for maintenance of sinus
rhythm in AF patients over 21 months.[23] Amiodarone was better
for prevention of longer AF episodes. Propafenone was slightly inferior to both amiodarone and flecainide. Flecainide has also been
used orally as pill-in-pocket therapy for acute onset AF.[24] This is particularly useful in patients with rare episodes of paroxysmal AF. The
strategy is successful in 84%–94% of episodes and the mean conversion time is 2 hours, although up to 8 hours may be required. Occasionally, atrial flutter with rapid ventricular rate can occur, and
therefore it is recommended that the first trial of such therapy be

performed in a medically supervised environment (such as an emergency room). There is a boxed warning in the package insert against use of flecainide in chronic sustained AF.

Dose. For atrial arrhythmias, flecainide is usually started at 50 mg orally BID and increased in 50-mg increments until therapeutic effect or when limited by side effects. The maximum daily dose is 300–400 mg. For ventricular arrhythmias, the dose may be started at 100 mg BID. For the pill in pocket approach, a single dose of 200–300 mg may be given, usually in conjunction with a fast-acting, low-dose β-blocker (like metoprolol 12.5–25 mg). ECG should be monitored once flecainide is initiated for any QRS prolongation—if the QRS is prolonged >25%, then the dose should be reduced/discontinued. Performance of exercise stress testing prior to drug initiation to rule out coronary disease is reasonable. Stress testing on drug to look for use-dependent QRS prolongation may also be useful but does not preclude proarrhythmic risk. Flecainide should almost always be coadministered with a concomitant AV nodal blocker (β-blocker, nondihydropyridine calcium channel blocker) to avoid increased ventricular conduction as atrial arrhythmias slow (Fig. 9.2). For creatinine clearance <35 mL/min, the dose should be reduced to once daily. IV flecainide is not approved in many jurisdictions but can be dosed as 2 mg/kg (maximum 150 mg) administered over 10 minutes.

Side effects. The major side effect of flecainide is ventricular proarrhythmia and sudden death. The cardiac proarrhythmic effects of flecainide include aggravation of ventricular arrhythmias and threat of sudden death as in the CAST study (Fig. 9.3).[1] The proarrhythmic effect is related to nonuniform slowing of conduction, and the risk is greatest in patients with prior MI, especially those with significant ventricular ectopy. Patients at risk of AMI are probably also at increased risk. Monitoring the QRS interval is logical but "safe limits" are not established. Furthermore, as shown in the CAST study, late proarrhythmic effects can occur. In patients with preexisting sinus node or atrioventricular (AV) conduction problems, there may be worsening of arrhythmia. Flecainide increases the endocardial pacing threshold and should therefore be used with some caution in pacemaker-dependent patients—particularly if the thresholds are elevated at baseline. Pacing thresholds should be checked at baseline and after 1 week. Atrial proarrhythmia occurs when the drug decreases the atrial rate, which can allow for increased AV nodal conduction and a paradoxical increase in the ventricular rate (Fig. 9.2). This can precipitate VT or VF and could be fatal. This is why class IC agents are always coadministered with an AV blocking drug such as a β-blocker or nondihydropyridine calcium channel blocker (like diltiazem). Digoxin is generally not used, since it is less effective for AV blockade in high catecholamine states. Central nervous system reactions (visual disturbance, dizziness, paresthesias, headache) occur in 1%–3% of patients. Rash can occur in 1% and nausea in 6% of patients.

Drug interactions and combination. Neurological toxicity is increased when other CYP2D6 inhibitors are used (like older SSRIs paroxetine and sertraline). QT-prolonging drugs should also be avoided (Fig. 9.5). Kinase inhibitors, which can increase the risk of AF, can be used in combination with flecainide but with careful monitoring. See Table 9.4.

Propafenone

Pharmacokinetics. In keeping with its class IC effects, propafenone blocks the fast-inward sodium channel, has a potent membrane stabilizing activity, and increases PR and QRS intervals without effect on the QT interval (Table 9.3). It also has mild β-blocking and calcium (L-type channel) antagonist properties, especially at higher doses. It is estimated that the β-blockade effect is approximately 1/40th that of propranolol,[25] so the effect is quite weak and does not preclude the possibility of causing increased ventricular rates as the atrial rates are slowed for atrial flutter or AF. Because of its short half-life, the drug requires two to three times daily dosing. Propafenone is primarily metabolized by the liver. Note that in 7% of white patients, the hepatic cytochrome isoenzyme CYP2D6 is genetically absent, so that propafenone breakdown is much slower. Propafenone is also metabolized partially via the p-glycoprotein mechanism. For further pharmacokinetics, drug interactions, and combinations, see Tables 9.2 to 9.4.

Clinical use. Indications are very similar to flecainide: (1) PSVT including paroxysmal atrial flutter or fibrillation and WPW arrhythmias, and always only in patients without structural heart disease; and (2) life-threatening sustained VT in which benefit outweighs proarrhythmic risks. Like flecainide, propafenone is primarily used for maintenance of sinus rhythm after cardioversion of AF and less commonly for control of premature ventricular beats in patients with structurally normal hearts. Propafenone is contraindicated in patients with coronary ischemia, structural heart disease, and in patients with right bundle branch block and left anterior hemiblock unless a pacemaker is implanted. It is also contraindicated in the sick sinus syndrome and when the left ventricle is depressed and in the postinfarct state. Oral propafenone may be the same as (or slightly inferior to) flecainide in terms of efficacy for maintenance of sinus rhythm in AF patients, but may be less well tolerated.[22,23] Propafenone has also been used orally as pill-in-pocket therapy for acute-onset AF.[25] This is particularly useful in patients with rare episodes, of paroxysmal AF. The strategy is successful in 94% of episodes and the mean conversion time is 113 minutes, although up to 8 hours may be required.[26] Occasionally, atrial flutter with rapid ventricular rate can occur, and therefore it is recommended that the first trial of such therapy be performed in a medically supervised environment (such as an emergency room).

Dose. For atrial and ventricular arrhythmias, propafenone is usually started at 150 mg orally BID and increased to 300 mg TID until therapeutic effect or when limited by side effects. The maximum daily dose is 900 mg. Where available, the sustained-release formula can be dosed 225–425 mg BID. For the pill-in-pocket approach, a single dose of 450–600 mg may be given, usually in conjunction with a fast-acting, low-dose β-blocker (like metoprolol 12.5–25 mg). Renal adjustment is not required, but hepatic dysfunction may require decreasing to once or twice daily. ECG should be monitored once propafenone is initiated for any QRS prolongation—if the QRS is prolonged >25%, then the dose should be reduced/discontinued. Performance of exercise stress testing prior to drug initiation to rule out coronary disease is reasonable. Stress testing on drug to look for use-dependent QRS prolongation may also be useful but does not preclude proarrhythmic risk. Propafenone should almost always be coadministered with a concomitant AV nodal blocker (β-blocker, nondihydropyridine calcium channel blocker) to avoid increased ventricular conduction as atrial arrhythmias slow (Fig. 9.2). For creatinine clearance <35 mL/min, the dose should be reduced to once daily.

Side effects. The major side effect of propafenone is ventricular proarrhythmia and sudden death. The cardiac proarrhythmic effects of flecainide include aggravation of ventricular arrhythmias and threat of sudden death as in the CAST study.[1] In patients with preexisting sinus node or AV conduction problems, there may be worsening of arrhythmia. Atrial proarrhythmia occurs when the drug decreases the atrial rate, which can allow for increased AV nodal conduction and a paradoxical increase in the ventricular rate (Fig. 9.2). This can precipitate VT or VF and could be fatal. This is why class IC agents are always coadministered with an AV-blocking drug such as a β-blocker or nondihydropyridine calcium channel blocker (like diltiazem). Digoxin is generally not used, since it is less effective for AV blockade in high catecholamine states. Propafenone often causes a change in taste (bitter or metallic). Central nervous system reactions (fatigue, headache, insomnia, and abnormal dreams) occur in 1%–3% of patients. Rarely, drug-induced lupus erythematosus and agranulocytosis have also occurred (see Procainamide for details). Hepatotoxicity has also been reported. Like flecainide, propafenone can also alter pacing thresholds, although usually not as profoundly.

Drug interactions and combination. CYP2D6 inhibitors can profoundly increase propafenone levels. Propafenone can also increase colchicine levels. Because of its mild β-blockade effects, propafenone can potentiate the bradycardia caused by concomitant β-blockers. Propafenone is also metabolized partially via the p-glycoprotein mechanism so it can increase serum levels of edoxaban and dabigatran. These oral anticoagulants should be avoided. QT-prolonging drugs should also be avoided (Fig. 9.5). See Table 9.4.

Class ID: Ranolazine

While there is officially no "class ID" in the Vauhgan Williams classification, ranolazine does not fit into one of the other three class I categories. It inhibits the late inward sodium current (I_{Na}) but also inhibits I_{Kr}, which can cause some QT prolongation. By inhibiting the late sodium current, it inhibits intracellular calcium levels and leads to reduced wall tension and decreased oxygen requirements. It may also stimulate myogenesis. Therefore, this drug has predominantly been used as an antianginal medication. However, ranolazine does have some antiarrhythmic effects.[27] It may promote conversion of AF to sinus, especially during acute coronary syndromes, and may also inhibit ventricular arrhythmias in patients with or without implantable defibrillators. It can be used in patients with heart failure. It is metabolized by CYP3A and inhibits CYP2D6. It should be avoided in patients with severe liver disease.

Class II Agents: β-Adrenoceptor Antagonists

Whereas class I agents are increasingly suspect from the long-term point of view, β-blockers have an excellent track record. The general arguments for β-blockade include (1) the role of tachycardia in precipitating some arrhythmias, especially those based on triggered activity; (2) the increased sympathetic activity in patients with sustained VT and in patients with AMI; (3) the fundamental role of the second messenger of β-adrenergic activity, cyclic AMP, in the causation of ischemia-related VF; and (4) the associated antihypertensive and antiischemic effects of these drugs. As a result, these drugs have demonstrated clear mortality benefits in patients post-MI[28] and in patients with heart failure with left ventricular dysfunction.[29]

Pharmacokinetics. These agents act on the β receptors. β-1 are found primarily in heart muscle, so inhibition causes decreased heart rate, contractility, and AV node conduction. β-2 are mostly in bronchial and peripheral vascular tissue, so inhibition of these can cause bronchospasm and vasoconstriction. β-3 are found in adipose tissue and the heart and can reduce thermogenesis. Typically, the more β-1 selective agents are better antiarrhythmics with fewer side effects. β-blockers may also inhibit both the α-1 and α-2 receptors, which can inhibit smooth muscle contraction in the GI tract and bladder and cause vasodilation (α-1) but also inhibit platelet activation and cause impotence (α-2). β-blockers also inhibit the current I_f, now recognized as an important pacemaker current (Fig. 9.8) that also promotes proarrhythmic depolarization in damaged heart tissue. β-blockers can also inhibit the inward calcium current, I_{Ca-L}, which is indirectly inhibited as the level of tissue cyclic adenosine monophosphate (cAMP) falls. Metoprolol and propranolol are predominantly eliminated by the liver, while atenolol and sotalol are mostly eliminated by the kidneys. Bisoprolol is metabolized by a mixture of both kidney and liver and carvedilol is metabolized by liver and excreted in the bile. Cardio-selectivity refers to agents that more selectively inhibit β-1 receptors in the heart. Bisoprolol is the most cardioselective followed by metoprolol and atenolol and nadolol. Propranolol is not as selective. Labetolol and carvediolol have both α and β blockade properties and therefore may cause some associated vasodilation in addition to the typical β-1 effects. Acebutolol and pindolol have intrinsic sympathomimetic activity (ISA) that can produce some mild β-1 agonism at rest while antagonizing more with activity. Such activity may reduce profound bradycardia at rest, although at higher doses

β & I_f EFFECTS ON SA NODE

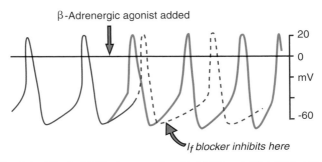

Fig. 9.8 Effect of β-blockers on sinoatrial (SA) nodal function. Action potential of SA node, with effect of β-adrenergic stimulation and of inhibition of current I_f. (Figure © L.H. Opie, 2012.)

the ISA effect may be lost. Details on cardioselectivity and ISA are provided. *Esmolol* is a selective β_1 antagonist but has a very short half-life (9 minutes) with full recovery from its β-blockade properties at 18 to 30 minutes.[30] Esmolol is quickly metabolized in red blood cells, independently of renal and hepatic function. Because of its short half-life, esmolol can be useful in situations in which there are relative contraindications or concerns about the use of a β-blocker: e.g., patient with arrhythmia and associated chronic obstructive airway disease or decompensated LV dysfunction.

Indications. Indications for β-blockade for coronary disease and heart failure are covered elsewhere. For antiarrhythmic therapy, β-blockade is indicated for the following: (1) inappropriate sinus tachycardia; (2) for paroxysmal atrial tachycardia provoked by emotion or exercise; (3) treatment of reentrant atrial arrhythmias, such as AV nodal reentrant or AV reentrant tachycardia (Fig. 9.9); (4) prevention of postoperative atrial fibrillation; (5) rate control for atrial fibrillation/flutter; (6) for exercise-induced ventricular arrhythmias, particularly catecholaminergic VT; (7) ventricular arrhythmias in the structurally normal heart, particularly from the right ventricular outflow tract; and (8) in the hereditary prolonged QT syndrome to prevent torsades de pointes. β-blockers are often used as first-line agents for AF (not postoperative), but they generally have a very mild antiarrhythmic effect in this setting and are generally more useful for rate control when the patient has an AF recurrence. These agents should be avoided in preexcited AF because by blocking the AV node selectively, they can create faster ventricular conduction as the arrhythmia preferentially conducts down the accessory pathway (Fig. 9.4). This may even precipitate ventricular fibrillation.

β-blockers are also effective as monotherapy in severe recurrent VT not obviously ischemic in origin in patients with cardiomyopathy with or without implantable defibrillators. β-blocker therapy improved survival in patients with VF or symptomatic VT not treated by specific antirrhythmics in the AVID trial.[30,31] They can also reduce implantable defibrillator shocks in patients with recurrent ventricular tachyarrhythmias. β-blockers in combination with amiodarone have a synergistic effect to significantly reduce cardiac mortality.[32] β-blockers with amiodarone may be effective in treating episodes of "electrical storm."[30]

Dose. Dosing for β-blockers can be found in Table 9.5. Metoprolol can be given 6.25–100 mg BID. Bisoprolol is given 1.25–10 mg once daily. Nadolol is given 10–240 mg once daily. Propranolol is given 10–40 mg TID or QID. Carvedilol is given 3.125–50 mg BID but is often not used for antiarrhythmic effects. Patients with heart failure on carvedilol who develop ventricular arrhythmias are frequently changed to bisoprolol or another cardioselective

AV NODAL RE-ENTRY VERSUS WPW

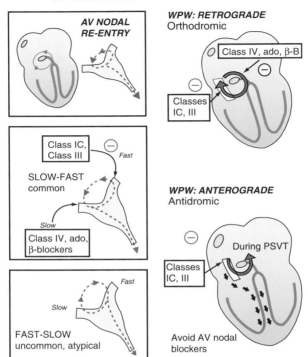

Fig. 9.9 Atrioventricular *(AV)* nodal reentry and Wolff-Parkinson-White *(WPW)* or preexcitation syndrome. The *top left panel* shows AV nodal reentry without WPW. The common pattern is slow-fast *(middle panel)*, whereas fast-slow conduction *(bottom left panel)* is uncommon. The slow and fast fibers of the AV node are artificially separated for diagrammatic purposes. The *right panel* shows WPW with the bypass tract as a white band. During paroxysmal supraventricular tachycardia *(PSVT)*, when anterograde conduction occurs over the AV node and retrograde conduction most commonly through the accessory pathway, the QRS pattern should be normal (orthodromic supraventricular tachycardia [SVT], *top right panel*). Less commonly, the accessory pathway is used as the anterograde limb and the AV node (or a second accessory pathway) is the retrograde limb (antidromic SVT, *bottom right panel*). The QRS pattern shows the pattern of full preexcitation. In such preexcited atrial tachycardias, agents that block the AV node may enhance conduction over the accessory pathway to the ventricles *(red downward arrows)*, leading to rapid ventricular rates that predispose to ventricular fibrillation. Sites of action of various classes of antiarrhythmics are indicated. *Ado,* Adenosine; *β-B,* β-blocker. (Figure © L.H. Opie, 2012.)

Table 9.5

Drug loading and maintenance regimens for control of ventricular rate in atrial fibrillation		Acute intravenous therapy	Chronic oral therapy
β-blockers[a]	Metoprolol	2.5–5 mg every 5 min up to 15 mg	12.5–100 mg BID
	Propranolol	0.15 mg/kg (1 mg every 2 min)	10–60 mg QID
	Esmolol	0.5 mg bolus, then 0.05–0.2 mg/kg per min	NA
	Bisoprolol	NA	2.5–10 mg/day
	Atenolol	5 mg over 5 min, repeat in 10 min	25–100 mg/day
	Nadolol	NA	20–80 mg/day
Calcium-channel blockers	Verapamil	0.075–0.15 mg/kg over 2 min; 0.005 mg/kg per min	120–480 mg/day
	Diltiazem	0.25–0.35 mg/kg followed by 5–15 mg/hour	120–480 mg/day

BID, Twice daily; *NA*, not available; *QID*, four times daily.

[a]Other β-blockers in addition to those listed may also be useful.

β-blocker for improved antiarrhythmic effect. IV metoprolol can be given in 2.5–5 mg IV boluses every 5 minutes until desired effect is reached. IV propranolol can be given as a 1–3 mg bolus until 5 mg is reached and then repeated until the desired effect is reached. IV esmolol is very short acting, and dosing is provided in Table 9.5.

Side effects. Given the substantial benefit provided by β-blockers for coronary disease and heart failure, relative contraindications should not prevent administration of this therapy. However, main cardiovascular side effects include hypotension, bradycardia (sinus), AV block, and cold extremities. Neurologic side effects are common (2%–10%) with dizziness, fatigue, insomnia, nightmares, and temporary insomnia. Impotence and decreased libido occur in up to 5% of men. Bronchospasm occurs in about 1% of patients. Blurred vision and pruritis can also occur rarely. β-blockers can inhibit sensation of hypoglycemia in diabetics. They should also never be used in patients with pheochromocytoma unless concomitant α-blockade is also on board.

Mixed Class III Agents: Amiodarone and Sotalol

As the evidence for increased mortality in several patient groups with class I agents mounted, attention shifted to class III agents. Two widely used agents with important class III properties are amiodarone and sotalol. Both amiodarone and sotalol are mixed, not pure, class III agents, a quality that may be of crucial importance. The *intrinsic problem* with class III agents is that these compounds act by lengthening the APD and must inevitably prolong the QT interval to be effective (Table 9.3). In the presence of hypokalemia, hypomagnesemia, bradycardia, or genetic predisposition, QT prolongation may predispose to torsades de pointes (Fig. 9.3). This may especially occur with agents such as sotalol that simultaneously cause bradycardia and prolong the APD. However, amiodarone and sotalol have additional properties that modify conduction—amiodarone being a significant sodium and calcium channel inhibitor and sotalol a β-blocker. Amiodarone, for example, makes the action potential pattern more uniform throughout the myocardium, thereby opposing EP heterogeneity that underlies some serious ventricular arrhythmias. The incidence of torsades with amiodarone is much lower than expected from its class III effects. Because of their mixed effects, both sotalol and amiodarone have better efficacy than the class I agents. In the ESVEM trial,[33] sotalol was better than six class I antiarrhythmic agents (Table 9.2). Amiodarone, in contrast to class I agents, exerts a favorable effect on a variety of serious arrhythmias both atrial and ventricular.[34-40] Yet both agents have significant limitations which prevent their broad application.

Amiodarone

Pharmacokinetics. Amiodarone is a unique "wide-spectrum" antiarrhythmic agent, chiefly class III but also with powerful class I activity and ancillary class II and class IV activity. It blocks sodium, calcium, and repolarizing potassium channels. The class III activity means that amiodarone lengthens the effective refractory period by prolonging the APD in all cardiac tissues, including bypass tracts. It also has a powerful class I antiarrhythmic effect inhibiting inactivated sodium channels at high stimulation frequencies (Table 9.2 and 9.3). Its benefits in AF may be explained at least in part by prolongation of the refractory periods of both the left and right superior pulmonary veins,[41] and inhibition of the AV node (see Fig. 9.10). Furthermore, it is "uniquely effective" against AF in experimental atrial remodeling.[42] Amiodarone noncompetitively blocks α- and β-adrenergic receptors (class II effect), and this effect

AMIODARONE FOR ATRIAL FIBRILLATION

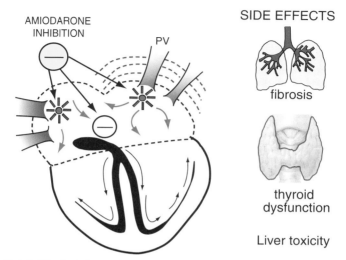

Fig. 9.10 Amiodarone inhibition of atrial fibrillation. Benefits must be balanced against risks of pulmonary fibrosis, thyroid dysfunction, and other side effects. *PV,* pulmonary vein. (Figure © L.H. Opie, 2012.)

is additive to competitive receptor inhibition by β-blockers.[43] The weak calcium antagonist (class IV) effect might explain bradycardia and AV nodal inhibition and the relatively low incidence of torsades de pointes. Furthermore, there are relatively weak coronary and peripheral vasodilator actions. There are some differences between IV and oral amiodarone because of the extensive first-pass effect of liver metabolism, particularly for the oral drug. IV amiodarone has more class I and nonselective class II effects, while PO amiodarone has more of the class III effect when it is converted to desethylamiodarone.

The pharmacokinetics of this highly lipid-soluble drug differ markedly from other cardiovascular agents.[43] After variable (30%–50%) and slow GI absorption, amiodarone distributes slowly but very extensive into adipose tissues.[43] Because of this, amiodarone must fill an enormous peripheral-tissue depot to achieve adequate blood and cardiac concentrations, accounting for its slow onset of action. In addition, when oral administration is stopped, most of the drug is in peripheral stores unavailable to elimination systems, causing very slow elimination with a very long half-life, up to 6 months.[44] The onset of action after oral administration is delayed and a steady-state drug effect (*amiodaronization*) may not be established for several months unless large loading doses are used. Even when given intravenously, its full EP effect is delayed,[45] although major benefit can be achieved within minutes as shown by its effect on shock-resistant VF.[46] Amiodarone is lipid soluble, extensively distributed in the body, and highly concentrated in many tissues, especially in the liver and lungs. It undergoes extensive hepatic metabolism to the pharmacologically active metabolite desethylamiodarone. A correlation between the clinical effects and serum concentrations of the drug or its metabolite has not been clearly shown, although there is a direct relation between the oral dose and the plasma concentration, and between metabolite concentration and some late effects, such as that on the ventricular functional refractory period. The therapeutic range is not well defined but may be between 1 and 2.5 mg/mL, almost all of which (95%) is protein-bound. Higher levels are associated with increased toxicity.[43] Amiodarone is not excreted by the kidneys, but rather by the lachrymal glands, the skin, and the biliary tract. For recurrent AF, amiodarone may be strikingly effective with little risk of side effects.[47,48] Amiodarone can increase serum creatinine levels by 5%–15% but this is not due to any negative impact on glomerular filtration rate or renal function, but rather decreased tubular excretion of creatinine. This resolves once the drug is discontinued.

Clinical use. Amiodarone is particularly well suited for both atrial and ventricular arrhythmias. Amiodarone is useful for a variety of ventricular arrhythmias including frequent, symptomatic premature ventricular beats; symptomatic nonsustained VT; sustained VT/VF and/or electrical storm; prevention of ICD shocks due to ventricular or atrial arrhythmias;[49] and primary and secondary prevention of sudden death when an ICD cannot be implanted. In the prophylactic control of life-threatening ventricular tachyarrhythmias (especially post-MI and in association with congestive cardiac failure), or after cardiac surgery,[50] amiodarone has been regarded as one of the most effective agents available.[51]

Amiodarone is probably the most effective of the available drugs to prevent recurrences of paroxysmal AF or flutter,[47,48,52,53] and is an entirely reasonable choice for patients especially with structural cardiac disease or CHF where class I agents cannot be used.[54] Even very low doses (100 mg daily)[53] of amiodarone can be effective with relatively fewer toxicities, especially in older, smaller patients. In the CTAF trial, amiodarone was twice as effective in maintaining sinus rhythm when compared to sotalol or propafenone.[48] Over 16 months, 65% of patients with amiodarone maintained sinus rhythm, although more patients on amiodarone were forced to withdraw from treatment because of side effects compared to the other two drugs (18% over 16 months).

Generally, IV amiodarone is used for 48 to 96 hours while oral amiodarone is instituted. In the ARREST study, amiodarone was better than placebo (44% versus 34%, $P = 0.03$) in reducing immediate mortality.[54] Similar data were obtained when amiodarone was compared with lidocaine for shock-resistant VF.[46] For the acute conversion of chronic AF, IV amiodarone is not acutely very effective[55] and often is delayed beyond 6 hours, thereby limiting its usefulness. However, by 24 hours, the efficacy of IV amiodarone for acute AF conversion is similar to that of IV class IC agents or IV procainamide.

Unlike all of the class I agents and even sotalol, amiodarone can be used in a variety of structural heart disease, including coronary disease, ischemic and nonischemic cardiomyopathy, and heart failure. While amiodarone does not improve mortality in these patients, it also does not seem to increase the risk of mortality and decreases the risk of sudden death as demonstrated by the CAMIAT and EMIAT trials.[34,35]

Dose. See Tables 9.2, 9.6. When reasonably rapid control of an urgent ventricular arrhythmia is needed, the initial loading regimen is up to 1600 mg daily in two to four divided doses usually given for 7–14 days, which is then reduced to 400–800 mg/day for a further 1–3 weeks. By using a loading dose (about 6–10 g), sustained VT can be controlled after a mean interval of 5 days. Practice varies widely, however, with loading doses of as low as 600 mg daily being used in less urgent settings. Maintenance doses for VT vary. Previously, many patients with ventricular arrhythmias were maintained on 400 mg daily or more, but the risk of side effects is substantial over time. Therefore, even for ventricular arrhythmias, maintenance doses should not typically exceed 200 mg daily unless absolutely required. Maintenance doses of 50–100 mg daily may be quite useful and prevent many unwanted side effects, particularly in smaller, elderly patients. Downward dose adjustment of the maintenance dose should always be attempted if the patient's ventricular arrhythmia is under good control.

For prevention of recurrent AF, one loading regimen used was 600 mg daily for 7–14 days, 400 mg daily for the next 14–21 days, and then 100–200 mg daily thereafter.[55] The target loading dose for atrial arrhythmias may be on the lower end of the 6–10 g target typically used for ventricular arrhythmias and even loads of 4 g may be sufficient. Downward dose adjustment of the maintenance dose should always be tried long term if the atrial arrhythmia is under good control. Maintenance doses for atrial flutter or fibrillation

Table 9.6

Recommended antiarrhythmic drug doses for pharmacologic cardioversion and prevention of recurrences of atrial fibrillation

		IV or oral therapy for rapid conversion	Chronic oral drug therapy to prevent recurrence[a]
Class IA	Procainamide	500–1200 mg IV over 30–60 min	500–750 mg QID
Class IC	Flecainide	1.5–3.0 mg/kg IV over 10 min[b]; 200–400 mg orally	50–200 mg BID
	Propafenone	1.5–2 mg/kg IV over 10–20 min[b] 300–600 mg orally	150–300 mg TID
Class III	Ibutilide	1 mg IV over 10 min, repeat once	Not available
	Sotalol		40–160 mg BID
	Amiodarone	5–7 mg/kg IV over 30 min, then 1.2–1.8 g/day	400–1200 mg/day for 7 days, then taper to 50–300 mg/day
	Dofetilide	Insufficient data	125–500 µg BID

BID, Twice daily; *IV*, intravenous; *QID*, four times daily; *TID*, three times daily.

[a] Initiation of oral therapy without loading may also result in conversion.
[b] Not available in North America.

are generally lower than for ventricular arrhythmias (100–200 mg daily), and even very low doses of 50–100 mg daily may be effective and used in smaller, elderly patients.[53,56-58] Amiodarone is also an excellent rate control agent for chronic, persistent AF, and contrary to flecainide and dronedarone, there are no contraindications for use of amiodarone for long-term rate control except for the risk of side effects. There is generally no dose adjustment for renal or hepatic dysfunction.

IV amiodarone may be used for intractable arrhythmias (Tables 9.2, 9.6). The aim is an infusion over 24 hours. Start with 150 mg/10 minutes, then 360 mg over the 6 next hours, then 540 mg over the remaining time up to a total of 24 hours, to give a total of 1050 mg over 24 hours Boluses may be repeated while the infusion is running if intractable arrhythmia continues. Boluses of amiodarone can cause hypotension, so the 150 mg may be given over a longer period of time (20–30 minutes) to avoid this problem. The maintenance infusion could be maintained at a rate of 0.5 mg/minute instead of reducing it after the initial 6 hours if the arrhythmias continue. For shock-resistant cardiac arrest, the IV dose is 5 mg/kg of estimated body weight, with a further dose of 2.5 mg/kg if the VF persists after a further shock.[54] Once the arrhythmias have come under acute control and a sufficient load has been obtained (6–10 g), transition to oral therapy may be performed. This is typically done by overlapping IV and PO amiodarone for at least 2 days. For intractable ventricular arrhythmias, PO and IV amiodarone may be coadministered for a longer time, since they have different EP effects: IV amiodarone has more class I and nonselective class II effects, while PO amiodarone has more of the class III effect.

Side effects. *Contraindications* to amiodarone are severe sinus node dysfunction with marked sinus bradycardia or syncope, second- or third-degree heart block, known hypersensitivity, cardiogenic shock, and probably severe chronic lung disease. The most common side effects are sinus bradycardia, especially in older adults, and QT prolongation with, however, a very low incidence of torsades (<0.5%).[43] Serious adverse effects, listed in a thorough review of 92 studies, include optic neuropathy/neuritis (≤1%–2%), blue-gray skin discoloration (4%–9%), photosensitivity (25%–75%), hypothyroidism (6%), hyperthyroidism (0.9%–2%), pulmonary toxicity (1%–17%), peripheral neuropathy (0.3% annually), and hepatotoxicity (elevated enzyme levels, 15%–30%; hepatitis and cirrhosis, <3%, 0.6% annually).[42] Recommended preventative actions are baseline and 6-monthly thyroid function tests and liver enzymes and baseline and yearly ECG and chest radiograph with physical examination of skin, eyes, and peripheral nerves if symptoms develop. Corneal microdeposits (>90%) are usually asymptomatic.

Thyroid side effects. Amiodarone has a complex effect on the metabolism of thyroid hormones because it contains iodine and shares a structural similarity to thyroxin. It can inhibit the peripheral conversion of T4 to T3 with a rise in the serum level of T4 and a small fall in the level of T3. It also has a direct toxic effect on thyroid follicular cells which can result in a destructive thyroiditis. In most patients, thyroid function is not altered by amiodarone. However, in 6%, hypothyroidism may develop during the first year of treatment. Hypothyroidism can easily be managed with oral levothyroxine and rarely requires discontinuation of therapy.[59] Hyperthyroidism is less common, developing only in 0.9%,[45] but has a very poor prognosis.[60] It is much more common in iodine-deficient areas (20% versus 3% in normal iodine areas).[60] Hyperthyroidism may precipitate recurrent ventricular and atrial arrhythmias and should always be excluded if new arrhythmias appear during amiodarone therapy. Amiodarone-induced hyperthyroidism has two types: type I occurs in patients who already have an underlying thyroid problem (Grave's, multinodular goiter), while type II occurs due to a direct destructive thyroiditis. Ultrasound of the thyroid may help distinguish between the two types. Since amiodarone has a long half-life, inhibits peripheral conversion of T4 to T3, and may be used for life-threatening arrhythmias, it does not have to be stopped immediately upon diagnosis of hyperthyroidism. Stopping may actually cause a temporary exacerbation. Treatment may include corticosteroids and methimazole to get acute control followed by radioiodine ablation (if possible) or surgical thyroidectomy. Definitive removal or ablation of the thyroid could allow for safe reintroduction of amiodarone.

Pulmonary side effects. In higher doses, there is an unusual spectrum of toxicity, the most serious being interstitial pneumonitis, potentially leading to pulmonary fibrosis and occurring in 10% to 17% at doses of approximately 400 mg/day. Pulmonary toxicity can be fatal in 10% of those affected. Meta-analysis of double-blind amiodarone trials suggests that there is an absolute risk of 1% of pulmonary toxicity per year, with some fatal cases. Of note, pulmonary toxicity is likely dose-related, and very rarely occurs with low doses of 200 mg daily or less.[42,58,61] Preexisting pulmonary disease does not increase the risk of toxicity, but these patients have reduced reserve in case toxicity occurs. Nonproductive cough and dyspnea are the symptoms. White blood cell counts, lactic acid dehydrogenase, and C-reactive protein may all be elevated. Chest x-ray often shows new diffuse or localized opacities. Pulmonary function tests may be an early sign of toxicity when the diffusing capacity for carbon monoxide (DLCO) is reduced by 20% or more. Pulmonary complications usually regress if recognized early and if amiodarone is discontinued. Symptomatic therapy may include steroids with a slow taper. Generally, amiodarone can never be used again.

Other extracardiac side effects. Central nervous system side effects like proximal muscle weakness, peripheral neuropathy, and other neural symptoms (headache, ataxia, tremors, impaired memory, dyssomnia, bad dreams) occur with variable incidence. Optic neuropathy is rare but can cause blindness. GI side effects were uncommon in the GESICA study.[62] Yet nausea can occur in 25% of patients with CHF, even at a dose of only 200 mg daily; exclude increased plasma levels of liver function enzymes. These effects usually resolve with dose reduction. Hepatotoxicity with a 25% increase in liver enzymes occurs in 10%–25% of patients. Drug should only be discontinued if the enzymes are elevated more than twofold. Since amiodarone is often used in situations of cardiogenic shock, elevation in liver enzymes may be due to the shock and not due to amiodarone. Liver toxicity appears to be dose related (>150–200 mg daily). Testicular dysfunction may be a side effect, detected by increased gonadotropin levels in patients on

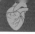

long-term amiodarone. Less serious side effects are as follows: Corneal microdeposits develop in nearly all adult patients given prolonged amiodarone. Symptoms and impairment of visual acuity are rare and respond to reduced dosage. Macular degeneration rarely occurs during therapy, without proof of a causal relationship. A photosensitive slate-gray or bluish skin discoloration may develop after prolonged therapy, usually exceeding 18 months. Avoid exposure to sun and use a sunscreen ointment with ultraviolet A (UVA) and UVB protection. The pigmentation regresses slowly on drug withdrawal. Finally, amiodarone may increase both pacing and defibrillation thresholds, and these should be considered and, if necessary, tested when amiodarone is initiated, particularly at higher doses.

Dose-dependency of side effects. A full and comprehensive meta-analysis of the side effects of amiodarone showed that even low doses may not be free of adverse effects.[61] However, thyroid, pulmonary, and hepatic side effects all seem to be dose related with a far smaller incidence occurring at doses ≤200 mg daily. Duration of therapy is also critical with longer durations associated with higher side effects. Most side effects take months to a year to present. When amiodarone must be withdrawn for toxicity, the plasma concentration falls by 50% within 3 to 10 days, and then the tissue stores deplete slowly, which can take 6 months or more.

Drug interactions and combination. See Table 9.4. The most serious interaction is an additive proarrhythmic effect with other drugs prolonging the QT interval (Fig. 9.5), such as class IA antiarrhythmic agents, phenothiazines, tricyclic antidepressants, thiazide diuretics, and sotalol. Amiodarone may increase quinidine and procainamide levels (these combinations are not advised). With phenytoin, there is a double drug interaction. Amiodarone increases phenytoin levels while at the same time phenytoin enhances the conversion of amiodarone to desethylamiodarone. A serious and common interaction is with warfarin. Amiodarone prolongs the prothrombin time and may cause bleeding in patients on warfarin, perhaps by a hepatic interaction; decrease warfarin by about one-third and retest the international normalized ratio (INR) within 3–7 days. Amiodarone increases the plasma digoxin concentration, predisposing to digitalis toxic effects (not arrhythmias because amiodarone protects); decrease digoxin by approximately half and re-measure digoxin levels. Amiodarone, by virtue of its weak β-blocking and calcium antagonist effect, tends to inhibit nodal activity and may therefore interact adversely with β-blocking agents and calcium antagonists. However, the antiarrhythmic efficacy of amiodarone is generally increased by coprescription with β-blocking drugs.[63] Amiodarone is metabolized, in part, by the p-glycoprotein mechanism, so drugs dependent on this mechanism may be affected. Colchicine, dabigatran, and edoxaban levels may all be increased, requiring dose reduction or even therapy modification.

In cases of severe ventricular arrhythmia/electrical storm, IV amiodarone can be easily combined with IV lidocaine. However, amiodarone may increase lidocaine blood levels, so the maintenance infusion of lidocaine should be titrated to as low as possible to avoid neurologic toxicity.

Sotalol

Phamacokinetics. Sotalol is a racemic mixture of dextro and levo isomers, and these differ in their EP effects. Although these agents have comparable class III activity, the class II activity arises from l-sotalol (Table 9.3).[64] The pure class III investigational agent d-sotalol increased mortality in postinfarct patients with a low ejection fraction (EF) in the SWORD study.[65] This result suggests that the class III activity, perhaps acting through torsades, can detract from the positive β-blocking qualities of the standard dl-sotalol. In practice, class III activity is not evident at low doses (<160 mg/day) of the racemic drug. In humans, class II effects are sinus and AV node depression. Class III effects are prolongation of the action potential in atrial and ventricular tissue and prolonged atrial and ventricular refractory periods, as well as inhibition of conduction along any bypass tract in both directions. APD prolongation with, possibly, enhanced calcium entry may explain why it causes proarrhythmic after-depolarizations and why the negative inotropic effect is less than expected. It is a noncardioselective, water-soluble (hydrophilic), nonprotein-bound agent, excreted solely by the kidneys, with a plasma half-life of 12 hours. Dosing every 12 hours gives trough concentrations half of the peak values. Because sotalol is completely cleared by the kidneys, it must be used with great caution in patients with impaired renal function and avoided in patients with more severe renal impairment. Sotalol demonstrates "reverse use dependence," which means that the prolongation of refractoriness increases at lower heart rates. Antiarrhythmic agents that exhibit reverse use-dependence are more efficacious at preventing a tachyarrhythmia than converting someone into normal sinus rhythm. However, it also means that at low heart rates, class III antiarrhythmic agents may paradoxically be more arrhythmogenic. Ibutilide and dofetilide also show reverse use dependence.

Clinical use. Because of its combined class II and class III properties, sotalol is active against a wide variety of arrhythmias, including sinus tachycardia, PSVT, WPW arrhythmias with either antegrade or retrograde conduction, recurrence of AF,[48] ischemic ventricular arrhythmias, and recurrent sustained VT or VF. In ventricular arrhythmias, the major outcome study with sotalol was the ESVEM trial[33] in which this drug in a mean dose of approximately 400 mg daily was better at decreasing death and ventricular arrhythmias than any of six class I agents. Unlike the class I agents, sotalol can be given to patients with coronary artery disease and with structural heart disease, although it needs to be used with caution in patients with EF <40% where it may increase the risk of mortality as demonstrated by the SWORD trial.[65] However, sotalol is often used in patients with low EF's and arrhythmias who have ICDs in order to avoid use of amiodarone. The increased risk of torsades or other ventricular arrhythmias is mitigated by the presence of the ICD.

Of the wide indications, the major current use is in maintenance of sinus rhythm after cardioversion for AF,[48] for which sotalol is about as effective as flecainide or propafenone, with the advantages that it can be given to patients with structural heart disease, particularly coronary disease and mild degrees of LV dysfunction >40% and can be given without an additional agent to slow AV-nodal conduction (Fig. 9.7). However, the efficacy of all three is outclassed by amiodarone.[44,47,48] Sotalol is also known to decrease both pacing and defibrillation thresholds and is sometimes used for this purpose in ICD patients with high defibrillation thresholds.

Dose. See Tables 9.2, 9.6. For patients with a history of AF or atrial flutter or ventricular arrhythmias, the dose is often started at 80 mg BID although doses as small as 40 mg BID can be used in smaller, elderly patients with mild degrees of renal impairment. The dose can be increased to 160 mg BID, although the ECG must be checked within 1 week of initiating therapy to check for QT prolongation (>500 milliseconds). If the QTc is not >500 milliseconds, the dose may be titrated upward until a therapeutic effect is reached. The risk of torsades de pointes is 0.3% at 320 mg/day but goes up to 3.2% at higher doses when used for AF or flutter. Doses of 320 to 480 mg per day may be needed to prevent recurrent VT or VF, especially in patients with ICDs where the risk of proarrhythmia may be offset by the protective presence of the ICD. When given in two divided doses, steady-state plasma concentrations are reached in 2 to 3 days. In patients with renal impairment or in older adults, or when there are risk factors for proarrhythmia, the dose should be reduced, and the dosing interval increased. When the creatinine clearance is >60 mL/min, the dose can be given BID, from 40–60 mL/min it can be given once daily, and when <40 mL/min, the drug is contraindicated.

In the United States, the label recommends that the initial treatment in patients with recurrent AF or flutter be performed in hospital with at least 3 days of monitoring while the dose is increased. In other jurisdictions, outpatient initiation of sotalol is the norm.

Side effects. Side effects are those of β-blockade, including fatigue (20%) (which appears to be more of a problem in younger patients), bradycardia (13%), and dyspnea (5%) which can be due to bronchospasm. Sleep disorders, depression, impotence, and cold extremities also can occur as for other β-blockers. The drug should be avoided in patients with serious conduction defects, including sick sinus syndrome, second- or third-degree AV block (unless there is a pacemaker), in severe bronchospastic disease, and when there are evident risks of proarrhythmia. Torsades occurs in 1%–4% of patients (see previous). Groups at highest risk for torsades are the elderly, females, those on diuretics (prone to hypokalemia), patients with severe LV failure, and those with a dose >320 mg/day.[65] The drug is contraindicated in patients with reduced creatinine clearance < 40 mL/minute (renal excretion).

Drug interactions and combination. See Tables 9.2, 9.4. Cotherapy with class IA drugs, amiodarone, or other drugs prolonging the QT interval should be avoided (Fig. 9.5). In pregnancy, the drug is category B. It is not teratogenic but does cross the placenta and may depress fetal vital functions. Sotalol is also excreted in mother's milk.

Dronedarone

Pharmacokinetics. Dronedarone was designed to be amiodarone without the side effects. It is a noniodinated congener of amiodarone and because of the lack of the iodinated molecules, it was expected (and is true) that dronedarone would lack the thyroid toxicity of amiodarone. Like amiodarone, dronedarone is a class III agent that also has class II (β-blocking) and class IV (calcium blocking) effects. The risk of torsades is mitigated by the combined effects. The half-life is also much shorter—only 24 hours compared to 50 days for amiodarone. However, dronedarone is not nearly as potent an antiarrhythmic as amiodarone. In fact, it may be less effective than even sotalol and the class IC agents, and most of its beneficial effect may be through rate control and its class II effect. Dronedarone can increase serum creatinine levels by 5%–15%, but this is not due to any negative impact on glomerular filtration rate or renal function, but rather decreased tubular excretion of creatinine. This resolves once the drug is discontinued.

Clinical use. The main use of this drug is for maintenance of sinus rhythm in patients with paroxysmal AF or those with persistent AF after cardioversion (Fig. 9.7). Dronedarone is not nearly as potent an antiarrhythmic as amiodarone and is likely inferior to sotalol and the class IC agents according to data from the DIONYSOS trial.[66] Although dronedarone is a potent rate control medication, the PALLAS study suggested an increased risk of mortality in patients with chronic AF using dronedarone strictly for rate control.[67] Dronedarone should also be avoided in heart failure patients or those with an EF <35%–40% because of the ANDROMEDA trial showing increased mortality risk in this patient population.[68] There is no role for dronedarone in the treatment of ventricular arrhythmias.

Dose. There is only one approved dose of dronedarone, which is 400 mg BID orally.

Side effects. Unlike amiodarone, dronedarone is not associated with an appreciable risk of thyroid dysfunction. Although the risk of pulmonary toxicity is lower than that of amiodarone, it has still been reported and the quantification of the risk is not well known. Liver toxicity has also been reported and usually occurs within 6 months of drug initiation. The risk appears to be lower than that of amiodarone. Torsades de pointes has not been reported with any frequency. The usual class II side effects such as bradycardia and heart block can occur.

Drug interactions and combination. Dronedarone significantly increases serum digoxin concentrations and should be used very cautiously in patients taking digitalis.[67,68] Digoxin doses may need to be reduced by 50%. Dronedarone is an inhibitor of CYP3A4 and CYP2D6 and should be avoided when combined with other inhibitors of these enzymes (like erythromycin type antibiotics and verapamil). The drug is also cleared by the p-glycoprotein system, and therefore, drugs also cleared by that system will have profound interactions. For example, colchicine, dabigatran, and edoxaban levels may all be significantly increased requiring cessation of these drugs.

Pure Class III Agents: Ibutilide, Dofetilide, and Vernakalant

The effectiveness of class III antiarrhythmic drugs such as amiodarone and sotalol has prompted the development of purer class III agents. Two such drugs, ibutilide and dofetilide, are presently in clinical practice. The efficacy of ibutilide and dofetilide in the acute conversion of atrial flutter is noteworthy because prior to their introduction, other antiarrhythmics have not been found to be efficacious in the acute cardioversion of atrial flutter (AFL) or AF. Ibutilide is primarily used for acute, IV conversion of AF/AFL while dofetilide is for chronic oral therapy (Tables 9.2, 9.6). Both agents are limited by QTc prolongation and the risk of torsades (Table 9.4 and Fig. 9.5). Despite the promising efficacy of dofetilide for AF in a variety of patients with heart failure and depressed EF, its broader implementation has been limited by a requirement for hospitalization for drug initiation.

Ibutilide

Pharmacokinetics. Ibutilide is a methanesulfonamide derivative, which prolongs repolarization primarily by inhibition of the delayed rectifier potassium current (I_{Kr}). Ibutilide has no known negative inotropic effects. It is available only as an IV preparation because it undergoes extensive first-pass metabolism when administered orally. The pharmacokinetics of ibutilide are linear and are independent of dose, age, sex, and LV function. Its extracellular distribution is extensive, and its systemic clearance is high. The elimination half-life is variable, 2 to 12 hours (mean of 6), which reflects considerable individual variation.[69] See Table 9.3.

Clinical use. See Table 9.6. This drug is efficacious in the termination of atrial flutter and, to a lesser extent, AF.[70] It is at least as effective as IV amiodarone for cardioversion of AF.[70,71] In patients who had persistent AF or atrial flutter, ibutilide had a conversion efficacy of 44% for a single dose and 49% for a second dose.[71] The mean termination time was 27 minutes after the start of the infusion. The efficacy of ibutilide in the cardioversion of atrial flutter is related to an effect on the variability of the cycle length of the tachycardia.[72] Like sotalol, ibutilide exhibits the phenomenon of reverse use dependence in that prolongation of refractoriness becomes less pronounced at higher tachycardia rates. After cardiac surgery, ibutilide has a dose-dependent effect in conversion of atrial arrhythmias with 57% conversion at a dose of 10 mg.[73] Ibutilide pretreatment facilitates direct-current (DC) cardioversion of AF but must be followed with 3 to 4 hours of ECG monitoring to exclude torsades.[74]

Dose. The recommended dose is 1 mg by IV infusion over 10 minutes. If the arrhythmia is not terminated within 10 minutes, the dose may be repeated. For patients who weigh less than 60 kg, the dose should be 0.01 mg/kg. Pretreatment with IV magnesium (2 g) prior to ibutilide administration can reduce QT prolongation during administration of the drug and may enhance efficacy. See Tables 9.2, 9.6.

Side effects. See Table 9.4. QT- and QT$_c$-interval prolongation is a consistent feature in patients treated with Ibutilide (Fig. 9.3). QT prolongation is dose-dependent, maximal at the end of the infusion, and returns to baseline within 2 to 4 hours following infusion.[75] Torsades de pointes (polymorphic VT with QT prolongation) occurs in approximately 4.3%[75] and may require cardioversion (in almost 2% of patients). Torsades tends to occur during or shortly after the infusion period (within 1 hour).[75] Patients should be continuously monitored for at least 4 hours after the start of the ibutilide infusion. To avoid proarrhythmia, higher doses of ibutilide and rapid infusion are avoided; the drug is not given to those with preexisting QT prolongation (>440 milliseconds); it should be avoided in patients with advanced or unstable heart disease; and the serum K must be greater than 4 mmol/L.

Drug interactions and combination. Theoretically, other cardiac and noncardiac drugs, which prolong the QT interval, may increase the likelihood of torsades and ibuitilide should be avoided in these patients (Table 9.4 and Fig. 9.5). Interestingly, in one study, prior therapy with sotalol or amiodarone did not appear to provoke torsades.[75]

Dofetilide

Pharmacokinetics. Like ibutilide, dofetilide (Tikosyn) is a methanesulfonamide drug. Dofetilide prolongs the APD and QT_c in a concentration-related manner (Table 9.3). Dofetilide exerts its effect solely by inhibition of the rapid component of the delayed rectifier potassium current I_{Kr}. Like ibutilide and sotalol, dofetilide exhibits the phenomenon of reverse use dependence. Antiarrhythmic agents that exhibit reverse use dependence are more efficacious at preventing a tachyarrhythmia than converting someone into normal sinus rhythm. However, it also means that at low heart rates, class III antiarrhythmic agents may paradoxically be more arrhythmogenic. Dofetilide has mild negative chronotropic effects, is devoid of negative inotropic activity, and may be mildly, positively inotropic. Whereas ibutilide is given only intravenously, dofetilide is given only orally. After oral administration, dofetilide is almost completely (92% to 96%) absorbed and mean maximal plasma concentrations are achieved roughly 2.5 hours after administration. Twice-daily administration of oral dofetilide results in steady state within 48 hours. Fifty percent of the drug is excreted through the kidneys unchanged and there are no active metabolites.

Clinical use. Dofetilide has good efficacy in the cardioversion of AF[76] and is even more effective in the cardioversion of atrial flutter (Table 9.6 and Fig. 9.7). Indications include (1) cardioversion of persistent AF or atrial flutter to normal sinus rhythm in patients in whom cardioversion by electrical means is not appropriate and in whom the duration of the arrhythmic episode is less than 6 months, and (2) maintenance of sinus rhythm (after conversion) in patients with persistent AF or atrial flutter (Fig. 9.7). Because dofetilide can cause ventricular arrhythmias, it should be reserved for patients in whom AF and atrial flutter is highly symptomatic and in whom other antiarrhythmic therapy is not appropriate. In addition, dofetilide may also be active against ventricular arrhythmias although it was not approved for this purpose. Dofetilide decreases the VF threshold in patients undergoing defibrillation testing prior to ICD implantation, and suppresses the inducibility of VT.

Dofetilide is as effective as sotalol against inducible VT, with fewer side effects.[77] In patients with depressed LV function both with and without a history of MI,[78] dofetilide has a neutral effect on mortality. Therefore, like amiodarone, dofetilide may be administered in patients with heart failure, cardiomyopathy with depressed ejection fraction, and coronary disease.

Dose. See Tables 9.2, 9.6. The dose must be individualized by the calculated creatinine clearance and the QT_c. Furthermore, patients must be admitted to hospital for a minimum of 3 days for initiation of the drug for continuous ECG monitoring to detect and manage any serious ventricular arrhythmias. Torsades de pointes most commonly occurs within the first 3 days after initiation. For patients with creatinine clearance of >60 mL/min, the dose is started at 500 µg BID. For 40–60 mL/min, the dose is 250 µg BID. For 20–39 mL/min, the dose is 125 µg BID and <20 mL/min use is contraindicated. If the increase in the QT_c is more than 15%, or if the QT_c is more than 500 milliseconds, the dose of dofetilide should be reduced. ECG to measure QTc should be performed at baseline and 2–3 hours after each dose.

Side effects. The major significant adverse effect is torsades de pointes in 3% of patients.[78] The risk of torsades de pointes can be reduced by normal serum potassium and magnesium levels, and by avoiding the drug (or reducing its dosage according to the manufacturer's algorithm) in patients with abnormal renal function, or with bradycardia, or with baseline QT prolongation (QT_c should be less than 440 milliseconds).[78] Eighty percent of torsades events occur within the first 3 days of therapy. Headache is the other main side effect occurring in about 10% of patients.

Drug interactions and combination. See Table 9.4. Drugs that increase levels of dofetilide should not be coadministered. These include ketoconazole and other inhibitors of cytochrome CYP 3A4, including macrolide antibiotics, fluoroquinolone antibiotics, protease inhibitors such as the antiviral agent ritonavir, verapamil, and cimetidine. Coadministration of drugs that prolong QTc should be avoided (see Fig. 9.5). Check for QT_c prolongation in scenarios prone to hypokalemia, such as with diuretics or chronic diarrhea. Dofetilide may be cautiously given in combination with β-blockers but care must be taken to avoid bradycardia which can increase the risk of torsades. Diltiazem can increase dofetilide levels but can be used cautiously. Verapamil has a significant interaction and should be avoided completely.

Vernakalant

Pharmacokinetics. Vernakalant blocks the I_{Kr} current just like other class III agents, but it is more selective for the ultra-rapid

I_{Kur} current, which is much more selective for the atrium versus ventricular tissue (Figs. 9.1, 9.11). It also blocks another potassium current I_{KAch}, which is also selective for the atrium (Fig. 9.11). The agent also blocks the I_{to} which is the transient outward potassium current, but the blockade occurs more as the heart rate increases. Therefore, unlike dofetilide, ibutilide, and sotalol, vernakalant does not demonstrate reverse use dependence. In other words, it is most potent when the heart rates are high versus low. Vernakalant also is a weak I_{Na} blocker, which is also more potent at higher rates, as with the class IC agents (which show use dependence). However, the I_{Na} blockade is relatively weak compared to the potassium channel blockade. QT prolongation is not a major feature of vernakalant in contrast to other class III agents. The drug has a short half-life (3.1 hours) and is metabolized mainly through CYP2D6. It is not protein bound. Because of its very short half-life, it is only administered intravenously for acute termination of atrial arrhythmias.

Clinical use. The main use of vernakalant is for acute pharmacologic cardioversion of AF and/or atrial flutter.

Dose. The dose is given as an initial bolus of 3 mg/kg over 10 minutes. If sinus rhythm does not occur after 15 minutes, a second dose of 2 mg/kg over 10 minutes may be given. No more than 5 mg/kg should be given within 24 hours.

Side effects. Hypotension may occur with the infusion—if the drop is sudden and/or symptomatic, the infusion should be stopped. Hypotension occurs in 4%–13% of patients. Abnormal taste may occur in about 10%–20% of patients. Sneezing can occur in 10%–15% of patients. The drug should be avoided in patients with a prolonged QT or significant bradycardia or decompensated heart failure.

Drug interactions and combination. The drug should be avoided in combination with any drug that can prolong the QT interval (Fig. 9.5).

Class IV Agents

Class IV agents are calcium channel blockers. They have been used extensively in a number of areas including for hypertension, management of angina, and, of course, the management of arrhythmias. The dihydropyridine calcium channel blockers, like nifedipine and amlodipine, have more vascular selectivity and less direct cardiac effects, so they are generally used in the management of hypertension and do not play a major role in arrhythmias. The nondihydropyridine agents, like diltiazem and verapamil, are more cardioselective and are the main agents utilized for arrhythmia management (Table 9.5). While amlodipine has demonstrated neutral safety in patients with heart failure, the nondihydropyridine

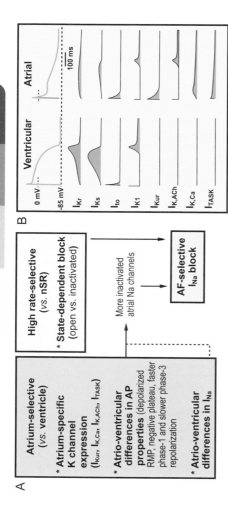

Fig. 9.11 Atrial-selective currents in humans. Current antiarrhythmics for atrial arrhythmias nonselectively target channels that are present in both atrial and ventricular myocardial cells. The result is that while agents may be very effective in controlling atrial arrhythmias, they also carry the risk of ventricular proarrhythmia (e.g., dofetilide, flecainide). Targeting channels/currents that are present predominantly in atrial tissue offers an opportunity to design atrial-selective antiarrhythmics that may not have the risk of ventricular proarrhythmia. Vernakalant, for example, targets both I_{Kur} and I_{KACh}, which are both found predominantly in atrial tissue. There are also differences in atrial repolarization between atrial and ventricular tissue and if blockade of this channel can occur preferentially in the activated state, such as during atrial fibrillation, it could be an ideal antiarrhythmic agent. I, current; Ca, calcium; K_{ACh}, acetylcholine activated inward-rectifying potassium channel (atrial selective); K_r, rapid component of repolarizing potassium current; K_{ur}, ultra-rapid repolarizing potassium current (atrial selective); K_s, slow component; K_1, inward rectifier potassium current; $TASK$, TWIK-related acid sensitive potassium channels; Na, sodium; nSR, normal sinus rhythm; t_o, transient outward.

agents should generally be avoided in patients with significant left ventricular dysfunction.

Pharmacokinetics. Calcium channel blockers mainly affect myocardial cells that are driven by slow action potentials mediated by calcium currents as opposed to cells that have faster action potentials driven by sodium currents. Generally, the SA and AV nodes depend more on calcium currents, so the class IV agents preferentially have their effects on these areas. In the setting of AMI/ischemia, diseased ventricular myocardium and Purkinje fibers may develop slower action potentials that are more sensitive to calcium channel blockade. Like class I agents, these agents demonstrate use dependence, which means these agents have a more pronounced effect at higher rather than slower heart rates.

Clinical use. Because verapamil and diltiazem slow the responses in both the SA and AV nodes, the medications are used mostly for (1) management of supraventricular tachycardias that require the AV node for reentry (AV nodal reentrant tachycardia, AV reentrant tachycardia) or (2) for rate control of atrial arrhythmias like AF, atrial flutter, and atrial tachycardia (Table 9.5). They are also particularly effective for treatment of multifocal atrial tachycardia that occurs in the setting of chronic obstructive lung disease. They can effectively rate control this arrhythmia without worsening bronchospasm, which may occur with β-blockers. Calcium channel blockers can be administered both orally—for chronic management—but also intravenously for acute management. These agents should be avoided in preexcited AF because by blocking the AV node selectively, they can create faster ventricular conduction as the arrhythmia preferentially conducts down the accessory pathway (Fig. 9.4). This may even precipitate ventricular fibrillation.

Class IV agents are considered contraindicated for ventricular arrhythmias because they cause myocardial depression and peripheral vasodilation, which can be fatal when given to patients with VT. Although class IV agents should be avoided in VT patients, there are four notable exceptions: (1) they may be effective for ventricular arrhythmias precipitated by coronary vasospasm; (2) they can be used to treat catecholaminergic VT due to mutations in the ryanodine receptor RyR2; (3) they can suppress frequent PVCs and nonsustained VT in patients with VT and structurally normal hearts (like right ventricular outflow tract VT); and (4) they may be effective in fascicular VTs or Belhassen tachycardia, which is characterized by a right bundle branch block VT with left axis deviation. The latter is sometimes referred to as "verapamil-sensitive VT."

Dose. See Table 9.5. Sustained-release verapamil can be given at a starting dose of 120 mg daily and increased in 120 mg increments to 360 mg daily. IV verapamil is not widely available but can be given as a 0.075–0.115 mg/kg bolus over 2 minutes followed by a continuous infusion at 5 mg/hour. Short-acting diltiazem can be given starting at 30 mg QID and increased until a total of 90 mg TID. Long-acting diltiazem is dosed starting at 120–180 mg once daily and increased in increments to 360–480 mg daily. IV diltiazem is widely available and is bolused at 0.25 mg/kg over 2 minutes (usually 20 mg), which can be repeated after 15 minutes and then a continuous infusion at 5–15 mg/hour.

Side effects. The main side effect of the calcium channel blockers is associated hypotension, which occurs, in up to 5% of patients. Heart block and sinus bradycardia can also occur so class IV agents should be avoided in patients with a history of significant bradycardia. Constipation occurs in about 5% and peripheral edema can occur in 5%–15%, although it is usually much less common than with the dihydropyridine agents. Verapamil specifically can cause gingival hyperplasia in about 15% of patients, and dyspepsia is more common compared to other calcium channel blockers.

Drug interactions and combination. See Table 9.4. Diltiazem should be avoided in the presence of strong inhibitors of CYP3A4. It can increase dofetilide levels but can be used cautiously. Verapamil has a number of important drug interactions, and administration of this drug should always be cross-checked with other medications. Verapamil inhibits CYP3A4 and can therefore increase the serum levels of many drugs. It also inhibits the p-glycoprotein pathway and therefore increases drugs metabolized by this route too. In particular, antiseizure medications, colchicine, dofetilide, dabigatran, edoxaban can all have increased serum levels with verapamil and should generally be avoided.

Class V Agents: Adenosine

Adenosine

Pharmacokinetics. Adenosine binds the adenosine receptor (especially A1), which inhibits adenylyl cyclase, reduces intracellular cAMP, and increases potassium influx via the adenosine-sensitive inward rectifier potassium channel. This inhibits the calcium current, which selectively occurs in both SA and AV myocytes (Fig. 9.12). Therefore, adenosine is a profound AV nodal blocker. It has a very short half-life, however, which is less than 10 seconds. It also causes vasodilation, in particular of the coronary arteries, which can cause coronary steal and chest pain. It is why adenosine is sometime used for chemical myocardial stress testing.

Clinical use. It is a first-line agent for terminating narrow complex PSVTs.[79] By inhibiting the AV node, it can terminate supraventricular tachycardias that are dependent on the AV node,

ADENOSINE INHIBITION OF AV NODE

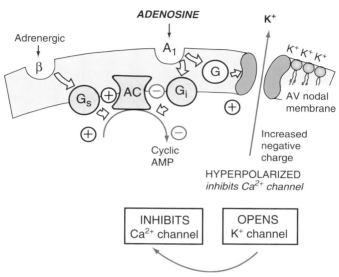

Fig. 9.12 Adenosine inhibits the atrioventricular *(AV)* node by effects on ion channels. Adenosine acting on the adenosine 1 *(A₁)* surface receptor opens the adenosine-sensitive potassium channel to hyperpolarize and inhibit the AV node and also indirectly to inhibit calcium channel opening. *AC*, Adenylate cyclase; *AMP*, adenosine monophosphate; β, β-Adrenoreceptor; *G*, G protein, nonspecific; *Gᵢ*, inhibitory G protein; *Gₛ*, stimulatory G protein. (Figure © L.H. Opie, 2012.)

such as AV nodal reentrant tachycardia and AV reentrant tachycardia (Fig. 9.9). By causing heart block, it can also be useful for the diagnosis of atrial flutter to bring out the flutter waves that are not obviously seen when the ventricular rate is also rapid. It is also used in the diagnosis of wide-complex tachycardia of uncertain origin. Supraventricular tachycardia with aberrancy may terminate if it is AV node dependent, or block may help bring out underlying flutter waves. Ventricular tachycardia, on the other hand, will not be affected. Since the half-life is so short, there is no adverse hemodynamic compromise as would be caused by the class IV agents. In the electrophysiology lab, adenosine can be administered to bring out subtle or latent preexcitation by blocking conduction through the AV node and forcing it through the antegrade accessory pathway.[80] Adenosine is also used to reveal concealed pulmonary vein conduction in an otherwise "isolated" pulmonary vein as a means of testing the completeness of pulmonary vein isolation for AF ablation.

Dose. Adenosine is given as an initial rapid IV bolus of 6 mg followed by a saline flush to obtain high concentrations in the heart.[79] If it does not work within 1 to 2 minutes, a 12-mg bolus is given that may be repeated once. At the appropriate dose, the anti-arrhythmic effect occurs as soon as the drug reaches the AV node, usually within 15 to 30 seconds. The initial dose needs to be reduced to 3 mg or less in patients taking verapamil, diltiazem, or β-blockers or dipyridamole, or in older adults at risk of sick sinus syndrome. Boluses of 18–24 mg can be given if heart block, or the desired effect is not noted with the smaller doses.

Side effects. Side effects ascribed to the effect of adenosine on the potassium channel are short lived, such as headache (via vasodilation), chest discomfort, flushing, nausea, and excess sinus or AV nodal inhibition. The precipitation of bronchoconstriction in asthmatic patients is of unknown mechanism and can last for 30 minutes. Transient new arrhythmias can occur at the time of chemical cardioversion. Because of abbreviating effects on atrial and ventricular refractoriness, adenosine may cause a range of proarrhythmic consequences, including atrial and ventricular ectopy, and degeneration of atrial flutter or PSVT into AF. Contraindications are as follows: asthma or history of asthma, second- or third-degree AV block, and sick sinus syndrome.

Drug interactions and combination. Dipyridamole inhibits the breakdown of adenosine, and therefore the dose of adenosine must be markedly reduced in patients receiving dipyridamole. Methylxanthines (caffeine, theophylline) competitively antagonize the interaction of adenosine with its receptors, so that it becomes less effective. See Table 9.4.

Other Agents

Ivabradine

Phamacokinetics. Ivabradine is a selective inhibitor of the I_f current, which is a current that modulates the slow depolarization phase of the action potential in the SA node (see Fig. 9.13 for details).

Clinical use. The drug was initially studied for the treatment of patients with heart failure and reduced EF with persistently elevated heart rates. The SHIFT trial showed that in patients with an EF <35% and a sinus rate >70 bpm, ivabradine was associated with a significant reduction in the composite of cardiovascular death and heart failure hospitalization.[81] Death was also significantly reduced.

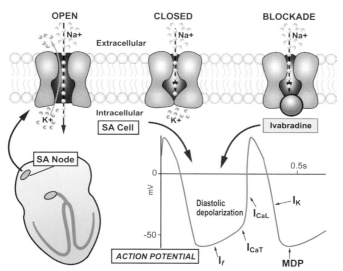

Fig. 9.13   Funny current and blockade by ivabradine. The funny current (I_f) is a mixed sodium–potassium current that activates during phase IV of the action potential in sinoatrial cells *(top panel)*. At the end of a sinoatrial action potential, the membrane repolarizes and then activates the I_f, which supplies inward current. This, in turn, is responsible for starting the diastolic depolarization phase, which is then mediated by calcium currents (I_{CaT} and I_{CaL}). The potassium current (I_K) then causes repolarization. Ivabradine blocks the I_f current and therefore delays phase IV depolarization in sinoatrial cells, therefore selectively lowering the sinus rate *(bottom panel)*.

Because of its selectivity for the SA node, the main arrhythmic application is for inappropriate sinus tachycardia. As it turns out, it is particularly effective for this indication.

Dose. Ivabradine is dosed at 5–7.5 mg BID orally

Side effects. The main adverse reaction is that of bradycardia, which occurs in 5%–10% of patients. There is also a small increase in the risk of AF (5%–8%). Visual scotomata (such as seeing flashing light) can also occur in 3% of patients supposedly due to blocked of hyperpolarization channels in the photoreceptors of the retina. These changes are not permanent and resolve upon discontinuation of the drug.

Drug interactions and combination. These drugs can potentiate the sinus bradycardia effect of class II or IV agents. While ivabradine can be used in combination with class II and IV agents, it should be done cautiously and only in cases of refractory inappropriate sinus tachycardia. Patients in the SHIFT trial with heart failure were often cotreated with both ivabradine and β-blockade.

Intravenous magnesium

IV magnesium weakly blocks the calcium channel and also inhibits both sodium and potassium channels. The relative importance of these mechanisms is unknown. It can be used to slow the ventricular rate in AF but is poor at terminating PSVTs. It may be the agent of choice in torsades de pointes by helping to shorten the QT interval. It has an additional use in refractory VF, which is resistant to combination antiarrhythmic therapy. It is usually given intravenously 1–2 g over 15 minutes. A continuous infusion can be maintained at 0.5–1.0 g/hour. The main side effect is muscle relaxation, particularly in patients with myasthenia gravis and also hypotension.

Inhaled Agents

Because of the ability to rapidly absorb certain antiarrhythmic compounds through the intranasal or intraoral inhaled routes and obtain therapeutic serum levels quickly, interest has increased over the use of inhaled preparations for acute termination of arrhythmias. Nasally inhaled etripamil, a calcium channel blocker, demonstrated high termination rates of PSVT dependent on the AV node. In one phase II study,[82] termination rates of SVT were between 65%–94% of patients depending on the dose given. Doses of 70–140 mg were associated with the highest conversion rate, but the highest dose had a small risk of hypotension and heart block. Ongoing phase III studies will more fully assess the efficacy and safety of this very promising approach.

Orally inhaled flecainide is also being assessed in phase II studies for acute conversion of AF. In a randomized study, 30–60 mg inhaled doses are being compared to placebo to assess conversion from AF to sinus rhythm after 240 minutes. The 60-mg dose is actually administered as two separate 30-mg doses in rapid succession to one another. QRS duration appears to be minimal, and the elimination half-life is about 10 hours.[83] Further data is being collected on the potential efficacy of this approach for termination of AF episodes.

New Developments in Antiarrhythmics

The development of novel antiarrhythmic agents has been very challenging. Recent accomplishments, such as dronedarone, were followed by rapid discovery of increased mortality in heart failure and chronic AF patients leading to significant restriction in the use of these agents.[67,68] Many antiarrhythmics have seen their development terminated after initially promising phase I results failed to produce any clinically meaningful results in phase II or beyond (for example, azimilide, celivarone, eleclazine, and tedisamil). Two novel I_{Kur} blockers also stopped development after discovery of unforeseen toxicity (such as pulmonary toxicity). Thus, there is a natural reluctance on the part of pharmaceutical companies to actively perform research in this area despite the desperate need for more effective and safer agents. Furthermore, an explosion in nonpharmacologic therapy for arrhythmias, specifically cardiac ablation for both atrial and ventricular arrhythmias, is decreasing the need for long-term antiarrhythmic therapy.

Having said that, there remain many potential targets for antiarrhythmic drug therapy, many of which are well outlined in the excellent new proposed classification system by Lei et al.[8] The ultra-rapid delayed rectifier current (I_{Kur}) and acetylcholine-activated inward rectifier current (I_{KAch}) are both atrial selective and could be exploited for treatment of AF with theoretically few ventricular effects (Fig. 9.11). Vernakalant is the only approved example and is only available in IV form. Several oral preparations have undergone phase I and II evaluation, although many have been abandoned due to lack of efficacy or unforeseen toxicity. The two-pore K current (I_{K2P}) consists of K channels that are regulated by stretch, temperature, and other factors. Blockade of this would be similar to the class III effect and could cause QT prolongation. However, TASK-1 is one such channel and is atrial selective, so it could be exploited for atrial arrhythmias with little ventricular proarrhythmia (Fig. 9.11). TREK-1 is expressed in both atrial and ventricular tissue. These channels may be downregulated in heart failure and therefore, agents targeting these may not be as effective in those patients. The late Na current (I_{NaL}) can promote prolonged repolarization and development of early after depolarizations which can be proarrhythmic. Blockage of this current could be antiarrhythmic. Ranolazine blocks this current but is not a potent antiarrhythmic (see drug description). Eclazine was a more selective I_{NaL} blocker, but development was stopped because of lack of efficacy. The ryanodine receptor underlies triggered activity in both atrial and ventricular tissue. It is involved in catecholaminergic VT. Dantrolene can inhibit ryanodine receptors and is being examined for potential antiarrhythmic benefit. Small conductance calcium- activated K currents (ISK) also have predominant atrial expression and could prolong atrial effective refractory period. Transient receptor potential channels (TRP) are expressed in the heart and alter calcium influx. Inhibition of these may have direct EP effects but also inhibit fibrosis, which can promote reentry.

Promotion of gap junctions via rotigaptide, inhibition of the sodium calcium exchanger (NCX), and ATP-sensitive potassium channel blockade could also reduce the risk of arrhythmogenesis.[84] To date, there are no new therapies that are imminently on the clinical horizon, but hope remains for the future.

Antiarrhythmic Choice for Arrhythmias

Supraventricular Tachycardia (AV nodal reentry, AV reentry, atrial tachycardia)

Acute therapy.
- IV adenosine
- IV calcium channel blocker (diltiazem, verapamil)
- IV β-blocker (metoprolol)

Chronic therapy
- Oral calcium channel blocker (diltiazem, verapamil) (first line)
- Oral β-blocker (bisoprolol, metoprolol, atenolol) (first line)
- Oral class IC drugs + β-blocker or calcium channel blocker (second line)
- Class III agents (last resort)

Catheter ablation now used as first-line therapy for most SVTs

Atrial Fibrillation

Acute conversion
- IV ibutilide
- IV vernakalant
- IV procainamide
- IV amiodarone (takes longer than above-mentioned agents)
- Oral "pill in pocket" class IC agent (flecainide, propafenone)— (takes longer than above-mentioned agents)

Electrical cardioversion can be used as an alternative, particularly when there is hemodynamic instability.

Acute rate control
- IV calcium channel blocker (should be normal LV)
- IV β-blocker

- IV amiodarone
- IV digoxin (particularly for decompensated heart failure)

Chronic maintenance of sinus rhythm

Normal heart function, no coronary disease

- Flecainide + β-blocker or calcium channel blocker
- Propafenone + β-blocker or calcium channel blocker
- Sotalol
- Dronedarone
- Dofetilide, amiodarone (second line agents when others fail)

Normal heart function, coronary disease

- Sotalol
- Dronedarone
- Dofetilide, amiodarone (second line agents when others fail)
    Hypertrophic cardiomyopathy
- Dofetilide
- Amiodarone
- Sotalol (may be used with caution, especially if patient has ICD)

Heart failure, left ventricular dysfunction (may be used in selected heart failure/LV dysfunction patients with ICD)

- Dofetilide
- Amiodarone

Increasingly catheter ablation is being used to avoid second line antiarrhythmics, like amiodarone, and even being used increasingly in heart failure patients.

Chronic rate control

- Oral calcium channel blocker (should be normal LV)
- Oral β-blocker
- Combination calcium channel blocker + β-blocker
- Oral digoxin (not effective as monotherapy, ideal for heart failure)
- Oral amiodarone (very effective, but limited by side effects)

Patients with persistent AF are increasingly being considered for catheter ablation of AF to maintain sinus rhythm as opposed to rate control; it depends on factors such as age, symptoms, left atrial size.

Preexcited Atrial Fibrillation

Acute therapy

- IV procainamide

- IV amiodarone

Often, electrical cardioversion is required—AVOID selective AV nodal blockers.

Chronic therapy

- Catheter ablation is therapy of choice to eliminate the accessory pathway causing preexcitation
- Oral amiodarone if ablation not desired or cannot be done

Atrial Flutter

Similar approach as for AF for acute and chronic therapy.
However, flutter often more difficult to rate control and ibutilide is drug of choice for acute pharmacologic cardioversion.
Ablation often used for long-term management of typical atrial flutter, even as first-line treatment.

Ventricular Arrhythmias (VT, VF)

Acute therapy

- Electrical cardioversion if hemodynamically unstable
- IV amiodarone

IV amiodarone can be combined with IV lidocaine for refractory ventricular arrhythmias ("storm")

- IV lidocaine
- IV procainamide

Chronic therapy (in patients with structural heart disease)

- Oral β-blocker (cardio-selective)

β-blocker, amiodarone and mexitiline can be combined for refractory ventricular arrhythmias

- Amiodarone
- Mexiletine
- Sotalol (may be used with caution, especially if patient has ICD)
- Flecainide (used with extreme caution in patients with ICD, second line)
- Dofetilide (not approved for this purpose)

Increasingly, catheter ablation is being used for recurrent ventricular arrhythmias.

Chronic therapy (in patients with no structural heart disease)

- Oral β-blocker (cardio-selective)

- Oral calcium channel blocker (diltiazem, verapamil)
- β-blocker + calcium channel blocker
- Flecainide + β-blocker
- Propafenone + β-blocker
- Sotalol
- Amiodarone (second line)

Many ventricular arrhythmias in structurally normal hearts are quite amenable to catheter ablation, particularly when very high burden, symptomatic, or causing LV dysfunction.

Torsades de pointes

Acute therapy

- Withdrawal of inciting drug (if present)
- IV/oral potassium if hypokalemic
- IV magnesium
- IV isoproterenol (raises heart rate, decreases QT interval)
- Temporary cardiac pacing (raise heart rate, decrease QT interval)

Chronic therapy

- If patient has long QT syndrome, long acting β-blocker—propranolol, nadolol, bisoprolol (metoprolol not as good)
- For selected LQTS, mexiletine and flecainide may be useful (see sections for each drug)

Summary

1. **Antiarrhythmic drug classification.** These are grouped into at least five classes: class I sodium channel blockers; class II β-adrenergic blockers; class III repolarization blockers; class IV those agents that block the calcium current in the AV node; and class V adenosine. Other classes are proposed in more novel classification schemes,[8] which will allow for more novel agents to be included if and when they are developed. Other agents, like ivabradine, do not fit in the traditional Vaughan Williams classes.

2. **Usage of antiarrhythmic drugs.** Class I agents are not often used because of adverse long-term effects. However, IV lidocaine or procainamide still remain effective for VT; oral agents flecainide and propafenone are useful for AF in the absence of structural heart disease. Class II, the β-blockers, are especially effective in hyperadrenergic states such as chronic heart failure,

some repetitive tachycardias, and ischemic arrhythmias. Among class III agents, amiodarone is a powerful antiarrhythmic agent, acting on both supraventricular and ventricular arrhythmias, but potentially quite toxic. Lower dosing regimens are recommended for long-term treatment although toxicity can still occur. Dofetilide is also very useful for AF in both the presence and absence of structural heart disease but the risk of torsades is significant and requires hospitalization for loading. Sotalol is less effective than amiodarone or dofetilide but with less toxicity and moderately lower risk of torsades. Class IV agents are excellent in arresting acute supraventricular tachycardias (adenosine is preferred), treating SVTs chronically, and also reduce ventricular rates in chronic AF (verapamil and diltiazem). Some older agents (like quinidine, mexiletine, and flecainide) have found new purpose for treatment of specific genetic variants of Brugada syndrome, long QT syndrome, and catecholaminergic VT.

3. **Current and future trends in arrhythmia therapy.** The complexity of the numerous agents available and the ever-increasing problems with side effects and proarrhythmia have promoted a strong trend toward intervention by ablation or devices for most arrhythmias. Inhaled versions of existing therapies may provide novel ways to terminate arrhythmias with potentially fewer side effects. New antiarrhythmic drug investigations have been limited by the discovery of agents with either limited efficacy, similar toxicity to existing agents, or discovery of unanticipated side effects. It remains to be seen whether more novel targets can be exploited successfully for a new generation of antiarrhythmics.

References

Complete reference list available at www.expertconsult.com.

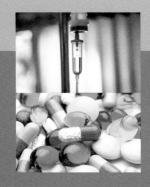

第10章
血管医学药物

外周动脉疾病的定义广泛,涵盖了冠状动脉循环以外的动脉闭塞性疾病,但通常指动脉粥样硬化性闭塞性疾病。因为非动脉粥样硬化性闭塞性疾病(如与纤维肌发育不良和血管炎相关的疾病)相对少见,所以本章将重点关注动脉粥样硬化性疾病。

本章重点介绍了戒烟药物治疗、降血压和抗血栓药物治疗、降低低密度脂蛋白和其他调脂治疗、降血糖治疗等。另外,本章还涉及扩血管药物、代谢类药物及使用血管生成因子治疗外周动脉疾病的实验性治疗方案。

另外,本章涵盖了静脉血栓栓塞症的药物治疗,包括胃肠外抗凝药、口服抗凝药及长期二级预防方案;主动脉瘤及主动脉夹层的治疗方案,包括主动脉夹层的初始处理及长期治疗,以及马方综合征的治疗;血管炎的药物治疗,如糖皮质激素、类固醇节约剂等药物的使用。同时,本章还介绍了雷诺现象及其药物治疗。

陈安天

Vascular Medicine Drugs

MARC P. BONACA

Overview

Drugs for Patients With Peripheral Artery Disease

Peripheral artery disease (PAD) is broadly defined as arterial occlusive disease outside of the coronary circulation and generally refers to atherosclerotic occlusive disease.[1,2] While nonatherosclerotic occlusive disease including that related to fibromuscular dysplasia and vasculitis does exist, it is relatively uncommon relative to atherosclerotic disease, and the focus of the current chapter will be on the latter. The most common manifestation of PAD is in the lower extremities and in some contexts PAD as a term is used to specifically describe lower extremity atherosclerotic occlusive disease. Overall it is estimated that over 10 million people in the United States and over 200 million globally have lower extremity PAD (referred to as PAD going forward).[3,4]

Patients with PAD are at heightened risk of atherothrombosis including systemic events, also referred to as major adverse cardiovascular events (MACE), such as myocardial infarction (MI), stroke, and cardiovascular death (CV death).[1,2] In addition, by nature of atherosclerosis of the limbs, patients with PAD suffer significant morbidity related to limb ischemia. This morbidity spans from functional limitations due to impaired limb perfusion to limb threatening events such as chronic critical limb ischemia (CLI), acute limb ischemia (ALI), and related ischemic tissue loss, the latter two are commonly referred to as major adverse limb events or MALE (Fig. 10.1).[1,2,5]

Medical therapy for the patients with PAD therefore has three key goals: to reduce the risk of MACE, to reduce the risk of MALE,

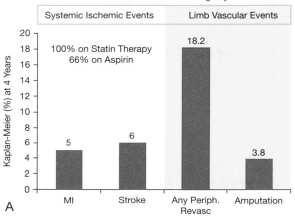

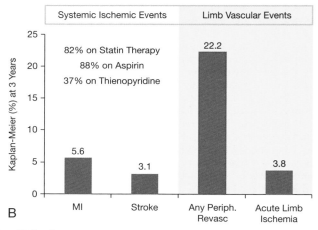

Fig. 10.1 Outcomes in patients with symptomatic peripheral artery disease at 4 years in the (A) REACH registry and the (B) TRA2P-TIMI 50 trial. (From Bonaca MP, Creager MA. Medical Treatment of Peripheral Artery Disease. In: *Vascular Medicine: A Companion to Braunwald's Heart Disease.* Philadelphia: Elsevier; 2020: Fig. 19.1.)

and to improve function (Fig. 10.2).[6,7] Because the risk of MACE and MALE are driven by atherothrombosis, preventive therapy overlaps with those for ischemic heart disease (Chapter 1) and specifically with antihypertensive therapies (Chapter 2), diabetes drugs (Chapter 4), lipid-modifying drugs (Chapter 6), and antithrombotic drugs (Chapter 8). The efficacy and safety, however, in PAD particularly with regard to limb outcomes is unique to this population (Fig. 10.3). In addition, two important risk factors for incident PAD and risk markers for adverse outcomes in PAD are smoking and diabetes, therefore medical therapy related to these issues is particularly important for prevention. It must also be noted that patients with PAD and concomitant coronary disease, described as polyvascular disease, may be particularly high risk and have greater absolute benefits of preventive therapies.[8,9] Finally, a large body of data supports the efficacy of exercise to improve function in PAD and, as such, exercise receives a class I indication in clinical practice guidelines.[1,2] Because this is not a medical therapy it will

Asymptomatic Low ABI Without Symptomatic Vascular Disease	Symptomatic PAD or Asymptomatic Low ABI With Concomitant Symptomatic Vascular Disease

Prevention of Progression to Symptomatic Disease

Reduction of MACE Risk

• Risk high in patients with symptomatic PAD

• Risk highest in patients with polyvascular disease, particularly concomitant coronary disease

Reduction in MALE Risk

• Risk highest in patients with prior peripheral revascularization

Prevention of Progression to Symptomatic Disease

Functional Improvement

• Symptoms most evident in patients with typical claudication

• Most patients with low ABI have some degree of functional impairment

Fig. 10.2 Markers of risk and goals of prevention in patients with peripheral artery disease *(PAD)* diagnosed by ankle-brachial index *(ABI)* and symptoms. *MACE*, Major adverse cardiovascular events; *MALE*, major adverse limb events. (From Bonaca MP, Creager MA. Medical Treatment of Peripheral Artery Disease. In: *Vascular Medicine: A Companion to Braunwald's Heart Disease.* Philadelphia: Elsevier; 2020: Fig. 19.4.)

	BP Lowering	Glucose Lowering	LDL-C Lowering	Anti-thrombotic	Anti-inflammatory
MACE Risk	Data strongest for ACEi	Mixed — SGLT-2 inhibitors (CVD/HF) & GLP1 agonists (MACE). Possibly with long-term therapy through other mechanisms	Risk reduction consistent to very low levels of achieved LDL-C	Monotherapy beneficial in symptomatic PAD. More potent strategies with clearest benefit in polyvascular disease (PAD+CAD)	Through inhibition of IL-1. Other mechanisms not proven to have benefit
MALE Risk	No benefit or harm demonstrated	Canagliflozin. No benefit or harm demonstrated with other targets	Risk reduction consistent to very low levels of achieved LDL-C	More potent strategies with greatest benefit in prior revascularization	No benefit or harm demonstrated
Microvascular Disease					

Fig. 10.3 See legend on facing page.

not be reviewed in this chapter; however, it should be a core aspect in the appropriate medical care of patients with PAD.

While there are a number of pharmacotherapies that have demonstrated efficacy in reducing rates of MACE and/or MALE in PAD, rates of utilization of these therapies remains low overall and especially when compared to patients with coronary artery disease (CAD).[10] Efforts to improve guideline dissemination and implementation of preventive therapies are needed.[10]

Drugs for Smoking Cessation

Smoking is strongly associated with the development of incident PAD.[11] In addition, continued smoking in patients with PAD is associated with accelerated disease progression and poor outcomes.[1,2,6] Smoking cessation in PAD is associated with improvement in function as measured by walking time as well as lower rates of the need for peripheral revascularization, CLI, and MACE. In spite of clear evidence of the harms of smoking,[12] the success rate of a strategy of physician advice for cessation low and estimated to be in the range of 5%–7%.[1,2] Randomized counseling interventions have increased success to ~20%; however, persistence is poor with almost 80% of those that quit returning to smoking by 6 months.[13] The coupling of pharmacologic therapy with counseling holds promise for improved rates of smoking cessation

Drug Class Overview and Guidelines

Current guidelines give a class I recommendation for the assistance in developing a plan for quitting including pharmacotherapy.[1,2] Three medication options include varenicline, bupropion, and/or nicotine replacement therapy.

Fig. 10.3, Cont'd Axes of therapy (columns) and effects on major adverse cardiovascular events *(MACE)*, major adverse limb events *(MALE)*, and microvascular disease in patients with peripheral artery disease *(PAD)* with or without diabetes (glucose-lowering therapies relevant for patients with diabetes). *ACEi*, Angiotensin-converting enzyme inhibitor; *BP*, blood pressure; *CAD*, coronary artery disease; *CVD/HF*, cardiovascular death/heart failure; *GLP1*, glucagon-like peptide-1; *IL-1*, interleukin-1; *LDL-C*, low-density lipoprotein cholesterol; *SGL T2*, sodium glucose transporter 2. (From Bonaca MP, Creager MA. Medical Treatment of Peripheral Artery Disease. In: *Vascular Medicine: A Companion to Braunwald's Heart Disease*. Philadelphia: Elsevier; 2020: Fig. 19.13.)

Mechanisms of Action

Varenicline is a partial agonist of the nicontinic acetylcholine receptor (nAchR) α4β.[14] Bupropion works by inhibiting the reuptake of selected neurotransmitters including dopamine, serotonin, and norepinephrine, and reduces the severity of withdrawal symptoms. Nicotine replacement is nicotine in noncigarette formulations and can come in several forms including gum and patches.[7]

Data for Use

Bupropion has been studied both alone and in combination with a nicotine patch, with both strategies showing benefits relative to placebo.[15] At 12 months, relative to placebo, bupropion increased the likelihood of quitting smoking by ~60% but with 20% remaining abstinent at 1 year.[16,17] Varenicline has been shown to increase the likelihood of abstinence at 1 year relative to placebo by threefold in patients with cardiovascular disease.[14] Overall it appears to be more efficacious than bupropion alone or in combination with nicotine replacement. Nicotine replacement appears to be efficacious with 50%–70% improvements in rates of quitting relative to placebo regardless of form (gum, transdermal patch, nasal spray, inhaler, oral).[18]

Side Effects

Varenicline has a number of associated side effects including sleep disturbance, nausea, skin reactions, and flatulence.[14] Both varenicline and bupropion are associated with neuropsychiatric side effects, and labels for both agents include black box warnings for observing changes in mood, behavior, and/or the development of suicidal ideations.[1,2] Bupropion should not be used in patients with seizure disorders, some eating disorders, or in those at high risk of seizure (e.g., those stopping benzodiazepine or antiseizure medications.) Nicotine side effects in part depend on the mode of use, but common side effects described include local irritation, dizziness, headache, nausea, palpitations, and sleep disturbance.[1,2]

Drug interactions. Bupropion should not be used within 14 days of stopping a MAO inhibitor, and there are interactions with a number of other drugs for depression or bipolar disorder. Varenicline may interact with ranolazine. Nicotine is a stimulant and therefore may interact with other stimulants, such as caffeine.

Antihypertensive Therapies

Antihypertensive therapies are covered in Chapter 2 in detail. The diagnosis and treatment of hypertension for patients with PAD mirrors general guidelines for hypertension including thresholds and selection of therapy.[19] Current guidelines recommend treating patients with established cardiovascular disease, including patients with PAD, to a blood pressure target below 130/80 mmHg.[19] The ESC guidelines note that in patients with PAD, an SBP below 110–120 mg may be associated with risk due to the J-shape relationship between SBP and CV events observed in PAD patients in the International Verapamil-SR/Trandolapril (INVEST).[1,20] Although there is theoretic concern in reducing blood pressure to low targets in patients with marginal limb perfusion, other trials have demonstrated benefit with achieving such targets and with an acceptable safety profile.[21] The Appropriate Blood Pressure Control in Diabetes (ABCD) trial that randomized 950 patients with diabetes to enalapril or nislodipine observed a reduction in MACE in patients with PAD receiving intensive treatment (mean BP 128/75 mmHg), with greater benefits in those with more severe occlusive disease as represented by lower ankle brachial index (ABI).[22] Similar findings were shown in the International Verapamil-SR/Trandolapril study, which observed a reduction in MACE with a target of <130/80 mmHg in the subgroup with PAD.

With regard to specific agents, angiotensin-converting enzyme inhibitors (ACEi) and angiotensin receptor blockers (ARBs) are preferred in PAD (class II in guidelines) due to consistent benefits observed in large PAD subgroups in trials demonstrating benefits of these therapies.[1,2] The benefits of these therapies for reducing MACE have been demonstrated robustly. In contrast, small studies describing improvements in function and limb outcomes have not been substantiated. The Heart Outcomes Prevention Evaluation Trial (HOPE) randomized patients to ramipril 10 mg daily or placebo and followed for 5 years observing significant reductions in MACE with the intervention arm.[23] A large subgroup of ~4000 patients had PAD, and benefits were consistent in this subgroup. The EUROPA trial similarly observed benefits of perindopril versus placebo with consistent benefits in the subgroup with PAD.[24] The Ongoing Telmisartan Alone and in Combination With Ramipril Global Endpoint Trial (ONTARGET) randomized patients to telmisartan, ramipril, or both and observed similar outcomes with either agent, including in a subgroup of 3000 patients with PAD.[25]

Theoretic concerns regarding the risk of worsening limb outcomes in PAD with β-blockade therapy have been raised. Although not a first choice in PAD, these therapies may be indicated in patients with concomitant CAD or arrythmia such as atrial fibrillation. The concern for harm is based on the theoretical decrease in cardiac output and/or unopposed α-agonism with nonspecific agents that could lead to worsening limb malperfusion. In spite of these concerns, no harm in randomized studies or meta-analyses have been reported, and current guidelines do not recommend against their use.[26,27]

A detailed description of mechanism of action, side effects, and drug interactions are included in Chapter 2. Experimental therapies with blood pressure–lowering effects in PAD have been studied with the question of whether vasodilator therapy may improve limb symptoms and limb outcomes. There are no current data to support the use of vasodilator therapy for limb outcomes in PAD and ongoing trials are discussed under the section titled "Vasodilators."

Antithrombotic Therapies

Antithrombotic drugs are covered in detail in Chapter 8. The data supporting specific antithrombotic strategies in PAD will be discussed in this section. Current guidelines only assign single antiplatelet therapy (SAPT) a class I indication in symptomatic PAD.[1,2] It is not recommended in asymptomatic PAD if identified through screening ABI. Since publication of the current guidelines there have been new data supporting the benefits of more intensive strategies in selected patients but with associated increased bleeding. These data will be incorporated into subsequent iterations of the guidelines.

Antiplatelet Monotherapy

Aspirin is an antiplatelet drug that works through irreversible inhibition of cyclooxygenase (COX)-1 through acetylation of the hydroxyl of a serine residue.[6,7] The most robust dataset evaluating the efficacy and safety of aspirin in PAD is the Antithrombotic Trialists Collaborative (ATT) meta-analyses including patients with primary and secondary prevention including a subgroup of the later of ~9000 with PAD.[28,29] Overall aspirin was associated with consistent benefits in secondary prevention with a 23% reduction in MACE in those with PAD at a cost of a 60% excess in major extracranial bleeding. Patients with PAD included in the ATT were symptomatic, including those with history of intervention. Subsequent studies have investigated broadening the use of aspirin to populations with no evidence vascular disease and marginally low ABI (called asymptomatic PAD). The prevention of Progression of Arterial Disease with Diabetes (POPADAD) trial randomized patients with diabetes and an ABI <0.99 to aspirin 100 mg or placebo.[30] At 7 years there was no benefit of aspirin in this population for MACE or limb outcomes. The Aspirin for Prevention of Cardiovascular Events in a General Population Screened for a low Ankle-Brachial Index (AAA) enrolled 3350 patients with an ABI ≤0.95 and randomized to aspirin or placebo.[31] At ~8 years, event rates were low and there was no significant differences in MACE or MALE with aspirin versus placebo, but there was a ~70% excess in bleeding.

Inhibitors of the platelet $P2Y_{12}$ receptor have been studied in patients with PAD both as monotherapy and as an adjunct to other agents, primarily aspirin. One of the earliest trials to evaluate this class of therapies in PAD was the Swedish Ticlopidine Multicenter Study (STIMS) evaluating MACE with Ticlopidine versus placebo in 687 patients with claudication over approximately 5 years.[32] Overall there was a 51% reduction in the need for lower extremity revascularization and a 30% reduction in all-cause mortality. Clopidogrel, a second-generation $P2Y_{12}$ inhibitor, was studied head to head against aspirin in the Clopidogrel versus Aspirin in Patients at Risk of Ischemic Events trial (CAPRIE), which enrolled more than 19,000 patients with stable atherosclerosis for a primary outcome of MACE.[33] Overall, clopidogrel was superior to aspirin with an 8.7% relative risk reduction; however, there was statistical heterogeneity of benefit based on qualifying disease state, with the 6452 patients with symptomatic PAD (ABI $\leq$0.85 and history of claudication or prior intervention for ischemia) deriving a greater (23.8%) benefit. Clopidogrel was subsequently tested directly against the third-generation agent, ticagrelor, in over 12,000 patients with symptomatic PAD (ABI $\leq$0.85 and history of claudication or prior intervention for ischemia) in the A Study Comparing Cardiovascular Effects of Ticagrelor and Clopidogrel in Patients with Peripheral Artery Disease (EUCILD) trial.[34] Ticagrelor was not superior, and overall outcomes both for efficacy and safety appeared similar between treatment arms.

More Intensive Antiplatelet Therapy

Several more recent trials have studied more intensive antiplatelet therapy in patients with PAD. The Clopidogrel for High Atherothrombotic Risk and Ischemic Stabilization, Management and Avoidance (CHARISMA) randomized 15,603 patients with stable atherosclerosis or risk factors to the addition of clopidogrel to aspirin (dual antiplatelet therapy or DAPT) versus aspirin alone and evaluated MACE over long-term therapy.[35] Overall there was no statistically significant benefit of DAPT; however, in a post hoc analysis of those patients with atherosclerosis, similar to those randomized in the CAPRIE trial, there was a 17% lower rate of MACE with DAPT.[36] In the 2383 patients with symptomatic PAD, there was no significant reduction in MACE; however, DAPT was associated with lower rates of hospitalization and MI, raising the hypothesis of potential benefits in this subgroup.[37] The CASPAR trial tested the same comparison in 851 patients with PAD undergoing lower extremity bypass and showed no benefit.[38] An analogous trial after endovascular intervention called CAMPER was launched but was terminated after failing to enroll enough participants.[6,7] A novel mechanism for platelet inhibition through antagonism of the protease-activated receptor (PAR) for thrombin was tested in the Trial to Assess the Effects of Vorapaxar in Preventing Heart Attack and Stroke in Patients with Atherosclerosis (TRA2°P-TIMI 50). The agent vorapaxar, a PAR-1 antagonist, was tested against placebo on a background or aspirin and/or clopidogrel in patients with symptomatic atherosclerosis for the reduction of MACE. In the 26,449 patients randomized, including patients with symptomatic PAD, vorapaxar reduced MACE by 13% and increased GUSTO moderate or severe bleeding.[39] There appeared to be heterogeneity for harm in terms of bleeding and intracranial hemorrhage, with a greater risk in patients with prior stroke. Consequently, the drug was approved for use in patients with a history of MI or symptomatic PAD. A novel aspect of this trial was the prospective definition, ascertainment, and adjudication of ALI as an endpoint.[40,41] In patients with PAD (ABI ≤ 0.90 or prior revascularization for ischemia) there was a 15% reduction in MACE, a 30% reduction in MALE, and a 42% reduction in ALI with the greatest absolute benefit for MACE in those with concomitant CAD, and the greatest absolute benefit for MALE in those with prior lower extremity revascularization.[42]

The use of DAPT (aspirin and a $P2Y_{12}$ inhibitor) has also been studied in patients with PAD and CAD, also called polyvascular disease. This population has been shown to be at higher risk of MACE than PAD or CAD alone.[9] A subgroup analysis of the PEGASUS-TIMI 54 trial, which randomized more than 21,000 patients with prior MI to ticagrelor 90 mg twice daily, ticagrelor 60 mg twice daily, or placebo all on a background of aspirin, demonstrated that DAPT with ticagrelor reduced MACE as well as was associated with lower rates of cardiovascular death and all-cause mortality.[43] In addition, ticagrelor reduced MALE by 35% with greater absolute benefits for both MACE and MALE in those with versus without PAD. Overall ticagrelor increased major bleeding by more than twofold, with the risk similar in those with and without PAD. Similar observations were published from the PRODIGY trial, which randomized patients after coronary intervention to shorter versus longer durations of DAPT with clopidogrel.[44] In patients with concomitant PAD, longer DAPT was associated with reductions in MACE as well as lower rates of all-cause mortality with similar risks of bleeding regardless of PAD status. MALEs were not reported in PRODIGY. The Study Comparing Cardiovascular Effects of Ticagrelor Versus Placebo in Patients With Type 2 Diabetes Mellitus (THEMIS) trial compared DAPT with ticagrelor versus aspirin alone in patients with CAD and type 2 diabetes mellitus (T2DM) but no history of MI.[45] Overall, ticagrelor reduced MACE but increased major bleeding, and the subgroup that appeared to derive the greatest benefit relative to risk was those with prior coronary revascularization. The composite of ALI or major amputation for vascular cause was defined as MALE, and there was a significant 54% reduction with ticagrelor relative to placebo.

Full Dose Anticoagulation

The use of anticoagulation as an adjunct to antiplatelet therapy has also been studied in PAD. The Warfarin Antiplatelet Vascular Evaluation (WAVE) trial randomized 2161 patents with PAD to warfarin, with an international normalized ratio (INR) target of 2–3 or placebo on a background of aspirin.[46] Overall there was no benefit of warfarin for MACE or MALE, but there was a greater than three-fold increase in life-threatening bleeding. The Dutch Bypass Oral Anticoagulants or Aspirin (BOA) Study Group trial randomized 2690 patients with PAD undergoing lower extremity bypass to the same two arms and similarly observed no benefit for MACE or MALE but did observed a 3.48-fold hazard of hemorrhagic stroke and a two-fold increase in major bleeding.[47]

Low-Dose Anticoagulation

The Rivaroxaban for the Prevention of Major Cardiovascular Events in Coronary or Peripheral Artery Disease (COMPASS) trial evaluated regimens of rivaroxaban 2.5 mg twice daily added to aspirin and rivaroxaban 5 mg twice daily alone and compared them each to aspirin monotherapy in high-risk patients (polyvascular, at least two risk factors, or older age) with CAD and/or PAD for MACE.[48] Overall the trial was terminated early for efficacy with a mean follow-up of 23 months. The rivaroxaban 2.5 mg twice daily plus aspirin arm was superior to aspirin alone for MACE, but rivaroxaban 5 mg twice daily alone was not. Overall this strategy significantly reduced MACE as well as the secondary outcomes of MALE and major amputation.[49] Rates of cardiovascular death and all-cause mortality were lower with rivaroxaban 2.5 mg twice daily as well. Bleeding with the regimen was increased, including a 70% increase in ISTH major bleeding. Benefits were consistent in the 4129 with symptomatic lower extremity PAD; however, due to enrichment, approximately 70% had concomitant CAD.[50] Subsequent analysis demonstrated that rivaroxaban 2.5 mg twice daily reduced MALE in patients with PAD (defined as ALI, urgent revascularization or amputation) by 46% with the greatest absolute benefit in patients with prior lower extremity revascularization.[49] The Efficacy and Safety of Rivaroxaban in Reducing the Risk of Major Thrombotic Vascular Events in Subjects With Symptomatic Peripheral Artery Disease Undergoing Peripheral Revascularization Procedures of the Lower Extremities (VOYAGER PAD) trial is evaluating rivaroxaban 2.5 mg twice daily versus placebo on a background of aspirin

100 mg daily as well as clopidogrel at the discretion of the treating physician.[51] Outcome from this trial will clarify the benefit and risk of this strategy in a dedicated PAD population, in the post-interventional period, and with regard to background $P2Y_{12}$ inhibition.

Summary: Antiplatelet monotherapy with either aspirin or clopidogrel remains the only antithrombotic therapy currently with a class I recommendation in PAD guidelines. Recent data demonstrate that more intensive regimens including the combination of aspirin and a $P2Y_{12}$ inhibitor, aspirin and/or clopidogrel with vorapaxar, and aspirin and rivaroxaban 2.5 mg twice daily reduce MACE in patients largely with PAD and CAD (polyvascular disease) as well as MACE and MALE in patients with prior revascularization. Full-dose anticoagulation with vitamin K antagonists have largely been harmful in this population, and there are no data to support other doses of factor Xa inhibitors. Ongoing trials will better define the optimal anti-thrombotic strategies after peripheral intervention. A personalized approach to antithrombotic therapy is recommended (Table 10.1).

Lipid-Modifying Therapies

A full overview of lipid-modifying therapy is provided in Chapter 6. The following section will focus on the evidence and indications in patients with peripheral artery disease. The epidemiologic data supporting the relationship of dyslipidemia to MACE is well established. Although relationships between several lipid parameters and outcomes have been described, the most robust literature for therapeutic intervention involves lowering low-density lipoprotein cholesterol (LDL-C). A number of large trials have established the benefits of LDL-C lowering through a variety of mechanisms in patients with atherosclerosis, with several showing consistency in patients with PAD. More recently, data describing the relationship of LDL-C and both the need for peripheral revascularization and MALE have been published, more clearly elucidating the role of LDL-C lowering in PAD. Finally, icosapent ethyl has been shown to be beneficial in terms of reducing MACE in patients with atherosclerosis and high triglycerides; however, the exact mechanisms are debated and the effect on MALE is not currently known.

Low-Density Lipoprotein Lowering

One of the first trials to robustly assess the effect of LDL-C lowering with statin therapy in patients with atherosclerosis, including PAD, was the Heart Protection Study (HPS), which randomized 20,536 patients to simvastatin or placebo and demonstrated a 24% reduction in MACE over a period of approximately 5 years.[52] The HPS trial

Table 10.1

Risk stratification and considerations for antithrombotic therapy in patients with PAD

Antithrombotic regimens studied in PAD	Patient risk profiles in PAD				
	Low Risk for MACE and MALE	High risk for MALE and low risk for MACE	High risk for MACE and low risk for MALE	High risk for MACE and MALE	
Monotherapy with aspirin or P2Y$_{12}$ inhibitor (n.b. clopidogrel monotherapy FDA approved for PAD)	Standard	Consider if high bleeding risk	Consider if high bleeding risk	Consider if high bleeding risk	
Aspirin and P2Y$_{12}$ inhibitor (n.b. DAPT with ticagrelor FDA approved for patients with prior MI or for CAD and diabetes mellitus including those with concomitant PAD)			Consider in PAD patients with high MACE risk (e.g. prior MI)	Consider in PAD patients with high MACE risk (e.g. prior MI) with benefit for MALE reduction	
Aspirin or clopidogrel + vorapaxar (n.b. vorapaxar FDA approved in PAD added to aspirin or clopidogrel)		Consider if at low bleeding risk	Consider if at low bleeding risk	Consider if at low bleeding risk	
Aspirin + rivaroxaban 2.5 mg twice daily		Consider if at low bleeding risk if approved in PAD	Consider if at low bleeding risk if approved in PAD	Consider if at low bleeding risk if approved in PAD	

DAPT, dual antiplatelet therapy; *FDA*, US Food and Drug Administration; *MACE*, major adverse cardiovascular events; *MALE*, major adverse limb events; *MI*, myocardial infarction; *PAD*, peripheral artery disease.

From Bonaca MP, Creager MA. Medical Treatment of Peripheral Artery Disease. In: *Vascular Medicine: A Companion to Braunwald's Heart Disease.* Philadelphia: Elsevier; 2020: Table 19.2.

included 6748 patients with PAD, and in this subgroup the benefit of simvastatin was consistent (22% reduction).[53] In addition, simvastatin was associated with a 20% reduction in the need for noncoronary revascularization; however, detailed data on the impact on MALE events was not described. Although several nonrandomized studies have observed lower rates of MACE and MALE with statin versus no statin or with high-versus low-intensity statins, there have been few other robustly powered randomized trials reporting outcomes in PAD.

Although some guidelines had previously focused on statin therapy for risk reduction, the Examining Outcomes in Subject With Acute Coronary Syndrome: Vytorin (Ezetimibe/Simvastatin) versus Simvastatin (IMPROVE-IT) trial demonstrated that further LDL-C lowering with the addition of the nonstatin therapy, ezetimibe, to statin therapy reduced the risk of MACE in patients with acute coronary syndromes (ACS). The subgroup with concomitant PAD and polyvascular disease was subsequently observed to have higher risk, particularly when combined with concomitant diabetes as well as greater absolute benefit with a number needed to treat (NNT) of 11 at 7 years in those with both features.[54] The IMPROVE-IT trial demonstrated that LDL-C lowering, even with nonstatin therapies, reduced risk in patients with atherosclerosis with consistent relative risk reductions in those with PAD.

Another mechanism of lowering LDL-C is through inhibition of the proprotein convertase subtilisin kexin type 9 (PCSK9), which acts as a chaperone carrying the LDL receptor from the surface of the liver to its destruction, thereby reducing the ability of the liver to uptake LDL-C and resulting in higher LDL-C levels. Two antibodies, evolocumab and alirocumab, have demonstrated sustained reductions in LDL-C and resulting reductions in MACE in patients with stable atherosclerosis (evolocumab) and ACS (alirocumab).[55,56]

Both the Further Cardiovascular Outcomes Research with PCSK9 Inhibition in Subjects With Elevated Risk (FOURIER) trial with evolocumab and the Evaluation of Cardiovascular Outcomes After an Acute Coronary Syndrome During Treatment With Alirocumab (ODYSSEY Outcomes) trial with alirocumab have reported data on patients with PAD and polyvascular disease. The FOURIER trial included 3642 patients with PAD and observed a consistent 60% reduction in LDL-C (from 92 mg/dL to 30 mg/dL) as well as a consistent relative risk reduction for MACE regardless of PAD status at baseline. Due to their higher risk, however, patients with PAD were observed to have a more robust absolute risk reduction (3.5% at 2.5 years, NNT 29).[57] Similarly, in ODYSSEY OUTCOMES, patients with polyvascular disease were higher risk, and the absolute risk reductions were greater with each increment in symptomatic vascular bed (ARR 3 years 1.4% one vascular bed, 1.9% two vascular beds, 13.0% three vascular beds, ARR interaction 0.0006).[58]

In patents with symptomatic PAD only (no prior MI or stroke), in FOURIER, the evolocumab for MACE were consistent; however, even without polyvascular disease, there was a robust risk reduction at 2.5 years (ARR 4.5%, NNT 21).[57] A novel aspect of this trial was the formal assessment of MALE as defined as the composite of ALI, urgent revascularization, or major vascular amputation. Treatment with evolocumab reduced MALE by 42% overall, and when combined as a composite of MACE or MALE in PAD without prior MI stroke, there was a 6.3% absolute risk reduction at 2.5 years translating into an NNT of 16.[57] The relationship of achieved LDL-C to risk of MALE as linear down to an LDL-C of less than 10 mg/dL (Fig. 10.4).

Other Lipid-Modifying Agents

The Fenofibrate Intervention and Event Lowering in Diabetes (FIELD) trial randomized patients with diabetes to fenofibrate or placebo. Although there was no significant reduction in MACE, there were lower rates of secondary endpoints including the need for peripheral revascularization. A subsequent analysis from this study also reported a 36% reduction in amputations. Ongoing studies of fibrate therapies are investigating their benefit in terms of reductions in MACE and limb outcomes.[59]

Several studies have evaluated polyunsaturated fatty acids and outcomes in peripheral artery disease; however, no consistent benefit for function or symptoms was observed. The Japan EPA Lipid Intervention Study (JELIS) was an open-label randomized trial of eicosapentanoic acid (EPA) in 18,645 patients with coronary artery disease. A small subgroup (n = 223) had PAD at baseline and were observed to be at higher risk for MACE and to drive a benefit from EPA (HR 0.44, 95% CI 0.19-0.97, $P = 0.041$).[60] A highly purified dose of EPA at 4 g daily was studied in the multicenter, randomized, double-blind, placebo-controlled study of AMR101 to Evaluate Its Ability to Reduce Cardiovascular Events in High Risk Patients With Hypertriglyceridemia and on Statin (REDUCE-IT) trial. The REDUCE-IT trial randomized 8179 patients with established cardiovascular disease or diabetes with other risk factors on statin therapy, and with fasting triglycerides of 135–499 mg/dL to EPA (4 g daily) or placebo. Overall there were significant reductions in MACE and cardiovascular death with benefits across the range of baseline triglycerides as well as for first and total events.[61-63] Novel therapies using small interfering RNA (siRNA) to lower LDL-C as well as therapies targeting other lipoproteins (e.g., lipoprotein[a] or Lp[a]) are under investigation. Genetic studies have suggested

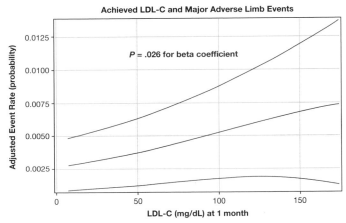

Fig. 10.4 The probability of major adverse limb event in patients randomized in the FOURIER trial by achieved low-density lipoprotein cholesterol (LDL-C) at month 1. Analyses adjusted for significant ($P < 0.05$) predictors of LDL-C at 1 month after randomization including age, body mass index, LDL-C at baseline, male sex, race, randomized in North America, current smoker, and high-intensity statin. (From Bonaca MP, Creager MA. Medical treatment of peripheral artery disease. In: *Vascular Medicine: A Companion to Braunwald's Heart Disease*. Philadelphia: Elsevier; 2020: Fig. 19.6.)

that the latter may be associated specifically with both incident PAD and PAD outcomes.[64]

Summary: Dyslipidemia, particularly LDL-C and Lp(a), are associated with incident PAD and higher risk of MACE and MALE in patients with PAD. Therapies to reduce LDL-C have demonstrated robust benefits in reducing both MACE and MALE in patients with PAD regardless of polyvascular disease. The risk and benefit of therapeutic intervention are reflected in current guidelines specifically identifying PAD as a high-risk condition for intensive lipid lowering. In addition, novel therapies such as icosapent ethyl, siRNA, and targeted therapies for Lp(a) hold promise for further risk reductions in PAD.

Glucose-Lowering Therapies

Drugs for diabetes are discussed in Chapter 4 in detail. The current section will focus on the evidence in patients with PAD including for limb outcomes.

Diabetes is a potent risk factor for the development of PAD. In addition, concomitant diabetes is associated with worse outcomes in PAD both for MACE and MALE. Diabetes and PAD are synergistic in their risk for outcomes such as amputation, as both macro- and microvascular disease independently contribute to risk.

Glycemic Targets in PAD

Data supporting the benefits of intensive glucose lowering for reducing macrovascular events in PAD are derived largely from broader trials of treatment in diabetes and cardiovascular disease and have been largely mixed. The Action to Control Cardiovascular Risk in Diabetes (ACCORD) trial investigated more versus less intensive glucose lowering to achieve a lower glycated hemoglobin in patients with cardiovascular disease ($\sim$1/3 with PAD) or risk factors, and the more intensive strategy demonstrated higher cardiovascular risk.[65] Similarly, the United Kingdom Prospective Diabetes Study (UKPDS) study randomized patients with T2DM to dietary restriction or intensive medical therapy, and while microvascular complications were reduced, there was no benefit for macrovascular outcomes. At 10-year follow-up, however, there appeared to be lower associated risks of MACE, suggesting that the benefits may only emerge after longer-term treatment.[66] Guidelines regarding glucose lowering in patients with vascular disease, and specifically PAD, generally follow recommendations for other patients with established cardiovascular disease. Clinicians should, however, pay even greater attention to foot hygiene, as patients with PAD and T2DM are at higher risk of not only amputation but also limb infections compared to patients with T2DM and no PAD.

Target Specific Glucose-Lowering Therapies

There are currently two classes of drugs that were designed to lower blood glucose and have specific impact for patients with vascular disease. The first is the class of inhibitors for sodium glucose cotransporter 2 (SGLT-2). The second are agonists of the glucagon-like peptide-1 (GLP-1).

SGLT-2 Inhibitors

There are three SGLT-2 inhibitors commercially available for which there are data to support use in patients with established atherosclerotic vascular disease. The first with outcomes data, empagliflozin, was found in the EMPA-REG trial to reduce ischemic events (myocardial infarction, stroke, and cardiovascular death or MACE) by about 14%.[67] In addition to benefits for MACE, there were robust reductions in hospitalization for heart failure and all-cause mortality. The population in EMPA-REG was characterized by known atherosclerotic vascular disease including peripheral artery disease.[68] In the subgroup of ~1400 patients with PAD, the benefits of empagliflozin were consistent, including significant reductions in cardiovascular and all-cause mortality. Limb outcomes were not prospectively adjudicated, but subsequent exploratory analyses showed no benefit or harm for amputation.

The CANVAS program studied the agent canagliflozin in a broader population including those with atherosclerotic vascular disease and those with risk factors.[69] Canagliflozin reduced MACE and the effects appeared most robust in those with cardiovascular disease versus those with risk factors only. An unexpected finding was a roughly twofold increase in amputations with canagliflozin with similar relative risks for major and minor amputation and for this with and without PAD; however, the greatest absolute risks were seen in patients with PAD and particularly those with prior amputation.[70] The excess in amputation risk was not seen in the subsequent CREDENCE trial that evaluated canagliflozin in patients with diabetes and chronic kidney disease; however, patients at high risk for amputation were excluded, and if a condition that put a patient at risk developed during the study, the drug was to be interrupted. In addition, the protocol called for excellent foot hygiene.[71] Whether the amputation risk with canagliflozin is a true finding or not, CREDENCE suggests that good foot hygiene and careful management in the small subset of patients at high risk for amputation would attenuate any such risk.

The third agent is dapagliflozin, which was studied in the DECLARE-TIMI 58 trial. Of the three outcomes trials this included the most patients with risk factors only and had coprimary endpoints of MACE and hospitalization for heart failure.[72] The benefits for heart failure were statistically significant and consistent in those with and without atherosclerotic vascular disease, effectively expanding the benefits to a broader population. Limb outcomes and specifically amputations were prospectively collected and reviewed by a blinded vascular specialist, and overall no imbalance in amputations was seen with dapagliflozin.

GLP1 Agonists

The glucagon-like peptide-1 (GLP1) agonists are a second class of agents that have demonstrated cardiovascular benefits. As opposed to the SGLT-2i, which appear to have the greatest benefit in terms of reductions in heart failure and mortality, the GLP1 agonists appear to have their greatest benefits for reducing ischemic risk.[73,74] Although early agents have been delivered parentally by injection, oral drugs are also available. The risks and benefits of this class are described in detail in Chapter 4. Of particular interest in the care of patients with PAD are observations that this class of therapy may reduce the risk of amputations.[75] Although confirmatory data are needed, lower rates of amputation have been observed in studies of at least one GLP1 agonist, and there have been no data to suggest any harm in terms of limb events.

Summary: Diabetes is a frequently comorbid condition with peripheral artery disease, and therefore diabetes management may be of particular interest for the vascular clinician. Glycemic control reduces the risk of microvascular complications such as neuropathy, which may predispose to lower extremity wounds and ultimately amputation. Both the SGLT-2 inhibitors and GLP1 agonists have shown consistent benefits in subgroups with PAD and should be considered in patients with PAD and diabetes. Deciding which to prioritize may be driven by comorbidities, with preference for SGLT-2i in patients with concomitant heart failure or at high risk of heart failure while GLP1 agonists may be preferred in patients at high ischemic risk and in those at high risk of amputation. Good foot hygiene is critical in patients with PAD and diabetes to reduce the risk of lower extremity infections and amputation.

Therapies for Symptoms

There are two approved pharmacotherapies for symptoms of claudication in patients with PAD. Both cilostazol and pentoxifylline are approved and available, although use overall is modest.

Cilostazol is an inhibitor of phosphodiesterase-3 (PD-3) and has been described as having effects on platelet aggregation, smooth muscle cell proliferation, and vasoactivity.[76-78] The exact mechanism by which cilostazol improves function is not known, although all of these effects may alone or in part have benefits in PAD. Several trials have evaluated the efficacy of cilostazol. A meta-analysis including 1258 patients with claudication found that cilostazol significantly increased maximal walking distance relative to placebo (50.7% versus 24.3%) with an absolute increase in walking distance of approximately 42 meters.[79] A subsequent meta-analysis of 3718 patients with claudication showed consistent benefits for claudicants.[76] Benefits appear sustained even after endovascular intervention.[80] Collectively these data demonstrate that cilostazol is superior to placebo at improving walking distance and delaying onset of pain in PAD.

There are, however, tolerability issues observed including gastrointestinal side effects, headache, and dizziness, which may limit or shorten use.[77,78,81,82] Although cilostazol is used more than pentoxifylline for this indication, most PAD cohorts describe use at 10% or less of patients. In addition, due to safety issues with other phosphodiesterase inhibitors, cilostazol is contraindicated in patients with heart failure. This is not due to any harm observed with cilostazol, but rather due to a warning across the class of agents. Because patients with PAD have class I indications for anti-platelet therapy, and in the post-intervention setting DAPT is often used, the question of bleeding risk with cilostazol may be of concern to the physician treating the vascular patient. Cilostazol does have antiplatelet and antithrombotic effects, but large outcomes trials powered for ischemic and bleeding events have not been conducted. Therefore, the interaction between therapies is not well characterized.[77,78,81,82] Large trials, however, of novel antithrombotics have not prohibited cilostazol and have not reported any heterogeneity in safety in those taking or not taking cilostazol. Therefore, a personalized approach should be taken, although cilostazol is generally not prohibited in patients on more potent antithrombotic regimens.

Cilostazol is prescribed at 100 mg twice daily. Patients may be started on 50 mg twice daily for 2–4 weeks to assess tolerability, with the dose titrated to 100 mg twice daily. In addition, patients taking drugs that are CYP3A4 or CYP2C19 inhibitors may reduce the dose to 50 mg twice daily. There is no dose adjustment recommended for patients with hepatic or renal impairment.

Pentoxifylline is a xanthine derivative that is a competitive nonselective phosphodiesterase inhibitor.[83,84] It has several downstream effects including inhibition of adenosine 2 receptors, increases in cyclic AMP, inhibition of tumor necrosis factor, and leukotriene synthesis reducing inflammation. It has also been described that exposure to pentoxifylline improves blood cell deformability and reduces viscosity as well as having a modest antiplatelet effect. For the vascular patient, pentoxifylline may be used on label for claudication symptoms and is sometimes used off label for the healing of chronic venous leg ulcers.

The data supporting the efficacy of pentoxifylline in PAD is modest. Meta-analyses have found that the individual studies are of low quality and with large variability and have concluded that the role in claudication remains uncertain.[85] A three-arm trial of cilostazol, pentoxifylline, and placebo was conducted and demonstrated that cilostazol improved function but pentoxifylline was similar to placebo.[86] Overall studies of pentoxifylline have shown that it is well tolerated. Contraindications include hypersensitivity to xanthine derivatives or recent retinal or cerebral hemorrhage, and there are cautions for patients at high risk of bleeding. Dosing is generally 400 mg every 8 hours, but the dose can be decreased to twice daily if gastrointestinal or other side effects occur. Dose modification to twice daily is also recommended for patients with a creatinine clearance less than 30 mL/min.

Summary: Claudication, and related functional limitation, is a major morbidity in PAD. Cilostazol and pentoxifylline are available and should be offered to appropriate patients with limiting claudication. Of the two, data supporting the efficacy of cilostazol are stronger and it is preferred as a first choice by practice guidelines.

Experimental Therapies for Peripheral Artery Disease

Vasodilator Drugs

Although the notion that dilation of the conduit arteries of the legs would lead to improved perfusion and improved symptoms in PAD is attractive, there are little data to support efficacy in this population. The lack of efficacy stands in contrast to that seen for angina in patients with coronary disease. There have been several studies evaluating the efficacy and safety of prostaglandin therapy in patients with claudication or CLI. Therapies evaluated include prostaglandin E1 (PGE1), prostacycline (PGI2), betaprost, and iloprost. These agents have been investigated as delivered both intraarterially and intramuscular. Although there are ongoing trials, completed studies have not observed benefits for CLI or function with these agents. A review of 33 trials and over 4000 patients randomized to therapy or placebo showed no benefit for amputation and higher risk of adverse events.[87] Trends suggesting small effects on rest pain and ulcer healing require validation in future studies.

Metabolic Drugs

Functional abnormalities in PAD are due to limitations in perfusion but also to maladaptation and metabolic dysfunction in affected muscle beds. Therefore, investigations into therapies that may improve metabolic efficiency and function have been conducted. Two such agents are L-carnitine and its derivative propionyl-L-carnitine. It has been hypothesized that by providing increased levels of carnitine, these agents will improve the Krebs cycle enhancing glucose and oxidative metabolism. Studies in claudicants, however, have shown no convincing benefit, and these agents remain largely investigational.[88] The piperazine derivative ranolazine induces metabolic effects that improve the efficiency of oxygen use. Ranolazine is effective and available for reducing angina in patients with coronary artery disease. A single-center pilot study observed benefits in function versus placebo as measured by pain-free walking time.[89] These findings require validation, and ranolazine is not currently approved for use in treating symptoms of claudication.

Angiogenic Growth Factors

Agents stimulating or promoting angiogenesis have been studied with the hypothesis that they may improve development of collateral vessels thereby improving overall perfusion. This improvement in perfusion may be beneficial for symptoms as well as treatment of CLI. This class includes vascular endothelial growth factor (VEGF), fibroblast growth factor (FGF), hepatocyte growth factor (HGF), and hypoxia-inducible factor 1 α (HIF-1α). Trials of these agents have not shown convincing benefit, although there have been promising signals for validation in smaller nonrandomized studies that require validation. A systematic review and meta-analysis found overall no benefit for gene therapy for angiogenesis for amputation, wound healing, or function PAD patients with claudication or CLI.[90] Currently these therapies are not recommended in patients with PAD.

Drugs for Venous Thromboembolism

Anticoagulant drugs are covered in detail in Chapter 8. The following chapter gives a focused review of their use in venous thromboembolism.

The mainstay of therapy for venous thromboembolism is anticoagulation. This can be delivered parenterally or orally. The strategy for initial treatment, switching, and long-term treatment is determined by the patient, comorbidities, and their risk in the acute and chronic settings.[91]

Parenteral Anticoagulants

Heparins are commonly used anticoagulants and can be delivered as unfractionated heparin (UFH), a sulfated glycosaminoglycan obtained from pig mucosa, or low-molecular-weight heparin (LWMH). The latter is more specifically directed at factor Xa and has greater bioavailability, a more predictable dose response, and longer half-life, all of which make it suitable for subcutaneous administration even at therapeutic doses, while UFH requires intravenous administration and frequent monitoring. Patients with impaired renal function require dose adjustment with LMWH, and dosing may be complex in patients with morbid obesity. The utility of titrating LMWH dosing to anti-Xa levels remains uncertain. A further derivative is the pentasaccharide fondaparinux. This injectable is an effective anticoagulant and has been administered in patients at risk for heparin-induced thrombocytopenia (HIT), although such use is off label. Two parenteral direct thrombin inhibitors can be used, bivalirudin and argatroban, but, their use in this setting is generally reserved for patient with or at risk for HIT.[92]

Oral Anticoagulants

As noted, these agents are covered in detail in Chapter 8. Available therapies include vitamin K antagonists (VKA) and the direct oral anticoagulants dabigatran, rivaroxaban, apixaban, and edoxaban (Box 10.1). Of particular relevance in the patient with acute VTE is the timing of initiation and dosing regimen. Dabigatran, a direct thrombin inhibitor, has been studied in the acute setting after a 5-day course of a parenteral agent and has not been studied as initial therapy.[93] Dosing for this indication after appropriate parenteral therapy is 150 mg twice daily, and it should not be used in patients with a creatinine clearance less than 30 mL per minute.

Edoxaban, an anti-Xa agent, was similarly studied after 5 days of parenteral therapy.[94] In this setting edoxaban should be given at 60 mg once daily. The dose should be adjusted to 30 mg once a day for patients with a creatinine clearance between 30 mL and 50 mL per minute, patients with a body weight ≤60 kg, or those receiving potent inhibitors of P-glycoprotein. For patients with creatinine clearance less than 30 mL per minute, edoxaban should not be used.

Rivaroxaban is another DOAC that is an anti-Xa agent. Its dosing in VTE is 15 mg twice daily for three week and then a maintenance dose of 20 mg daily.[95] There is no dose adjustment for renal function, but it should not be used in patients with a creatinine clearance <30 mg/dL.

Apixaban is a third anti-Xa and in its pivotal trial for VTE it was started without prior parenteral therapy and can be utilized in this manner for appropriate patients.[96] Dosing for this indication is 10 mg twice daily for 7 days followed by 5 mg twice daily. There

---

Box 10.1   Direct oral anticoagulants for acute venous thromboembolism

- Dabigatran 150 mg twice daily with a large breakfast and dinner—after 5 days of parenteral anticoagulation
- Rivaroxaban 15 mg twice daily for 3 weeks, then 20 mg once daily with the dinner meal
- Apixaban 10 mg twice daily for 1 week, then 5 mg twice daily
- Edoxaban 60 mg once daily (reduced to 30 mg once daily with low body weight or severe chronic kidney disease)—after 5 days of parenteral anticoagulation

From Goldhaber SZ, Piazza G. Management of venous thromboembolism. In: *Vascular Medicine: A Companion to Braunwald's Heart Disease.* Philadelphia: Elsevier; 2020: Box 52-3.

is no dose adjustment for renal dysfunction, but it should not be used in patients with a creatinine clearance <25 mL per minute.

Long-Term Secondary Prevention

Trials and observational studies have demonstrated that patients with VTE, even some with provoked VTE, remain at heightened risk of recurrent VTE. Careful patient selection is necessary in selecting an optimal duration. Options for long-term prevention include aspirin, which was studied in two randomized trials with a total of 1224 patients showing that versus placebo aspirin reduces the risk of VTE by 32% versus placebo.[97]

In addition to aspirin, oral anticoagulants can be used and have been studied at lower doses. Apixaban was studied in the AMPLIFY-EXTEND trial, which found that the 2.5 mg twice-daily dose was as efficacious for long-term prevention as the higher dose but with an excellent safety profile.[98] The EINSTEIN-CHOICE trial tested extended treatment with rivaroxaban 10 mg or 20 mg versus aspirin, with a significant reduction in recurrent VTE with both doses of rivaroxaban versus aspirin.[99]

Summary: Anticoagulant choice depends on the patient, setting, and VTE risk. Parenteral agents are often the first agents utilized, particularly in the hospital setting and when intervention is considered. In cases where an oral agent is desired as the initial agent, rivaroxaban and apixaban have trial data to support that strategy. Careful attention to dosing and timing is required in the setting of VTE and the dose adjustments that apply to other settings (e.g., atrial fibrillation) may not apply in VTE. Growing data supports the use of long-term prevention even in some patients with provoked VTE, and lower doses of apixaban and rivaroxaban have demonstrated efficacy and safety.

Drugs for Aortic Aneurysm and Dissection

Drugs for aortic dissection and aneurysm are largely directed at blood pressure and heart rate control and are discussed in detail in Chapter 2. In addition, smoking is a potent risk factor particularly for abdominal aortic aneurysm (AAA), and therefore, therapies discussed in the "Drugs for Smoking Cessation" section should be considered. Finally, AAA is associated with atherosclerosis, and therefore antiplatelet therapy and lipid-lowering therapies should generally be considered in patients with this condition, not with the aim of impacting the progression of AAA, but rather to reduce the risk of other major adverse cardiovascular events.

Initial Medical Management of Aortic Dissection

Rapid hemodynamic control is needed in patients presenting with acute aortic syndromes (AAS) unless there are contraindications such as shock or pericardial effusion. Aortic wall strain is a function of left ventricular (LV) contraction velocity (or change in pressure over time also called dP/dT); agents that reduce both heart rate and contractile force are first line in AAS. β-blocking drugs are preferred, although nondihydropyridine calcium channel blockers could be used in the small subset of patients with true contraindications to β-blockers. Importantly, vasodilators to reduce blood pressure should not be started prior to ß-blockade, as they may lead to a reflex tachycardia and actually increase dP/dT.[100]

Initial approaches to β-blockade are generally parenteral (Table 10.2). Options include metoprolol tartrate, which is B1 specific and has a half-life of ∼4 hours. It is dosed at 5 mg every 4 hours, and this dose as IV is generally equivalent to 25 mg orally. Doses of 5–10 mg every 4 hours are generally given as IV administration. For patients with significant systolic hypertension requiring more intensive blood pressure lowering, the mixed α and β-blocker labetalol is a common choice.[101] This agent has a half-life of ∼6 hours and is given as a 10–20 mg bolus at either interval dosing or an IV infusion

Table 10.2

Intravenous β-adrenergic receptor antagonists for the management of acute aortic dissection		
Therapy	**Dose**	**Receptor selectivity and half-life**
Metoprolol	5 mg bolus every 5 min for three doses; additional doses of 5–10 mg every 4–6 h as needed	$\beta_1 > \beta_2$ 3–6 h
Labetolol	10–20-mg bolus, repeat 20–40-mg bolus every 10–15 min as needed. Maintenance infusion 1–2 mg/min; maximum total dose of 300 mg	α_1-, β_1-, and β_2 ∼ 5.5 h
Esmolol	0.5-mg/kg bolus, then 50 µg/kg/min infusion	β_1 9 min
Propranolol	0.05 – 0.15 mg/kg every 4–6 h as needed	$\beta_1 \approx \beta_2$ 5–7 h

From Carroll BJ, Maron BA, O'Gara PT. Pathophysiology, clinical evaluation, and medical management of aortic dissection. In: *Vascular Medicine: A Companion to Braunwald's Heart Disease*. Elsevier; 2020: Table 32.1.

of 1–2 mg/min. The maximal daily dose is 300 mg. In contrast, for patients for whom there is concern about hemodynamic stability or tolerability of β-blockers, IV esmolol is notable for its short-acting properties. It is generally administered as a 0.5 mg/kg bolus and then 50 μg/kg/min as an infusion, and with its half-life of ~10 minutes it can be stopped quickly in patients with hemodynamic instability. Therapy should be titrated to a heart rate goal of ≤60 beats per minute as allowed by blood pressure.

Patients who require additional blood pressure lowering generally benefit from added vasodilator therapy. The target systolic blood pressure is <120 and ideally 110 mm/Hg. Sodium nitroprusside is a preferred agent in this setting and is started at 25 μg/min by continuous infusion. Doses can be titrated, but at a rate greater than 2 μg/kg/min, toxicity can occur due to cyanide concentrations, and measuring thiocyanate levels should be considered to prevent this toxicity. Of note, patients with renal insufficiency may be at increased risk, and alternative vasodilators such as nicardipine (calcium channel blocker), enalaprilat (ACE inhibitor), or hydralazine can be utilized.

Long-term Therapy in Aortic Dissection and Aneurysm

Patients with dissection who survive to discharge should be treated with a long-acting β-blocker. For patients treated with metoprolol tartrate as an inpatient, conversion to metoprolol succinate is recommended. For patients on labetalol, the longer-acting α and β-antagonist carvedilol can be considered. Change from short- to long-acting therapies improves adherence and avoids changes in heart rate and blood pressure associated with extended dosing intervals that go beyond drug half-life (e.g., twice-daily labetalol). ACEi are commonly used for additional blood pressure control, particularly in patients with other indications (e.g., atherosclerotic vascular disease, diabetes).[100] Long-acting dihydropyridine calcium channel blockers may also be used for blood pressure control.

Outpatient monitoring of blood pressure is critical in the dissection patient. Initial presentation is often characterized by a heightened sympathetic state requiring high doses of therapies. These may not be well tolerated as patients are followed long-term, and tapering may be required. Home blood pressure monitoring should be considered in order to optimize hemodynamic control.

In patients with AAA there is experimental and early clinical data suggesting that the antibiotics doxycycline and roxithromycin may reduce aneurysm growth rates. These findings require validation in larger trials and are not currently standard care.

Patients With Marfan Syndrome

Patients with Marfan are at heightened risk of aneurysm and dissection. Typically, β-blocker medications are utilized or, alternatively, nondihydropyridine calcium channel blockers. Animal models suggest a specific benefit of ARBs such as losartan due to their inhibition of transforming growth factor β (TGF-β); however, trials have not demonstrated benefits beyond blood pressure reduction and similar outcomes as atenolol in children and young adults with Marfan's syndrome.

Summary: Drugs for aortic aneurysm and dissection are centered around hemodynamics to reduce aortic wall stress. β-blockade and vasodilators are often used in combination to achieve heart rate and blood pressure targets. In patients with concomitant atherosclerosis, antiplatelet monotherapy and lipid-lowering therapies are used in accordance with practice guidelines for patients with atherosclerotic vascular disease.

Drugs for Vasculitis

Medical therapies for vasculitis generally fall into the class of drugs called immunosuppressive agents and should be prescribed and monitored by physicians familiar with their use. A broad spectrum of therapies has been used for vasculitis (Box 10.2). (See Box 10.3.)

Glucocorticoids

The glucocorticoids are often utilized in the acute setting of active vasculitis to stabilize the disease. They may be given orally or parenterally, and they may be given at a high, "pulse dose" with an aim of rapidly controlling disease. Long term, however, these agents carry significant toxicity that may result in immunosuppression, weight gain, osteoporosis, and other metabolic abnormalities. Therefore, for long-term control, other agents are often used along with or instead of glucocorticoids as "steroid-sparing agents."

Steroid Sparing Agents

A number of therapies can be used for long-term immunosuppression and treatment of vasculitis.[102,103] Cyclophosphamide is considered effective and is commonly utilized but has common toxicities including cytopenias and malignancy.[104] Alternative options include methotrexate, azathioprine, and cyclosporine. Few randomized or comparative trials exist, and choice should be based on the patient, comorbidities, and the disease being treated. Trials of rituximab have demonstrated efficacy for ANCA-associated vasculitis and have become part of standard therapy.[105,106]

Box 10.2   Treatments for inflammatory vasculitis

Commonly used medications/treatments
- Aspirin
- Glucocorticoids
- Cyclophosphamide
- Azathioprine
- Methotrexate
- Mycophenolate mofetil
- Cyclosporine and tacrolimus (FK506)
- Antiviral agents
- Plasmapheresis
- Intravenous immunoglobulin

Newer and/or experimental agents
- Rituximab (anti-CD20)
- Inhibitors of tumor necrosis factor-α
- Tociluzumab (anti–IL-6)
- Mepolizumab (anti–IL-5)
- Abatacept (CTLA4-Ig)
- Other experimental biologics

Surgical/invasive treatments
- Balloon angioplasty
- Intravascular stents ($\pm$ drug-eluting coating)
- Vascular bypass or replacement grafts
- Reconstructive surgery

From Markel PA. Overview of vasculitis. In: *Vascular Medicine: A Companion to Braunwald's Heart Disease.* Philadelphia: Elsevier; 2020: Box 39.2.

Box 10.3   Raynaud phenomenon

Conservative measures
- Warm clothing
- Avoidance of cold exposure
- Abstinence from nicotine
- Remove offending drug (if present)
- Behavioral therapy

Pharmacological interventions

Calcium channel blockers
- Nifedipine
- Diltiazem
- Felodipine
- Isradipine
- Amlodipine

> **Box 10.3   Raynaud phenomenon** (Continued)

Sympathetic nervous system inhibitors
- Prazosin
- Doxazosin
- Terazosin

Organic Nitrates
- Topical nitrates

Phosphodiesterase type-5 inhibitors
- Sildenafil
- Tadalafil

Classes of drugs with uncertain efficacy
- Selective serotonin reuptake inhibitors
- Vasodilator prostaglandins
- Thromboxane inhibitors
- Angiotensin-converting enzyme inhibitors
- Angiotensin receptor antagonists
- Endothelin receptor antagonists

Sympathectomy
- Stellate ganglionectomy
- Lumbar sympathectomy
- Digital sympathectomy

Botulinum Toxin Injection

From Henkin S, Creager MA. Raynaud Phenomenon. In: *Vascular Medicine: A Companion to Braunwald's Heart Disease.* Philadelphia: Elsevier; 2020: Box 46.3.

Raynaud Phenomenon

The episodic vasospastic ischemia of the digits is described as Raynaud Phenomenon. It generally occurs in two forms: primary, or idiopathic; and secondary, which occurs in the setting of an underlying associated disease state (e.g., collagen vascular disease, neurologic disorders, drug, toxins). Treatment includes conservative measures such as avoidance of cold and removal of associated drugs or toxins and pharmacotherapy (Box 10.3 from Vascular Medicine).[107]

Pharmacotherapies

A range of vasodilator therapy has been used for Raynaud Phenomenon.[108] The most commonly used therapies are of the calcium channel blocker class (see chapter on Drugs for Hypertension) including dihydropyridine agents.[109,110] These drugs can cause hypotension, which can limit dose titration. Other vasodilators including ACEi, angiotensin II receptor blockers, endothelin antagonists, nitrates, phyosphdiesterase Type 5 inhibitors, and vasodilator prostaglandins have all been described as potential therapies for Raynaud's. Sympatholytic agents affecting the nervous system are also utilized, including α blockers such as prazosin, doxazosin and terazosin.[111]

Other therapies that can be used as an alternative to or in conjunction with vasodilator therapy include selective serotonin reuptake inhibitors; however, only small studies describe efficacy, and additional trials are needed.[112] Botulinum toxin can be injected, and sympathectomy presents a surgical approach to the condition. In general, when vasodilator therapy is insufficient, consultation with a specialist is recommended.

References

Complete reference list available at www.expertconsult.com.

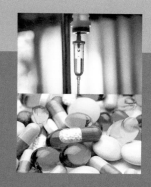

第11章
肺动脉高压药物

肺动脉高压是一类罕见的、异质性的、以肺血管系统发生病理性重塑并引起肺动脉压力升高，最终可导致右心衰竭、缺氧和死亡为特点的疾病。肺动脉高压被认为是脉管系统自身的原发性疾病，可由结缔组织病、药物、毒素、感染、遗传等一系列病因引起。另外，肺动脉高压约40%为特发性。

本章涵盖了肺动脉高压的病理学特点、临床分类、最新进展，并对药物治疗进行了详细介绍，还讲解了肺动脉高压治疗的"前世今生"。现有可用或已批准的药物类别包括前列环素类药物、内皮素拮抗剂、5型磷酸二酯酶抑制剂和钙通道阻滞剂等，并阐述其相关作用机制、药物不良反应及相互作用等。同时，本章阐述了不同种类药物的区别，如前列环素类药物中前列醇分类下的Flolan与Veletri、依前列醇与肠外曲前列环素、吸入曲前列环素与吸入伊洛前列素等。

本章覆盖了相关治疗指南，内容包括肺动脉高压的治疗原则、风险分层、血管反应阳性患者、无症状患者、初始联合治疗、初始单药治疗、序贯治疗等，还介绍了试验药物。

自从治疗肺血管扩张的药物面世以来，其不仅能够有效治疗肺血管扩张，而且肺动脉高压患者的预后也得到了极大改善。然而，对于患者和临床医师来说，肺动脉高压仍然是一个巨大挑战，并且仍然存在缓解这一疾病症状的需求。在强调精准医疗的当下，对肺动脉高压分子层面的新见解有望使下一代血管重塑药物成为可能。

　　　　　　　　　　　　　　　　陈安天

Drugs for Pulmonary Hypertension

STEPHEN Y. CHAN · MICHAEL V. GENUARDI

Drug Class Overview and Guidelines

Pulmonary arterial hypertension (PAH) is a rare, heterogenous family of disease states marked by pathologic remodeling of the pulmonary vascular system, leading to increased pulmonary artery pressure and ultimately right ventricular failure, hypoxia, and death.[1] Unlike the majority of pulmonary hypertension in the United States, which is secondary to either chronic lung disease or chronic left ventricular dysfunction,[2,3] PAH is thought to be a primary disease of the vasculature itself, triggered by an array of etiologic agents, including connective tissue disease, drugs or toxins, infections, genetic triggers among others, or is idiopathic in approximately 40% of cases.[4,5]

Pathobiology of Pulmonary Arterial Hypertension

Historically neglected due to its relatively rare prevalence, insights into the pathophysiology of PAH have led to a steady influx therapies for patients over the past two decades. Most of these therapies that primarily work by specific pulmonary vasodilation have been developed based on a now classical view of PAH characterized by a mismatch between vasodilatory and vasoconstrictive molecules in the pulmonary arteriolar tree. An important vasodilator, nitric oxide (NO), has long been identified as a key regulatory molecule in PAH.[6] NO is decreased in the pulmonary artery endothelial cells (PAECs) of diseased patients. A lack of NO triggers both loss of vasorelaxation mediated by cyclic guanosine monophosphate (cGMP) as well as smooth muscle cell proliferation.[7,8] Endothelin-1 (ET-1), a vasoconstricting small peptide is a second molecule implicated in PAH pathobiology. ET-1 has been shown to be overexpressed in PAECs of PAH patients.[9,10] Prostacyclin, a potent vasodilatory prostanoid, is a third important vasoactive small molecule. Prostacyclin, via cyclic adenosine monophosphate (cAMP), normally vasodilates smooth muscle cells but is decreased in afflicted patients.[11]

Most of the mainstays of modern PAH pharmacologic therapy operate via one of the pathways previously discussed. More recently, discoveries in the basic science of the disease are driving interest in new drug classes aimed at targeting the disordered and proliferative aspects of diseased arterioles in PAH. Development of these drugs are in various stages of implementation.

Updates in the Clinical Classification of PAH

The World Health Organization (WHO) organized the first World Symposium on Pulmonary Hypertension (WSPH) in 1973.[12] Since that time, pulmonary hypertension has been invariably defined as a mean pulmonary artery pressure (mPAP) $\geq$25 mmHg. PAH, or WHO group 1 disease, requires not only mPAP $\geq$25 mmHg but also the presence of precapillary pulmonary hypertension with pulmonary vascular resistance >3 Wood units in the absence of alternative causes of precapillary disease such as chronic thrombo-embolic disease, lung disease, or select rare other causes not considered to be group 1 etiologic agents.[1] At the sixth WSPH in 2018, however, the definition of pulmonary hypertension and PAH was changed. It is now recommended that a lower mPAP cutoff of >20 mmHg now be used to define pulmonary hypertension and PAH.[13] This change was made to better reflect the understanding that the typical upper limit of normal for mPAP is lower than the traditional 25 mmHg as endorsed by the older definition[14] and mPAP >20 mmHg is associated with worse clinical outcomes. As of this writing, the American Heart Association and American College of Cardiology PAH guidelines have not been revised to reflect the new WHO-endorsed position.[15] It is also unclear whether this new definition should drive the use of pulmonary vasodilator drugs in this population of formerly "borderline" PAH patients.

In addition to the change in PAH definition, three new oral agents have become available for treatment of PAH since 2013. Riociguat is a first-in-class soluble guanylate cyclase (sGC) stimulator that was approved in 2013. Riociguat achieves its augmented vasodilation via the NO-cGMP pathway. Later that same year, the United States Food and Drug Administration (FDA) approved an oral form of the prostanoid treprostinil (treprostinil diolamine) for use in PAH patients. Finally, in 2015, selexipag, a nonprostanoid oral prostacyclin (PGI_2) receptor (IP receptor) agonist, was approved for use to delay disease progression and reduce risk of hospitalization in PAH.

Currently Available/Approved Drug Classes

History and the Modern Era of PAH Therapy

"I would comment now upon the clinical picture of pure right ventricular failure. Usually one sees it secondary to failure of the left side, or the case is one of mitral disease with embarrassment of the pulmonary circulation... It is rare in my experience to witness such a pure and rapidly progressive failure of the right ventricle."

— Dr. Terence East, London, 1940, describing a series of three young women with rapidly fatal PAH.[16]

PAH was traditionally an invariably progressive and often fatal condition. Although it remains incurable (except by lung transplantation), PAH has become viewed in more recent years a more manageable chronic condition that can be marked by long periods of clinical stability. This is in large part due to the number of agents now available for patients with PAH and the expansion of dedicated PAH comprehensive care centers with expert multidisciplinary teams dedicated to this disease.

The modern era of PAH therapy began in the mid-1990s with the remarkable success of intravenous prostacyclin. In a landmark 1996 study including 81 patients with PAH followed for only 12 weeks, intravenous epoprostenol was associated with a reduction in pulmonary vascular resistance, 6-minute walk test (6MWT) distance, and mortality—100% of epoprostenol patients were alive at study end versus 80% in the control group.[17] Prior to the epoprostenol era, registry data of patients with idiopathic PAH showed a 1-year and 5-year survival of 68% and 34%, respectively.[18,19] These figures have slowly improved over the years. Over a decade later, results from the Registry to Evaluate Early and Long-term Pulmonary Arterial Hypertension Disease Management (REVEAL Registry) showed that the 1- and 5-year survival for idiopathic PAH patients had improved to 91% and 65%, respectively.[20]

Prostanoids

The first truly efficacious therapy in PAH, the prostanoid class of medications has now grown to include medications available in four routes of administration: intravenous, subcutaneous, inhaled, and oral.

Approved in 1996 on the basis of the randomized trial described previously, *epoprostenol* is the prototypical example of a vasodilatory agent used in PAH. Available only in intravenous formulation, epoprostenol has two available preparations: Flolan and Veletri, the latter designed to have enhanced room temperature stability.

Treprostinil is a synthetic prostanoid that is now available for use intravenously or subcutaneously (Remodulin), via inhalation

(Tyvaso), or orally (Orenitram). Like epoprostenol, treprostinil is a potent pulmonary vasodilator. It is distinguished from epoprostenol by its much longer half-life (4 hours versus 2.7 minutes for epoprostenol) and greater flexibility with respect to route of administration.

Approved in 2004, and only available in inhaled formation, *Iloprost* is the third currently available prostanoid for the treatment of PAH. It is marketed under the trade name Ventavis.

While not a true prostanoid by molecular structure, *Selexipag* (Uptravi) is an IP receptor antagonist, administered orally, and approved for use since 2015.

Endothelin Receptor Antagonists (ERAs)

With action against the ET-1 receptor, there are three ERAs currently available for use: *bosentan* (Tracleer), *ambrisentan* (Letaris), and *macitentan* (Opsumit). All are oral agents and have been proven efficacious in improving hemodynamics and symptoms in PAH.

Phosphodiesterase Type 5 Inhibitors (PDE-5is)

Orally taken, the PDE-5is vasodilate the pulmonary circulation via augmentation of the cGMP pathway. Two agents are available for use in the US, *sildenafil* (Revatio) and *tadalafil* (Adcirca). Vardenafil has been studied for use in a PAH population but is not approved for use in PAH by the FDA.

Closely related to PDE-5is are the sGC stimulators, of which the recently approved oral agent *riociguat* (Adempas) is the only approved agent.

Calcium Channel Blockers (CCBs)

Off-label use of CCBs, particularly *diltiazem* and *nifedipine*, and occasionally *amlodipine*, has long had a role in PAH, specifically in those with a positive vasoreactivity study on right heart catheterization.[21] To perform such a study, an operator with experience in PAH would place a pulmonary artery catheter in position, then administer a vasodilator, typically inhaled NO, intravenous epoprostenol, adenosine, or sodium nitroprusside. A drop in mPAP of ≥ 10 mmHg to a mPAP of ≤ 40 mmHg with stable cardiac output is defined as a positive vasoreactivity test. Approximately 5%–10% of treatment naïve patients will have a positive vasoreactivity test—a figure that may be higher in idiopathic PAH patients.[22–24] A 2010 analysis of approximately 2400 registry patients showed that 8.7% took CCBs specifically for PAH, a number that is consistent with the expected prevalence of positive vasoreactivity studies.[25]

Guidelines

Rationale and General Principles

In general, more aggressive therapy, including parental medications, is reserved for patients with more advanced and higher-risk disease. Correctly matching PAH therapy to a patient requires a careful and complete physiologic and historical assessment. Diligent evaluation of PAH patients, both at index presentation and longitudinally, is essential. The most important historical element is the patient's level of functioning. Often referred to as the WHO functional class (FC), it is modeled on the frequently used New York Heart Association functional status.[26] Briefly, FC I patients have no functional limitation. FC II patients have a slight impairment in physical activity, where ordinary causes symptoms such as dyspnea, chest pain, fatigue, or presyncope. FC III patients recall symptoms with less than ordinary daily activity, and FC IV patients are either symptomatic at rest, often with signs of overt right heart failure.

Patients with PAH often suffer from delayed diagnosis, meaning it is not unusual for PAH patients to first present with severe disease and advanced symptoms. In one study, a series of retrospective interviews with PAH patients revealed that patients averaged 5.3 general practitioner visits and 3.0 specialist visits prior to being seen in a PAH referral center—a process that took 47 months on average.[27] In REVEAL, 61% of patients were FC III at the time of diagnostic right heart catheterization and 12% suffered from FC IV.[25]

Initial workup of PAH will include detailed history and physical examination to determine the WHO functional class and assess for signs of right ventricular failure, including syncope, ascites, and edema. An electrocardiogram and echocardiogram are included in the initial evaluation of all patients.[28] At times, cardiac magnetic resonance imaging (MRI) can be helpful in quantifying the level of right ventricular dysfunction.[29-31] In patients in whom initial evaluation raises concern for PAH, and in patients with established disease but a change in clinical status, a right heart catheterization is required.[1,15]

Risk Stratification

The evaluation of the PAH patient should allow for risk stratification. Patients with more significant functional limitation are higher risk. In addition, patients with so-called "sentinel events" such as hospital admission, intensification of PAH therapy, decrease in 6MWT distance by 15%, or worsening WHO FC should be given heightened scrutiny, as these morbidity events have been shown to be predictive of incident mortality.[32]

The 2015 European Society of Cardiology/European Respiratory Society (ESC/ERS) guidelines proposed a simple low/moderate/high risk framework based on history, laboratory, and hemodynamic assessment (Table 11.1). Patients in the highest risk category should be considered for aggressive escalation of therapy.

Patients With Positive Vasoreactivity Studies

Guidelines support vasoreactivity testing during right heart catheterization in select patients with an initial diagnosis of PAH.[1,15,33] Contraindications include low blood pressure, reduced cardiac output, a diagnosis of pulmonary vasoocclusive disease, or pulmonary capillary hemangiomatosis (PVOD or PCH), as these patients may not tolerate an acute vasodilator challenge. Patients with FC IV would not be candidates for a trial of CCB even if vasoreactivity test were positive; therefore, it is of questionable utility to proceed with such testing in these patients.

For the 5%–10% of patients who do respond to vasodilator challenge and have FC II or III symptoms, current guidelines suggest a trial of CCB as initial therapy, with early repeat catheterization in 3 months to assess for response. Required doses are typically high; up to 240 mg for nifedipine, 20 mg for amlodipine, and 720 mg for diltiazem. Verapamil is not typically used or recommended for use in this indication, mostly over concern (perhaps based more on experience than data[34]) that verapamil is more potent negative inotrope than the other CCBs, including diltiazem.

Multiple concerns have been voiced for the use of long-term CCB in the PAH population. Most acutely, there is concern for the lack of direct evidence of benefit in the modern vasodilator therapy era, along with the theoretical risk of worsening inotropy on high-dose CCBs.[22,23]

Asymptomatic Patients

Patients without symptoms (WHO FC I) at diagnosis represent a rare clinical scenario. Current guidelines suggest close monitoring for the development of symptoms while withholding active therapy.[33] In such cases, careful examination, history, and functional testing may be required to determine if patients are truly asymptomatic. Occasionally, cardiopulmonary exercise testing, either invasive or noninvasive, may be considered to provide an objective assessment of severity of functional limitation and may be of use in borderline cases.[35]

Initial Combination Therapy

From the early 1990s until 2004, all PAH clinical drug trials tested single drug regimens against placebo or alternatives.[36] It was not

Table 11.1

Low/moderate/high risk assessment framework for patients with pulmonary arterial hypertension

Risk category est. 1-year mortality	Low <5%	Moderate 5%–10%	High >10%
Clinical signs of right heart failure[a]	Absent	Absent	Present
Progression of symptoms	Stable symptoms	Slow	Rapid
Syncope	Absent	Occasional; orthostatic or with heavy exercise	Frequent; especially with minimal activity
Functional class[b]	I, II	III	IV
6-minute walk test distance	>440 m	165–440 m	<165 m
CPET			
Peak VO$_2$	>15 mL/min/kg	11–15 mL/min/kg	<11 mL/kg/min
% Predicted	>65% predicted	35%–65% predicted	<35% predicted
VE/CO$_2$ slope	<36	36–45	≥45
BNP level	<50 ng/L	50–300 ng/L	>300 ng/L
NT-pro BNP level	<300 ng/L	300–1400 ng/L	>1400 ng/L
Imaging	RA area <18 cm^2	RA area 18–26 cm^2	RA area >26 cm^2
	No pericardial effusion	Trivial pericardial effusion	Pericardial effusion
Hemodynamics			
RA pressure	<8 mmHg	8–14 mmHg	>14 mmHg
Cardiac index	≥2.5 L/min/m^2	2.0–2.4 L/min/m^2	<2.0 L/min/m^2
Mixed venous SvO$_2$	>65%	60%–65%	<60%

CPET, Cardiopulmonary exercise test; BNP, brain natriuretic peptide; RA, right atrium.
[a]Signs of right heart failure include peripheral edema, hepatic congestion, decreased urine output, and ascites.
[b]Functional class I: no limitations; II: symptoms with ordinary activity; III: symptoms with less than ordinary activity; IV: symptoms with any activity or at rest.
Adapted from Galiè N, Humbert M, Vachiery JL, et al. 2015 ESC/ERS Guidelines for the diagnosis and treatment of pulmonary hypertension: The Joint Task Force for the Diagnosis and Treatment of Pulmonary Hypertension of the European Society of Cardiology (ESC) and the European Respiratory Society (ERS): Endorsed by: Association for European Paediatric and Congenital Cardiology (AEPC), International Society for Heart and Lung Transplantation (ISHLT). Eur Heart J 2016;37(1):67–119.

until the BREATHE-2 trial, which compared epoprostenol plus bosentan to epoprostenol plus placebo in patients with WHO FC III or IV, that initial combination therapy was rigorously tested.[37] Although it did not show significant difference in hemodynamics or clinical status, BREATHE-2 was an important first step toward initial combination therapy in treatment naïve individuals, and led the way for the AMBITION trial, published in 2015.[38] Comprised of patients with WHO FC II and III on no current PAH therapy, AMBITION was a three-armed protocol that randomized patients to ambrisentan plus tadalafil combination therapy or to each drug (plus placebo) alone. In contrast to BREATHE-2, AMBITION showed a marked reduction in a combined clinical endpoint of all-cause mortality, PAH hospitalization, and disease progression.

The 2015 ESC/ERS guidelines make no value judgment on starting combination therapy versus monotherapy in treatment naïve patients presenting with FC II or III,[1] citing the possible benefit of combination therapy seen in AMBITION but also the potential for increased drug interactions and side effects with upfront combination therapy. In contrast, the 2019 update to the American College of Chest Physicians (ACCP) guideline now recommends initial combination ambrisentan plus tadalafil for patients with FC II and III,[33] reflecting the advancing acceptance of the overall benefit profile of upfront combination therapy. This represents a change from the 2014 guidelines[39] and is given a grade of weak recommendation with moderate quality of evidence. Tables 11.2[1,40] and 11.3 outline selected regimens for initial combination therapy as supported by current guidelines and expert consensus.

Initial Monotherapy

Starting monotherapy in treatment naïve PAH patients, then adding additional agents sequentially based on patient response and tolerability is the more traditional approach to the management of PAH—albeit a decreasingly popular choice in light of the AMBITION trial data. In general, patients presenting with WHO FC II or III symptoms are recommended to begin with oral therapy; parenteral therapy is reserved for WHO functional class IV patients and those with high-risk features (Table 11.4). In the 2019 ACCP guidelines, the same therapy might have several different recommendation grades for a particular WHO FC, as the guidelines' authors may provide a separate recommendation grade for multiple outcomes. For example, there may be two recommendations provided for one particular drug: one for the endpoint of improving 6MWT and one for improving functional class. The summary information in Table 11.4 records the strongest recommendation given for each drug.

Table 11.2

Strength of recommendation and level of evidence schema in ESC/ERS and ACCP guidelines

European Society of Cardiology/European Respiratory Society (ESC/ERS)

STRENGTH OF RECOMMENDATION		LEVEL OF EVIDENCE	
Class I	Is recommended. Evidence or general agreement of benefit.	A	Data from multiple randomized controlled trials.
Class IIa	Should be considered. Weight of evidence or opinion is in favor of usefulness.	B	Data from a single randomized controlled trial or from high-quality observational studies.
Class IIb	May be considered. Usefulness/efficacy is less well established	C	Consensus opinion and/or evidence from small studies, registries, and other nonrandomized studies.
Class III	Not recommended. Evidence or agreement of lack of efficacy or harm		

American College of Chest Physicians (ACCP)

1A	Strong recommendation, high-quality evidence: Benefits clearly outweigh risks, evidence from multiple randomized trials or overwhelming evidence from nonrandomized studies.
1B	Strong recommendation, moderate quality evidence: Benefits clearly outweigh risks, evidence from randomized trials with limitations or high-quality nonrandomized studies.
1C	Strong recommendation, low-quality evidence: Benefits clearly outweigh risks, evidence from observational studies or case series only.
2A	Weak recommendation, high-quality evidence: Benefits closely balanced with risks, evidence from multiple randomized trials or overwhelming evidence from nonrandomized studies.
2B	Weak recommendation, moderate quality evidence: Benefits closely balanced with risks, evidence from randomized trials with limitations or high-quality nonrandomized studies.
2C	Weak recommendation, low-quality evidence: Benefits closely balanced with risks, evidence from observational studies or case series only.
UC	Ungraded, consensus-based statement of recommendation

Adapted from Galiè N, Humbert M, Vachiery JL, et al. 2015 ESC/ERS Guidelines for the diagnosis and treatment of pulmonary hypertension: The Joint Task Force for the Diagnosis and Treatment of Pulmonary Hypertension of the European Society of Cardiology (ESC) and the European Respiratory Society (ERS): Endorsed by: Association for European Paediatric and Congenital Cardiology (AEPC), International Society for Heart and Lung Transplantation (ISHLT). *Eur Heart J.* 2016;37(1):67–119; and Guyatt G, Gutterman D, Baumann MH, et al. Grading strength of recommendations and quality of evidence in clinical guidelines: Report From an American College of Chest physicians task force. *CHEST* 2006;129(1):174–181.

Table 11.3

Selected initial combination therapy for treatment naïve patients with pulmonary arterial hypertension, summary of professional society guidelines

Therapy	WHO FC	ESC/ERS, 2015[1] class/level of evidence	ACCP, 2019 update[33] grade
Ambrisentan + tadalafil	II	1/B	2B
	III	1/B	2B
	IV	IIb/C	–
Other ERA + other PDE-5i	II	IIa/C	–
	III	IIa/C	–
	IV	IIb/C	–
Bosentan + sildenafil + IV epoprostenol	III	IIa/C	–
	IV	IIa/C	–
Bosentan + IV epoprostenol	III	IIa/C	–
	IV	IIa/C	–
Inhaled prostanoid + PDE-5i + ERA	IV	–	UC[a]

[a]For patients unable or unwilling to manage parenteral prostanoids.
ACCP, American College of Chest Physicians; *ERA*, endothelin receptor antagonist; *ESC/ERS*, European Society of Cardiology/European Respiratory Society; *PDE-5i*, phosphodiesterase type 5 inhibitor; *UC*, ungraded consensus-based statement of recommendation; *WHO FC*, World Health Organization Functional Class.

Several key differences exist among the presently offered expert guidelines. The ACCP currently recommends starting an intravenous or subcutaneous prostanoid (epoprostenol or treprostinil) in patients with FC IV and issue no recommendation for oral agents in this scenario. The ESC/ERS guidelines do issue recommendations for specific oral agents as monotherapy in FC IV; however, these guidelines also make a statement recommending upfront combination therapy that includes an intravenous or subcutaneous prostanoid in such patients.

Sequential Therapy

For patients already started on initial monotherapy, a common strategy for treatment of PAH consists of short interval reassessment of symptoms and risk (Table 11.1) with consideration of sequential addition of therapies. This has been the approach often taken in the trial literature as well, where novel agents are often tested when added to established medications.

Table 11.4

Selected initial monotherapy for treatment naïve patients with pulmonary arterial hypertension, summary of professional society guidelines

Therapy	WHO FC	ESC/ERS, 2015[1] Class/Level of evidence	ACCP, 2019 Update[33] Grade
Calcium channel blockers[a]	II	1/C	UC
	III	1/C	UC
Ambrisentan	II	1/A	1C
	III	1/A	1C
	IV	IIb/C	–
Bosentan	II	1/A	UC
	III	1/A	1B
	IV	IIb/C	–
Macitentan	II	1/B	UC
	III	1/B	UC
	IV	IIb/C	–
Sildenafil	II	I/A	1C
	III	I/A	1C
	IV	IIb/C	–
Tadalafil	II	I/B	UC
	III	I/B	UC
	IV	IIb/C	–
Riociguat	II	I/B	UC
	III	I/B	UC
	IV	IIb/C	–
Epoprostenol, IV	III	1A	UC[b]
	IV	1A	UC
Treprostinil, IV	III	IIa/C	UC[b]
	IV	IIb/C	UC
Treprostinil, SC	III	I/B	UC[b]
	IV	IIb/C	UC
Treprostinil, oral	III	IIb/B	–
Selexipag	II	I/B	–
	III	I/B	–

[a]Only for use in patients with a positive vasoreactivity test
[b]In patients with WHO FC III symptoms but with rapid progression or other markers of poor prognosis
ACCP, American College of Chest Physicians; *ESC/ERS*, European Society of Cardiology/European Respiratory Society; *IV*, intravenous; *SC*, subcutaneous; *UC*, ungraded, consensus-based statement of recommendation; *WHO FC*, World Health Organization Functional Class.

In patients who continue to be symptomatic on stable doses of an ERA or PDE-5i, the addition of inhaled iloprost or inhaled treprostinil is guideline-supported. Riociguat is recommended as an addition to bosentan, ambrisentan, or inhaled prostanoid. Macitentan receives a recommendation as an addition to symptomatic patients on stable doses of a PDE-5i or inhaled prostanoid, and tadalafil as add-on therapy to ambrisentan.

In practice, drugs within a class are often substituted for each other, based on side effect profiles, availability or formulary access, and cost. This is done with the presumption that class effects may be interchangeable to varying degrees, but evidence does exist regarding the specific nature of activity of single drugs independent of drug class as well.

Mechanisms of Action

A mechanistic overview for important pathways of action for PAH drugs is shown in Fig. 11.1.

Prostanoids

Prostanoids were first indirectly described in the 1960s upon the discovery of a vasoactive substance that was downregulated by administration of aspirin.[41] Prostanoids were subsequently characterized as a family of 20-carbon eicosanoids (from the Greek είκοσι—"twenty") derived from arachidonic acid via oxygenation by cyclooxygenase (COX). The prostanoid family includes PGI_2, thromboxane A_2, and the prostaglandins, among other molecules. Most prostanoids share a five-carbon ring base with attached fatty-acid derived chains.[42] In the pulmonary hypertension literature, the term "prostanoid" refers almost exclusively to PGI_2, or epoprostenol, and a number of synthetic stable PGI_2 analogues, including treprostinil and iloprost. PGI_2 was discovered in 1976, and within 5 years its use was described in a patient with idiopathic PAH.[42] The potent vasodilatory properties of PGI_2 were recognized early on,[43] but a wealth of evidence now exists suggesting that beyond providing vasodilation to improve pulmonary vascular resistance, prostanoids have a wide array of other disease modifying effects.[44]

PGI_2 and its analogues bind the IP receptor on the cell surface membrane. Once engaged, the IP receptor couples the G-protein Gs and activates adenylyl cyclase, producing cyclic adenosine monophosphate (cAMP) and leading to relaxation in smooth muscle cells and antithrombosis in platelets.[44] Like PGI_2, treprostinil engages the IP receptor, but also demonstrates strong affinity to the EP_2 and DP_1 cell surface receptors. Ex vivo study indicates that

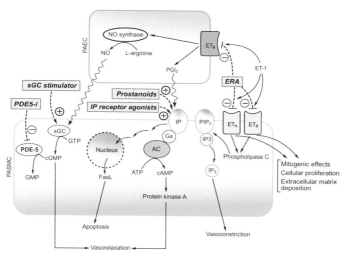

Fig. 11.1 Mechanisms of action for currently approved drugs for pulmonary arterial hypertension in the pulmonary artery smooth muscle cell (PASMC) and pulmonary artery endothelial cell (PAEC). Both prostanoids and prostacyclin receptor agonists engage the prostacyclin receptor (IP), which couples with the G-protein *Gs* to activate adenylyl cyclase *(AC)*, thus converting adenosine triphosphate *(ATP)* into cyclic adenosine monophosphate *(cAMP)* and causing vasorelaxation via activated protein kinase A. Moreover, prostanoids may provide proapoptotic effect via upregulation of transcription of the gene *FasL*. Both the phosphodiesterase type 5 inhibitors *(PDE-5is)* and soluble guanylyl cyclase *(sGC)* stimulators enhance vasorelaxation via the nitric oxide-cyclic guanosine monophosphate *(NO-cGMP)* pathway. Stimulated sGC increases production of cGMP from guanosine triphosphate (GTP), and inhibition of PDE-5i prevents hydrolysis of cGMP to guanosine monophosphate (GMP). The endothelin receptor antagonists (ERAs) oppose the action of endothelin-1 *(ET-1)* on its receptors, ET_A and ET_B. Both endothelin receptors have mitogenic and proliferative effects in PASMCs. Additionally, vasoconstriction is promoted via the production of inositol trisphosphate *(IP$_3$)* from hydrolysis of the phospholipid *PIP$_2$*. In the PAEC, ET_B is vasodilatory via the NO and prostacyclin *(PGI$_2$)* pathways; however, the net effect of ET_B activation in the pulmonary vasculature is vasoconstrictive.

the latter may have an increased role in dilation of pulmonary veins in addition to arteries; the clinical relevance of this finding is unclear.[45] Iloprost has also been shown to have action at the EP_4 receptor, an additional pathway of vasodilation.[46] Such a finding may be important therapeutically, as there is some evidence that patients with PAH have downregulated IP receptors, perhaps reducing their susceptibility to treatment with prostacyclin/epoprostenol.[47]

Beyond vasodilation, PGI_2 also has proapoptotic properties via the IP receptor.[48] This is particularly important given the recent attention given to the "cancer theory" of PAH. BMPR2, the most important gene identified in hereditary PAH,[49–51] has been implicated in dysregulation and proliferation (antiapoptosis) in diseased pulmonary artery endothelial cells.[52,53] Important activities are also held by the growth factors PDGF and VEGF, as well as a shift from oxidative metabolism to glycolysis in processes mirroring cancer pathogenesis.[54,55] There is evidence that prostanoids may directly interrupt some of these processes and may enhance apoptosis.[48] Treprostinil, for example, has been shown to reduce PDGF-related proliferative signaling.[56]

While not a prostanoid, selexipag also exerts its effects via the IP receptor. Selexipag is an orally available prodrug of MRE-269, a highly selective IP receptor agonist with a half-life of approximately 8 hours.[56] Unlike epoprostenol, treprostinil, and iloprost, selexipag does not appear to engage prostanoid receptors other than the IP receptor.[44,57,58]

Phosphodiesterase Type 5 Inhibitors

Selective PDE-5is leverage the action of endogenous NO in the cells of smooth muscle and other tissues. NO is produced in endothelial cells from L-arginine via NO synthase.[59] A small molecule, NO diffuses into smooth muscle adjacent to endothelial cells where it binds to sGC, stimulating production of cGMP from guanosine triphosphate. cGMP has potent vasodilatory effects by decreasing intracellular calcium concentration, leading to lower smooth muscle tone. It is rapidly hydrolyzed by PDE-5. The two currently approved PDE-5is for the treatment of PAH, sildenafil and tadalafil, both function to selectively inhibit PDE-5, thus augmenting the availability of cGMP and leading to vasorelaxation.[60]

PDE-5is can cause a certain degree of nondiscriminate vasodilation in both arterial and venous systems in healthy subjects.[61] However, affinity for the pulmonary circulation has been described in patients with PAH.[62] An early hemodynamic study found, for example, that pulmonary systolic pressures decreased over twice as much as systemic systolic pressures (14 mmHg versus 5.9 mmHg) after 3 months of sildenafil treatment in PAH patients.[63] The underlying reason for this is only partially clear. It has been proposed that atrial natriuretic peptide, found in increased concentration in PAH patients, may act synergistically with the NO-cGMP pathway to selective vasodilate the pulmonary circulation.[64,65]

Like prostanoids, there is evidence that PDE-5is have important disease-modifying effects outside of vasodilation. One intriguing possibility is that PDE-5is may improve dysfunctional signaling in PAH patients with abnormal bone morphogenetic protein (BMP). Pulmonary artery smooth muscle cells carrying loss-of-function mutations in *BMPR2* tend to become proproliferative via decreased and/or altered BMP and SMAD 1/5/8 signalling.[52,66,67] In a *BMPR2* knockout animal model, sildenafil has been shown to prevent development of PAH and partially restore SMAD signaling.[68]

Riociguat, the only available sGC stimulator, has a mechanism closely related to PDE-5is, in that it is active directly via the NO-cGMP pathway. The original synthesis of riociguat was propelled by the discovery in the 1990s that YC-1, a related compound originally discovered as a synthetic benzylindazole antiplatelet agent, had sGC stimulatory properties.[69,70] Riociguat binds sGC and increases production of cGMP from GTP in a NO-independent manner. Synergism with NO is also possible. *In vitro*, sGC activity is increased 122-fold by riociguat in the presence of NO, and 73-fold when riociguat acts alone.[71]

Endothelin Receptor Antagonists

A potent vasoconstrictor, ET-1 is a 21-amino-acid peptide overexpressed in patients with PAH.[9] ET-1 is produced mainly in endothelial cells—it is not stored and both transcription its mRNA and ET-1 itself have relative short half-lives (10–20 minutes), meaning that ET-1 levels may fluctuate in response to a myriad stimulators.[72] Notable stimuli include hypoxia, ischemia, shear stress. ET-1 has two cellular targets relevant to PAH therapeutics. Endothelin receptor A (ET_A) is found on the surface of pulmonary artery smooth muscle cells, while endothelin receptor B (ET_B) is found both on pulmonary artery smooth muscle cells and endothelial cells.[60]

ET-1 has mitogenic properties via both ET_A and ET_B; the overall effect is to increase extracellular matrix proliferation as well as potentiation of growth factors such as TGF-β.[73,74] On the smooth muscle cell, the binding of ET-1 to both ET_A and ET_B activates phospholipase C and promotes vasoconstriction via production of inositol triphosphate, which raises intracellular calcium. The vasoactive effects of ET_B on endothelial cells are more complex. ET-1 binding endothelial cells may increase NO production, leading to vasorelaxation. However, the vasodilatory properties of ET-1, acting at the ET_B receptor, appear to be impaired in PAH-afflicted patients.[60] In sum, the net effect of ET-1 on the pulmonary circulation is vasoconstriction and cellular proliferation.[75,76]

Differences Among Drugs in Class

The full list of currently available PAH-specific drug therapies approved for use in the United States is presented in Table 11.5. Specific and important intraclass differences between agents are discussed later.

Prostanoids

With three agents, four routes of administration, and multiple formulations available for epoprostenol, prostanoids may lead to some confusion among patients and providers not accustomed to PAH therapy. Prostanoids are available in oral, intravenous, subcutaneous, and inhaled forms, making it the only class of PAH medications that is available with more than one route of administration. Table 11.6[17,77–91] compares pharmacologic profiles of available agents in this class.

Epoprostenol: Flolan Versus Veletri

Epoprostenol is available in two formulations, usually referred to by their US trade names, Flolan (GlaxoSmithKline) and Veletri (Actelion).[92] Epoprostenol as a PAH therapy was approved in 1995. Formulated with glycine-mannitol excipients, reconstituted Flolan has stability at room temperature for up to 8 hours. This can be extended for up to 24 hours with the use of ice packs; however, the need for refrigeration beyond this time causes some logistical difficulties with administration, especially for patients on home therapy.[93] Veletri, which uses arginine-mannitol excipients at a higher pH, was approved by the FDA in 2008 on the basis of having an identical active ingredient to Flolan. Although rigorous pre-approval testing of the new formulation was not required prior to approval, small postmarketing studies have shown equivalence of Flolan and Veletri with respect to tolerability, effect, and bioavailability.[94,95]

Epoprostenol Versus Parenteral Treprostinil

The synthetic prostanoid treprostinil has a similar mechanism of action and side effect profile to epoprostenol.[96] Initially formulated as a subcutaneous infusion to reduce risk associated with indwelling central catheters and approved in 2002, treprostinil is additionally distinguished from epoprostenol by its much longer half-life. Since initial approval, an intravenous form has been made available. Reconstituted treprostinil has excellent stability at room temperature and may be stored for up to 14 days once mixed with

Table 11.5

Drug therapies currently approved for use in pulmonary arterial hypertension

Drug	US trade name(s)	Route	Mechanism of action	Notable class-wide side effects	High-level evidence
Prostanoids					
Epoprostenol	Flolan, Veletri	IV	Stimulation of IP and other prostanoid receptors. Effects vasodilation and antiproliferation.	Nausea, headaches, diarrhea, flushing, hypotension, high-output heart failure, bleeding. Injection site pair and/ or infection where applicable.	Barst et al.[17]
Iloprost	Ventavis	Inhaled			Olschewki et al.[77] TRUST[78]
Treprostinil	Remodulin	IV SC			Simonneau et al.[79]
	Tyvaso	Inhaled			TRIUMPH-I[80]
	Orenitram	Oral			FREEDOM-C[81] FREEDOM-C2[82]
IP receptor agonists					
Selexipag	Uptravi	Oral	Direct stimulation of IP receptor.	Headache, diarrhea, nausea, flushing. Avoid in severe hepatic impairment.	GRIPHON[83]

Continued on following page

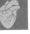

Table 11.5

Drug therapies currently approved for use in pulmonary arterial hypertension (Continued)

Drug	US trade name(s)	Route	Mechanism of action	Notable class-wide side effects	High-level evidence
Phosphodiesterase type 5 inhibitors					
Sildenafil	Revatio	Oral	Inhibition of PDE-5, leading to increased NO-cGMP pathway activation and vasodilation.	Hypotension, flushing, diarrhea, priapism	SUPER[84] PHIRST[85] PHIRST2[86]
Tadalafil	Adcirca	Oral			
Guanylate cyclase stimulators					
Riociguat	Adempas	Oral	Direct stimulation of sGC leading to cGMP production	Headache, dyspepsia, dizziness, nausea, diarrhea, hypotension	PATENT-1[87]
Endothelin receptor antagonists					
Bosentan	Tracleer	Oral	ET$_A$ and ET$_B$ antagonism, preventing ET-1 mediated vasoconstriction and proliferation	Hepatotoxicity, anemia, pulmonary edema, peripheral edema, nasal congestion, sinusitis	Channick, et al.[88] BREATHE-1[89]
Ambrisentan	Letairis	Oral			ARIES[90]
Macitentan	Opsumit	Oral			SERAPHIN[91]

IV, intravenous; *PDE-5*, phosphodiesterase type 5; *NO-cGMP*, nitric oxide- cyclic guanosine monophosphate; *sGC*, soluble guanylate cyclase; *SC*, subcutaneous.

Table 11.6

Prostanoids: available agents and drug characteristics

Drug	US trade name	Route of administration	Typical dose range	Half-life	Comments	Metabolism
Epoprostenol	Flolan	IV	2–40+ ng/kg/min	6 min	Stable for 8 hours at room temperature or 24–48 hours if refrigerated at 2–8°C	Spontaneous degrades. Metabolites are primarily recovered in urine.
	Veletri	IV			Stable for 48–72 hours at room temperature or 8 days if refrigerated at 2–8°C	
Iloprost	Ventavis	Inhaled	2.5–5 µg; 6 to 9 times daily	20–30 mins		Inactivated by β-oxidation and excreted in urine.
Treprostinil	Remodulin	IV	1.25–100+ ng/kg/min	4.5 hours	IV and SC have dose equivalency in normal therapeutic dose ranges	Hepatic metabolism via CYP2C8 and excreted in urine. Clearance significantly impaired in liver dysfunction.
	Remodulin	SC				
	Orenitram	Oral	0.25–16 mg BID			
	Tyvaso	Inhaled	3–9 breaths QID	4.5 hours		

IV, intravenous; *SC*, subcutaneous.

proper dilutents.[97] At the molecular level, epoprostenol and treprostinil have similar structure and engage similar targets.

The half-life of treprostinil is approximately 4.5 hours, but the effective half-life may be shorter.[96,98] Based on bioavailability studies, it appears that subcutaneous and intravenous treprostinil have dosing equivalence through the normal therapeutic range (up to 125 ng/kg/min).[99] There may be some depot effect from subcutaneous administration of treprostinil such that the drug serum concentration takes longer to decline as compared to intravenous administration, but this difference does not appear to be clinically meaningful.

Unlike epoprostenol, which is spontaneously metabolized, treprostinil is extensively cleared by the cytochrome P450 system in the liver. Strong modifiers of CYP2C8 should be used with caution in patients receiving treatment with treprostinil. Intravenous and subcutaneous treprostinil should be dose-reduced in patients with mild to moderate hepatic impairment; no studies have been done in patients with severe hepatic impairment.[97] Patients with liver dysfunction are more vulnerable to toxicity with treprostinil diolamine (oral treprostinil) due to lack of normal first past metabolism. As a result, treprostinil diolamine should be dose-reduced in patients with Child-Pugh A hepatic dysfunction and should be avoided and is contraindicated in Child-Pugh B and C disease.[100,101]

Inhaled Treprostinil Versus Inhaled Iloprost

Inhaled iloprost is designed to be administered in a specially made delivery device. For patients who self-administer iloprost at home, some dexterity is required in order to break the vials storing the medication and pipette the contents into the delivery device, which may need to be done several times per day depending on dosage.[102] Inhaled treprostinil is delivered via an ultrasonic pulsed-delivery device that meters out 6 µg of drug per inhalation. The device is loaded each morning with treprostinil from an ampule by the patient.[103] The longer half-life of treprostinil allows for QID dosing, as compared to up to nine times daily for iloprost.[100]

Phosphodiesterase Type 5 Inhibitors

Table 11.7 summarizes the important differences between the two available PDE-5is. The primary difference between sildenafil and tadalfil is pharmacokinetics and elimination half-life. Sildelafil is extensively metabolized by the liver, mostly by CYP3A4, and to a lesser extent CYP2C9.[104] Its half-life of 4 hours is substantially short than that of tadalfil (15 hours). Both PDE-5is are metabolized by the liver, predominantly by CYP3A4. While use of both appear safe in

Table 11.7

Properties of available phosphodiesterase type 5 inhibitors

Drug	US trade name	Route of administration	Typical dose range	Half-life	Comments	Metabolism
Sildenafil	Revatio	Oral[a]	5–20 mg TID	4 hours		Hepatically metabolized by CYP3A4, CYP2C9
Tadalafil	Adcirca	Oral	10–40 mg daily	15 hours		Hepatically metabolized by CYP3A4

[a]An injectable form of sildenafil is available for patients on sildenafil therapy who are temporarily unable to take oral medications.

patients with mild or moderate hepatic dysfunction, use in patients with Child-Pugh C liver disease has not been established.[105]

Endothelin Receptor Antagonists

Key considerations in the use of the three available ERAs are summarized in Table 11.8. Bosentan, the first ERA to market in the United States, is dosed twice daily, with a shorter half-life than either ambrisentan or macitentan. While all three drugs are hepatically metabolized, only bosentan is both a substrate and inducer of the cytochrome P450 system, specifically CYP2C9 and CYP3A4, leading to significant concern for drug-drug interactions.[106] All three drugs should be used with caution in severe hepatic impairment due to metabolism. In addition, bosentan has been associated with risk of true hepatotoxicity, a concern which may or may not be associated with ambrisentan and macitentan. A recent meta-analysis of clinical trials of ERAs supported this unique risk of bosentan, with a risk ratio for abnormal liver function tests of 3.8 [95% CI, 2.4, 5.9] compared to placebo.[107] Monthly monitoring of liver function tests was formerly suggested for all patients on ERAs,[15] but currently only applies to bosentan in the US.[1]

Bosentan is a nonselective inhibitor of both ET_A and ET_B. However, due to the partial vasodilatory effects of ET_B, there was considerable interest in finding an ET_A-selective ERA, leading to the development and subsequent approval of ambrisentan in 2007.[106] Macitentan, the newest ERA on the market, is a dual (ET_A/ET_B) antagonist with high-affinity ET_A in particular. It was developed with the goal of improved safety in a dual-receptor ERA.[108]

Data for Use

The modern drug therapy era for PAH began with the demonstration of a mortality benefit for patients treated with epoprostenol in 1996, published via a randomized trial by Barst and colleagues.[17] Since that time, while the prognosis has improved for PAH patients treated with epoprostenol suggesting improvement in overall mortality,[20] no other drug has been proven to offer a definitive mortality benefit for patients across any FC and diagnosis subtype. This may be attributable to improvement in nonpharmacologic management or diminishing returns for each additive therapy. Perhaps most notably, as PAH disease progression has slowed in the current era of drug therapy, it becomes more challenging to power a randomized trial for a mortality endpoint. Since regulatory agencies increasingly have been willing to base approval on surrogate (yet

Table 11.8

Properties of available endothelin receptor antagonists

Drug	US trade name	Route of administration	Typical dose range	Half-life	Comments	Metabolism
Bosentan	Tracleer	Oral	62.5–125 mg BID	5 hours	Nonselective antagonist of both ET_A and ET_B. Inducer of CYP2C9 and CYP3A4.	Hepatic: CYP2C9 and CYP3A4
Ambrisentan	Letairis	Oral	5–10 mg daily	13.6–16.5 hours	Selective ET_A antagonist.	Hepatic: UGT, CYP3A4, CYP2C19
Macitentan	Opsumit	Oral	10 mg daily	17 hours	Nonselective ERA but with significant affinity for $ET_A > ET_B$.	Hepatic: primarily CYP3A4

ERA, endothelin receptor antagonist; ET_A, endothelin receptor A; ET_B, endothelin receptor B;

still patient-centered) outcomes such as 6MWT time or worsening of WHO FC, incentives have decreased for drug developers and other investigators to design trials with an endpoint of mortality. Selected discussion of key trials leading to medication approval or clinical practice change are discussed in this section. A summary of high-level evidence is presented in Table 11.5.

Combination Therapy

Tadalafil and Ambrisentan

Upfront combination in treatment naïve PAH patients with WHO FC II or III symptoms is now recommended as the first choice by the 2019 ACCP guideline.[33] This recommendation is based largely on the AMBITION trial, published in 2015.[38] In this study, 500 participants with treatment naïve PAH and FC II or III symptoms were randomized, in 2:1:1 ratio, to combination ambrisentan and tadalafil versus each drug as monotherapy. In the combination therapy group, 18% of participants reached a primary endpoint event (a composite of death, hospitalization for worsening PAH, or disease progression) compared to 31% in the pooled monotherapy group (Fig. 11.2).

Monotherapy and Sequential Therapy

Prostanoids

Barst and colleagues demonstrated the efficacy of intravenous epoprostenol in 81 patients with PAH and WHO FC III or IV symptoms as compared to placebo. After just 12 weeks of epoprostenol therapy, patients randomized to epoprostenol demonstrated improved 6MWT distance, lower mPAP, and lower pulmonary vascular resistance. In addition, there were eight deaths in the control group (20%) and none in the active therapy group.[17]

Continuous subcutaneous treprostinil infusion was demonstrated to be effective by Simonneau and colleagues in 2002.[79] In addition to background therapy (which notably did not include modern ERAs or PDE-5is), infusion of subcutaneous treprostinil lead to improved hemodynamics and 6MWT distance versus placebo in 470 patients with PAH and WHO FC II, III, or IV symptoms.

Treprostinil diolamine (orally administered treprostinil) was tested in the FREEDOM series of trials.[81,82,109] In FREEDOM-C and FREEDOM-C2, the addition of treprostinil diolamine to background therapy including ERA and/or PDE-5i did not improve 6MWT, the primary outcome, compared to placebo. However, in the FREEDOM-M investigation of treprostinil diolamine in patients not currently on ERA of PDE-5i therapy, patients assigned to treprostinil showed an

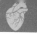

COMBINATION THERAPY VS. POOLED MONOTHERAPY

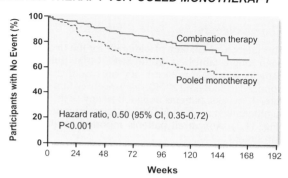

No. at Risk								
Combination therapy	253	229	186	145	106	71	36	4
Pooled monotherapy	247	209	155	108	77	49	25	5

Fig. 11.2 **Upfront combination therapy with ambrisentan and tadalafil versus monotherapy in treatment naïve pulmonary arterial hypertension (PAH) patients with functional class II or III symptoms, from the AMBITION trial.** In this placebo-controlled, randomized trial, 500 patients with PAH and not previously treated were assigned, in 2:1:1 ratio, to initial combination therapy with 10 mg of ambrisentan plus 40 mg of tadalafil (combination-therapy group), 10 mg of ambrisentan plus placebo, or 40 mg of tadalafil plus placebo. Freedom from the primary combined endpoint is shown in the figure for the combination therapy group versus the two monotherapy groups combined. The primary combined endpoint was any of following: death of any cause, hospitalization for worsening PAH, disease progression, or unsatisfactory clinical response, the latter two assessed via functional class and 6-minute walk test distance. (Modified from Galiè N, Barberà JA, Frost AE, et al. Initial use of ambrisentan plus tadalafil in pulmonary arterial hypertension. *N Engl J Med* 2015;373(9):834–844.)

increase in 6MWT of 23 meters. Results from the FREEDOM-EV study, quantifying mortality and morbidity outcomes of oral treprostinil on top of initial monotherapy, await formal release.

IP Receptor Agonists

The novel oral IP receptor agonist selexipag was tested in the multicenter GRIPHON study of patients who were either treatment-naïve (20% of enrollees) or on stable background therapy of an ERA, PDE-5i, or both.[83] This study, conducted in 1156 patients, demonstrated a 40% reduction in a composite endpoint of death or worsening PAH for selexipag versus placebo. The vast majority of patients were WHO FC II or III at enrollment. A slight majority of the study population (56%) had idiopathic PAH.

Phosphodiesterase Type 5 Inhibitors

The safety and efficacy of sildenafil for the treatment of PAH have been long established. In the SUPER trial, published in 2005, 278 patients with PAH not currently on vasodilator therapy were randomized to sildenafil 20, 40, or 80 mg three times daily or placebo.[84] After 12 weeks, patients assigned to any of the sildenafil arms had significantly improved 6MWT distance from baseline over placebo (Fig. 11.3). Almost all patients reported FC II or III symptoms at enrollment.

Tadalafil was tested in the multicenter PHIRST trial, which randomized 405 patients with PAH to tadalafil 2.5, 10, 20, or 40 mg daily or placebo.[85] Patients were either treatment naïve or on stable background therapy with full dose bosentan (125 mg twice daily).

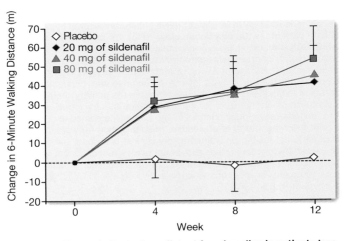

Fig. 11.3 Change in 6-minute walk test from baseline in patients treated with sildenafil versus placebo from the SUPER trial. In a placebo-controlled randomized clinical trial, 278 patients with pulmonary arterial hypertension (PAH) were randomly assigned 1:1:1:1 to monotherapy with sildenafil 20, 40, or 80 mg three times daily or placebo. Figure shows the change from baseline 6-minute walk test distance at week 12 for each of the four arms. There was significant improvement compared to baseline in all active arms; in contrast, no difference was seen in patients taking placebo. (Modified from Galiè N, Ghofrani HA, Torbicki A, et al. Sildenafil citrate therapy for pulmonary arterial hypertension. *N Engl J Med* 2005;353(20):2148–2157.)

Tadalafil 10, 20, and 40 mg daily (but not 2.5 mg) showed efficacy in improving 6MWT distance over placebo. In addition, the high-dose group (40 mg daily) showed significantly improved time to clinical worsening over placebo.

Soluble Guanyl Cyclase Stimulators

The sGC stimulator riociguat was proven efficacious in the 443 patient PATIENT-1 trial.[87] Included patients suffered from PAH and were either taking no background therapy (50% of participants) or were taking stable doses of an ERA and/or a prostanoid (excluding intravenous prostanoid). Participants were randomized to placebo or riociguat, individually adjusted, up to 2.5 or 1.5 mg three times daily. After 12 weeks, the mean difference in 6MWT between the 2.5 mg riociguat group and placebo was 36 meters. This was accompanied by hemodynamic improvements, including lower pulmonary vascular resistance, lower mPAP, and higher cardiac output in the riociguat group.

Endothelin Receptor Antagonists

Bosentan was the first oral vasodilator proven to benefit patients with PAH. Compared to placebo in FC III and IV patients taking no other therapy, it was shown to improve symptoms and increase 6MWT (BREATHE-1).[89] The follow-up study, BREATHE-2, which randomized patients (approximately 75% FC III and 25% FC IV) to epoprostenol versus epoprostenol plus bosentan, did not show a significant difference in outcomes between the two groups.[37]

Monotherapy with ambrisentan was evaluated in the concurrent ARIES-1 and ARIES-2 studies, each testing several dosing alternatives to placebo in PAH patients with predominantly FC III presentations on no other therapy. Subjective dyspnea, as well as 6MWT distance, improved at the end of the 12-week study period.[90] SERAPHIN was a modern trial of macitentan, the newest ERA, for use as either monotherapy or add-on therapy in PAH.[91] Approximately two-thirds of the 250 patients randomized were taking a PDE-5i at randomization. Macitentan 10 mg daily was associated with a 45% reduction in the primary composite endpoint, a combination of death or disease worsening.

Side Effects

Almost invariably, PAH therapies are associated with side effects of vasodilation—generally with severity directly related to agent potency. Various class-wide side effects are shown in Table 11.5.

Prostanoids

Typical and nearly universal side effects of epoprostenol and treprostinil infusion therapy are jaw pain (trismus), flushing, nausea, and headaches. Frequency can range from over half of patients to nearly 90%.[17,79,93] Diffuse body aches, diarrhea, and vomiting can also occur. Side effects are typically dose-related, but they often improve with symptomatic support and time, without necessitating dose decrease. For patients using subcutaneous delivery devices for treprostinil, injection site pain is common occurrence, and can often be managed by rotating the infusion site. Fewer than 10% of patients may have to discontinue therapy due to injection site pain.[79] For patients receiving intravenous medication, central line infections are a serious concern, especially in PAH patients who, if requiring parenteral therapy, likely have little physiologic reserve. In one observational series of patients on long-term epoprostenol, there were 119-line infections, and 70 episodes of sepsis, in 162 over an average of 3 years of follow-up.[110]

All prostanoids inhibit platelet function;[41] thus bleeding is a common side effect of their use. This is particularly true of PAH patients on oxygen, among whom epistaxis is a common complaint.

Unintended hemodynamic consequences can be seen with virtually all PAH therapy. These include hypotension as well as high output heart failure, which may lead to pulmonary edema.

IP receptor agonists

Side effects with selexipag are similar to those for prostanoids: headache, diarrhea, jaw pain, nausea, and myalgia. Hyperthyroidism was more common among patients taking selexipag than placebo in a large clinical trial. The mechanism and implications of such thyroid dysfunction are currently unclear.[83]

Phosphodiesterase type 5 inhibitors

Class-related side effects of PDE-5is include hypotension, headache, and nausea. In a trial of sildenafil in a population of patients all with connective tissue disease associated PAH, epistaxis was more common (13%) than reported in other populations.[111] Priapism is not a common side effect of PDE-5is when used in PAH; however, a placebo-controlled trial of sildenafil for sickle cell anemia–associated pulmonary hypertension was stopped early due to an increase of adverse events in the active treatment arm, including priapism.[112]

Soluble Guanylyl Cyclase Stimulators

In clinical trials, riociguat was generally well tolerated. Major adverse events included headache, dyspepsia, dizziness, nausea, and vomiting.[87,113,114] Rare cases of drug-related syncope, gastritis, and renal failure have been reported among patients taking riociguat.

Endothelin Receptor Antagonists

Common class side effects of ERA therapy include headache and dizziness.[115] Idiosyncratic agent adverse effects, however, include risk of hepatotoxity, thought to be chiefly attributable to bosentan. In a trial of 213 patients randomized to bosentan or placebo, the incidence of abnormal liver function tests >five times the upper limit of normal. This occurred in 3% of participants taking placebo, 4% among patients taking 125 mg twice daily, but 14% among participants taking 250 mg twice daily.[89] Study drug was discontinued for aminotransferase >eight times the upper limit of normal in 2% of active drug patients and 0% of controls. In the ARIES trials of ambrisentan, no patients on active drug were reported to have serum aminotransferase concentrations greater than three times the upper limit of normal, compared to three patients (2.3%) taking placebo. Macitentan is generally very well tolerated, but headache, nasopharyngitis, and anemia have been seen with higher frequency in participants taking macitentan compared with controls.[91]

Drug Interactions

Prostanoids

The prostanoids are free of major drug-drug interactions that limit use. In all prostanoids, the antiplatelet and antithrombotic effects might be exacerbated in patients who receive anticoagulation for other indications. There has been some concern for decreased clearance of furosemide in patients administered both epoprostenol and furosemide, but the effect was small, found in only a single study, and may be statistical aberration.[116] Due to its metabolism by CYP2C8, treprostinil is susceptible to drug interactions by agents that induce (such as rifampin) or inhibit (e.g., gemfibrozil) this enzyme.[100]

IP Receptor Agonists

Like treprostinil, selexipag is extensive metabolized by CYP2C8. Coadministration with strong inhibitors of this enzyme, such as gemfibrozil, is not advised due to the risk of selexipag toxicity. Selexipag undergoes partial metabolism by CYP3A4, but it is not clear that there is a risk of significant drug-to-drug interactions between selexipag and agents that affect this enzyme.[117] Selexipag should not be used concurrently with prostanoids due to shared action site at the IP receptor.[1]

Phosphodiesterase Type 5 Inhibitors

Both sildenafil and tadalafil may cause lowering of systemic blood pressure, and so caution is advised when combining these agents with other antihypertensives. It should be noted, however, that the systemic blood pressure lowering effect of these agents is modest; in a preapproval hemodynamic study of healthy volunteers, administration of a high dose of sildenafil (50 mg three times daily) resulted in a systemic systolic blood pressure decrease of only 6 mmHg.[63] PAH patients with abnormal baseline hemodynamics may respond more dramatically however. Due to shared pathway of action on the NO-cGMP pathway, oral nitrates should never be coadministered with PDE-5is.

Sildenafil is metabolized via CYP3A4 and to a lesser extent CYP2C9 and should be avoided in patients taking the antiviral ritonavir and other potent CYP3A4 inhibitors—an important consideration in patients with HIV-associated PAH.[118] A similar interaction is seen with tadalafil, which is also extensively metabolized via CYP3A4.[119]

Pharmacodynamic studies have suggested that bosentan, an inducer of both CYP3A4 and CYP2C9, may lead to reduced serum levels of sildenafil in patients taking both.[120] Interestingly, this may explain why trials examining dual therapy with sildenafil and bosentan in PAH have been negative.[121,122]

Soluble Guanylyl Cyclase Stimulators

The sGC stimulator riociguat acts via the NO-sGC-cGMP pathway and thus should not be coadministered with a PDE-5i.[1] Use of riociguat along with strong CYP and P-glycoprotein/BCRP inhibitors (ketoconazole, itraconazole, ritonavir) may increase riociguat levels and risk of toxicity.[123]

Endothelin Receptor Antagonists

Bosentan is an inducer of CYP3A4 and CYP2C9, a finding that may have clinical relevance when coadministered with sildenafil, as discussed previously. Unlike bosentan, ambrisentan does not appear to share this risk.[120] However, ambrisentan is metabolized by

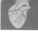

CYP3A4 and CYP2C19, and concomitant administration with strong inducers or inhibitors of those enzymes is discouraged. Macitentan is also metabolized by CYP3A4, but in vivo pharmacokinetic studies seem to support low risk of drug-to-drug interactions with macitentan.[106,124]

Experimental Drugs

Despite the many advances in the understanding of and care for patients with PAH in the years since the first PAH therapies became available, PAH remains a difficult disease to treat—it remains incurable and the field is lacking a complete molecular understanding of disease pathogenesis.[125] Although recently approved drugs, such as oral treprostinil, selexipag, and riociguat, represent exciting new drug formulations and/or oral therapy options, they are all active along established mechanistic and vasodilatory pathways. In fact, not since sildenafil in 2005 has a PAH drug been approved with an entirely new mechanism of action (Fig. 11.4). Additional agents leveraging established therapeutic pathways are currently under development. Ralinepag, a new IP receptor agonist,[126] is currently in phase III clinical trial (ClinicalTrials.gov Identifier: NCT03626688). A phase III randomized trial (NCT01908699) of the addition of the oral prostanoid beraprost-314d to inhaled treprostinil has completed with preliminary reports indicating that it did not meet its primary endpoint; official results are pending.[127]

Drugs with novel mechanisms of action are under development, as investigators work to transform new insights of pulmonary vascular remodeling and right ventricular dysfunction into the molecular basis of PAH into therapeutic targets. For example, pursuant to the discovery of multiple inflammatory pathways that initiate and sustain PAH pathogenesis, a number of candidate therapeutic agents are currently under evaluation that have antiinflammatory effects.[128,129] Bardoxolone methyl is an orally available triterpenoid that inhibits inhibitor transcription factor NF-κB[130] and is currently undergoing evaluation in patients with connective tissue disease-associated PAH (NCT02657356). Other specific antiinflammatory therapies, including the anti-CD20 inhibitor rituximab, are under study in planned or ongoing early phase trials. In addition to inflammation, *BMPR2*-related signaling is being targeted for new drug therapy, as are PAH-specific alterations seen in vascular metabolism,[53] stiffening, and peroxisome proliferator-activated receptor gamma (PPAR-γ) activity.[131,132] Such discoveries hold promise for new therapies under development.[133–135] Finally, rapid advances in new genetic associations with PAH will almost certainly lead to new molecular targets.[136–138]

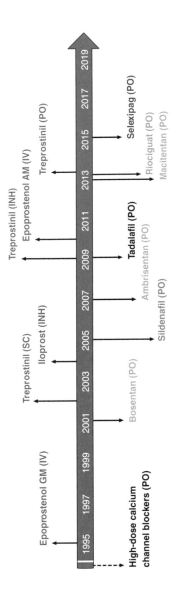

Fig. 11.4 Pulmonary arterial hypertension (PAH) drugs by year of approval by the US Food and Drug Administration, with routes of administration. Color represents medication class. *Blue:* prostanoid; *orange:* endothelin receptor antagonist; *red:* phosphodiesterase type 5 inhibitor; *green:* soluble guanylyl cyclase stimulator; *purple:* IP receptor agonist. High-dose calcium channel blockers were used off-label prior to approval of epoprostenol in 1995. *Epoprostenol GM,* epoprostenol with glycine-mannitol excipients (Flolan); *Epoprostenol AM,* epoprostenol with arginine-mannitol excipients (Veletri); *PO,* orally; *IV,* intravenous; *SC,* subcutaneous; *INH,* inhaled. (Modified from Perrin S, Chaumais M-C, O'Connell C, et al. New pharmacotherapy options for pulmonary arterial hypertension. *Expert Opin Pharmacother.* 2015;16(14):2113–2131.)

Conclusions

The prognosis in PAH has been greatly improved in the over two decades since potent pulmonary vasodilatory drugs became available. Yet, PAH continues to present great challenge to patients and clinicians alike, and a clear unmet need still exists for new disease-modifying therapies. New molecular insights into PAH hold promise for initiating the next generation of vascular remodeling drugs in the care for PAH.

References

Complete reference list available at www.expertconsult.com.